Management of Medical Technology

Butterworth–Heinemann's

BIOMEDICAL ENGINEERING SERIES

Series Editor: Joseph D. Bronzino, Ph.D., *The Verna Roosa Professor of Applied Science; Director, Biomedical Engineering Program, Trinity College / The Hartford Graduate Center, Hartford, Connecticut*

With the dramatic role technology has played in shaping health care, engineering professionals have become intimately involved in many medical ventures. As a result, the discipline of biomedical engineering has emerged as an integrating medium for two dynamic professions: medicine and engineering. This series is dedicated to exploring the evolution, development, and the latest in implementation in this rapidly expanding field.

Management of Medical Technology

A Primer for Clinical Engineers

Edited by

Joseph D. Bronzino, Ph.D., P.E.

The Vernon Roosa Professor of Applied Science
Director, Biomedical Engineering Program
Trinity College / The Hartford Graduate Center
Hartford, CT

Butterworth–Heinemann

Boston London Oxford Singapore Sydney Toronto Wellington

DEDICATION

This book is dedicated to the memory of my mother,
Antoinette Saporito Bronzino,
my greatest fan.

Every effort has been made to ensure that the drug dosage schedules within this text are accurate and conform to standards accepted at the time of publication. However, as treatment recommendations vary in the light of continuing research and clinical experience, the reader is advised to verify drug dose schedules herein with information found on product information sheets.This is especially true in cases of new or infrequently used drugs.

Recognizing the importance of preserving what has been written, it is the policy of Butterworth–Heinemann to have the books it publishes printed on acid-free paper, and we exert our best efforts to this end.

Library of Congress Cataloging-in-publication Data

Management of medical technology : a primer for clinical engineers /
edited by Joseph D. Bronzino
p. cm.
includes bibliographical references and index.
ISBN (invalid) 0-7506-9252-9 (alk. paper)
1. Biomedical engineering. I. Bronzino, Joseph D., 1937 – .
[DNLM: 1. Biomedical Engineering—methods. 2. Maintenance and Engineering, Hospital.
3. Technology, Medical—organization and administration. go 34 M266]
R856.M288 1992
610_.28—dc20
DNLM/DLC
for Library of Congress 92-21070
CIP

British Library Cataloging-in-Publication Data. A catalogue record for this book is available from the British Library.

Butterworth–Heinemann
80 Montvale Avenue
Stoneham, MA 02180

10 9 8 7 6 5 4 3 2 1

Printed in the United States of America

CONTENTS

CONTRIBUTORS

MATTHEW BARETICH, Ph.D.
Director of Bioengineering
University of Colorado
Health Science Center
Denver, CO

MONIQUE FRIZE, Ph.D, P.E.
Professor of Electrical Engineering
Institute of Biomedical Engineering
University of New Brunswick
Fredericton, N.B., Canada

MARK BRODY, M.S., C.C.E.
Director of Clinical Engineering
Baystate Medical Center
Springfield, MA

GERALD GOODMAN, M.S., C.C.E.
Associate Director of
Biomedical Engineering
Texas Children's Hospital
Houston, TX

YADIN DAVID, Ph.D., C.E., P.E.
Director of Biomedical Engineering
Texas Children's Hospital
Houston, TX

DENNIS MINSENT
Biomedical Equipment Support
Clinical Engineering and
Equipment Services Branch
U. S. Air Force Logistics Office
Frederick, MD

MARK ENGLISH, M.S., C.C.E.
Director of Clinical Engineering
Hartford Hospital
Hartford, CT

MAURICE WADE, Ph.D.
Associate Professor of Philosophy
Trinity College
Hartford, CT

PREFACE

During the late twentieth century, technological innovation has progressed at such a rapid pace that it has permeated almost every facet of our lives. This is especially true in the field of medicine and the delivery of health-care services. Although the art of medicine has a long history, the evolution of a health-care system capable of providing a wide range of positive therapeutic treatments in the prevention and cure of illness is a decidedly new phenomenon. Of particular importance in this evolutionary process has been the establishment of the modern hospital as the center of a technologically sophisticated health-care delivery system. From within the framework of this evolutionary process, the discipline of clinical engineering has emerged to assist health-care professionals in the effective utilization and management of the vast array of medical devices and technologies presently available. We define **clinical engineering** as that subspecialty of **biomedical engineering** that is devoted to the application of engineering methods and technologies in the delivery of health-care. As a result, today's clinical engineers are responsible for the management of the high-technology devices and systems used in modern hospitals, for the training of medical personnel in the safe use of medical devices and equipment, and for the design, selection, use, and maintenance of these devices for the safe and effective delivery of health-care services.

Over the past two decades, many hospitals have established centralized clinical/biomedical engineering departments to meet these responsibilities. In the process, clinical engineers are called upon to provide the hospital administration with objective and informed opinions regarding the assessment, acquisition, and utilization of medical technologies. Consequently, today's clinical engineer plays an increasingly integral role in the development and operation of a wide range of hospital programs, including quality assurance, risk management, and strategic planning.

The purpose of this text is to introduce and examine the functions and activities of clinical engineering within the medical environment of the modern hospital. The text is intended for use by senior or graduate level students in engineering, and others in the health-care community (administrators, clinicians, nurses, etc.) who are interested in technology management in the modern health-care system. With this in mind, the text has been organized to address those topics that will provide insight into the role that clinical engineers play in the management of medical technology.

Chapter 1 begins with a historical perspective of the evolution of clinical engineering as a specialized discipline, defines the job functions associated with this field, and reviews the professionalization of clinical engineering within the evolving health-care system.

Chapter 2 discusses safety in the clinical environment. In the process, the role of the clinical engineer in establishing and organizing electrical and medical device safety programs is presented. Because clinical engineers are concerned with more than electrical safety issues, an examination of radiation, laser, and infection control is also included.

One of the primary functions of clinical engineers is technology management. **Chapter 3** discusses this function in detail, highlighting the various types of equipment repair and maintenance services and the calculation of costs associated with these services.

Technology assessment and acquisition are increasingly becoming functions of the clinical engineer. **Chapter 4** examines methods and rationale for the assessment of medical technologies and provides detailed procedures for the establishment and operation of programs for acquisition, distribution, and utilization of technologies in the health-care environment.

Chapter 5 covers a traditional, but important topic for clinical engineers—Codes and Standards—and highlights the role of the federal government in regulating the development and use of medical devices. Included are discussions of the Safe Medical Devices Act of 1990, and the presentation of particular codes and standards such as NFPA 70: The National Electrical Code; NFPA 99: Standards for Health-care Institutions; NFPA 101: The Life Safety Code. Also discussed are the Joint Commission on Accreditation of Health Care Organizations (JCAHO) requirements for the accreditation of hospitals.

In today's health-care environment, clinical engineers are often required to engage in activities that closely involve facilities management (FM) and design. As a result, **Chapter 6** describes the fundamental operations of an FM department and presents, in some detail, those activities that are of particular interest to the clinical engineer. The second portion of this chapter presents concepts of particular significance to clinical engineers related to facilities design, discussing issues of both new construction and renovation. Specific examples include considerations for design of intensive care units, surgical suites, obstetrical facilities, and imaging suites.

Clinical engineers are, by virtue of their profession, managers of both people and machinery. Therefore, it is important that they be familiar with basic managerial concepts. **Chapter 7** presents a discussion of management concepts necessary to the operation of a clinical engineering department. Significant emphasis is placed on the preparation of a business plan for the clinical engineering department as a basis for organizing, leading, and controlling the various aspects of departmental activities.

Chapter 8 illustrates how the basic principles developed in Chapter 7 can be applied to develop effectively a clinical engineering program from the ground up. Processes related to this development, such as how to conduct a review of existing equipment, how to determine the services to be provided by the department, how to determine the resources required to provide these services, and how to present these issues and requests to administrators, are discussed in detail as are methods used to maintain continuous levels of service on a day-to-day basis.

The computer revolution continues to have a significant impact on almost every facet of human activity. Perhaps no single area illustrates the impact of computer technology better than the health-care field. **Chapter 9** reviews these computer applications of interest to clinical engineers. Highlighted topics include computers in clinical laboratory applications, computerized patient record systems, patient monitoring systems and diagnostic systems. Examples of computer-dependent medical imaging systems (e.g., radiology; i.e., computed tomography), ultrasound, and nuclear magnetic resonance are also presented. The use of expert systems in clinical care, especially as adjuncts of clinical decision making is discussed. Finally, the chapter reviews the use of clinical engineering management systems designed to assist the clinical engineering department in the management of technical and personnel resources, the scheduling and accounting of services rendered, and the documentation of activities as required by federal and state regulations and accreditation agencies.

Clinical engineers must be aware of the moral and ethical issues that surround the delivery of health-care in general, and the application of emerging medical technological innovations in particular. **Chapter 10** addresses these concerns, in terms both of the individual and society at large, and reviews basic ethical theory. This review is followed by a discussion of specific issues of importance to clinical engineers, including the definition of death, concepts of euthanasia, research and experimental applications of technology, and medical device use and regulation. Issues related to the allocation of medical care services and technology are also discussed with reference to the future directions of health-care delivery.

Because health is a central concern of all human beings, health-care delivery and the organization, management, and maintenance of systems required for that delivery process are activities that are carried out throughout the world. It seems appropriate, therefore, that this text end with a consideration of clinical engineering department functions in countries other than the United States. Thus, **Chapter 11** presents the results of an international comparative survey of clinical engineering programs and functions in the U.S., Canada, the Western European Community, and the Nordic countries and discusses these results in terms of the cultural ideals that drive particular aspects of the health-care delivery system within these countries.

ACKNOWLEDGMENTS

This book is a product of interactions between clinical engineering directors of the Greater Hartford (CT) Clinical Engineering Internship Program and members of the American College of Clinical Engineers (ACCE). In addition to the contributors already listed, special acknowledgments are made to Thomas Hayes (St. Francis Hospital), Nicholas Noyes and Robert Clawson (University of Connecticut Health Center), Frank Painter (Bridgeport Hospital), Larry Fennigkoh (St. Luke's Hospital), Alvin Wald (Columbia-Presbyterian Hospital) and Wayne Morse (SpaceLabs Medical, Inc.). Each of these individuals made special contributions to the development of this text.

Also, a special note of thanks to my research assistant from the Biomedical Engineering/Electrophysiology Laboratories at Trinity College, Robert J. Austin-LaFrance, for coordinating and organizing the presentation of text and figures for this manuscript.

A special thanks are due to MIT Press, publisher's of Dr. Bronzino's book *"Medical Technology and Society,"* for permission to use materials in this text.

CHAPTER 1

CLINICAL ENGINEERING: EVOLUTION OF A DISCIPLINE

In the twentieth century, technological innovation has reshaped the field of medicine and the delivery of health-care services. Although the art of medicine has a long history, advances in medical technology, primarily in this century, have provided a wide range of positive diagnostic, therapeutic, and rehabilitative tools that are now routinely used in the cure of specific diseases and illnesses. In the process, the modern hospital in the United States has evolved as the center of a technologically sophisticated health-care system serviced by a technologically sophisticated staff.

With the dramatic role technology has played in shaping medical care, engineering professionals have become intimately involved in many medical ventures. As a result, the discipline of **biomedical engineering** has emerged as an integrating medium for two dynamic professions: medicine and engineering. Today, biomedical engineers assist in the struggle against illness and disease by providing materials, tools, and techniques (such as biomaterials, medical imaging, and artificial intelligence) that can be utilized for research, diagnosis, and treatment by health-care professionals. In addition, one subset of the biomedical engineering community, namely **clinical engineers**, has become an integral part of the health-care delivery team by managing the utilization of medical equipment within the hospital environment. The purpose of this chapter is to provide a broad overview of technology's role in shaping our modern health-care system and to review the basic functions performed by clinical engineers within a hospital environment. This chapter also presents the status of the professionalization of clinical engineering (including certification), describes attributes of clinical engineering educational programs, and reflects upon the future of the discipline.

EVOLUTION OF THE MODERN HEALTH-CARE SYSTEM

Before 1900, medicine had little to offer the average citizen because its resources consisted mainly of the physician, his education, and his little black bag. In general, physicians seemed to be in short supply, but the shortage then had rather different causes than found today. Although the costs of obtaining medical training were relatively low, the demand for doctors' services was also very small because many of the services provided by the physician could also be obtained from experienced amateurs in the community. The home was typically the site for diagnosis, treatment, and recuperation, and relatives and neighbors constituted an able and willing nursing staff. Babies were delivered by midwives, and those illnesses not cured by home remedies were left to run their natural, albeit frequently morbid, course. The contrast with contemporary health-care practices, in which specialized physicians and nurses located within the hospital provide critical diagnostic and treatment services, is dramatic.

The changes that have occurred within medical science originated in the rapid developments that took place in the applied sciences (chemistry, physics, engineering, microbiology, physiology, pharmacology, etc.) at the turn of the century. This process of development was characterized by intense interdisciplinary cross-fertilization, which provided an environment in which medical research was able to take giant strides in developing techniques for the diagnosis and treatment of disease. For example, in 1903, Willem Einthoven, the Dutch physiologist, devised the first electrocardiograph to measure the electrical activity of the heart. In applying discoveries in the physical sciences to the analysis of a biological process, he initiated a new age in both cardiovascular medicine and bioelectrical measurement techniques.

New discoveries in medical technology followed one another like intermediates in a chain reaction. However, the most significant innovation for clinical medicine was the development of X-rays. These "new kinds of rays," as their discoverer W.K. Roentgen described them in 1895, opened the "inner man" to medical inspection. Initially, X-rays were used to diagnose bone fractures and dislocations. In the process, this "modern technology" became commonplace in most urban hospitals. Separate departments of radiology were established, and their influence spread to other departments throughout the hospital. By the 1930s, X-ray visualization of practically all organ systems had been made possible because of the inherent radiopacity of the body and the use of barium salts and a wide variety of radio-opaque materials.

X-ray technology gave physicians a powerful tool that, for the first time, permitted accurate diagnosis of a wide variety of diseases and injuries. Moreover, since X-ray machines were too cumbersome and expensive for local doctors' clinics, they had to be placed in hospitals. Once there, X-ray technology essentially triggered the transformation of the hospital from a passive receptacle for the sick poor to an active curative institution for all members of society.

For economic reasons, the centralization of health-care services became essential because of many other important technological innovations appearing on the medical scene. However, hospitals remained institutions to dread, and it was not until the introduction of sulfanilamide in the mid-1930s and penicillin in the early 1940s that the main danger of hospitalization, i.e., cross-infection among patients, was significantly reduced. With these new drugs in their arsenals, surgeons were permitted to perform their operations with reduced morbidity and mortality due to infection. Furthermore, even though the different blood groups and their incompatibility were discovered in 1900 and sodium citrate was used in 1913 to prevent clotting, full development of blood banks was not practical until the 1930s when technology provided adequate refrigeration. Until that time, "fresh" donors were bled, and the blood was transfused while it was still warm.

Once these surgical units were established, employment of the available medical technology assisted in further advancing the development of complex surgical procedures. For example, the Drinker respirator was introduced in 1927, and the first heart-lung bypass was accomplished in 1939. By the late 1940s, medical procedures heavily dependent upon medical technology, such as cardiac catheterization and angiography (the use of a cannula threaded through an arm vein and into the heart with the injection of radio-opaque dye for the X-ray visualization of heart vessels and valves), were developed. As a result, accurate diagnoses of congenital and acquired heart disease became possible, and a new era of cardiac and vascular surgery was established.

Following World War II, the development of medical devices accelerated rapidly and the medical profession benefitted greatly from this rapid surge of technological finds throughout the next four decades.

Since it is impossible to cover all of the medical innovations that occurred during this period, consider just a few examples:

- **Advances in electronics** made it possible to map the subtle electrical behavior of the fundamental unit of the central nervous system—the neuron—and to monitor various physiological functions of patients in intensive care units (ICUs) by utilizing such diagnostic tools as the electrocardiogram (ECG) and the electroencephalogram (EEG). (Figure 1.1)
- **Nuclear medicine,** an outgrowth of the atomic age, emerged as a powerful and effective approach to applying radioactive materials (tracers) to medical diagnosis and treatment. Activities in this area have included (a) the creation and use of radiopharmaceuticals; (b) the design and application of appropriate nuclear instrumentation to detect and display the activity of these radioactive elements; and (c) the determination of the relationship between the activity of radioactive tracers and specific physiological processes.
- **"Spare parts" surgery** became commonplace. Technologists were encouraged to provide prosthetic devices, such as artificial heart valves and artificial blood vessels, and the artificial heart program was launched to develop a replacement for a defective or diseased human heart (Figure 1.2).
- **Computers,** similar to those developed to control the flight plans of the *Apollo* capsule, were used to store, process, and cross-check medical records, monitor patient status in intensive-care units, and provide sophisticated statistical diagnosis of potential diseases correlated with specific sets of patient symptoms (Figure 1.3).

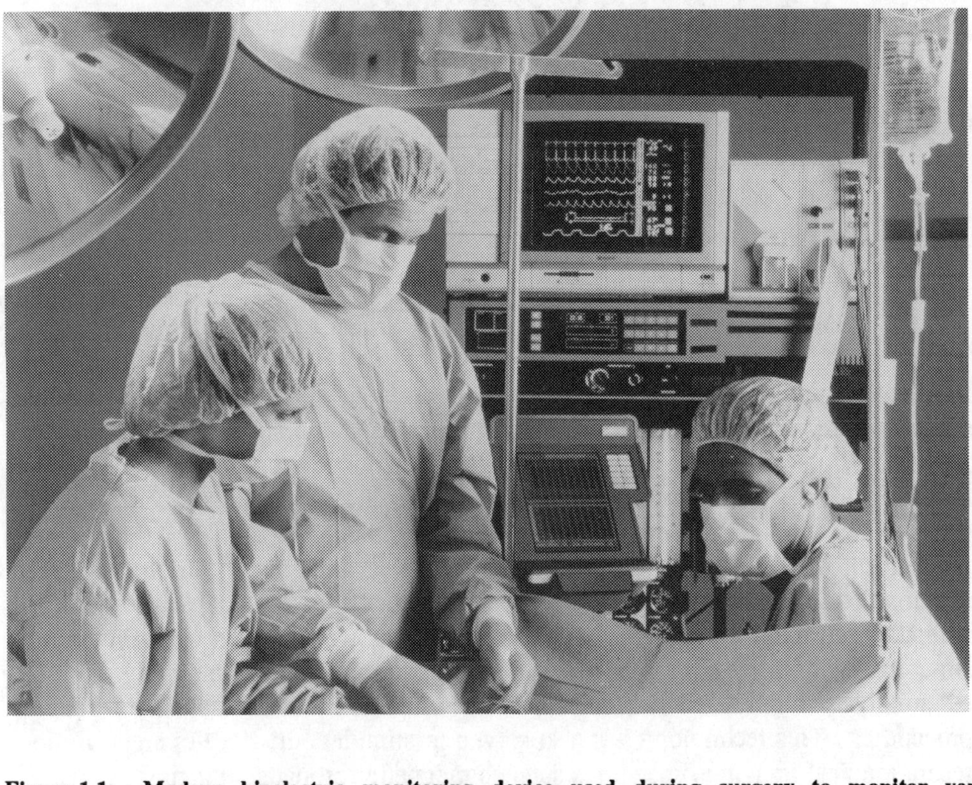

Figure 1.1: Modern bioelectric monitoring device used during surgery to monitor various physiological signals. (Courtesy of SpaceLabs Medical, Inc. Redman, WA)

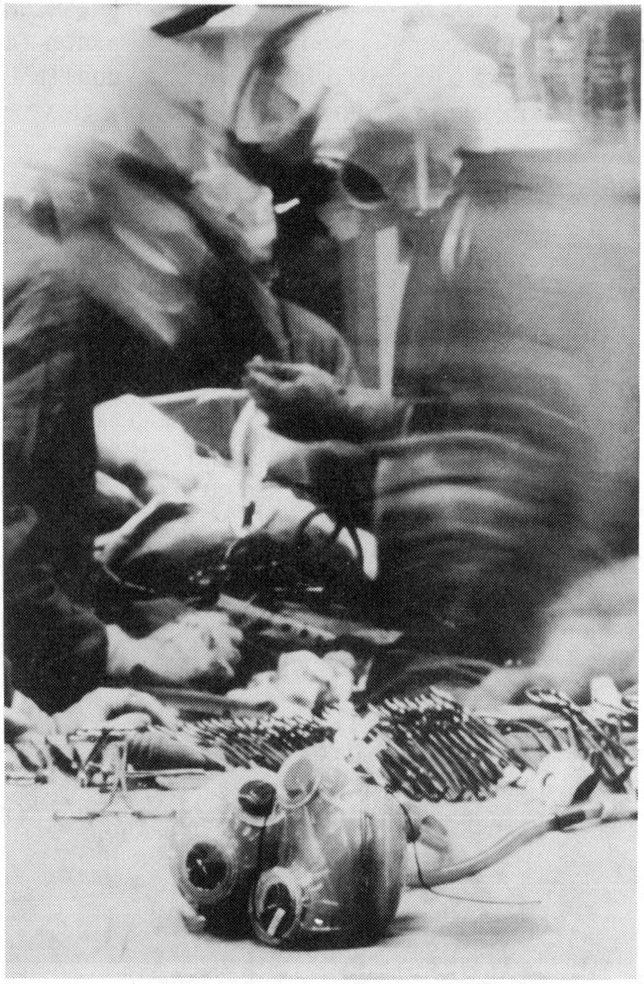

Figure 1.2: Jarvik VII artificial heart (foreground) and surgical team preparing for implantation into a human patient.

- **Medical imaging** became a vital part of patient diagnostic systems. For example, diagnostic ultrasound based on sonar techniques has been so widely accepted that ultrasonic studies are now part of the routine diagnostic workup in many medical specialties. In fact, diagnostic ultrasound studies are often the method of choice because they provide information otherwise unavailable. For example, ultrasound images of the fetus are especially useful in evaluating the status of fetal development. Development of the first computer-based medical instrument, the computerized axial tomography (CAT) scanner has permitted the visualization of structures and masses in otherwise inaccessible regions of the body and has essentially revolutionized clinical approaches to non-invasive diagnostic imaging procedures. This technology has also served to stimulate the development of more recent medical imaging procedures such as magnetic resonance imaging (MRI) and positron emission tomography (PET).

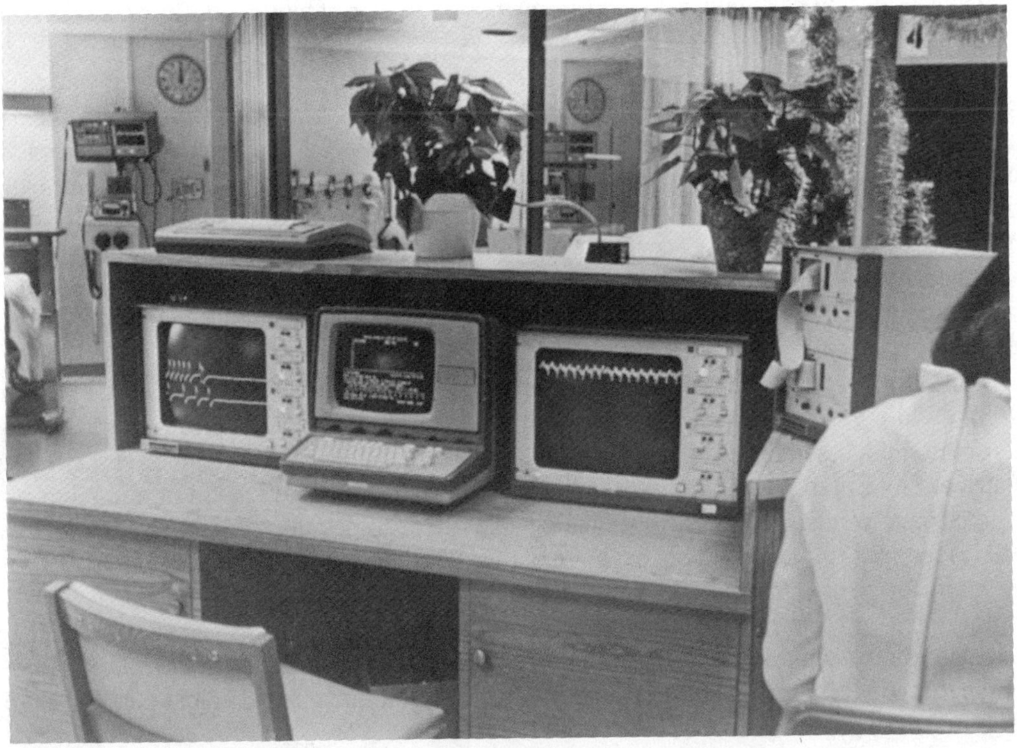

Figure 1.3: Centralized computer monitoring of patients in an ICU. Physiological data from any patient in the ICU can be monitored by the duty nurses at this station.

The effect of these discoveries and many others has been profound. The health-care system that existed at the turn of the century, consisting primarily of the "horse-and-buggy" physician, has disappeared forever. It has been replaced by a clinical staff that consists of physicians, nurses, and other professional allied- health specialists and operates primarily in hospitals. The clinical staff now stands as the fundamental component of the American health-care system (Crichton, 1970; Knowles, 1973; Bronzino, 1977; Vogel, 1980; Bronzino, 1986; Bronzino et al., 1990).

WHAT IS CLINICAL ENGINEERING?

Many of the problems confronting health professionals today are of extreme interest to engineers because they involve the design and practical application of medical devices and systems—processes that are fundamental to **engineering practice**. These medically related design problems can range from very complex, large-scale constructs, such as the design and implementation of automated clinical laboratories, multiphasic screening facilities (i.e., centers that permit many clinical tests to be conducted), and hospital information systems, to the creation of relatively small and "simple" devices, such as recording electrodes and transducers that may be used to monitor the activity of specific physiological processes in either a research or a clinical setting. Furthermore, these problems often involve addressing the many complexities found in specific clinical areas, such as emergency vehicles, operating rooms, and intensive-care units. The American health-care system, therefore, presents significant challenges and opportunities to those members of the engineering profession called **biomedical engineers.**

Since the field of biomedical engineering involves applying the concepts, knowledge, and approaches of virtually all engineering disciplines (e.g., electrical, mechanical, and chemical engineering) to solve specific health-care-related problems, the opportunities for interaction between engineers and health professionals are many and varied. As a result, biomedical engineers may become involved in the design of a new medical imaging modality or the development of new medical prosthetic devices to aid the handicapped. Although what is included in the field of biomedical engineering is considered to be quite clear, many conflicting opinions concerning the field can be traced to disagreements about its definition. For example, consider the terms **biomedical engineering, bioengineering,** and **clinical (or medical) engineering,** which are defined in the *Bioengineering Education Directory* (Pacela, 1990). While Pacela defines "bioengineering" as the broad umbrella term used to describe this entire field, bioengineering is usually defined as a basic research-oriented activity closely related to biotechnology and genetic engineering; that is, the modification of animal or plant cells, or parts of cells, to improve plants or animals or to develop new microorganisms for beneficial ends. In the food industry, for example, this has meant the improvement of strains of yeast for fermentation. In agriculture, bioengineers may be concerned with the improvement of crop yields by treatment of plants with organisms to reduce frost damage. It is clear that bioengineers of the future will have a tremendous impact on the quality of human life; the full potential of this specialty is difficult to imagine. Typical pursuits include the following:

- Development of improved species of plants and animals for food production.
- Invention of new medical diagnostic tests for diseases.
- Production of synthetic vaccines from clone cells.
- Bioenvironmental engineering to protect human, animal, and plant life from toxins and pollutants.
- Study of protein-surface interactions.
- Modeling of the growth kinetics of yeast and hybridoma cells.
- Research in immobilized enzyme technology.
- Development of therapeutic proteins and monoclonal antibodies.

The term "biomedical engineering," in my opinion, however, has the most comprehensive meaning. Biomedical engineering is an interdisciplinary branch of engineering with a foundation based in both engineering and the life sciences. It ranges from theoretical, nonexperimental undertakings to state-of-the-art applications. It can encompass research, development, implementation, and operation. Accordingly, like medical practice itself, it is unlikely that any single person can acquire expertise that encompasses the entire field. As a result, there has been an explosion of biomedical engineering specialists to cover this broad spectrum of activity. Yet, because of the interdisciplinary nature of this activity, there is considerable interplay and overlapping of interest and effort. For example, biomedical engineers engaged in the development of biosensors may interact with those interested in prosthetic devices to develop a means to detect and use bioelectric signals to power a prosthetic device. Those engaged in automating clinical chemistry instrumentation may collaborate with those developing expert systems to assist clinicians in making clinical decisions based upon specific laboratory data. The possibilities are endless. Biomedical engineers apply electrical, chemical, mechanical, and other engineering principles to understand, modify, or control biological (i.e., human and animal) systems. When biomedical engineers work within a hospital or clinic, they are more properly called **clinical engineers.** However, this theoretical distinction is not always observed in practice, since many professionals working in U.S. hospitals today continue to be called "biomedical engineers." Unfortunately, this inconsistency within the profession has caused a great deal of confusion among clinicians, nurses, and hospital administrators.

In the field of biomedical engineering there are seven major career areas (Bronzino, 1991):

1. Application of engineering system analysis and modeling (computer simulation) to biological problems.
2. Measurement or monitoring of physiological signals.
3. Diagnostic interpretation via signal-processing techniques of bioelectric data.
4. Therapeutic and rehabilitation procedures and devices.
5. Prosthetic devices for replacement or augmentation of body functions.
6. Computer analysis of patient-related data.
7. Medical imaging—the graphic display of anatomical detail or physiological function.

Typical pursuits of biomedical engineers include these:

- Design of instrumentation for research in human physiology.
- Monitoring of astronauts and maintenance of life in space.
- Research on new materials for implanted artificial organs and prosthetic devices.
- Development of new diagnostic instruments for blood analysis.
- Computer modeling of human heart function.
- Writing software for analysis of medical research data.
- Analysis of medical device hazards for the United States government and consumers of medical technology.
- Monitoring of animal physiological functions.
- Development of new diagnostic imaging systems.
- Design of telemetry systems for patient monitoring
- Design of biomedical sensors for measuring multiple variables of human physiological systems.
- Research on artificial intelligence (AI) and development of expert systems for diagnosis of disease.
- Design of closed-loop control systems for drug administration.
- Modeling of the physiological systems of the human body.
- Design of instrumentation for sports medicine.
- Development of new dental materials.
- Design of computers and communication aids for the handicapped.
- Research in pulmonary fluid dynamics.
- Study of the biomechanics of the human body.

This list is not intended to be all-inclusive, but rather to illustrate the types of activities of interest to biomedical engineers. There are many other applications that utilize the talents and skills of the biomedical engineer. In fact, the list of activities of biomedical engineers depends upon the medical environment in which they work. This is especially true for the clinical engineer.

The universal acceptance of a definition for "clinical engineer" is important. In recent years, a number of organizations have attempted to provide an appropriate definition (Schaffer and Schaffer, 1992). For example, the AHA defines a clinical engineer as

- "*a person who adapts , maintains, and improves the safe use of equipment and instruments in the hospital,*" (AHA, 1986).

The American College of Clinical Engineering defines a clinical engineer as

- "*a professional who supports and advances patient care by applying engineering and managerial skills to health-care technology,*" (Bauld, 1991).

The definition which the AAMI originally applied to board certified practitioners describes a clinical engineer as

- "*a professional who brings to health-care facilities a level of education, experience, and accomplishment which will enable him to responsibly, effectively, and safely manage and interface with medical devices, instruments, and systems and the user thereof during patient care . . . ,*" (Goodman, 1989).

For the purpose of internal certification, the Board of Examiners for Clinical Engineering Certification considers a clinical engineer to be

- "*an engineer whose professional focus is on patient-device interfacing; one who applies engineering principles in managing medical systems and devices in the patient setting,* (ICC, 1991).

Finally, the *Journal of Clinical Engineering* has defined the distinction between a biomedical engineer and a clinical engineer by suggesting that the biomedical engineer

- "*applies a wide spectrum of engineering level knowledge and principles to the understanding, modification or control of human or animal biological systems,* (Pacela, 1991).

For the purposes of this book, we will define a clinical engineer as

- *an engineer who has graduated from an accredited academic program in engineering or who is licensed as a professional engineer or engineer-in-training and is engaged in the application of scientific and technological knowledge developed through engineering education and subsequent professional experience within the health-care environment in support of clinical activities.*

The clinical environment is that portion of the health-care system in which patient care is delivered. Clinical activities include direct patient care, research, teaching, and public service activities intended to enhance patient care.

Engineers were first encouraged to enter the clinical scene during the late 1960s in response to concerns about patient safety as well as the rapid proliferation of clinical equipment, especially in academic medical centers. In the process, a new engineering discipline—clinical engineering—evolved to provide the technological support necessary to meet these new needs. During the 1970s, a major expansion of clinical engineering occurred, primarily due to the following events (Bronzino and Hayes, 1988):

- The Veterans' Administration (VA), convinced that clinical engineers were vital to the overall operation of the VA hospital system, divided the country into biomedical engineering districts, with a chief biomedical engineer overseeing all engineering activities in the hospitals in that district.
- Throughout the United States, clinical engineering departments were established in most large medical centers and hospitals and in some smaller clinical facilities with at least three hundred beds.
- Clinical engineers were hired in increasing numbers to help these facilities use existing technology and incorporate new technology.

Having entered the hospital environment, routine electrical safety inspections exposed the clinical engineer to all types of patient equipment that were not being properly maintained. It soon became obvious that electrical safety failures represented only a small part of the overall problem posed by the presence of medical equipment in the clinical environment. This equipment was neither totally understood nor properly maintained. Simple visual inspections often revealed broken knobs, frayed wires, and even evidence of liquid spills. Investigating further, it was found that many devices did not perform in accordance with manufacturers' specifications and were not maintained in accordance with manufacturers' recommendations. In short, electrical safety problems were only the tip of the iceberg. By the mid-1970s, complete performance inspections before and after use became the norm and sensible inspection procedures were developed (Newhouse et al., 1989). Clinical engineering departments became the logical support center for all medical technologies. As a result, clinical engineers assumed additional responsibilities, including the management of high-technology instruments and systems used in hospitals, the training of medical personnel in equipment use and safety, and the design, selection, and use of technology to deliver safe and effective health-care.

Figure 1.4 illustrates the multi-faceted role played by clinical engineers. They must successfully interface with clinical staff, hospital administrators, regulatory agencies, etc., to ensure that the medical equipment within the hospital is safely and effectively utilized.

Hospitals that have established centralized clinical engineering departments to meet these responsibilities use clinical engineers to provide the hospital administration with an objective opinion of equipment function, purchase, application, overall system analysis, and preventive maintenance policies. With the in-house availability of such talent and expertise, the hospital is in a far better position to make more effective use of its technological resources (Jacobs, 1975; Bronzino, 1977, 1986). It is also important to note that competent clinical engineers, as part of the health-care system, can help create a more unified and predictable market for biomedical equipment. By providing health professionals with needed assurance of safety, reliability, and efficiency in using new and innovative equipment, clinical engineers can identify poor quality and ineffective equipment much more readily. These activities, in turn, can lead to a faster, more appropriate utilization of new medical equipment and provide a natural incentive for greater industrial involvement—a step that is an essential prerequisite to widespread utilization of any technology (Newhouse et al., 1989).

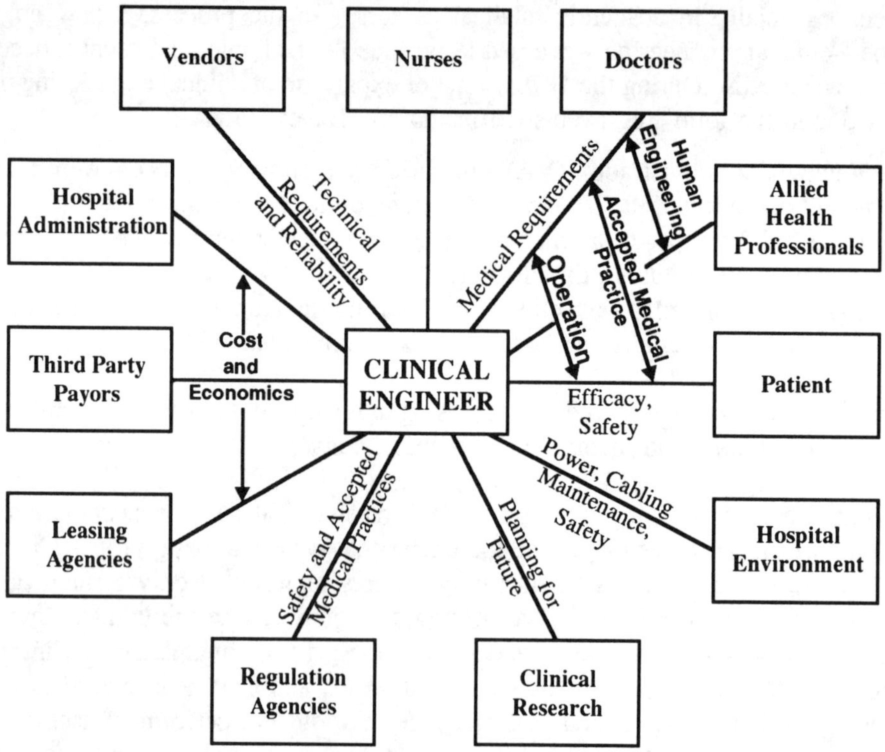

Figure 1.4: **Diagram illustrating the range of interactions in which a clinical engineer may be required to engage in a hospital setting.**

Typical pursuits of clinical engineers therefore include the following:

- Supervision of a hospital clinical engineering department that includes clinical engineers and biomedical equipment technicians (BMETs).
- Prepurchase evaluation and planning for new medical technology.
- Design, modification, or repair of sophisticated medical instruments or systems.
- Cost-effective management of a medical equipment calibration and repair service.
- Safety and performance testing of medical equipment by BMETs.
- Inspection of all incoming equipment (new and returning repairs).
- Establishment of performance bench marks for all equipment.
- Medical equipment inventory control.
- Coordination of outside services and vendors.
- Training of medical personnel in the safe and effective use of medical devices and systems.
- Clinical applications engineering, such as custom modification of medical devices for clinical research, evaluation of new noninvasive monitoring systems, etc.
- Biomedical computer support.
- Input to the design of clinical facilities where medical technology is used, e.g., operating rooms (ORs), intensive-care units, etc.
- Development and implementation of documentation protocols required by external accreditation and licensing agencies.

Clinical engineers thereby provide extensive engineering services for the clinical staff and, in recent years, have been increasingly accepted as valuable team members by physicians, nurses, and other clinical professionals. The acceptance of clinical engineers in the hospital setting has led to different types of engineering–medicine interactions, which in turn have improved health-care delivery. For example, clinical engineers serve as a significant resource for the entire hospital. They possess in-depth knowledge regarding available in-house technological capabilities and the technical resources available from outside firms. The availability of such talent enables the hospital to make effective and efficient use of all of its technological resources.

HOSPITAL ORGANIZATION AND THE ROLE OF CLINICAL ENGINEERING

In the hospital, management organization has evolved into a diffuse authority structure that is commonly referred to as the "triad model." The three primary components are the governing board (trustees), hospital administration (CEO and administrative staff), and the medical staff organization. The role of the governing board and the chief executive officer are discussed in detail to provide some insights regarding their individual responsibilities and their interrelationship (Bronzino and Hayes, 1988).

Governing Board (Trustees)

The **Joint Commission on the Accreditation of Healthcare Organizations** summarizes the major duties of the governing board as "adopting by-laws in accordance with its legal accountability and its responsibility to the patient." The governing body, therefore, requires both medical and paramedical departments to monitor and evaluate the quality of patient care, which is a critical success factor in hospitals today.

To meet this goal, the governing board essentially is responsible for establishing the mission statement and defining the specific goals and objectives that the institution must satisfy. Therefore, the trustees are involved in the following functions:

- Establishing the policies of the institution.
- Providing equipment and facilities to conduct patient care.
- Ensuring that proper professional standards are defined and maintained (i.e., providing quality assurance).
- Coordinating professional interests with administrative, financial, and community needs.
- Providing adequate financing by securing sufficient income and managing the control of expenditures.
- Providing a safe environment.
- Selecting qualified administrators, medical staff, and other professionals to manage the hospital.

In practice, the trustees select a hospital chief administrator who develops a plan of action that is in concert with the overall goals of the institution.

Hospital Administration

The hospital administrator, the chief executive officer of the medical enterprise, has a function similar to that of the chief executive officer of any corporation. The administrator represents the governing board in carrying out the day-to-day operations to reflect the broad policy formulated by the trustees. The duties of the administrator are summarized as follows:

- Preparing a plan for accomplishing the institutional objectives, as approved by the board.
- Selecting medical chiefs and department directors to set standards in their respective fields.
- Submitting for board approval an annual budget reflecting both expenditures and income projections.
- Maintaining all physical properties (plant and equipment) in safe operating condition.
- Representing the hospital in its relationships with the community and health agencies.
- Submitting to the board annual reports that describe the nature and volume of the services delivered during the past year, including appropriate financial data and any special reports that may be requested by the board.

In addition to these administrative responsibilities, the chief administrator is charged with controlling cost, complying with a multitude of governmental regulations, and ensuring that the hospital conforms to professional norms, which include guidelines for the care and safety of patients.

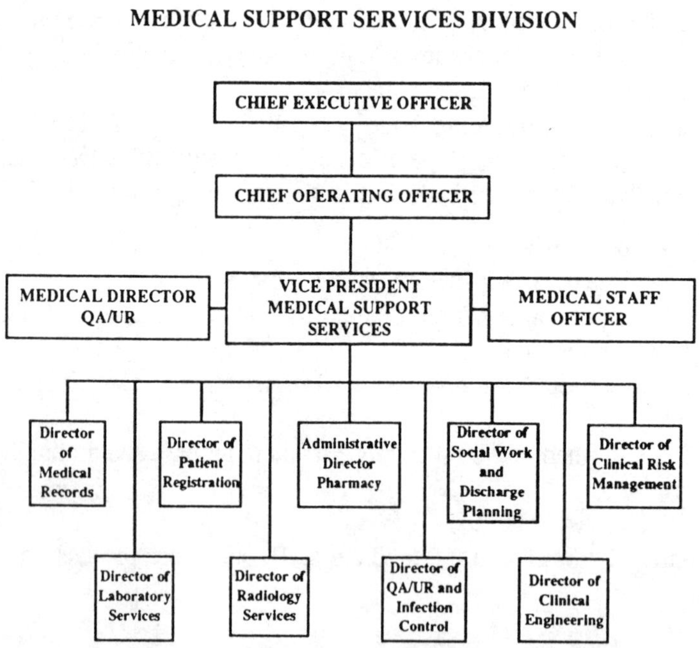

Figure 1.5: Organizational chart of medical support services division for a typical, major medical facility. This organizational structure points out the critical interrelationship between the clinical engineering department and the other primary services provided by the medical facility.

Clinical Engineering Program

In many hospitals, administrators have established clinical engineering departments to manage effectively all the technological resources, especially those relating to medical equipment, that are necessary for providing patient care. The primary objective of these departments is to provide a broad-based engineering program that addresses all aspects of medical instrumentation and systems support.

Figure 1.5 illustrates the organizational chart of the medical support services division of a typical major medical facility. Note that within this organizational structure, the director of clinical engineering reports directly to the vice-president of medical support services. This administrative relationship is extremely important since it recognizes the important role clinical engineering departments play in delivering quality care. It should be noted, however, that in the more common organizational structure, clinical engineering services fall under the category of "facilities," "materials management," or even just "support services."

In practice, there is an alternative capacity in which clinical engineers can function. They can work directly with clinical departments, thereby bypassing much of the hospital hierarchy. In this situation, clinical departments can offer the clinical engineer both the chance for intense specialization and, at the same time, the opportunity to develop a personal relationship with specific clinicians based on mutual concerns and interests (Wald, 1989).

Establishment of a Clinical Engineering Department

The establishment of a clinical engineering department requires the following three major administrative steps. First, the hospital administration appoints a qualified individual as director. Directors of clinical engineering usually function at the department-head level in the organizational structure of the institution and are provided with sufficient authority and resources to perform their duties efficiently and in accordance with professional norms. According to the **World Health Organization** (WHO)(Issakov et al., 1990), the job title for **clinical engineering director** is as follows.

General Statement. *The clinical engineering director, by his or her education and experience, acts as a manager and technical director of the clinical engineering department. The individual designs or directs the design of equipment modifications that may correct design deficiencies or enhance the clinical performance of medical equipment. The individual may also supervise the implementation of those design modifications. The education and experience that the director possesses enables him or her to analyze complex medical or laboratory equipment for purposes of defining corrective maintenance and developing appropriate preventive maintenance or performance assurance protocols. The clinical engineering director works with nursing and medical staff to analyze new medical equipment needs and participates in both the prepurchase planning process and the incoming acceptance testing process. This individual also participates in the equipment management process through involvement in the system development, implementation, maintenance and modification processes.*

Duties and Responsibilities. *The director of clinical engineering has a wide range of duties and responsibilities. For example, this individual:*

- *Works with medical and nursing staff in the development of technical and performance specifications for equipment required in the medical mission.*

- *Once equipment is specified and the purchase order developed, generates appropriate testing of the new equipment.*
- *Does complete performance analysis on complex medical or laboratory equipment and summarizes results in brief, concise, easy-to-understand terms for the purposes of recommending corrective action or for developing appropriate preventive maintenance and performance assurance protocols.*
- *Designs and implements modifications that permit enhanced operational capability. May supervise the maintenance or modification as it is performed by others.*
- *Must know the relevant codes and standards related to the hospital environment and the performance assurance activities. (Examples in the U.S. are **NFPA 99**, **UL 544**, and **JCAHO**, and internationally, **IEC-TC 62**. See Chapter 5 for details of these codes and standards.)*
- *Is responsible for obtaining the engineering specifications (systems definitions) for systems that are considered unusual or one-of-a-kind and are not commercially available.*
- *Supervises in-service maintenance technicians as they work on codes and standards and on preventive maintenance, performance assurance, corrective maintenance, and modification of new and existing patient care and laboratory equipment.*
- *Supervises parts and supply purchase activities and develops program policies and procedures for same.*
- *Sets department goals, develops budgets and policy, prepares and analyzes management reports to monitor department activity, and manages and organizes the department to implement them.*
- *Teaches measurement, calibration, and standardization techniques that promote optimum performance.*
- *In equipment-related duties, works closely with maintenance and medical personnel. Communicates orally and in writing with medical, maintenance, and administrative professionals. Develops written procedures and recommendations for administrative and technical personnel.*

Direction Received and Supervisory Responsibility. *The director of clinical engineering functions with a minimum of supervision and often supervises or directs the work of biomedical equipment maintenance technicians and clinical engineers with less seniority.*

Working Conditions. *The work site is within the hospital and includes patient areas where the employee may be exposed to sick patients and to research projects.*

Minimum Qualifications. *A bachelor's degree (four years) in an electrical or electronics program or the equivalent is required (preferably with a clinical or biomedical adjunct). A Master's degree is desirable. A minimum of three years experience as a clinical engineer and two years in a progressively responsible supervisory capacity is needed. Additional qualifications are as follows:*

- *Must have some business knowledge and management skills that enable him or her to participate in budgeting, cost accounting, personnel management, behavioral counseling, job description development, and interviewing for hiring or firing purposes. Knowledge and experience in the use of microcomputers is desirable.*

- *Must be able to use conventional electronic trouble-shooting instruments such as multimeters, function generators, oscillators, and oscilloscopes. Should be able to use conventional machine shop equipment such as drill presses, grinders, belt sanders, shears, brakes, and standard hand tools.*
- *Must possess or be able to acquire a knowledge of the techniques, theories, and characteristics of materials, drafting and fabrication techniques in conjunction with chemistry, anatomy, physiology, optics, mechanics, and hospital procedures.*
- *Clinical engineering certification or professional engineering registration are required.*

In the second step in the establishment of a clinical engineering department, the hospital administration, in conjunction with the director of clinical engineering, prepares a mission statement which defines the dimension and scope of responsibility of the clinical engineering department. The mission statement and list of objectives must conform to the overall strategic plan of the hospital. For example, consider the following (Simmons and Wear, 1988).

Mission Statement. *It is the policy of the hospital clinical engineering department to provide technical and management professional clinical engineering support to hospital administration, hospital engineering department, medical, surgical, nursing, and other allied health professional departments, and staff medical professionals. The clinical engineering department will perform a primary role in the assurance of compliance to relevant laws, statutes, regulations, and standards by the establishment and implementation of effective instrumentation control programs. These programs will ensure the efficacious and safe use of medical instrumentation for the benefit of the patients and hospital employees alike. It is the policy of the clinical engineering department to augment this program by the continued development and presentation of educational materials through the use of in-service education and training sessions for clinical personnel.*

Objective 1. To define, develop, and implement the hospital clinical engineering program which will provide scientific, technical, and management support to hospital administration, clinical departments, and medical staff.

Objective 2. To develop and issue all necessary programs, technical procedures, and documentation with the concurrence of appropriate personnel.

Objective 3. To determine and provide those professional scientific and technical consultation services that will be provided by the hospital clinical engineering department to the clinical and medical staffs.

Objective 4. To define program education and training needs for clinical department employees, medical staff, and clinical engineering personnel.

Objective 5. To establish communication methods for status reporting of program implementation both in management and in technical areas.

Objective 6. To optimize program costs in such a way so as to provide maximum improvement in patient care as a result of this program while attempting to minimize costs. No compromise will be made in the area of employee safety, as required by applicable laws, codes, and standards.

Finally, the clinical engineering department determines and requests adequate work space, personnel, test equipment, and supplies to accomplish its specified objectives in compliance with established codes and standards. A detailed discussion on how a clinical engineering department may be established is provided in Chapter 8.

Major Functions of a Clinical Engineering Department

The role of the clinical engineer in today's hospital can be both challenging and gratifying because the care of patients requires a partnership between medical staff and modern technology. As previously discussed, this interchange has led to a close working relationship between the clinical engineer and many members of the medical and hospital staff. The team approach is key to the successful operation of any clinical engineering program. Figure 1.6 illustrates the degree of teamwork and interdependence required to maintain constructive interrelationships. In this matrix presentation, it is important to note that the health-care team approach to the delivery of patient care creates both vertical and lateral reporting relationships. Although clinical engineers report hierarchically to their hospital administrator, they also interact with hospital staff to meet patient requirements.

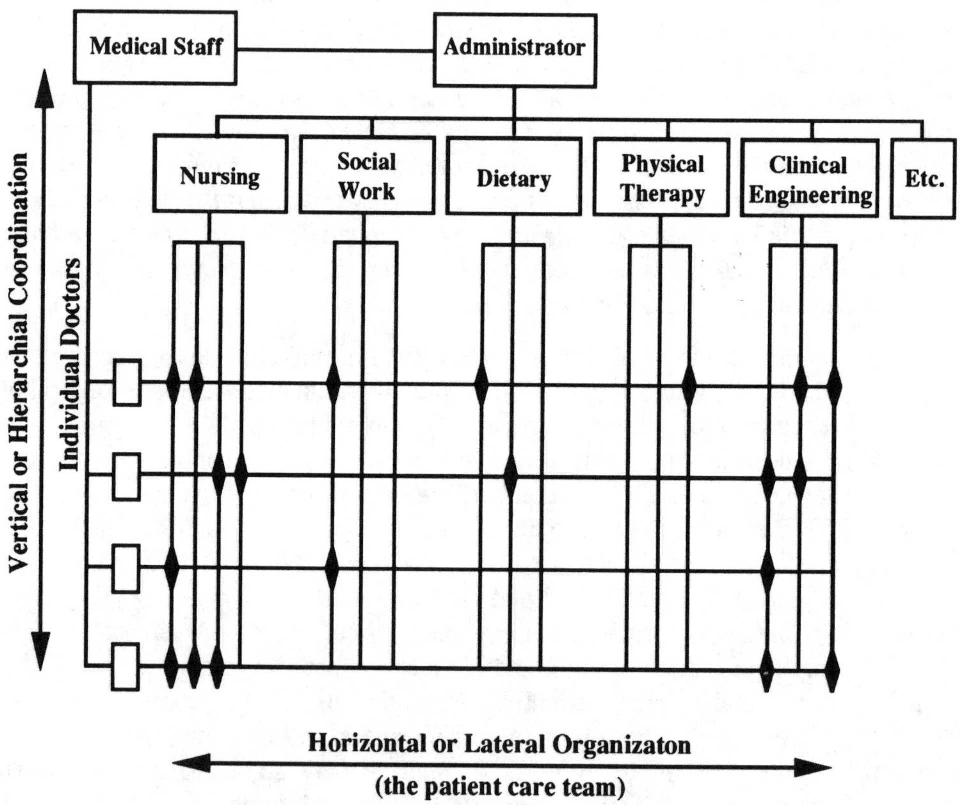

Figure 1.6: Matrix diagram illustrating the bi-directional interdependence and degree of teamwork required to maintain effective interaction between the members of the health-care delivery team.

As a result of the wide-ranging scope of interrelationships within the medical setting, the duties and responsibilities of clinical engineering directors are extremely diversified. Yet, a common thread is provided by the very nature of the technology they manage.
Directors of clinical engineering departments are usually involved in the following areas:

- Developing, implementing, and directing equipment management programs. Specific tasks include evaluating and selecting new technology, accepting and installing new equipment, and managing the inventory of medical instrumentation, all in keeping with the responsibilities and duties defined by the administrator. The director advises the administrator of the budgetary, personnel, space, and test equipment requirements necessary to support this equipment management program.
- Advising administration and medical and nursing staffs in areas such as safety, the purchase of new medical instrumentation and equipment, and the design of new clinical facilities.
- Evaluating and taking appropriate action on incidents attributed to equipment malfunction or misuse. The director summarizes the technological significance of each incident and document the findings of the investigation. He or she submits a report to the appropriate hospital authority and, according to the **Safe Medical Devices Act of 1990**, to the device manufacturer, the **Food and Drug Administration** (FDA) or both.
- Selecting departmental staff and training them to perform their functions in a professional manner.
- Establishing departmental priorities, developing and enforcing departmental policies and procedures, and supervising and directing departmental activities. The director takes an active role in leading the department to achieve its overall technical goals.

The core functions of clinical engineers are as follows:

1. Technology management.
2. Risk management.
3. Technology assessment.
4. Facilities design and project management.
5. Quality assurance.
6. Training.

PROFESSIONAL STATUS OF CLINICAL ENGINEERING

Upon careful review of our definition of clinical engineering and the responsibilities and functions that clinical engineers assume within the hospital, it is clear that the term clinical engineer must be associated with individuals who can provide engineering services, not simply technical services. Clinical engineers, therefore, must be individuals who have a minimum of a four-year bachelor's degree in an engineering discipline. They must be well versed in the design, modification, and testing of medical instrumentation, skills that fall predominantly in the field of engineering practice. Only with an engineering background can clinical engineers assume their proper role working with other health professionals to use available technological resources effectively and to improve health-care delivery.

By clearly linking clinical engineering to the engineering profession, a number of important objectives are achieved. First, it enables hospital administrators to identify qualified individuals to serve as clinical engineers within their institutions and to understand better the wide range of functions that clinical engineers can perform, while making it clear that this role cannot be assumed by technicians. Second, from this foundation it is possible for the profession of clinical engineering to mature. It has been pointed out that professional activities exist if "a cluster of roles in which the incumbents perform certain functions valued in the society in general" can be identified (Parsons, 1954; Courter, 1980; Goodman, 1989). Clearly, this goal has been achieved for the clinical engineer.

Professionals have been defined as an aggregate of people finding identity in sharing values and skills absorbed during a common course of intensive training. Parsons (1954) stated that one determines whether or not individuals are professionals by examining whether or not they have internalized certain given professional values. Friedson (1971) redefined Parsons's definition by noting that a professional is someone who has internalized professional values and is to be recruited and licensed on the basis of his or her technical competence. Furthermore, he pointed out that professionals generally accept scientific standards in their work, restrict their work activities to areas in which they are technically competent, avoid emotional involvement, cultivate objectivity in their work, and put their clients' interests before their own.

The concept of a profession that manages technology encompasses three occupational models; science, business, and profession. Of particular interest is the contrast between science and profession. Science is seen as the pursuit of knowledge, its value hinging on providing evidence and communicating with colleagues. Profession, on the other hand, is viewed as providing a service to clients who have problems they cannot handle themselves. Science and profession have in common the exercise of some knowledge, skill, or expertise. However, while scientists practice their skills and report their results to knowledgeable colleagues, professionals—such as lawyers, physicians, and engineers—serve lay clients. To protect both the professional and the client from the consequences of the layperson's lack of knowledge, the practice of the profession is regulated through such formal institutions as state licensing. Both professionals and scientists must persuade their clients to accept their findings. Professionals endorse and follow a specific code of ethics to serve society. On the other hand, scientists move their colleagues to accept their findings through persuasion (Goodman, 1989).

Consider, for example, the medical profession. Its members are trained in caring for the sick, with the primary goal of healing them. These professionals not only have a responsibility for the creation, development, and implementation of that tradition, they are expected to provide a service to the public, within limits, without regard to self-interest. To ensure proper service, the profession itself closely monitors licensing and certification. Thus, medical professionals themselves may be regarded as a mechanism of social control. However, this does not mean that other facets of society are not involved in exercising oversight and control of physicians in their practice of medicine.

A final attribute of professionals is that of integrity (Parsons, 1954). Physicians tend to be both permissive and supportive in relationships with patients and yet are often confronted with moral dilemmas involving the desires of their patients and the social interest. For example, how to honor the wishes of terminally ill patients while not facilitating the patients' deaths is a moral question that health professionals are forced to confront. A detailed discussion of the moral issues posed by medical technology is presented in Chapter 10.

One can determine the status of professionalization by noting the occurrence of six crucial events: (1) the first training school; (2) the first university school; (3) the first local professional association; (4) the first national professional association; (5) the first state license law; and (6) the first formal code of ethics (Wilensky, 1964; Goodman, 1989).

The early appearances of the training school and the university affiliation underscore the importance of the cultivation of a knowledge base. The strategic innovative role of the universities and early teachers lies in linking knowledge to practice and creating a rationale for exclusive jurisdiction (Wilensky, 1964). Those practitioners pushing for prescribed training then form a professional association. The association defines the tasks of the profession: raising the quality of recruits; redefining their function to permit the use of less technically skilled people to perform the more routine, less involved tasks; and managing internal and external conflicts. In the process, internal conflict may arise between those committed to established procedures and newcomers committed to change and innovation. At this stage, some form of professional regulation, such as licensing or certification, surfaces because of a belief that it will ensure minimum standards for the profession, enhance status, and protect the layperson in the process (Wilensky, 1964; Goodman, 1989).

The last area of professional development is the establishment of a formal code of ethics, which usually includes rules to exclude the unqualified and unscrupulous practitioners, rules to reduce internal competition, and rules to protect clients and emphasize the ideal service to society. A code of ethics usually comes at the end of the professionalization process.

Now let us consider the present status of clinical engineering. The progression towards professionalism is clearly underway. Consider the following: (1) there is continued discussion about the educational needs of existing, as well as beginning, professionals; (2) there is now a professional society, the **American College of Clinical Engineering**, which should be effective in establishing the knowledge base on which the profession is to develop; (3) there is a credentials process that reflects the needs of this new profession; and (4) there is a code of ethics, which has been developed by the American College of Clinical Engineering for use by all in the profession.

This process toward professionalization will certainly continue in the years ahead as this new professional society seeks to define and control certification activities, to define the educational process required for these new professionals, and to promote the status of clinical engineering to hospital administrators and society as a whole.

CERTIFICATION FOR CLINICAL ENGINEERS

One of the key factors in assessing professionalism is the ability of a responsible group to monitor and control entry into the profession. This is usually accomplished through the process of licensing or certification. Since certification is presently a desired goal of all clinical engineering professionals, let us explore this process.

According to Frank Painter (1989), certification is a means by which an individual can indicate to the general public, co-workers, and employers that a nongovernmental, impartial, nationally recognized organization has determined that he or she has met certain minimum standards of education, experience, and technical knowledge. In this way, individual recognition is obtained by allowing the certified individuals to establish that they have met a bench-mark of proficiency in the skills required in their profession. This recognition, in turn, enables employers to quantify achievement levels in the field and to select individuals that meet an established standard.

Certification of clinical engineers and biomedical equipment technicians began in the early 1970s. At that time, two separate organizations were certifying clinical engineers, and one was certifying biomedical equipment technicians. When these groups were first formed, certification was offered to those who met the criteria for education and experience, without requiring them to take an examination (referred to as "grandfathering"). In May 1983, the organizations merged to form one body to certify clinical engineers (CEs) and biomedical equipment technicians (BMETs). The new organization, the **International Certification Commission (ICC) for Clinical Engineering and Biomedical Technology (ICC)**, manages the certification programs in several countries, including the U.S. and Canada. In each country, boards of examiners exist for both clinical engineering and biomedical equipment technology. The ICC certifies clinical engineers in nine countries, including the U.S.A., Singapore, Jordan, Canada, Saudi Arabia, South Africa, Poland, Brazil and the former U.S.S.R.

The ICC consists of representatives of 15 health-care organizations and the chair of each board of examiners. The organizations, which all have an interest in the advancement of health-care and the certification of CEs and BMETs, include the **Association for the Advancement of Medical Instrumentation (AAMI)**, **American College of Clinical Engineering (ACCE)**, **Canadian Medical and Biological Engineering Society**, **IEEE/Engineering in Medicine and Biology Society (EMBS)**, **Joint Commission for the Accreditation of Healthcare Organizations**, and **Veterans' Administration.**

Each board of examiners is chosen by election for a three-year term and consists only of individuals who have previously been certified by the board. Each board of examiners is responsible for the following:

- Evaluation of applications.
- Administration of written and oral exams.
- Management of requests for appeals.
- Preparation and revision of the application, written exam, operating procedures, and bylaws of the board as needed.
- Recommendation to the ICC of activities and programs that will enhance the certification process, the professional specialty, and the profession. For example, the ICC is presently considering a renewal process that would require continuing education units (CEUs) or some other evidence of continuing competence.

Clinical engineers must meet at least one of the following requirements in order to be eligible as a candidate for certification:

- Have at least a bachelor's (four-year) degree in engineering or electronics technology from an accredited program and have at least three years of clinical engineering experience.
- Be a registered professional engineer and have at least three years of clinical engineering experience.
- Have a bachelor's degree in basic science from an accredited program or a bachelor's degree in electronics technology from a non–accredited program, have passed the Engineer in Training (EIT) examination, and have at least four years of clinical engineering experience.

- Have established standing in the clinical engineering profession, have been a practicing clinical engineer for at least 15 years, and have been in a position of responsible for at least six years.

The examination process consists of filing an application with the secretariat, providing the names of five professional references, and submitting a certified copy of the transcript. The next step is taking a written exam consisting of 150 multiple choice questions (Figure 1.7). The written exam must be passed with a minimum score of 60 percent. The final part of the exam is an oral interview with two members of the board of examiners.

CLINICAL ENGINEERING EDUCATION

Having identified the roles clinical engineers play, and the types of knowledge and experience they must possess, it is now possible to identify the types of programs necessary to provide the appropriate training and education for future clinical engineering professionals. In the 1990s, students interested in clinical engineering should begin their education by obtaining a bachelor's degree in an engineering discipline such as biomedical, chemical, electrical, or mechanical engineering. Upon completion of the undergraduate degree program, the individual should proceed to work in a hospital and gain direct professional experience. An appropriate alternative would be to enter a master's degree program in biomedical engineering that includes a clinical engineering internship. There are a number of such programs in the United States, including California State University at Sacramento, Case Western Reserve University, Drexel University, and the Clinical Engineering Internship Program established in the region of greater Hartford, Connecticut.

Academic Plan for Graduate Study

It is important to emphasize that the academic component of a clinical engineer's knowledge base is essentially found within the biomedical engineering curriculum. Therefore, a typical plan of graduate study in clinical engineering follows that of a normal master's degree program in biomedical engineering. For example, in the clinical engineering program in the greater Hartford area, involving Trinity College and the Hartford Graduate Center, three core courses are included:

- Anatomy and physiology.
- Bioinstrumentation.
- Clinical engineering fundamentals.

In addition, at least four electives from the following set of biomedical engineering courses are required:

- Electrophysiology of the central nervous system.
- Biomaterials.
- Biological control systems.
- Musculoskeletal biomechanics.
- Expert systems in medicine.
- Computer applications in medical technology.
- Medical imaging.
- Biofluid dynamics.

1. The S.A. node is normally the pacemaker because of its

(a) rate of impulses.
(b) location in the atrium.
(c) proximity to the A.V. node.
(d) magnitude of electrical impulse.

2. Ground fault circuit interrupters

(a) measure the resistance of the ground.
(b) protect the electrical ground against corrosion.
(c) monitor the difference between currents in two conductors.
(d) establish an auxiliary ground if the main ground is interrupted.

3. In accordance with JCAHO standards, hospital electrical power supplied by an emergency system must transfer from normal to emergency power in a minimum time of

(a) 1 millisecond.
(b) 1 second.
(c) 10 seconds.
(d) 1 minute.

4. The sum of the residual volume and the expiratory reserve volume is equal to

(a) vital capacity.
(b) total lung capacity.
(c) resting tidal volume.
(d) functional residual capacity.

5. The most frequent site for nosocomial infection is

(a) the skin.
(b) the blood.
(c) the urinary tract.
(d) the respiratory tract

6. The Swan-Ganz catheter is used in the

(a) monitoring of renal efficiency.
(b) monitoring of arterial pressure.
(c) measurement of cerebrospinal fluid viscosity.
(d) measurements of volume changes in body segments.

7. The temperature of pure saturated steam at 15 psi is

(a) 105 C.
(b) 110 C.
(c) 121 C.
(d) 125 C.

8. According to Beer's Law, optical density is

(a) directly proportional to concentration.
(b) inversely proportional to concentration.
(c) proportional to the square of the concentration.
(d) inversely proportional to the square of the concentration.

9. In diagnostic ultrasound, higher frequencies have

(a) better penetration and better resolution.
(b) poorer penetration and better resolution.
(c) poorer penetration and poorer resolution.
(d) better penetration and poorer resolution.

10. An X-ray grid is used to

(a) intensify the image.
(b) position the patient.
(c) control the tube current.
(d) reduce secondary radiation.

11. For compliance with NFPA Standard No. 56A, no conductive floor location shall have a resistance less than

(a) 10,000 Ω.
(b) 25,000 Ω.
(c) 1,000,000 Ω.
(d) 5,000,000 Ω.

12. In diagnostic ECG amplifiers, the minimum bandwidth between 3 dB points is

(a) 0.05 to 10 Hz.
(b) 1 to 100 Hz.
(c) 0.05 to 100 Hz.
(d) 10 to 100 Hz.

13. The third derivative of y with respect to x in the equation $y = 8x^3$ is

(a) 0.
(b) 48.
(c) 48x.
(d) $24x^2$.

14. Pair production, the photoelectric effect, and the Compton effect all produce different energies. The ascending energy order is

(a) pair production, Compton, photoelectric.
(b) Compton, photoelectric, pair production.
(c) pair production, photoelectric, Compton.
(d) photoelectric, Compton, pair production.

Figure 1.7: Sample questions used on Certification Examination (Painter, 1989).

Finally, at least two courses in an engineering discipline, e.g., electrical or mechanical engineering, and a six-credit-hour thesis/project, which is usually undertaken during the second year of the associated internship program, must be completed.

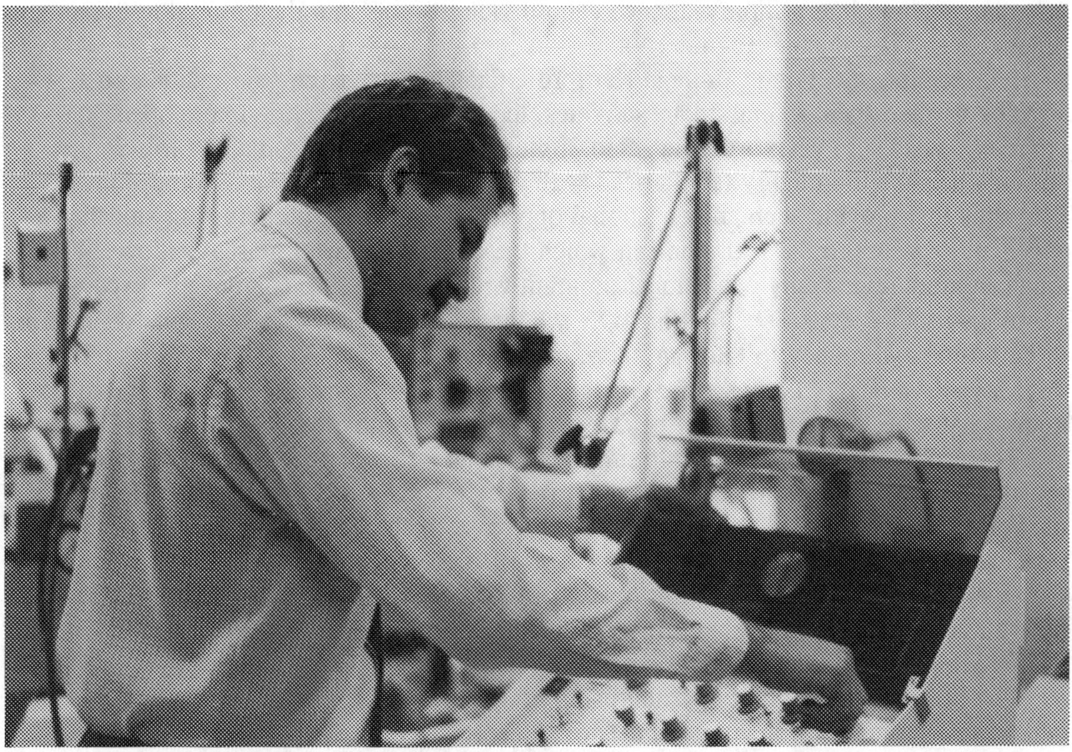

Figure 1.8: An intern conducting a performance assurance test on a ventilator.

The Internship Experience

In addition to the engineering courses required to provide the necessary fundamentals in specific biomedical engineering topics, it is necessary that students interested in clinical engineering be exposed to and work in the hospital environment (Figure 1.8). Such an experience permits these students to observe not only the operation of specific medical instruments, but also the environment in which they are used and the people who use them. The nature of this hospital experience may vary in terms of its duration and specificity, but an internship of some type is essential.

One way to obtain this experience is through an internship established as part of the individual's overall educational program. In the past, several biomedical engineering programs have attempted to meet this objective by initiating a required or optional internship program with a clinical institution (Cook et al., 1973; Cox et al., 1975; Peura et al., 1975; Cook and Rose, 1978; Bronzino et al., 1979; Potvin et al., 1981; Bronzino, 1985). Most of these programs have been based primarily within an academic institution and have provided internships of varying duration. For example, some institutions required students to engage in a hospital project for one to two months, while others have insisted on a one- or two-year experience.

Any internship experience should be designed to permit budding clinical engineers to assume a role analogous to that of their medical counterparts to learn the intricacies of their profession in a personal manner. Since specific clinical, organizational, and managerial skills needed by clinical engineers cannot be taught in a formal academic program, such an internship experience can provide insights into the profession that might otherwise be unattainable (Figure 1.9).

For example the Trinity College/Hartford Graduate Center program requires that, in addition to time spent in classroom activities, the clinical engineering intern spend the entire two academic years working 25 to 30 hours/week at the hospital. In this way, students become thoroughly familiarized with standard hospital operating procedure. Programs that provide such an educational opportunity offer the participating student excellent exposure to the real world in which the clinical engineer must function. When administrators review any educational program with an internship component, two questions usually arise. The first is *"Why the internship format?"* It is expensive in terms of both time and money to tutor an intern in a hospital setting. The second question is *"Why should a hospital pay for the education of clinical engineers?"* Hospitals want to know what their return will be if they invest in such a program.

The economics of the internship program depend on its organization. The fact that the clinical engineering intern begins as a graduate engineer and provides useful work is comforting to the hospital administrator. In the case of the Trinity College/Hartford Graduate Center program, the extent of the payoff depends on the success and value of the second-year project, which directly serves the needs of the hospital. According to hospital administrators, the key advantage of this internship is that it provides the hospital with engineering services it would otherwise do without.

The primary objective of any internship program is to provide a high-quality educational program for a small number of students. The internship approach is not appropriate for large numbers of students, nor is it desirable for large numbers of clinical engineers to be trained, as the market for this type of professional is still relatively small. However, the market may increase significantly as the value of these professionals is realized by the medical-device industry and by the insurance companies who underwrite hospital and malpractice insurance policies.

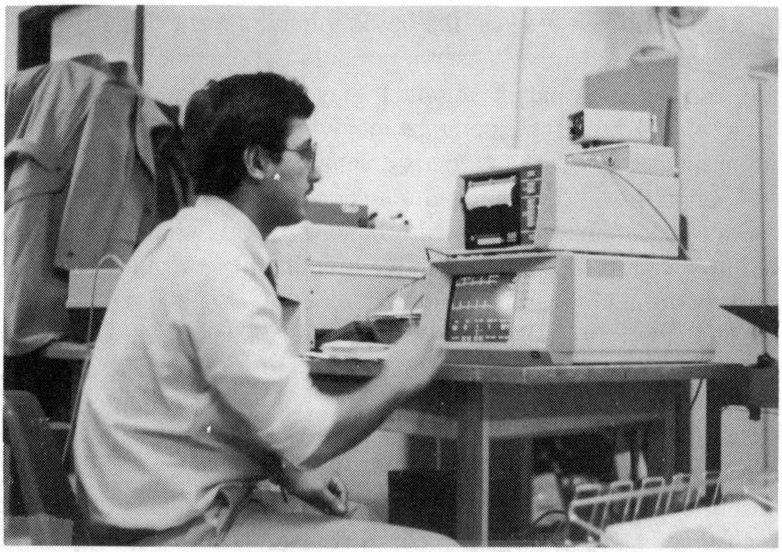

Figure 1.9: An intern trouble-shooting an elctrocardiograph (ECG) monitor.

Educational programs for clinical engineers, therefore, must include internship experiences. In the long run, this type of educational experience will be beneficial to individual clinical engineers, to the clinical engineering profession, and to the American health-care system.

FUTURE OF CLINICAL ENGINEERING

From its early days, when electrical safety testing and basic preventive maintenance were the primary concerns, to the present, the practice of clinical engineering has changed enormously. Yet, it is appropriate to use the cliche "The more things change, the more they stay the same." Today, hospital-based clinical engineers still have the following as their primary concerns: patient safety and good hospital equipment management. However, these basic concerns are being supplemented by new areas of responsibility, making the clinical engineer not only the chief technology officer, but also an integral part of the hospital management team (Newhouse et al., 1989).

In large part, these demands are due to the economic pressures that hospitals now face. To further complicate this financial situation, state-of-the-art, high-level instruments, such as MRI systems, surgical lasers, and other sophisticated devices, are now used as a matter of course in patient care. Because of the high cost and complexity of such instrumentation, the institution needs to plan carefully—at both a technical and a managerial level—for the assessment, acquisition, and use of this new technology.

With these needs in mind, hospital administrators have begun to turn to their clinical engineering staffs for assistance in operational areas. Clinical engineers now provide assistance in the application and management of many other technologies that support patient care, e.g., computer support, telecommunications, and facilities operations.

Computer Support

The use of personal computers (PCs) has grown enormously in the past decade. PCs are now commonplace in every facet of hospital operations, including data analysis for research, use as a teaching tool, and many administrative tasks. PCs are also increasingly used as integral parts of local area networks and hospital information systems (Schrenker, 1988).

Because of their technical training and experience with computerized patient record systems and inventory and equipment management programs, clinical engineers have extended their scope of activities to include personal computer support. In the process, the hospital has accrued several benefits from this involvement in computer servicing. The first is time: whether computers are used in direct clinical applications or in administrative work, downtime is expensive. In-house servicing can provide faster and often more dependable repairs than an outside group. Second, with in-house service, there is no need to send a computer out for service. This reduces the possibility that computer equipment will be damaged or lost. Finally, in-house service reduces costs by permitting the hospital to avoid expensive service contracts for computers and peripheral equipment (Ben-Zvi, 1985).

With all of these benefits, it might seem that every clinical engineering department should carry out computer servicing. However, the picture is not so simple. At the most basic level, the clinical engineering program must be sure it has the staff, money, and space to do the job well. To assist in making this determination, several questions should be asked: Will computer repair take too much time away from the department's primary goal—patient care-instrumentation? Is there enough money and space to stock needed parts, replacement boards, diagnostic software, and peripheral devices? For those hospitals that do commit the resources needed to support computer repair, clinical engineers have found that their departments can provide these services very efficiently, and they subsequently receive added recognition and visibility within the hospital (Schrenker, 1988).

Telecommunications

Another area of increased clinical engineering involvement is hospital-based telecommunications. In the modern health-care institution, telecommunications covers many important activities, the most visible of which is telephone service. Broadly speaking, however, telecommunications includes many other capabilities.

Until the 1970s, telephone systems were basically electromechanical, using switches, relays, and other analog circuitry. During the 1970s, digital equipment began to appear. This development allowed the introduction of innovations such as touch-tone dialing, call forwarding, conference calling, improved call transferring, and other advanced services. The breakup of the Bell System also changed the telecommunications field enormously by opening it to competition and diversification of services (John Diebold and Associates, 1986). Today, many hospitals use a private branch exchange (**PBX**), in which all switching equipment is located on-site. In comparison to the old PBX systems, which could fill an entire room, newer systems offer several advantages. They take up less space, they can be serviced in-house, and they are relatively easy to customize — all cost-saving features. For example, it is possible to limit long-distance capabilities for specific phones. PBX systems also handle more traffic, serve local area network functions, and tap into data networks.

Data transmission capability allows the hospital to send scans and reports to physicians at their offices or at other remote locations. Data, such as patient ECGs, can be transmitted from the hospital to a data analysis system at another location, and the results can be transmitted back. Hospitals are also making increased use of facsimile (FAX) transmission. This equipment allows documents, such as patient charts, to be sent via telephone line from a remote location and reconstructed at the receiving site in a matter of minutes.

Modern telecommunications equipment also allows the hospital to conduct educational conferences. This is accomplished through microwave links that allow video transmission of a conference taking place at a separate site. Some newer equipment allows pictorial information, such as patient slides, to be digitally transmitted via a phone line and then electronically reassembled to produce a video image (Newhouse et al., 1989).

Clinical engineers can play an important role in helping the hospital administrators develop plans for a new telecommunications system. They can provide technical support during the planning stage, can assist in the development of requests for proposals for a new system, and can help resolve any physical plant issues associated with installing the new system. Thereafter, the clinical engineer can assist in reviewing responses to the hospital's requests for quotations and can lend a hand during installation of the system.

Facilities Operations

Recently, some hospital administrators have begun to tap the high-level technical skills available within their clinical engineering departments to assist in other operational areas. One of these is facilities operations, which includes heating, ventilation, and air conditioning (HVAC), electrical supply and distribution (including isolated power), central gas supply and vacuum systems, and other physical plant equipment (Newhouse et al., 1989). This has occurred for a number of reasons. First, the modern physical plant contains microprocessor-driven control circuits, sophisticated circuitry, and other high-level technology. In many instances, facilities personnel lack the training needed to understand the engineering theory underlying these systems. Thus, clinical engineers can effectively work in a consultation role to help correct malfunctions in the hospital's physical plant systems. Another reason is cost; the hospital may be able to avoid expensive service contracts by performing this work in-house.

Clinical engineers can assist in facilities operations in other ways. For example, they can lend assistance when compressed gas or vacuum delivery systems need to be upgraded or replaced. While the work is taking place, the clinical engineer can serve as the administration's technical arm, ensuring that the job is done properly, is in compliance with code, and is done with minimal disruption (Newhouse et al., 1989).

Strategic Planning

Today's emphasis on health-care cost control requires that clinical engineers assist in containing costs associated with medical instrumentation. To accomplish this objective, clinical engineers are increasingly becoming involved in strategic planning, technology assessment, and purchase review. During assessment and purchase review, the clinical engineer studies a request to buy a new system or device and ensures that the purchase request includes (1) needed accessories, (2) warranty information, and (3) user and service training. This review process ensures that the device is, in fact, needed (or whether there exists a less-costly unit that meets the clinician's requirements) and will be properly integrated into the hospital's existing equipment and physical environment.

Clinical engineers can provide valuable assistance during the planning for and financial analysis of potential new services. If one considers the steps involved in planning for a new patient-care area, many design questions immediately come to mind; What is the best layout for the new area? What equipment will be used there? How many suction, air, oxygen, and electrical outlets will be needed? Is there a need to provide for special facilities, such as those needed for hemodialysis treatment at the bedside? With their knowledge of instrumentation and user needs, clinical engineers can help select reliable, cost-effective equipment to help ensure that the hospital obtains the best possible plan.

In the future, clinical engineering departments will need to concentrate even more heavily on management, with the goals of increased productivity and reduced costs. Clinical engineers will also need to keep up with the latest developments in medical instrumentation; computers and telecommunications systems; and other technologies that affect the financial operation of the hospital (Simmons, 1988). By expanding their horizons, clinical engineers can further contribute to the overall operation of the hospital and to ensure high-quality patient care at a reasonable cost.

EXERCISES

1. Select two medical devices that were invented after 1945, describe the fundamental principles of their operation, and discuss their impact on health-care delivery.

2. From the definition of "clinical engineering," select two key words and discuss their significance.

3. The three primary components in the organizational structure of a hospital are

   (a) the governing board.
   (b) the hospital administration.
   (c) the clinical engineering division.
   (d) the medical staff.

4. Provide specific examples of two of the responsibilities of the hospital administrator.

5. List the duties for the director of a clinical engineering department.

6. The core functions of a clinical engineering department include

   (a) litigation.
   (b) consulting.
   (c) technology management.
   (d) technology assessment.

7. How does nursing fit the definition of a profession?

8. The status of professionalization can be ascertained by noting

   (a) the enactment of the first state law.
   (b) the first graduate of a training school.
   (c) the appearance of a journal.
   (d) the first conference.

9. What requirements must clinical engineers meet in order to be certified?

10. As the director of the clinical engineering department you have been asked to provide a plan for the clinical engineering department you manage. Include in this plan a Mission Statement and a list of objectives for the department, identify the users of each of the services provided by the department and specify how you intend to market these services and how the department is to be evaluated. Include any other material you consider pertinent.

11. (a) Provide an organizational chart of a hospital in your community, depicting the reporting lines of the clinical engineering department. Discuss the strengths and weaknesses of this organization. Provide any modification that you believe would improve the operation of the CE department, and justify your changes.

    (b) Using the organizational chart outlined in Figure 1.5, describe the functions of each of the subsections of the CE department.

12. List the areas of knowledge necessary to practice clinical engineering. Identify where in the normal educational process one can acquire this knowledge. How best can the administrative skills be best acquired?
13. In addition to the new areas of activities for clinical engineers listed in this chapter, list some other activities that you think would be appropriate for clinical engineers to assume in the future.

REFERENCES

AHA. American Hospital Association Resource Center, *Hospital Administration Terminology*, 2nd ed., American Hospital Publishing, Washington, D.C., 1986.

Bauld, T.J. "The Definition of a Clinical Engineer," *J. Clin. Engin.*, 16:403–405, 1991.

Ben-Zvi, S. "In-House Servicing of Microprocessor-Based and Digital Patient Care Equipment," *J. Clin. Engin.*, 10:121–130, 1985.

Bronzino, J.D. *Technology for Patient Care*, C.V. Mosby, St. Louis, 1977.

Bronzino, J.D., et al. "A Regional Model for a Hospital-Based Clinical Engineering Internship Program," *J. Clin. Engin.*, 7:34–37, 1979.

Bronzino, J.D. "Clinical Engineering Internships: A Regional Hospital-Based Approach," *J. Clin. Engin.*, 10:235–239, 1985.

Bronzino, J.D. *Biomedical Engineering and Instrumentation: Basic Concepts and Applications*, PWS Publishing Co., Boston, 1986.

Bronzino, J.D. "Biomedical Engineering," in *Encyclopedia of Applied Physics* (G. Trigg, ed.), VCH Publishers, New York, pp. 513–548, 1991.

Bronzino, J.D., and Hayes, T.P. "Hospital-Based Clinical Engineering Programs," in *Handbook for Biomedical Engineering*, Academic Press, New York, pp. 565–595, 1988.

Bronzino, J.D., Smith, V., and Wade, M. *Medical Technology and Society*, MIT Press, Cambridge, 1990.

Cook, A.M., et al. "Graduate Bioengineering Assistantships in a Community Hospital," *Engineering Education*, 64:194–197, 1973.

Cook, A.M. and Rose, L.E. "Cost-Effective Clinical Engineering Internships in Community Hospitals," *J. Clin. Engin.*, 3:173–178, 1978.

Courter, S.S. "The Professional Development Degree for Biomedical Engineers," *J. Clin. Engin.*, 5:299–302, 1980.

Cox, J.E., et al. "Experience with a Training Program in Technology in Healthcare," *IEEE Transactions in Biomedical Engineering*, 22:129–133, 1975.

Crichton, M. *Five Patients — the Hospital Explained*, Alfred A. Knopf, New York, 1970.

Friedson, E. *Profession of Medicine*, Dodd, Mead & Co., New York, 1971.

Goodman, G. "The Profession of Clinical Engineering," *J. Clin. Engin.*, 14:27–37, 1989.

ICC. *International Certification Commission's Definition of a Clinical Engineer*, International Certification Commission Fact Sheet, ICC, Arlington, VA, 1991.

Issakov, A., Mallouppas, A., and McKie, J. "Manpower Development for a Healthcare Technical Service," report of the World Health Organization, WHO/SHS/NHP/90.4, 1990.

Jacobs, J.E. "The Biomedical Engineering Quandary," *IEEE Transactions in Biomedical Engineering*, 22:100–106, March 1975.

John Diebold and Associates. "John Diebold and Associates: Telecommunications Planning for Hospitals," American Hospital Association Technical Document Series, American Society for Hospital Engineering of the American Hospital Association, New York, 1986.

Knowles, J. "The Hospital," *Sci. Am.*, 229:128–137, September 1973.

Newhouse, V.L., et al. "The Future of Clinical Engineering in the 1990s," *J. Clin. Engin.*, 14:417–430, 1989.

Pacela, A. *Bioengineering Education Directory*, Quest Publishing Co. Brea, CA, 1990.

Pacela, A. "Career "Fact Sheets" for Clinical Engineering and Biomedical Technology," *J. Clin. Engin.*, 16:407–416, 1991.

Painter, F.R. "Clinical Engineering and Biomedical Equipment Technology Certification," World Health Organization meeting on Manpower Development and Training for Health Care Equipment, Management, Maintenance and Repair, WHO/SHS/NHP/90.4, pp. 130–185, 1989.

Parsons, T. *Essays in Sociological Theory*, rev. ed., Free Press, Glencoe, IL, 1954.

Peura, R.A., et al. "Organization and Function of a Hospital Biomedical Engineering Internship Program," *IEEE Transactions in Biomedical Engineering*, 22:134–139, 1975.

Potvin, A.R., et al. "Biomedical Engineering Education: Enrollment, Courses, Degrees and Employment," *IEEE Transactions in Biomedical Engineering*, 28:22–28, 1981.

Schaffer, M.J., and Schaffer, M.D. "The Professionalization of Clinical Engineering," *Biomed. Instr. Technol.*, 23:370–374, 1989.

Schaffer, M.J., and Schaffer, M.D. "What is a Clinical Engineer? Issues in Definition," *Biomed. Instr. Technol.*, July/August pp. 277–282, 1992.

Schrenker, A. "Clinical Engineering and Personal Computer Maintenance," American Hospital Association Technical Document Series, American Society for Hospital Engineering of the American Hospital Association, New York, 1988.

Simmons, D.A., and Wear, J.O. *Clinical Engineering Manual*, 3rd ed., Scientific Enterprises, North Little Rock, AR, 1988.

Simmons, D.A. "The Future of Hospital-Based Clinical Engineering," *Clin. Engin. Informat. Serv.*, 2:106–112, 1988.

Vogel, M.J. *The Invention of the Modern Hospital*, University of Chicago Press, Chicago, 1980.

Wald, A. "Clinical Engineering in Clinical Departments: A Different Point of View", *Biomed. Instr. Tech.*, 23:58–63, 1989.

Wilensky, H.L. "The Professionalization of Everyone," *Am. J. Sociol.*, 69:137–158, 1964.

CHAPTER 2

SAFETY IN THE CLINICAL ENVIRONMENT

Patients enter hospitals today with much the same feelings as they did years ago, that is with a mixture of hope and fear. They hope that modern medicine is capable of alleviating their physical distress, and entrust themselves to the care and ministrations of physicians and nurses. At the same time, however, they try to suppress the apprehension and fear they feel as they enter a rather complex and technologically sophisticated health-care delivery system. These concerns are real and appropriate, since patients today are likely to encounter a host of medical devices and systems that may be both potentially beneficial and hazardous to their well-being. Of particular concern here are the hazards associated with medical devices. These include the following (Webster and Cook, 1979):

- **Electrical hazards:** Patients are surrounded by and often connected to electrical devices. Some patients, because of their physical condition and the invasive nature of certain medical procedures, are particularly susceptible to low-level electrical hazards. Furthermore, in oxygen enriched environments and in those clinical areas where flammable anesthetic gases are used, electrical energy can be an ignition source.
- **Mechanical hazards:** Mechanical devices used for clinical purposes in the modern hospital include mobility aids, transfer devices, prosthetic devices, mechanical-assist devices, and patient-support equipment. Since each of these devices embodies numerous threats to patients as well as to hospital staff, they must be subjected to careful design review and failure indication, and specifications for safe use must be established.
- **Environmental hazards:** The hospital has its own ecosystem. The environment within the hospital includes such elements as solid wastes, noise, utilities (natural gas, water, etc.), and building structures which must be carefully controlled and managed to reduce hazards ranging from the spread of infection to injury from physical objects.
- **Biological hazards:** Infection control is a major factor in hospital safety today, especially in light of the AIDS (Aquired Immunodeficiency Syndrome) epidemic. Here, the term "safety" is used in its broadest sense because infection threatens the safety of staff members as well as patients. Infection control is accomplished by instituting and managing programs that identify exposures to, and eliminate sources of infection. Isolation, decontamination and sterilization, and appropriate methods of biological waste disposal are the primary tools of infection control.
- **Radiation hazards:** Radiation and radioactive materials have assumed a broad role in medical treatment. However, their use also may be hazardous to both patients and the medical staff. The health hazards from these devices and substances require the establishment of programs to control the use of diagnostic machines and therapeutic devices that release ionizing radiation and to monitor exposure of patients and medical staff. Control of radioactive waste is especially critical because of the extended periods during which these substances remain hazardous.

The presence of these and other hazards in the medical environment has made it essential for modern health-care facilities to have a clinical engineering department that is intimately involved in and responsible for establishing and maintaining a safe environment. While physicians, nurses, and other medical personnel are busily serving patients under their care, there is a distinct need for the clinical engineer to focus on those hazards that may disrupt or destroy the life-saving efforts of this medical team.

Since a detailed presentation of all aspects of safety within the hospital is not possible here, this chapter emphasizes those safety issues that are of particular relevance to clinical engineering departments, with special emphasis on electrical and medical device safety. However, following discussions of the implementation of safety plans to reduce the potential for electrical hazard and to increase quality assurance in the use of medical devices, this chapter also addresses concepts of radiation safety, laser safety, and programs for the control of biological hazards.

ELECTRICAL SAFETY

Due to the prevalence of electrical devices, electrical safety is a vital component of a hospital's comprehensive safety program. Concern for electrical safety in the patient care environment has a long history with particular relevance to the development of the clinical engineering profession.

Historical Background

During the late 1960s, there was intense publicity surrounding the electrical safety of hospital patients. This safety scare reached its peak when consumer activists, most notably Ralph Nader (1971), claimed that "*at the very least, 1,200 Americans are electrocuted annually during routine diagnostic and therapeutic procedures in hospitals.*" This concern was based primarily on the supposition that catheterized patients with a low-resistance conducting pathway from outside the body into blood vessels near the heart could be electrocuted by voltage differences well below the normal level of sensation. Although no statistical evidence has ever been developed to substantiate these claims (Bruner and Leonard, 1989), this outcry raised the level of consciousness of health-care professionals with respect to the safe use of medical devices.

In the process, a new industry—hospital electrical safety—arose almost overnight. Organizations, such as the **National Fire Protection Association (NFPA)**, wrote standards addressing electrical safety in hospitals; electrical safety analyzer manufacturers and equipment safety consultants became eager to serve the needs of various hospitals for a "safety fix"; and some companies, particularly those specializing in power distribution systems (most notably isolation transformers), deliberately preyed on the fears of hospitals. To alleviate these fears, the **Joint Commission on the Accreditation of Healthcare Organizations** (then known as the Joint Commission on Accreditation of Hospitals) turned to **NFPA** codes as the standard for electrical safety, and further specified that hospitals must inspect all equipment used on or near a patient for electrical safety at least every six months. To meet this new requirement, hospital administrators considered a number of options, including (1) paying medical device manufacturers to perform these electrical safety inspections, (2) contracting for the services of shared-services organizations, or (3) providing these services with in-house staff. As discussed in Chapter 1, when faced with this decision, most large hospitals opted for in-house service and created clinical engineering departments to provide the technological support to address these electrical safety concerns. Once in place, however, these clinical engineering pioneers began to play a more substantial role within the hospital. As new members of the hospital team, they became actively involved in developing cost-effective approaches to the use of medical technology. They immediately cautioned hospital administrators about purchasing millions of dollars worth of isolation transformers that added little, if any, additional protection against microshock hazards. They started to work with standards-writing organizations, utilizing modern scientific methods. As the electrical safety issue abated, they became so effective that clinical engineering departments gradually assumed a wider role in the daily operation of the hospital. Since the 1970s, however, dramatic changes have affected the hospital's approach to safety. Consider the following:

- Significant improvements have been made regarding the safe operation, better performance, and greater reliability of medical equipment.
- More realistic codes and standards have been developed that make more efficient use of hospital resources in minimizing electrical hazards.
- Clinical engineering departments have been effectively utilized to assist in the purchase, inspection, and preventive maintenance of medical equipment.

All of these factors have made it possible for clinical engineering departments to relegate the electrical safety issue to the status of an important but routine matter that is reasonably controlled by simple periodic measures.

Physiological Effects of Electrical Currents

For electricity to have any effect on the body, certain conditions must be satisfied:

- An electrical potential difference (or voltage) must be present.
- The individual must be part of the electrical circuit, permitting electrical current to flow through the body.

When these requirements are met, the actual effect of the electrical current passing through the body depends on the amount of current passed and the pathway the current takes through the body.

Figure 2.1 summarizes the physiological effects of one-second exposures to various levels of alternating current (AC) current (root mean squared, [RMS] values) at 60 Hz applied arm-to-arm (Olson, 1978). As can be seen, very little current (1 mA) is sufficient to produce an awareness of the presence of current within the body, and only 100 mA may result in a truly hazardous situation for the individual.

Since the magnitude of the current flowing in any circuit depends not only on the voltage between the connections, but also on the electrical resistance of the various pathways through the body, it is important to consider the values of resistance of biological tissues and how they may be changed. Most body tissues contain a high percentage of water (containing ions). Therefore, they are usually considered to be fairly good conductors of electricity. However, the surface resistance — that is the condition of the actual contact point — also affects the amount of current that flows through the body. For example, if contact is made directly on moist skin, there will be little surface resistance, and a considerable amount of current will flow directly into the body.

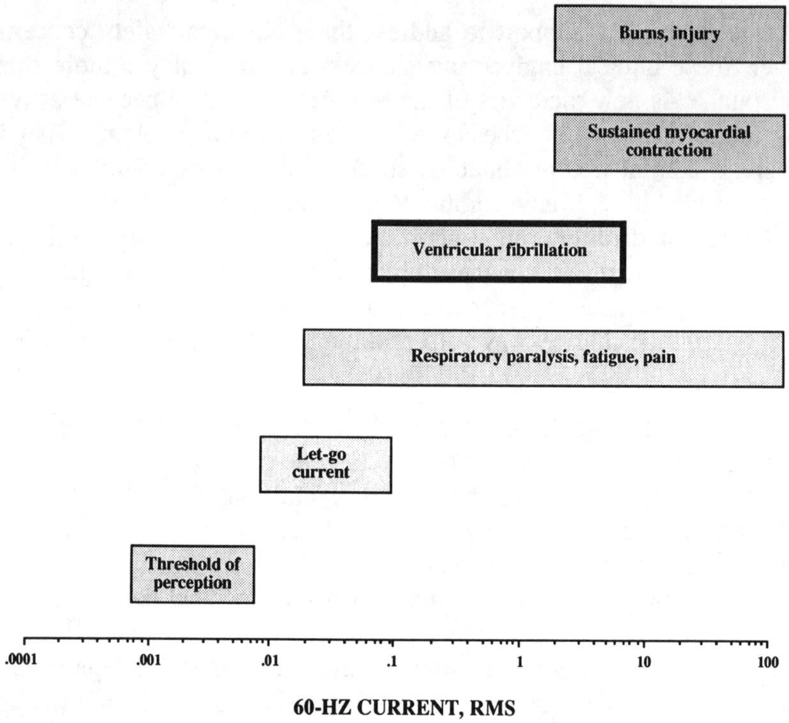

Figure 2.1: Physiological responses to electricity.

On the other hand, if there is no direct contact with body fluids (e.g., when the skin is dry or when contact is made against protective clothing), then the surface resistance will be quite high, and much less current will be able to find its way into body tissue. Table 2.1 indicates, for example, that the skin impedance at 60 Hz may vary from 200 Ω to 93 kΩ, depending on the condition of the skin (Spach, et al., 1966). Thus, the human body's first line of defense against electrical shock is its own protective covering—the skin. To illustrate exactly how these factors come into play, consider the following example.

Table 2.1: Impedance per cm² of skin tissue at 60 Hz

Condition	*Skin impedence*
Dry Skin	93 KΩ
Electrode gel on skin	10.8 KΩ
Penetrated skin	200 Ω

* note: values of impedance depend on the electrode gel used, skin properties, etc.

Example 2.1 — What is the RMS voltage (at 60 Hz) required to deliver a current of 10 mA between two gelled surface electrodes each having a cross-sectional area of 1.5 cm²? Assume that the visceral impedance is 200 Ω.

Solution. The impedance at each skin electrode is

$$Z_{SKIN} = (10.8\ k\Omega^{-cm2})\ /\ (1.5\ cm^2) = 7.2\ k\Omega$$

The total circuit impedance is

$$Z_{TOTAL} = 2(Z_{SKIN}) + (Z_{VISCERA}) = 14.6\ k\Omega$$

The voltage required to deliver 10 mA is

$$V = (Z_{TOTAL})(I) = 146\ volts$$

Keep in mind, however, that the physiological effect of this current will depend on the path the current takes through the body. Since the distribution of current flow is determined by the specific resistance of local tissue (i.e., a nonhomogeneous volume conductor), the electrical current tends to spread out. Consequently, there are a variety of pathways that the current may follow in its course through the body, depending on the resistance of the tissues involved. It should be apparent that it is possible for situations to arise in which an individual comes into contact with a relatively large voltage source but experiences only a minor electrical shock. Conversely, application of a relatively low voltage directly to the heart (e.g., during surgery or via the invasive components of certain diagnostic and therapeutic equipment) can produce ventricular fibrillation, a life-threatening arrhythmia. The danger in one's exposure to various electrical devices is not the voltage, but the magnitude and pathway of electrical current that flows through body tissue and major organs. In addition, for electrically sensitive organs such as the heart, physiological effects are also dependent on the frequency and waveform of the current.

If electrical current enters the body, it may also burn the tissue through which it passes. Whenever electrical current passes through any resistive element, some of the electrical energy is dissipated in the form of heat. As a result, damage to the biological tissue in the form of a burn will result when the temperature produced by this phenomenon is high enough to affect the tissue. This is especially true at the point of contact, where the current intensity is usually quite high and the pathway is limited to a relatively small area.

Consider the case of skin burns that may result when electrosurgical units are used in surgery to cut tissue or stop bleeding of small blood vessels. When these devices are used, a dispersive electrode is usually placed under the patient's shoulder or buttocks to ensure that high current densities occur only at the point of contact for the "active" electrode, controlled by the surgeon. If the dispersive electrode is too small there is a significant risk of skin burn at the contact point. The absence or presence of burns is directly related to the current density (**J = I/area**); i.e., for any given amount of current, the current density will vary depending upon the cross-sectional area of the dispersive electrode.

Electrical current can also affect the functioning of nerve and muscle tissue. In this situation, the current actually stimulates the nerve or muscle into activity. When individual nerve cells, or neurons, are activated, an action potential, or electrical pulse, is generated that travels along the axon, or nerve, to its synaptic connection with other cells. This electrical pulse can be stimulated, with some startling results, by an electrical current passing through the nerve. For example, if sensory nerves are stimulated, the result is a prickling sensation, which at sufficient intensity becomes unpleasant and even painful; if motor nerves or muscles are affected, severe muscular contraction can result. If an electrical current interferes with the functioning of heart muscle, ventricular fibrillation could result. If this occurs, the pumping action of the heart would stop, circulation of the blood would be interrupted, and the patient would be in critical condition. Thus, the introduction into the body of conductive materials, such as fluid-filled catheters and pacemaker leads, can drastically alter the electrical environment of the patient by creating direct low-impedance pathways to electrically sensitive organs.

Electrical shock hazards are usually classified as either macroshock or microshock. "Macroshock" is the term applied to high currents (on the order of milliamperes and above) that pass through the skin, typically from limb to limb (Figure 2.2). This type of electrical shock can result in burns and a wide variety of physiological consequences. Macroshock is a hazard to healthy people in everyday life as well as to patients in the clinical environment.

"Microshock" is the term applied to low currents (on the order of microamperes) that present a fibrillation hazard to patients who are electrically susceptible because of invasive diagnostic and therapeutic procedures (Figure 2.3). These categories of electrical shock differ not only in magnitude of electrical current but in their etiology and control.

Protection against Electrical Hazards

All electrical and electronic devices are sources of potentially harmful current. Most of this equipment is powered by electricity obtained from the building's power distribution system. In practice, electricity is usually generated at a power generator station, transmitted at very high voltages, and subsequently transformed to a much lower voltage for local distribution. This lower voltage is then further reduced for local use to 110–120 V or 220–240 V by power distribution transformers located at the electrical entrances to hospitals, industrial plants, and residential districts for local use.

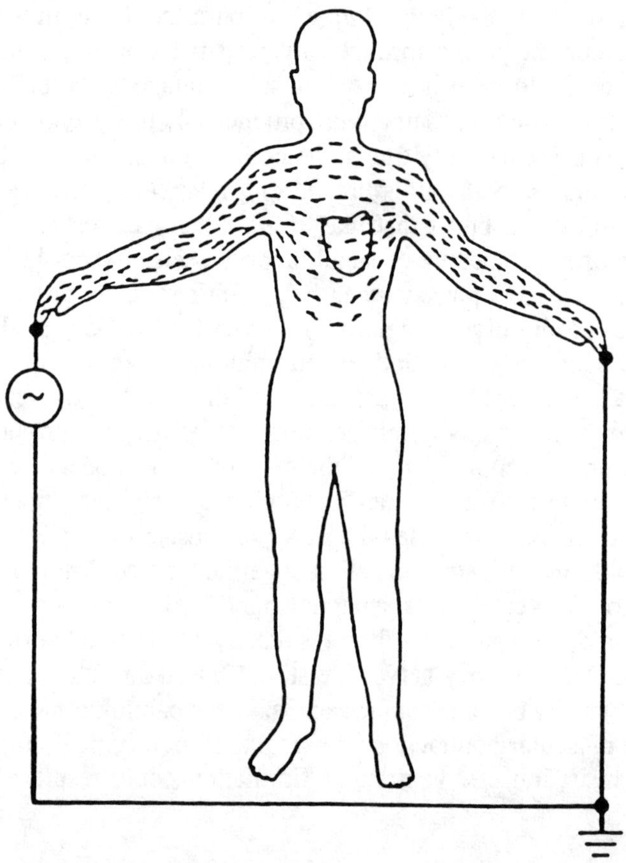

Figure 2.2: Macroshock current distribution.

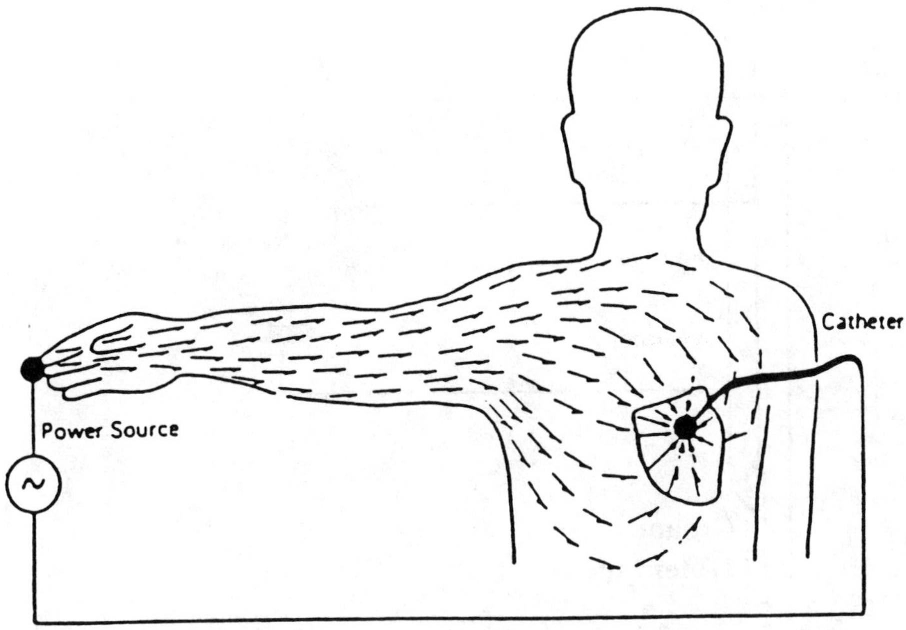

Figure 2.3: Microshock current distribution.

Heavy-duty electrical devices requiring larger amounts of current, such as large air conditioners, ovens, and X-ray equipment, operate on 230 V, while most wall receptacles receive 115 V. Today within the hospital, electrical power is provided by a three-wire system in which one of the wires (G) is at ground potential; another is called the "hot" wire (H), and the last is the return, or neutral, wire (N), which is also connected to ground (Figure. 2.4). The line voltage between the hot and neutral wires is either 115 or 230 V. The hot and neutral wires, respectively, carry current to and from equipment; the ground wire does not normally carry substantial currents. However, as we shall see, it serves as a first line of defense against electrical hazards.

Grounding and Leakage Current Limits. If electrical devices were perfect, the conventional (ground-referenced) electrical power distribution system described above would require only two conductors; all power current would be confined to those conductors and the electrical equipment that they supply. However, in practical applications, there are two major departures from this ideal case:

- If a fault occurs (i.e., through miswiring, insulation failure, electrical component failure, etc.), it is possible for an electrical potential to exist between an exposed conductive surface (the metal case of a device, for example) and a grounded surface (a wet floor, the grounded metal case of another device, etc.). Any person who bridges these surfaces is subject to macroshock.
- Even if a fault does not occur, imperfect insulation and electromagnetic coupling (capacitive or inductive) may produce an electrical potential relative to ground. An electrically susceptible patient who provides a path for this "leakage current" to flow to ground is subject to microshock.

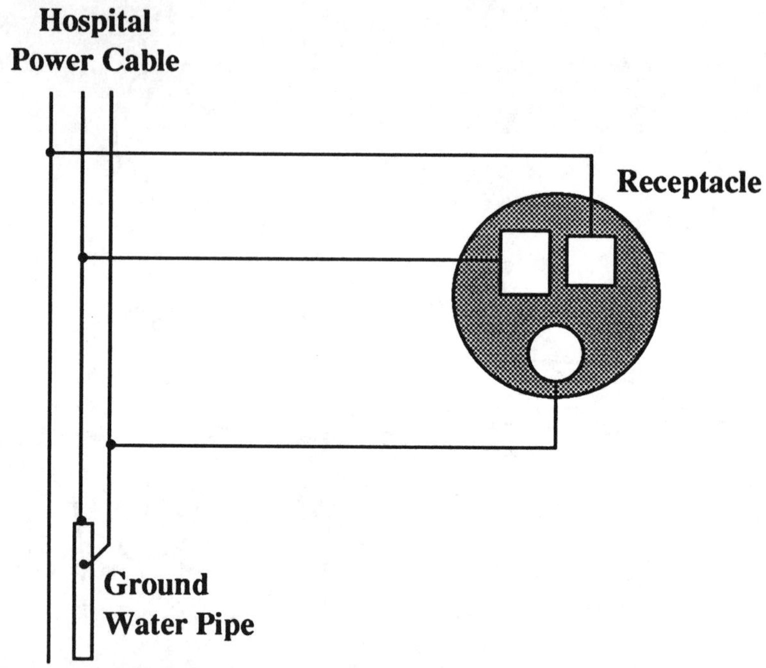

Figure 2.4: Conventional (grounded) electrical power distribution system.

To address these problems, all electrical power distribution systems in the clinical environment are required to have a third conductor (ground wire) that is directly connected to ground. All line-operated electrical devices (except those meeting strict "double-insulation" standards) use this ground wire to ground all external conductive surfaces. This produces the following effects:

- If an electrical fault occurs (for example, a short circuit between the "hot" power conductor and the metal case of the device), the resulting fault current will cause the circuit breaker to open (after a short delay) and remove power from the device. This method of reducing the macroshock hazard depends on the ability of the grounding system (ground connections within the device, the device power cord and the plug, the power distribution system receptacle and wiring) to conduct high currents to ground.
- If there is no fault, the ground wire serves to conduct leakage current safely back to the electrical power source. As long as the grounding system provides a low resistance pathway to ground, the microshock hazard caused by leakage current is greatly reduced.

To meet both objectives, the grounding system must have large-gauge, low-resistance conductors as well as high-integrity connections along the entire electrical pathway. The size and type of conductors is specified by the design standards for buildings and equipment. On the other hand, high-integrity connections require good design (the use of hospital-grade plugs and receptacles, for example) but also good maintenance (as discussed later in the chapter).

Because they are unique to the clinical environment, microshock hazards created by equipment leakage currents require additional consideration. Leakage current may occur in a variety of ways:

- **Capacitive coupling:** Since it is possible to establish a potential difference between any two metal conductors through the process of "separation of charge," leakage current will flow whenever anyone makes contact with both metal surfaces. This type of fault is frequency sensitive because as the frequency of the voltage increases or deceases, so does the capacitive coupling.

- **Inductive coupling:** In this case, the hazardous voltage difference is established by "transformer action" via the close proximity of motors, transformers, and other inductive devices. As in the case of capacitive coupling, inductive coupling is also frequency dependent.

The leakage current limits recommended by the Emergency Care Research Institute (ECRI) were established so that if the grounding of a device should fail, injuries would be avoided if a patient touched the chassis of that device while in contact with a grounded conductor (Table 2.2). Thus, these leakage current limits represent a redundant protection system. Therefore, in any electrical safety program, the values of leakage current for medical equipment in these areas must be verified to be below the limits specified in applicable codes and standards (Chapter 5).

Table 2.2 ECRI-recommended risk current limits for line-Powered, cord-connected equipment†

{These values are based on limited experimentation on humans and on the results of similar tests on animals using currents required to cause ventricular fibrillation.}

Type of Equipment	*Patient applied Parts or Leads*	*Chassis*
Patient equipment w/o patient connection.	NA	100 A *
Patient contact eqipment with nonisolated patient connections	50 A each lead or 100 A all leads together	100 A *
Patient contact eqipment with isolated patient connections	10 A each lead **	100 A *
Equipment located outside the patient vicinity and nonmedical appliances	NA	500 A

* The chassis leakage current criterion in NFPA 99-1990 is under appeal and may be modified to 500 A.

** An isolated patient connection must also pass an isolation test. The NFPA 99-1990 criterion for lead-to-groundmeasurements of isolated patient connections is 10 A with the ground intact and 50 A with the ground open.

† Reprinted from pp. 27–28 of *Electrical Safety Document 1.4, 1990*, with permission of Emergency Care Research Institute (ECRI).

Isolated Patient Connections. Most devices, such as ECG and blood pressure monitors, that are connected directly to the patient, have patient input isolation. An isolated patient connection not only limits leakage current levels from the patient contact points to very low levels, but it also reduces the amount of current that can flow into the patient connection from another (defective) device. It is recommended that equipment with isolated patient leads be used whenever the device is to be in contact with the heart or with a fluid-filled catheter located within the heart or great vessels.

A device designated as having an isolated patient connection must pass an isolation test from the patient connection (electrode). The test consists of applying a 120-V, 60-Hz, ground-referenced potential to each patient connection and measuring the resulting current (Figure 2.5). The maximum allowable current is 20 A when the voltage is applied to the distal end of the patient cable (connected to the device under test) and 10 A when the voltage is applied directly to the patient cable connector (with the patient cable removed) on the chassis of the device (ECRI, 1990). One also tests for leakage currents from the leads (standards for isolated and nonisolated inputs differ).

Isolated Power Systems. The conventional electrical power distribution system described above is "ground-referenced" in that the neutral wire (N) is connected to ground, and therefore, the hot wire (H) can serve as a source of current to any grounded conductor. An alternative scheme is to isolate both power-carrying lines from ground. In this scheme, called an "isolated power system," the two power-carrying wires are labeled L_1 and L_2 (rather than H and N) and are electrically identical. It is important to note, however, that isolated power systems still include a ground wire (G) that functions just like the ground wire in a conventional power distribution system (Figure 2.6).

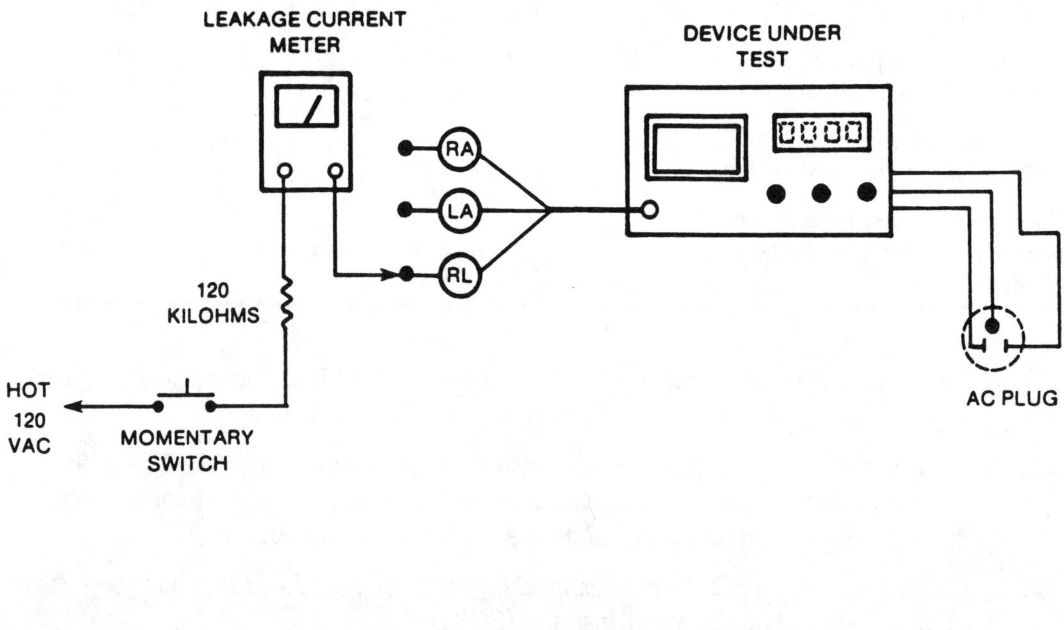

Figure 2.5: Patient lead input isolation test circuit. (Reprinted by permission of ECRI.)

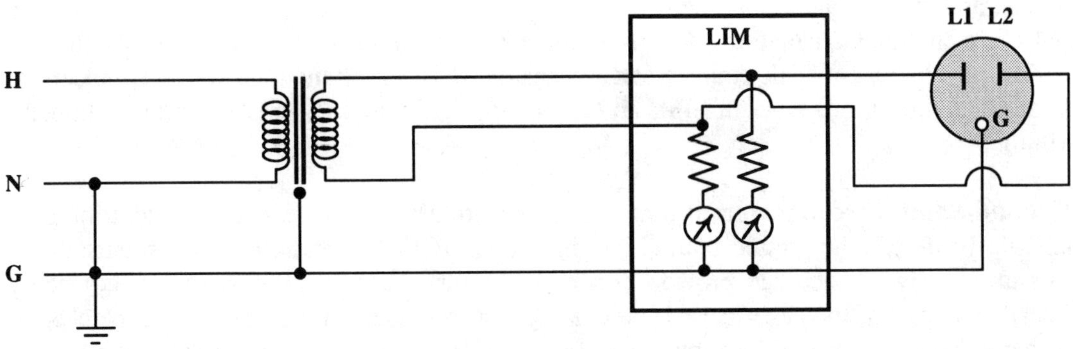

Figure 2.6: An isolation transformer connected to a line isolation monitor (LIM).

Although isolated power systems are expensive to install and maintain, they have three beneficial features:

- The perfect isolated power system would allow no current flow from either L_1 or L_2 to ground. However, because of imperfections in the transformers used to convert a ground-referenced system into an isolated system, some current does flow. In the early days of microshock hysteria, isolated power systems were recommended for use in intensive-care units to reduce microshock hazards. However, the degree of isolation is inadequate to be of significant benefit in this regard, and the use of isolated power systems in intensive-care units is no longer recommended.
- Isolated power systems, in conjunction with explosion-proof electrical outlets, can reduce the likelihood of arcing which could ignite flammable anesthetic gases. This hazard has become rare since the introduction of nonflammable inhalation anesthetics. In fact, explosive anesthetic agents are no longer used in the United States and Canada. Although many operating rooms have isolated power systems, they are not required in locations where flammable inhalation anesthetics are banned by institutional policy and signage.
- In the ground-referenced power distribution system, certain equipment faults result in opened circuit breakers and loss of power. In an isolated power system, such equipment may continue to operate without interruption. For example, in a ground-referenced system, a short circuit between the hot wire (H) to the grounded case of a device would cause the circuit breaker to open and the device to cease functioning. However, in an isolated system, a short circuit from L_1 (or L_2) to ground would not cause a current overload. In fact, the effect would be to functionally transform the isolated power system into a ground-referenced system. Thus, the isolated power system can allow equipment to function under certain "single-fault" conditions. Faults of this type are rare but sometimes occur in wet environments such as operating rooms. Coupled with the critical nature of equipment in the operating theater, this may justify the installation of an isolated power system.

In addition to special transformers, isolated power systems include line-isolation monitors (LIMs) to check the degree of electrical isolation in the system. In effect, LIMs "predict" the maximum amount of current that can flow from L_1 or L_2 to ground. This value increases as a result of either a degradation within the isolated power system or faulty equipment connected to the isolated power system. When the LIM indication exceeds a design set point, visible and audible alarms are activated. It is important to note that these alarms indicate only a reduction in isolation, which is not a hazard in itself; the alarm warns that an additional equipment fault could create a hazard. It is important for clinical engineers to understand the various types of LIMs and the appropriate responses to LIM alarms (Feinberg, 1986).

Ground-Fault Circuit Interrupters. Another protective device that can contribute to electrical safety is the ground-fault circuit interrupter (GFCI). Under certain circumstances, this inexpensive device can provide protection against macroshock hazards. It is usually installed as part of the electrical wiring that feeds a receptacle or a cluster of receptacles, or it may even be integrated into the power outlet itself. There are also portable, stand-alone GFCIs and devices with built-in GFCIs.

Figure 2.7 illustrates the circuit of a generic GFCI (Aston, 1990). It consists of a magnetic toroid around which the hot lead and the neutral wire are wound, each with the same number of turns, but in opposite directions. The GFCI continually senses the difference in current flow between the hot and neutral wires. Normally, the difference between these two currents is small, and the magnetic fields created by them are opposite and approximately equal, and will therefore cancel. However, under fault conditions, where some or all current returns to the generating source by some route other than the neutral wire (i.e., through a person in contact with the electrical device), the corresponding fluxes in the coil will be unequal, thereby producing a voltage that will be detected by the sensing amplifier. When this potential difference (proportional to the current imbalance) exceeds some critical value, power to the GFCI receptacle or device is shut off. It is important to note that although GFCIs protect against excessive exposure to ground fault currents, they do not limit these currents (i.e., a substantial fault current may flow for a brief period of time). Therefore, GFCIs are not intended to protect against leakage currents in the microshock range, but will help protect against macroshock. In some instances, they may be used to meet requirements for special protection against electrical shock in locations where fluids are frequently used or in designated wet locations, such as hydrotherapy tanks.

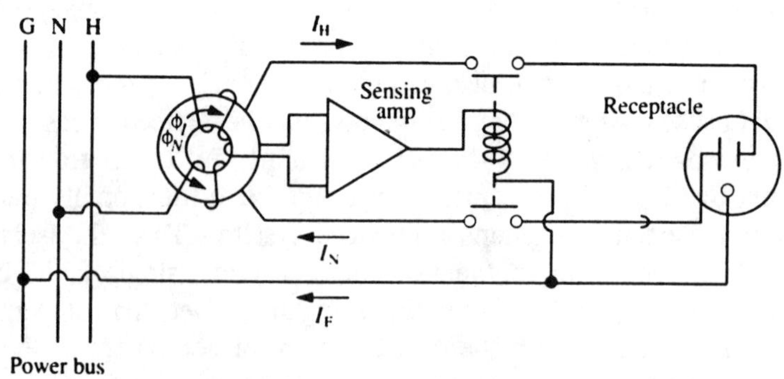

Figure 2.7: Schematic diagram of a generic ground fault circuit interrupter (GFCI). (Redrawn with permission from Aston, 1990.)

The choice of locations for the use of GFCIs in the hospital must be carefully considered because in the interest of preventing shock, GFCIs may cause a far greater hazard by shutting off power to critical or life-support patient-care equipment. For this reason, it is not recommended that such equipment be powered from a GFCI circuit. Instead, an isolated power system may be necessary. Isolated power systems and GFCIs are required by code only in areas designated as wet locations.

SAFETY PROGRAMS

This section describes the major safety programs in which clinical engineers are likely to be involved. Although in some hospitals the clinical engineering department may not have the entire responsibility for all of these programs, clinical engineers will be active participants and must be knowledgeable in each area.

Electrical Safety Programs

Electrical safety in hospitals today clearly requires that appropriate attention be paid to the electrical environment of the patient. To achieve this goal, it is necessary to develop a comprehensive safety plan. This involves implementing a periodic maintenance check of all line-operated equipment and establishing a good record-keeping scheme to keep track of the tests conducted and the relative status of the equipment tested. In providing such a safety program, the following three steps are required:

- Checking the environment.
- Checking the equipment before bringing it into the environment.
- Providing education and training in safety procedures.

Environmental Inspection. The hospital environment consists of a wide range of facilities, each of which requires special consideration from a safety perspective. Consider the following locations:

Anesthetizing Locations. These are areas normally used for the administration of an inhalation anesthetic agent. Traditionally, this term refers to operating rooms and delivery rooms; however, with the advent of changing patient populations and new technologies, delivery of anesthesia occurs in other areas, such as emergency and medical imaging sites (e.g., X-ray, magnetic resonance imaging).

- **Anesthetizing Location—Nonflammable** refers to anesthetizing locations that, by issuance of a hospital policy, are posted to be used only for nonflammable inhalation anesthetizing agents.
- **Anesthetizing Location—Flammable** must be labeled as such and be specifically designed with safeguards to allow for safe administration of flammable inhalation anesthetic agents.
- **Anesthetizing Locations—Mixed** refers to all anesthetizing sites that allow either flammable or nonflammable inhalation anesthetic agents. Hospital policies must insure that only properly designed equipment is used in these locations and must require both appropriate posting of signs on each room and labeling of equipment.

Critical Care Locations. These areas include all patient care areas classified as critical-care sites by hospital policy or where patients are subjected to invasive procedures and directly connected to line-operated medical devices. Typically, these include operating rooms, delivery rooms, and intensive care, cardiac care, and cardiac catheterization areas.

General Care Locations. These are the patient-care locations where patients are expected to come in contact with ordinary electrical appliances (lamps, beds, televisions, etc.) or be connected nonelectrically to medical devices. This does not include nursing stations.

Nonpatient Areas. These are areas in which patients are not normally cared for or treated, such as administrative offices, laboratories, nursing stations, storage areas, kitchens, or plant equipment areas.

Wet Locations. These include patient-care areas normally subject to wet conditions, including standing water on the floor, or routine dousing or drenching of the work area. Routine housekeeping procedures and incidental spillage do not constitute cause for designation as a wet location. Generally, this classification includes only hydrotherapy tanks in the physical therapy department, garbage storage areas, and certain food service areas.

In all these areas of the hospital, the use of proper "grounding" procedures to remove hazardous electrical currents from the patient environment is critical. A proposed or expected ground point must be verified as actually being at ground potential, thereby presenting a low resistance path to the common reference point at the service panel. The reason for this precaution should become clear when one is reminded of the numerous discontinuities that exist in the ground connections located throughout the building. It is at these discontinuities that electrical hazards may arise. A loose or disconnected wire is all that is required to remove a particular outlet or room from ground. Therefore, one must never simply assume continuity to ground—it must be tested.

Isolated power systems and GFCIs must also be checked periodically in accordance with some appropriate schedule. For example, Table 2.3 provides a list of specific equipment and the maximum interval between testing in anesthetizing, critical care, and ambulatory care locations. Similar schedules need to be developed for equipment in each of the areas mentioned above.

Equipment Inspection. Once the environment has been checked, it is necessary to test all electrical equipment brought into the patient environment. This means that the quality and continuity of ground between each instrument's chassis and the ground lug of its line cord must be verified. This is extremely important because defective ground lugs and wires in the plug are among the most common causes of shock hazard. Equipment grounding and leakage currents can be quickly measured by safety analyzers designed for this purpose.

Education of Clinical Staff. One of the key factors in preventing electrical accidents is the education of the hospital staff. Individuals who are well informed and knowledgeable about the causes and consequences of electrical hazards represent the best preventive measure any institution can have. This does not imply that any of the steps just discussed may be discarded, simply that only with proper training can these safety measures be effectively utilized. The extent to which a safe electrical environment is established within a hospital today is directly related to the support given by the clinical staff. These individuals can easily carry out the simple steps of electrical safety by using and interacting with user-friendly monitors and test equipment. Consequently, programs directed at the in-house training of medical personnel in the basics of electrical safety and safety instrumentation are absolutely necessary.

In the modern hospital, patient safety is considered by many to be a medical problem that requires the coordinated effort of the entire health-care delivery team. It is essential that medical personnel are properly trained to look for possible electrical defects before using line-operated equipment on patients. When these three steps (checking the environment, checking the equipment and educating the necessary personnel) are followed, patients will not only receive the best medical care possible, but will also be protected from the potential electrical hazards that may surround them.

Model Program. This section presents a model electrical safety program that deals with the electrical safety of patients, visitors, and employees. It applies to all electrical equipment used in the hospital, including equipment that has been purchased, leased, rented, or borrowed by the hospital; equipment brought into the hospital by clinical staff, patients, or visitors; equipment that is being demonstrated or is under evaluation for acquisition; and eqipment for research and investigation purposes.

Table 2.3: Periodic testing in anesthetizing, critical-care, and ambulatory-care locations.

(from G. Panagiotopoulus, Kaiser Permanente, *Electrical Safety Manual*, 1989)

MAXIMUM INTERVAL			
1 Month	*6 Months*	*12 Months*	*Periodic*
Isolated power systems with dynamic line isolation monitors	Duplex receptacles Ground fault circuit interrupters Duplex receptacles—grounding circuits Ground resistance Chassis leakage current Isolated patient connection leakage current Isolated power systems with dynamic line isolation monitors—with simulated faults	Inspection and calibration of isolated power systems Conductive flooring and anti-static accessories—in non-flammable anesthetizing locations with conductive floors	Input isolation of isolated patient connections—only during acceptance testing or following circuitry repairs

EQUIPMENT ACQUISITION PROGRAM

Prior to the acquisition of any new piece of equipment, a review of the requisition will be conducted by the appropriate engineering department as follows:

Clinical engineering—medical equipment

Facilities engineering—nonmedical equipment

If the manufacturer's technical specifications are not submitted with the requisition, the purchasing department will obtain and provide this information to the appropriate engineering department. Upon arrival at the hospital, all medical and nonmedical equipment will be inspected by clinical engineering to verify compliance with hospital standards and manufacturers' specifications before delivery to the requesting department.

SCHEDULED MAINTENANCE PROGRAM

All equipment to be used in critical-care units will be inspected quarterly by clinical engineering for adherence to safety and performance standards.

All equipment to be used in other patient-care areas will be inspected at least semiannually by clinical engineering for adherence to safety and performance standards.

All equipment in nonpatient areas will be inspected at least annually by clinical engineering for adherence to safety standards.

Upon completion of an inspection, an inspection label will be affixed to the equipment showing the date of the inspection and the initials of the technician who performed the inspection.

If a piece of equipment is found to be defective, the unit supervisor will be notified immediately and corrective action initiated. Written results of the testing program will be maintained by the inspecting department. At the conclusion of each inspection period, deficiencies and any action that is taken will be reported to the person responsible for the operation of the hospital unit inspected.

Equipment users will inspect all pieces of equipment before each use for physical damage and correct operation. If a hazard is suspected, clinical engineering personnel should be notified and corrective action initiated if necessary.

EQUIPMENT RESTRICTIONS

Three-to-two wire electrical adapters are prohibited, and extension cords are prohibited except in case of emergency. Modifications to the electrical distribution system will be made to ensure that these devices are unnecessary.

Special-purpose electrical adapters are to be avoided whenever possible. However, if adapters must be used to allow equipment fitted with distinctive plugs to be used with conventional grounded outlets, they will be inspected periodically by the appropriate engineering department to ensure continuity of all conductors.

Patient-owned, line-powered devices are prohibited from all critical-care areas. In other patient-care areas of the hospital, permission from the director of clinical engineering must be obtained prior to use. When such devices are permitted, they will be inspected before use and an inspection label will be affixed.

POWER DISTRIBUTION SYSTEMS TESTING PROGRAM

All electrical receptacles will be inspected periodically for polarity, ground conductor integrity, contact tension, and overall physical condition. Defective receptacles will be replaced with hospital-grade devices. Clinical engineering will perform testing in critical-care units; Facilities engineering will perform testing in other patient and nonpatient areas.

Line isolation monitor test switches will be actuated monthly. A thorough evaluation of isolated power systems will be performed semiannually by clinical engineering.

IN-SERVICE EDUCATION

All personnel who have contact with patients and work in patient-care areas will be instructed about potential electrical hazards that are present in their areas. This will be accomplished initially during new employee orientation and at regular intervals thereafter. Personnel in critical-care nursing areas will receive additional instruction as appropriate.

Medical Device Safety Programs

In today's health-care environment, medical device safety programs are critical to hospitals as a means of addressing the issues of risk control and quality assurance. Furthermore, these programs, which involve the collection of data concerning various hazards and incidents and their correction, belong in the domain of the clinical engineering department.

Hazard Alerts and Recalls. With this in mind, hospital clinical engineering departments must screen hazard alerts and recall notices pertaining to medical devices within their facilities. Hazard alerts and recall notices may be received from these sources:

- Equipment manufacturers.
- Food and Drug Administration enforcement report.
- Subscription services or publications.

The term "recall," as used by the FDA, does not necessarily mean that the defective products should be taken out of use. In the extreme, the manufacturer may suspend distribution of the product and request that all existing units in the field be returned or, in some cases, destroyed by the hospital. Other corrective actions include modification kits provided to the customer, relabeling, or on-site modification by the manufacturer. The FDA assigns each recall to one of three classes:

Class I: A reasonable probability exists that use of or exposure to the device will cause serious injury or death.

Example: A monitoring device (with alarm) for detecting and recording cardiac arrhythmias does not alarm during ventricular tachycardia or ventricular fibrillation.

Class II: Use of or exposure to the device may cause temporary or medically reversible health consequences, or the probability of serious adverse health consequences is remote.

Example: Wheeled stretchers without braking mechanisms were sold to hospitals.

Class III: Use of or exposure to the device is unlikely to cause adverse health consequences.

Example: Pneumatic transducers for pulmonary laboratory are found to be incorrectly calibrated.

Each hospital, through the clinical engineering department, should develop procedures to handle hazard and recall notices. Required steps usually include receiving notices, identifying those devices within the hospital, sequestering or modifying defective devices, notifying appropriate personnel, dealing with the manufacturer regarding refund or replacement, and documenting all of these activities. In such deliberations, careful consideration of all relevant information must occur before a device is removed from service. Consider, for example, the consequences of suspending all defibrillators from service and having a patient go into ventricular fibrillation. In certain cases the risk to patients may actually be lessened by using the device than by delaying or suspending treatment. However, any such decision must be carefully documented and approved by the appropriate hospital administration body.

A hospital is clearly negligent if it receives a recall notice and takes no action on it. The hospital may be liable if an injury is caused by a recalled device that has not been corrected. There are four types of action that may be required on a recalled device (ECRI, 1991a):

- Permanent removal from service.
- Modification of the device.
- Changes in instructions.
- Warnings to the users.

All actions must be documented for each recall notice received. Even if a hospital does not have the recalled device, the notice should be filed with an indication of this fact.

Incident Investigation. An "incident" is defined as an event in which equipment or procedure has caused injury to a patient, staff member, or visitor. Hospitals are almost always named in lawsuits when equipment-related incidents occur and a patient is injured. It makes little difference whether the incident is caused by specific equipment malfunction, user error, or a combination of the two. Even if the hospital itself is clearly not responsible, it must invest valuable staff time to minimize liability exposure.

The key to minimizing the hospital's liability exposure in equipment-related incidents is to increase the level of awareness of all hospital personnel involved in acquisition, maintenance, and use of equipment regarding medical device failure. This includes ensuring that they understand the basic causes of medical device failure and the mechanisms by which the failures cause harm. This increased knowledge—coupled with the effective management of medical devices within the hospital, including selection, acquisition, training, maintenance, and disposal of the device and thorough incident investigation procedures—will provide appropriate risk control measures, thereby limiting liability exposure.

Medical equipment-related failures may be classified as follows:

A. Defects related to the design or production of the item.
B. Random failure or premature wear of components, subassemblies, or mechanisms.
C. Failure to follow directions given in the operator's manual.
D. Failure of maintenance technicians to exercise appropriate care during the repair, or inspection.
E. Intentional tampering, sabotage, or malicious use.
F. Abnormal or unpredictable response by the patient.
G. Failure of the manufacturer to provide full information about possible use and misuse of the device.

The manufacturer would normally be held liable for incidents involving failures **A**, **B**, **G**, and possibly **D** if they perform the maintenance. Liability for failures **C**, **D**, and **E** would be born by the hospital. Failure **F** may be overlooked or misdiagnosed by health-care providers; however, a competent clinical engineer should be able to identify this failure.

Equipment-related incidents may lead to the following types of patient injury (Bruley, 1988):

- Overdose.
- Suffocation or barotrauma.
- Embolism (particulate or gas).
- Skin lesion (burns).
- Electrocution.
- Crushing.

While these outcomes demonstrate the physical results of an equipment-related incident, the events leading to these outcomes are a greater cause for concern. Effective investigation of a medical device–related incident is important. The director of the clinical engineering department should conduct a formal investigation in conjunction with the medical facility safety officer, or others as appropriate. A summary of this investigation should be documented on the **"hospital incident statement"** and provided to the risk manager. An investigation includes but may not be limited to:

- Preservation of evidence (i.e., impounding the equipment, recording the position of all controls, and noting any missing components or parts) and assessment of the overall condition of the equipment.
- Interviews with involved personnel.
- Identification of consumable supply items by lot number, date of manufacture, and any other pertinent data.
- Review of the maintenance history and test procedures run on the medical device.
- Review of the date and content of training given operators and maintenance technicians.

During the process of the investigation, it is important for the clinical engineering director to examine three basic interfaces and answer specific questions related to each.

1. **Operator/device interface.**

   (a) Was the device used appropriately?
   (b) Were control settings appropriate for the diagnostic or therapeutic procedure?
   (c) When was operator training accomplished and documented?
   (d) Were any facility utility problems identified prior to, during, or after the procedure (e.g., electrical, medical gas, water, or heating, ventilation and air conditioning, etc.)?

2. **Patient/device interface.**

   (a) How did the device respond when connected to the patient?
   (b) What medications was the patient receiving? Were there any sensitivities?

3. **Consumable supply/device interface.** Consumable supplies include leads, electrodes, plastic tubing, filters, reservoirs and breathing circuits.

   (a) Were the items designed for use with the affected device?
   (b) Were items properly interfaced to the device and the patient?
   (c) Were items reusable or intended for one-time use?

Such an investigation allows determination of the cause of an incident.. This knowledge can then be used to prevent similar occurrences in the future. The proper management of incident-related information can assist the hospital in ensuring patient safety, thus minimizing institutional liability.

As discussed earlier, the Safe Medical Devices Act of 1990 imposes new reporting requirements on "device-user facilities." The reporting requirements associated with this act require all health-care facilities, including hospitals, ambulatory-surgical facilities, nursing homes, and outpatient treatment facilities, to report information that "reasonably suggests" the probability that a medical device has caused or contributed to the death, serious injury, or serious illness of a patient at that facility. When such an incident has occurred, it must be reported to the Food and Drug Administration with a copy of the report sent to the manufacturer, if known, or to the distributor. These reports must be sent no later than ten working days after the facility becomes aware of the incident. The act also requires the device-user facility to provide the FDA with semiannual summaries (January 1 and July 1) of all such reports (ECRI, 1991c).

Radiation Safety Programs

Exposure of living organisms, especially mammals, to high levels of radiation can induce pathological conditions and even death. This fact, in turn, is utilized by specific medical devices to treat certain malignant diseases; the intention is to deliver a localized high-radiation dose to destroy undesirable tissue. Even exposure to lower levels of radiation is not safe. Although low-dose exposure may not show any apparent initial effect, other than some chromosomal breakage, it increases the long-term risks of cancer and, possibly, of genetic defects. These possible adverse effects from exposure to radiation impose the need for clinical engineers to understand the sources of the various types of radiation and how to minimize exposure to them.

Atomic Structure and Emissions. Bohr's model of the atom (Figure 2.8) suggested the existence of an atomic structure analogous to the solar system. In this system, electrons revolve in discreet orbits or shells around a nucleus consisting of neutrons and protons. The electrical charge carried by the electron is a fundamental property of matter, as is the mass of each particle. Since this is the smallest amount of electricity that can exist, it is usually expressed as a negative unit charge (−1). Expressing a unit charge in the metric system of units (meters, kilograms, and seconds), gives the value 1.6 10^{-19} coulombs. The charges carried by all other atomic particles are, therefore, some integral multiple of this value. Consequently, it is impossible for a particle to have, for example, a charge equal to two and one-half times that of the electron.

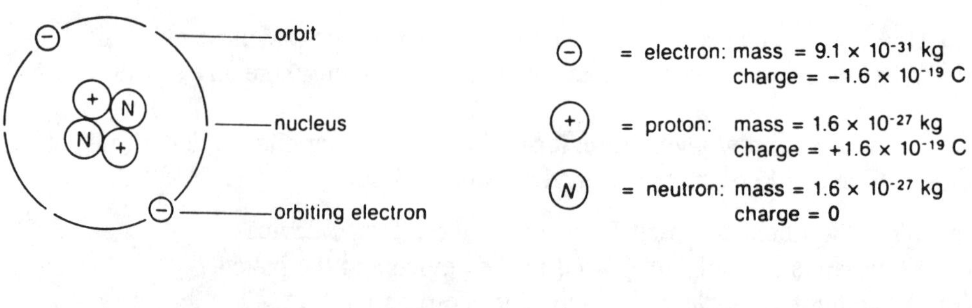

Figure 2.8: Planetary view of the structure of the atom. The primary mass is in the nucleus, which contains protons and neutrons. The nucleus has a net positive charge and is surrounded orbiting electrons. In stable atoms, the net charge of the electrons in orbit is equal and opposite to the net charge of the nucleus. The atom illustrated is helium.

Neutrons and protons exist together in the nucleus and have been given the collective name of "nucleons." The total number of nucleons in the nucleus of an element is called the "atomic mass," or mass number, and is represented by the symbol (A), whereas the number of protons alone is referred to as the "atomic number" (Z).

The various combinations of neutrons and protons that may exist in nature are illustrated by examining the composition of the nuclei of the three types of hydrogen atom (hydrogen, deuterium, and tritium). Although hydrogen has a nucleus consisting of a single proton, the combination of one proton and one neutron exists as a single particle called a "deutron," which is the nucleus of the atom called "heavy hydrogen," or deuterium. Extending this concept further, the combination of two protons and two neutrons forms a stable particle, the alpha particle, which in nature exists as the nucleus of the helium atom. Tritium, the third form of hydrogen, on the other hand, has a nucleus consisting of only one proton and two neutrons.

These three types of hydrogen are examples of atoms whose nuclei have the same number of protons and therefore the same atomic number (Z), and at the same time they may have a different number of neutrons and thereby a different atomic mass (A). Atoms exhibiting this characteristic called "isotopes" (from the Greek, meaning "same place"). This term has been widely used to refer to any atom, particularly a radioactive one. However, current usage favors the word "nuclide" to refer to a particular combination of neutrons and protons. Thus, isotopes are nuclides that have the same atomic number. In order to designate each individual atom specifically, certain symbols have been developed. Until recently in the United States, it was the practice to place the atomic number as a subscript before and the atomic mass as a superscript after the chemical symbol of the atom ($_{53}I^{131}$). Since the chemical symbol itself also specifies the atomic number, one often omits it and simply writes I^{131}. In Europe, on the other hand, the atomic mass was customarily written as a superscript prior to the chemical symbol (^{131}I). In an effort to achieve international standards, it was agreed in 1964 that the atomic mass should be placed as a superscript preceding the chemical symbol (^{131}I). When superscripts are not used, a more literal form of designation, such as Cobalt 60, is commonly used. Referring to Bohr's model of the helium atom illustrated in Figure 2.8, then, one simply writes $^{4}He_{2}$, where 4 is equal to the atomic weight (because of the aggregation of protons and neutrons in the nucleus), and 2 denotes the atomic number of the element.

The amount of energy required to eject an electron from its orbit is equivalent to the binding energy for that shell, which is highest for the electrons at the innermost shell. The energy required to move an electron from an inner shell to an outer shell is equal to the difference in binding energies between the two shells. This energy requirement represents one of the natural characteristics of an element. In the case of transition of an electron from an outer shell to an inner shell, energy is released as a photon or characteristic X-ray energy. However, if instead of the emission of a photon, the energy is transferred to another orbital electron, called an "Auger electron," it will be ejected from orbit.

All elements with an atomic number (Z) greater than 83, or atomic mass (A) greater than 209 are radioactive; that is, they decay spontaneously into other elements, and this decay causes the emission of active particles. These elements are called "radionuclides." In general, there are two classifications of radionuclides: natural and artificial. Naturally occurring radionuclides are those nuclides that emit radiation spontaneously and therefore require no additional energy from external sources. Artificial radionuclides, on the other hand, are essentially human-made, produced by bombarding so-called stable nuclei with high-energy particles.

All radioactive materials, whether they occur in nature or are artificially produced, decay by the same types of processes and usually involve the disintegration of one element into another. The rate of this decay process is spoken of in terms of disintegrations per unit time or its half-life (T , time for half the original number of atoms in a sample of a given radioactive element to disintegrate). Half-lives of radioactive elements range in value from thousandths of a second to millions of years. For example, ^{131}I has a half-life of 8.05 days, whereas ^{60}Co has a half-life of 5.24 years. Information regarding properties of some other radionuclides is presented in Table 2.4.

Sometimes, a radionuclide attains its final stable state in successive stages of transition. A radionuclide is often called the "parent," and the decay products are known as the "daughters." Broadly speaking, the modes or phases of transformation in the process of a radionuclide passage from an unstable to a stable condition may be divided into six categories (Spencer and Hosain, 1986):

- **Alpha (α) decay:** Alpha particles are ionized helium atoms moving at a high velocity. The emission of an alpha particle from the nucleus produces a different element by reducing Z by 2 and A by 4. A number of naturally occurring heavy elements undergo α decay. For example, radium (^{226}Ra) transforms to radioactive radon (^{222}Rn) by α decay. Alpha emitters are rarely used in nuclear medicine, although some of them have been considered for therapy.

Table 2.4: Physical data for some radionuclides used in nuclear medicine

Element	*Symbol*	*Atomic number*	*Atomic mass*	*Half-life**	*Principal gamma energy (Kev)*
Cesium	^{137}Cs	55	137	30y	662
Chromium	^{51}Cr	24	51	27.8d	322
Cobalt	^{57}Co	27	57	270d	122
Gallium	^{67}Ga	31	67	78h	93,184,296
Gold	^{198}Au	79	198	2.7d	412
Indium	^{113m}In	49	113m	104m	393
Iodine	^{123}I	53	123	13.3h	160
	^{125}I	53	125	56d	35
	^{131}I	53	131	8.1d	364
Iron	^{59}Fe	26	59	45d	191,1097,1289
Mercury	^{203}Hg	80	203	46.9d	279
Selenium	^{75}Se	34	75	120d	136,265,402
Strontium	^{85}Sr	38	85	65d	514
	^{97m}Sr	38	87m	2.8h	391
Technetium	^{99m}Tc	43	99m	6h	140
Xenon	^{133}Xe	54	133	5.27d	83
Ytterbium	^{169}Yb	70	169	32d	63,93,177

* = minutes, h = hours, d = days, y = years

- **Negatron (ß⁻) decay:** A negatron, or beta particle, is an electron that leaves the nucleus with a certain amount of kinetic energy. The $ß^-$ decay process produces a different element by increasing Z by 1, with A remaining constant. Phosphorus 32 is a typical example of a pure ß$^-$ emitter which has been used for therapy (^{32}P is transformed to ^{32}S). Most of the radionuclides undergoing ß$^-$ decay, however, also emit gamma rays almost simultaneously.

- **Positron (ß$^+$) decay:** Positrons are created in the nucleus: it is as if a proton were converted to a neutron and a positron. The positron decay produces a different element by decreasing **Z** by 1, with **A** remaining the same. For example, carbon 11 decays to the predominant stable isotope of boron (i.e., ^{11}C transforms to ^{11}B). Positron decay is also associated with gamma-ray emission beacause the positron, once emitted, is annihilated by a collision with an electron, which in turn produces a pair of photons, each moving in opposite directions.
- **Electron capture (EC), or K capture:** An orbital electron, usually from the inner shell (K shell), is captured by the nucleus (it is as if a proton captured an electron and converted itself to a neutron). An electron capture process produces a different element by decreasing Z by 1, with A remaining the same (similar to ß$^+$ decay). Some radionuclides have definite probabilities of undergoing either positron decay or electron capture (such as iron 52, which decays with about 42 percent EC and 58 percent ß$^+$ emission). Further, it is possible for gamma emission to be associated with electron capture. For example, ^{51}Cr transforms to ^{51}V (vanadium 51) with about 90 percent going directly to the ground state and the remaining 10 percent going to an excited state of ^{51}V, followed by transition to ground state with the emission of photons. An electron capture also causes a vacancy in the inner shell, which leads either to the emission of a characteristic X-ray or Auger electron.
- **Isomeric transition (IT) and internal conversion (IC):** When a radionuclide is unstable but has a relatively long half-life, it usually emits only gamma rays. The element remains the same with no change in A. For example, ^{99m}Tc (Technetium 99m) decays to ^{99}Tc. However, there is a definite probability that instead of a photon coming out, the energy may be transferred to an inner orbital electron. This is known as "internal conversion." For example, barium 135, when decaying by IT, emits about 84 percent IC electrons. This also creates a vacancy in the shell, consequently leading to the emission of characteristic X-rays and Auger electrons.
- **Nuclear fission:** Heavy nuclides usually break up into two nuclides of more or less equal fragments. This may happen spontaneously, but it is more likely to occur with the capture of a neutron. The uranium fission products mostly range between atomic numbers 42 and 56. A number of medically useful radionuclides are produced as fission products, such as xenon 133, which may be extracted by appropriate radiochemical procedures.

Detection of Radioactivity. It should be apparent by now that all radionuclides decay and in the process emit various types of radiation. However, since the emitted energy or particles usually occur in various combinations, it is difficult to measure them separately. As a result, measurement of radioactivity is usually accomplished by using one of the following techniques:

- Counting the number of disintegrations that occur per second in a radioactive material.
- Quantifying how effective this radiation is in producing ions possessing a net positive or negative charge.
- Measuring the energy absorbed by matter from the radiation penetrating it.

Included among the various indirect techniques to measure radioactivity are the following:

- **Photography:** The darkening of film when it is exposed to a specific type of X-ray radiation.
- **Ionization:** The passage of radiation through a volume of gas contained in the probe of a detector produces ion pairs. This type of detector counts the ion pairs produced. This technique has been most effective in measuring alpha radiation and least effective in measuring gamma radiation.
- **Luminescence:** The emission of light due to incandescence. Since the flash of light produced by the bombardment of a certain type of material with penetrating-type radiation can be detected and processed, this technique is extremely useful (Figure 2.9). Scintillation detectors, which use this principle, frequently measure all types of radiation.

Using these detection schemes, a number of radiation units have been established (Table 2.5). The curie (Ci) is defined as that amount of radioactive material that has the same number of disintegrations per second as 1 gram of radium. Thus, the curie is that amount of radioactive material in which there are 3.7×10^{10} nuclear transformations per second. Thirty-seven billion disintegrations per second is a large number; therefore, in practice, two subdivisions of the curie are used: the millicurie (mCi) and the microcurie (Ci). Attention should be paid to the fact that the curie defines the number of disintegrations per unit time and not the nature of the radiation, which may be alpha, beta, or gamma rays.

The roentgen and the radiation absorbed dose (RAD), on the other hand, are units based on the effect of the radiation on an irradiated object. Thus, while the curie measures a source of radiation, the roentgen and RAD measure the effect of radiation on an object. One of the major effects of irradiation by X-radiation or gamma radiation is the ionization of atoms, that is, the creation of atoms possessing a net positive or negative charge (ion pair). The roentgen value is determined by observing the number of ion pairs produced by X-radiation or gamma radiation of air at standard temperature and pressure conditions. One roentgen is defined as the amount of X-radiation or gamma radiation that produces sufficient ion pairs to establish an electrical charge separation of 2.58×10^{-4} coulombs per kilogram of air. The roentgen (or its subunit, the milliroentgen) is used in area surveys for radiation levels.

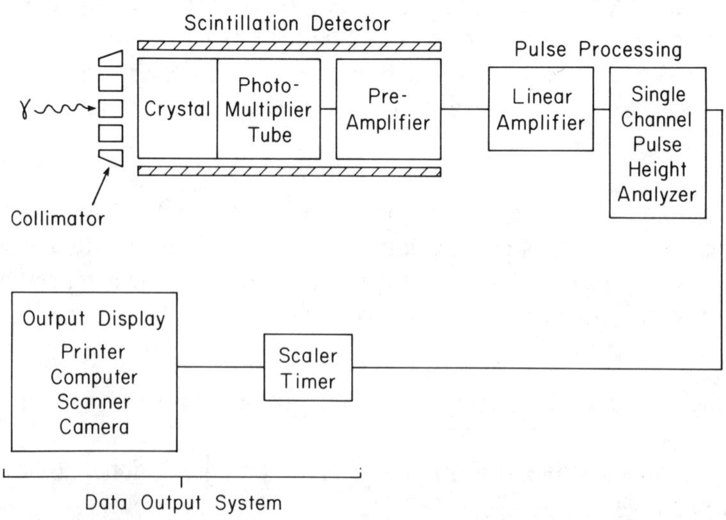

Figure 2.9: Basic scintillation detection system.

Table 2.5: Radiation measurement units.

Ci	(Curie) is a unit of *activity* of a radioactive nuclide that is equal to 3.7 $\times 10^{10}$ radioactive disintegrations per second.
R	(Roentgen) is a unit of *exposure* of x- or gamma radiation based on the ionization that these radiation produce in air. An exposure of one roentgen results in 2.584 $\times 10^{-4}$ coulomb per kilogram of air, or one esu per cc of air at at standard temperature and pressure.
Rad	is a unit of *absorbed dose* for any ionizing radiation. One rad equals 100 ergs absorbed per gram of any substance.
Rem	is a unit of *odse equivalent* which is numerically equal to the dose in rads multiplied by appropriate modifying factors such as RBE (or QF) or DF.
RBE	(Relative Biological Effectiveness) is a factor expressing the relative effectiveness of radiations with differing linear-energy-transfer (LET) values, in producing a given biological effect. This unit is now limited to use in radiobiology.
QF	(Quality Factor) is another name for a linear-transfer dependent factor by which absorbed doses are to be multiplied to account for the varying effectiveness of different radiations. This unit is used for purposes of radiation protection and is similar to the RBE unit used in radiobiology.
DF	(Dose Distribution Factor) is a factor expressing the modification of biological effect due to nonuniform distribution of internally deposited radionuclides.

Table 2.6: Effects caused by different doses of radiation (humans).

Dose (within a factor of 2 or 3)	*Effects and conditions*
100,000r	Spastic seizures; death within seconds; sperm motility stopped.
10,000r	Disruption of central nervous system function; death within minutes to hours.
1,000r	Necrosis of progenitive tissues; 100 percent in 30 to 60 days.
100r	Mild irradiation sickness;in part of the organism; no deaths.
10r	Few or no detectable effects.
10r/day	Debilitation in 3 to 6 weeks; death in 3 to 6 months (projected from animal data).
1r/day	Debilitation in 3 to 6 months; death in 3 to 6 years (projected from animal data).
0.1r/day	Permissible dose range 1930–1950.
0.01r/day	Permissible dose range 1957.
0.001r/day	Natural radiation level.

While the roentgen measures the effect of radiation in a standard material (air), the RAD measures the total energy absorbed by a particular irradiated material. For a material of interest, one RAD of exposure is equivalent to 0.01 joule of energy absorbed by a kilogram of the material. The RAD is used to measure the amount of exposure received, for example, by an organ of interest upon injection of a radiopharmaceutical.

Since human tissue is exposed to various types of radioactive materials in nuclear medicine, another unit of measure, the roentgen equivalent man (REM), is often used to specify the biological effect of radiation. The REM is used to measure, for example, the exposure values of personnel-monitoring devices such as film badges. The REM is also referred to as the Sievert (Sv).

Since the effects of nuclear radiation can be extremely harmful (Table 2.6), the **United States Nuclear Regulatory Commission** (**NRC**) has adopted a philosophy of implementation of principles and practices for keeping occupational radiation exposure at medical institutions as low as reasonably achievable. The regulatory maximum exposure limit for the general public has been set at 0.5 Sv per year. Limits for occupational exposure are 1.25 Sv over three months for the whole body, and 18.75 Sv over three months for the extremities.

The NRC has responsibility for issuing licenses authorizing the use of any material made radioactive by exposure to other nuclear material. It does not regulate the use of X-ray producing machines, fluoroscopic devices, or linear accelerators. Special and separate license applications are typically required for the following medical specialties:

- Nuclear medicine, where radioactive isotopes are used for imaging purposes and/or for the treatment of disease conditions.
- Radiation oncology, where external beam therapy (teletherapy) is applied via the use of cobalt 60, or internal radiation therapy is applied via the use of radioactive implants (brachytherapy).
- Cardiology, in those situations involving the implementation of nuclear-powered pacemakers, which require patient follow-up until the nuclear power source is ultimately recovered.
- Research, where radioactive isotopes are used as tracers for quantitative analysis.

All **NRC** regulations pertaining to the use of radiation are contained within Title 10, Chapter 1, of the **Code of Federal Regulations** (Nuclear Regulatory Commission, 1990). **Part 20**, titled "*Standards for Protection against Radiation*", is the document that lists all permissible radiation exposure levels in restricted and unrestricted areas for employees, patients, and visitors and outlines all requirements related to radiation surveys, documentation, reporting of incidents, and storage and disposal of radioactive waste.

Outlined in the **Code of Federal Regulations** there are many NRC regulatory guides applicable to management of a radiation safety program. These include (1) guide **10.8**, "*Guide for Preparation of Applications for Medical Program,*" (2) guide **8.23**, "*Radiation Safety Surveys at Medical Institutions,*" (3) guide **8.10**, "*Operating Philosophies for Maintaining Occupational Radiation Exposure as Low as Reasonably Achievable* (ALARA)," (4) guide **8.13**, "*Instructions Concerning Prenatal Radiation Exposure,*" and (5) guide **8.29**, "*Instruction Concerning Risks from Occupational Radiation Exposure.*" Combined, these regulations and guides provide stipulations or offer guidance in setting up a radiation safety program under the supervision of a radiation safety officer (**RSO**). Such a program is meant to ensure the safe use of radioactive materials in the health-care setting.

Duties and responsibilities of the RSO are clearly specified in Part 35 of the NRC regulations and include such things as implementation of a radiation safety program, investigations into overexposure and misadministration, development and enforcement of policy and procedures, management briefings, establishment of radiation exposure investigational levels, and statements for authority to manage such a program. The NRC must approve whomever the licensee identifies or specifies as the RSO. Training and experience requirements for the RSO include two-hundred hours of classroom and laboratory training in radiation physics, instrumentation, radiation protection, mathematics, radiation biology, and radiopharmaceutical chemistry or certification by the **American Board of Health Physics, American Board of Radiology, American Board of Nuclear Medicine, American Board of Science in Nuclear Medicine,** or **Board of Pharmaceutical Specialties in Nuclear Pharmacy**. Additionally, any authorized user (physician) who is identified on the license can get NRC approval to be the RSO. The activities of a radiation safety officer therefore involve the following:

- Routine assessment of personnel exposure.
- Monitoring of radioactive contamination in the work area.
- Evaluation of radiation shielding arrangements.
- Arrangements for appropriate disposal of radioactive waste.

Routine personnel monitoring is usually accomplished using film badges or other exposure-monitoring devices. Area surveys of radiation levels are carried out at regular intervals and following incidents of contamination. The common shielding material is lead, the appropriate thickness of which is dependent upon the level of gamma radiation (the most penetrating type of radiation). Finally, radioactive waste must be properly handled. To accomplish this, an appropriate plan for the collection, storage, and disposal of these wastes must be developed and implemented by each health-care institution.

In managing these services and related aspects of the radiation safety program, one must keep in mind that many of the related duties can be delegated to individuals other than the NRC-designated RSO. The clinical engineering department has extensive expertise in scheduling equipment inspections, maintaining records, performing and documenting equipment-related investigations, reporting to management, and dealing with various inspection agencies. The competent clinical engineer has also had formal training in mathematics, physics, instrumentation, and clinical applications of technology. This background and experience are exactly what are required to understand and manage a radiation safety program.

Delegation as the "radiation safety officer" should not be confused with other safety titles, such as "laser safety officer," "hospital safety officer," or "environmental safety officer." While many clinical engineers now serve dual roles by taking on these or similar titles, designation as the hospital's RSO requires NRC or state approval. Meeting the training and experience requirements requires that the proposed RSO attend special classes in health physics or take special training courses specifically designed to educate and prepare one for the duties of the RSO.

Many clinical engineering departments already have in place programs and responsibilities for X-ray equipment support, including repair, preventive maintenance, quality assurance, and patient exposure evaluation. Additional responsibilities for film badge management, employee exposure record review, radiation detection/counter equipment maintenance, and radiation surveys form the basis for inclusion of radiation safety program duties (Dickey, 1991).

Laser Safety Programs

The word "laser" began as an acronym for light amplification by the stimulated emission of radiation. In recent years, the medical and surgical use of lasers has grown dramatically, and because lasers can present a variety of hazards to patients and staff, laser safety programs have become increasingly important.

Types of Lasers. Several types of lasers are used in patient care. In technical terms, they differ in the frequency and power of the light they produce; in clinical terms, they differ in the types of physiological effects they have. The most common types of medical lasers use a variety of lasing media: carbon dioxide (CO_2), argon, neodymium:yttrium-aluminum-garnet (Nd:YAG), krypton, and various dyes (Absten, 1989). For purposes of a laser safety program, lasers can be divided into four categories:

- **Class I:** Enclosed lasers that do not inflict harm under normal circumstances. Emission levels are low, and warning labels are not required.
- **Class II:** Low-powered lasers that emit visible light at levels that are safe for momentary viewing. An intact aversion reflex provides adequate protection for the eye.
- **Class III:** Lasers with emission levels high enough to cause injury if viewed directly or if specularly reflected. Some low-power surgical lasers are in Class III.
- **Class IV:** Lasers with high emission levels that can cause fire, burns, and optical damage. Most surgical lasers are in Class IV.

The classes have been defined by the **American National Standards Institute** (ANSI), and further information can be found in ANSI Z136.1, "*Safe Use of Lasers*", and ANSI Z136.3, "*Safe Use of Lasers in Health Care Facilities*" (ECRI, 1991b).

Laser-Related Hazards. Although lasers can present a wide range of hazards, optical damage is of particular concern (Ben-Zvi, 1989). It is the combination of high power in surgical lasers and the sensitivity of the human eye to light of various colors that produces this unique potential for injury. Thus, the laser power level and wavelength are critical factors. There are two general approaches to controlling laser-related hazards:

- **Control of exposure**: Physical and visual access to rooms in which lasers are being used should be controlled. Clinical staff using lasers should be well trained and especially careful to avoid unnecessary exposure to themselves and others. Efforts should be made to reduce the potential for reflection as well as direct exposure.
- **Use of protective devices**: Safety glasses and goggles, when kept in good condition and used conscientiously, offer protection from laser light. However, it is important that the lenses be appropriate for the type of laser in use and that they do not interfere unnecessarily with vision.

The importance of safety precautions when working with and maintaining lasers cannot be overstated. Surgical lasers are as "sharp" as scalpels, and accidental contact with a laser beam can result in serious injury. Even low-power lasers can cause damage to human tissue. The eyes are most susceptible to damage from laser light. Never let a direct beam enter the eye.

An added safety problem is the invisibility of some laser radiation (CO_2, for example). Unless proper safety techniques are observed and care is exercised when handling invisible laser beams, the beams can be unintentionally directed or reflected, causing injury. Safety recommendations include the following (Duer, 1991):

- Cover windows, doors and reflective walls so that the beam will not be misdirected outside the room or be inadvertently reflected within the room.
- Place precautionary signs on all doors prior to performing laser maintenance or using a laser in surgical practice. Do not allow unauthorized personnel in the room when a laser is in use or being serviced.
- Do not work alone. If you must, make sure someone knows where you are.
- Use as little power as practicable when aligning and maintaining lasers.
- Use extreme caution when high power is being used.
- Beware of all components that may contain high voltages, and employ procedures which prevent the body from becoming a grounding path.
- Use caution when inserting instruments into the path of the beam to avoid random reflections. When possible, close the laser's aperture before inserting any instruments.
- Do not use reflective instruments. If anodized instruments are not available, use tape, liquid rubber, or another coating for safety.
- Be very careful that laser light is not directed or reflected into the eyes. Always wear safety glasses or goggles.

The last point merits further discussion. Safety glasses or goggles often block laser light completely, rendering a laser beam invisible. Technicians usually need to see the beam when aligning a laser and therefore remove the safety eye-wear for short periods of time during the process. An alternative to exposing the eyes to possible hazards is to obtain safety eye-wear with an optical density that is calculated to provide adequate protection to the eyes without completely obscuring the beam. In this way, removing safety eye-wear can be avoided.

Hospitals should consider appointing a laser safety officer and establishing a program to ensure the safe use of lasers. The duties and responsibilities of the laser safety officer would essentially parallel those of the RSO.

Infection Control Programs

Although the probability that clinical engineering personnel will be become infected as a result of servicing medical equipment is low, they should nevertheless take appropriate infection control precautions. Disease can be transmitted by several modes; contact transmission and, to a lesser extent, airborne transmission are the most likely modes. Contact transmission can occur through direct contact with an infected patient, droplet contact (i.e., from a cough or sneeze), or indirect contact (i.e., from handling equipment that is contaminated). Airborne transmission can occur through inhaling disease-causing microorganisms on dust particles or infectious residue on evaporated droplets (droplet nuclei). To protect against exposure to infectious diseases, clinical engineers should be familiar with basic infection control practices and disinfection, sterilization, and decontamination procedures that may be necessary before servicing medical devices (ECRI, 1990).

Clinical engineering personnel must also be able to give advise concerning the potential of cross-infection of patients through the use of improperly cleansed and disinfected equipment. Human immunodeficiency virus (HIV) and hepatitis-B are potentially the most hazardous diseases that might be encountered.

Basic Infection Control Practices. Good personal hygiene and common sense are instrumental in developing an effective infection-control program. Infection control practitioners should provide clinical engineering personnel with training that includes review of voluntary hepatitis-B virus (HBV) immunization and postexposure follow-up procedures.

The following are some basic infection-control practices that are appropriate for clinical engineering personnel (ECRI, 1990):

- Wash hands routinely—especially when hands are obviously soiled, after handling soiled equipment, after removing protective gloves, before eating, and before leaving the hospital.
- Do not eat, drink, smoke, or apply cosmetics in work areas.
- Wear a lab coat or other appropriate outer garment to prevent contaminating street clothing. Do not take lab coats home. Have them washed frequently in the hospital laundry.
- Wear gloves when touching contaminated objects, but do not touch "clean" items (e.g., door-knobs, telephones, test equipment, computer terminals, keyboards) with soiled gloves.
- Do not rub eyes or other mucous membranes.
- Inspect or repair devices that normally require cleaning, disinfection, or sterilization only after such procedures are completed. Clean, disinfect, or sterilize these devices again before returning them to patient-care areas.
- Use standard hospital procedures when entering, leaving, and working in areas that pose special infection-control problems (e.g., surgical suites, dialysis units, nurseries, neonatal ICUs, burn units, isolation rooms, and critical-care areas). Patients in these areas may be unusually susceptible to infection, and the inspector may be at a considerable risk as well.
- Treat as contaminated any device that is visibly soiled with patient material, even if dried. However, even if a device appears to be clean, do not handle in an unhygienic manner. Treat the following as contaminated devices:

a. Dialysis equipment. Units may be dedicated to patients with HBV; consider maintaining separate, dedicated tool sets for servicing these units.
b. All devices or items in the OR and ER at about the level of a surgical table or below, especially footswitches of devices used during surgery (e.g., electrosurgical units).
c. Any hand-held items or other items that can be found in beds (e.g., nurse call buttons, remote controls for TV sets, pillow speakers, blood pressure cuffs, telemetry transmitters).
d. Clinical laboratory instruments.
e. Centrifuges. Blood splashes and fragments of glass from broken blood collection tubes may be present; vacuuming the interior may be necessary.
f. Surgical instruments.
g. Reusable blood pressure transducers and breathing circuits.
h. Blood warmers.
i. In general, devices from any area where body fluids (especially blood) are spilled, splashed, or routinely handled, and devices that are in contact with or contain patient material. While device contact is usually limited to or contained within a disposable set, fluid squirts, leaks, spills, or handling by personnel whose hands are contaminated often result in device contamination (e.g., in dialysis equipment, blood warmers, autotransfusion units).

Decontamination and Sterilization. Decontamination, the process of reducing microorganisms to safe levels, can be accomplished by thorough cleaning followed by an appropriate disinfection or sterilization procedure.

Disinfection is the process of killing virtually all recognized pathogenic organisms, but not necessarily all forms of microbial life on inanimate objects. Disinfectants are classified in three levels (high, intermediate, or low), depending on their lethality. The effectiveness of a disinfectant depends on several factors, including the nature and number of contaminating microorganisms (especially the presence of spores), the concentration of the disinfectant, the length of the application period, the amount of organic soil present, the type and condition of the material to be disinfected, and the temperature. Thus, the effectiveness of disinfectants can range from sterility at one extreme to minimal reduction of microorganisms at the other.

Sterilization is the process of killing all microorganisms, including vegetative bacteria, viruses, fungi, and bacterial spores (dormant forms of microorganisms that are more resistant to heat and chemicals than their nondormant forms). In health-care settings, sterilization is generally accomplished by using physical agents (steam autoclaving) or chemical agents (ethylene oxide gas). These procedures require specialized equipment and should be performed only by personnel trained in sterile processing. For the purpose of decontamination, medical devices can be classified into three categories:

- **Visibly contaminated:** Devices soiled with blood, feces, urine, etc.
- **Very likely to be contaminated even though no visible contamination is evident:** Devices used for perfusion, hemodialysis units, autotransfusion devices, aspiration probes of clinical laboratory instruments, and any other devices that routinely come into contact with blood. Treat these devices as though they were contaminated.
- **Other:** Devices not visibly contaminated and not very likely to be contaminated (e.g., infusion pumps, bedside monitors). Although these devices may not require decontamination, handle them and all clinical equipment with care, and be aware of infection control issues.

Manufacturers are responsible for outlining decontamination procedures in the instruction manuals for their devices. Before purchasing equipment, insist that the manufacturer define appropriate decontamination procedures, and have the infection-control practitioner review them.

SUMMARY

An essential function for all clinical engineers is to ensure the safe use of medical instruments and systems. As a result, this chapter reviews electrical, environmental, biological, and radiation hazards. Because electrical safety is such an important area, it is presented in considerable detail. The physiological effects of electric current and steps that are taken to protect against electrical hazrds, including the use of isolated power supplies and ground-fault circuit interrupters and the development of electrical safety programs are covered.

The importance of a comprehensive medical device safety program is emphasized. With this in mind, the steps required to establish programs in radiation safety, laser safety, and infection control have also been presented in considerable depth. Finally, because clinical engineers must respond to medical device failures in accordance with specific federal, state, and local regulation, hazard alert, recall, and incident investigation procedures are also presented.

EXERCISES

1. Assume that 120 volts (RMS) is delivered between two gelled surface electrodes with cross-sectional areas of 3 cm^2

   (a) What is the resultant current?
   (b) What will be the physiological effect of this current?
   (c) What will be the effect of the cross-sectional area of the electrodes when reduced to 0.3 cm^2?

2. Distinguish between macroshock and microshock hazards. Give examples of each.

3. Define leakage current. Provide a circuit diagram to illustrate how to test for leakage current. What types of devices are available to test for and protect against leakage current? For two specific pieces of medical equipment, list the leakage current specified by the manufacturer.

4. About an hour after plugging an electrical device into a wall receptacle, smoke was observed rising from behind the receptacle cover plate. Name several faults that may have contributed to this condition. For each fault, design an inspection program to preclude future faults.

5. List at least ten types of electrical devices that patients would be likely to bring into the hospital. Assuming that the patient will not be in a critical-care area, decide which of the devices you would (a) ban entirely, (b) allow under certain conditions, and (c) allow without reservation. As you do this, imagine yourself as the patient (who would like the comfort of familiar items), the nursing unit manager (who has to tell the patient whether he or she can keep the device), and the director of clinical engineering (who interprets hospital policy). Now, write a policy regarding the use of patient-owned electrical devices.

6. Develop an outline for a half-hour lecture on equipment safety (not just electrical safety) to be delivered during the orientation of new nurses.

7. Isolated power systems have a number of beneficial features. Discuss two of them. What is the purpose of line-isolation monitors (LIMs)?

8. Discuss the steps required in establishing an electrical safety program.

9. Radiation safety requires, in part, monitoring radiation absorbed by the medical staff. Discuss how this monitoring activity should be conducted and what criteria should be used to alert personnel about unsafe levels of radiation.

10. Discuss the role of the radiation safety officer.

11. What steps can be taken to reduce the hazard of reflected laser light during surgery? What are some negative side effects of using safety glasses or goggles?

12. Disinfection and sterilization techniques have some negative side-effects. Obtain Material Safety Data Sheet (MSDS) information for some common hospital disinfectants such as ethylene dioxide, and provide exposure limits.

13. The infection-control activities of clinical engineers require understanding the procedures that may be necessary before servicing medical equipment. Discuss these procedures.

For the following multiple choice question circle all appropriate answers.

14. The danger in a patient's exposure to electrical devices lies in

    (a) the voltage.
    (b) the resistance of local tissue.
    (c) the magnitude of current.
    (d) the pathway that electrical current takes.

15. The absence or presence of skin burns is directly related to

    (a) magnitude of voltage.
    (b) skin resistance.
    (c) current density.
    (d) size of electrodes.

16. The electrical environment of the patient can be adversely affected if

    (a) conductive materials are placed in the body.
    (b) high currents are supplied to the body.
    (c) the skin is punctured.
    (d) high voltages are present.

17. A ground within a structure can be made to

    (a) a cold-water pipe.
    (b) the grounding conductor.
    (c) an electrical conduit, if used.
    (d) any of the above.

18. The ultimate ground for a structure is

    (a) the cold-water intake pipe to the structure.
    (b) the neutral wire of the electrical service to the structure.
    (c) the structural metal frame of the building.
    (d) a copper pipe, at least 20 feet in length, driven into damp earth.

19. A ground fault (as used in the National Electrical Code) refers to

    (a) a short between the neutral and ground conductors.
    (b) a current return to ground by any path other than the neutral line.
    (c) a break in the grounding system.
    (d) all of the above.

20. A ground-fault circuit interrupter

    (a) measures the resistance of the ground.
    (b) protects the ground against corrosion.
    (c) compares currents in the hot and neutral lines and disconnects power if the currents are not the same.
    (d) establishes an auxiliary ground if the main ground is interrupted.

21. Of the following, the most penetrating radiation is

    (a) alpha.
    (b) beta.
    (c) gamma.
    (d) neutrons.

22. The unit of radiation that tells you intensity of an X- or gamma beam is

    (a) roentgen.
    (b) roentgen/second.
    (c) curie.
    (d) curie/second.

23. The roentgen refers to

    (a) total ionization produced in irradiated matter.
    (b) ions/unit track length in irradiated matter.
    (c) total number of disintegrations occurring in the irradiated matter.
    (d) disintegration/second occurring in the radionuclide.

24. The measurement of radioactivity can be based on

    (a) the number of disintegrations occurring/second in a radioactive material.
    (b) the number of ions produced or energy released per unit track length.
    (c) the total number of ions produced in 1 cc of air.
    (d) any of the above.

25. The film badge

    (a) is sensitive only to alpha radiation.
    (b) is sensitive only to beta radiation.
    (c) is sensitive only to gamma radiation.
    (d) uses windows and filters to distinguish between radiation types.

26. The radiation most damaging biologically is

    (a) alpha.
    (b) beta.
    (c) gamma.
    (d) all are about the same.

REFERENCES

Absten, G.T. "Types of Surgical Lasers," in *Lasers in General Surgery* (S.N. Joffe, ed.), Williams and Wilkins, Baltimore, 1989.

Aston, R. *Principles of Biomedical Instrumentation and Measurement*, Merrill Publishing Co., Columbus, OH, 1990.

Ben-Zvi, S. "Laser Safety: Guidelines for Use and Maintenance," *Biomed. Instr. Technol.*, 23:360–368, 1989.

Bruley, M.E. "Medical Device Accidents: Causes, Prevention, Liability, and Investigation," Emergency Care Research Institute, Plymouth Meeting, PA, 1988.

Bruner, M.J.R., and Leonard, P.F. *Electricity, Safety, and the Patient*, Yearbook Medical Publishers, Chicago, 1989.

Dickey, D.M. "New Adventures in Biomedical Engineering: Radiation Safety Program Management," *Biomed. Instr. Technol.*, 25:380–384, 1991.

Duer, J. "Laser Maintenance and Safety," *Biomed. Instr. Technol.*, 25:374–377, 1991.

Emergency Care Research Institute. *Health Devices Inspection and Preventive Maintenance Systems*, 2nd ed., ECRI, Plymouth Meeting, PA, 1990.

Emergency Care Research Institute. "An Action Plan: Handling Medical Device Hazards and Recalls," Health Device Alerts, 1991a.

Emergency Care Research Institute. "ANSI Z136 Series Laser Safety Standards," *Health Devices*, 20:253, 1991b.

Emergency Care Research Institute. "Safe Medical Device Act Requires User Reporting," *Health Technology Management and Regulation*, 4, 1991c.

Feinberg, B.N. *Applied Clinical Engineering*, Prentice-Hall, Englewood Cliffs, NJ 1986.

Nader, R. "Ralph Nader's most shocking exposé," *Ladies' Home Journal* 88:98,176–179, 1971.

Nuclear Regulatory Commission. Office of the Federal Register National Archives and Records Service, General Services Administration. Code of Federal Regulations Title 10— Energy, Parts 0–199, Chapter 1, U.S. Government Printing Office, Washington, D.C., 1990.

Olson, W.H. "Electrical Safety," in *Medical Instrumentation: Application and Design* (J.G. Webster, ed.), Houghton Mifflin Co. Boston, 1978.

Panagiotopoulos, G. *Kaiser Permanente Electrical Safety Manual*, Kaiser Permanente, Berkeley, CA, 1989.

Spach, M.S., et al. "Skin-Electrode Impedance and its Effect on Recording Cardiac Potentials," *Circulation*, 34:649–656, 1966.

Spencer, R.P., and Hosain, J. "Basic Science and Practice of Nuclear Medicine," in *Biomedical Engineering and Instrumentation* (J.D. Bronzino, ed.), PWS Press, Boston, 1986.

Webster, J.G., and Cook, A.M., eds. *Clinical Engineering: Principles and Practices*, Prentice-Hall, Englewood Cliffs, NJ 1979.

CHAPTER 3

TECHNOLOGY MANAGEMENT

Technology management has been defined as an accountable, systematic approach to ensuring that cost-effective, efficacious, safe, and appropriate equipment is available to meet the demands of quality patient care (ECRI, 1989a). In most hospitals the importance of technology management is already well recognized and routinely accepted. Modern health-care institutions are increasingly coming to the view that technology is an integral part of all major policy and program-planning decisions. In many of these hospitals, technology management has become the responsibility of the clinical engineering department.

As discussed in Chapter 2, electrical safety concerns raised in the early 1970s stimulated the initial development of biomedical equipment maintenance programs under the guidance of clinical engineers and led to the creation of clinical engineering departments. From these beginnings, the levels of clinical engineering responsibility within the health-care environment have evolved to include traditional equipment maintenance functions such as electrical safety, equipment acquisition, repair and maintenance, supervision of service contracts, and computerized equipment control (Figure 3.1).

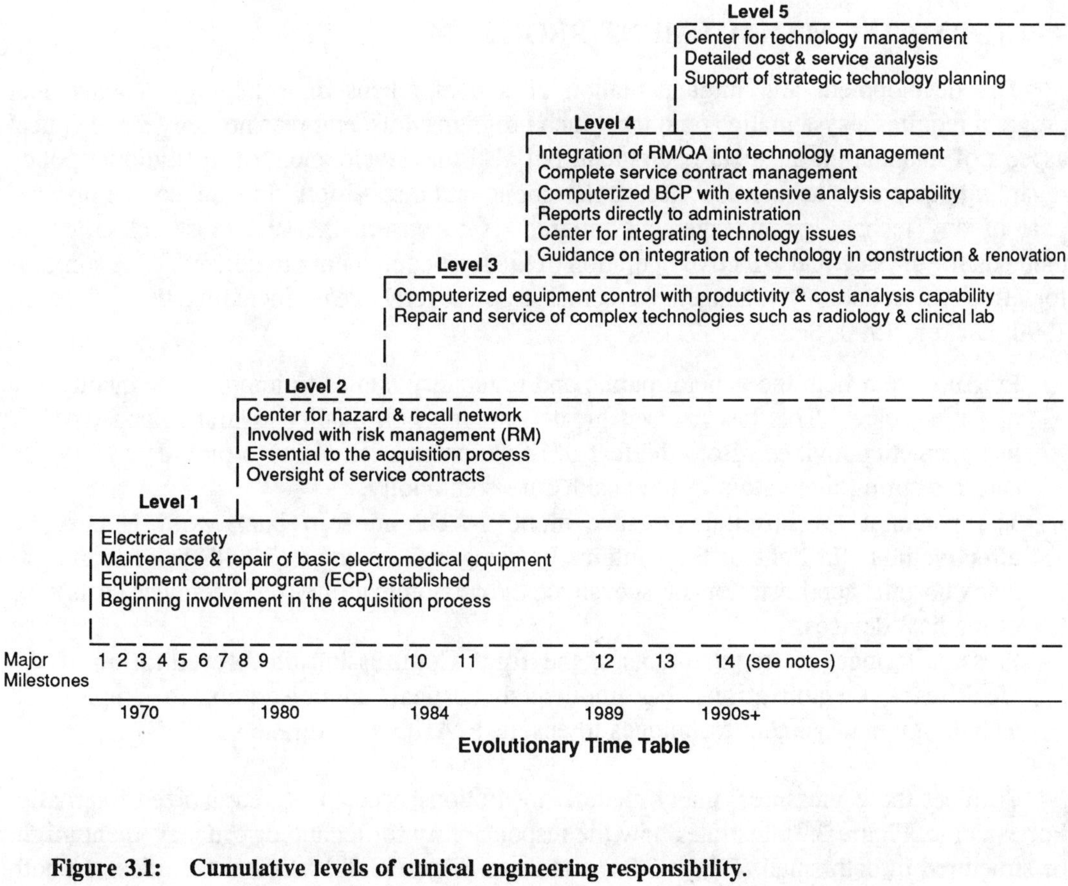

Figure 3.1: Cumulative levels of clinical engineering responsibility.

As we approach the twenty-first century, clinical engineering departments will be required to assume ever greater responsibilities, in areas such as technology assessment, strategic planning, and technology management, so that they can provide the hospital administration with information and guidance regarding the risks, cost effectiveness, reliability, and maintainability of a wide range of medical devices and equipment. These activities will enable hospitals to take fullest advantage of technology management's potential.

This chapter provides an overview of the major activities involved in establishing and supervising any technology management program. It presents the administrative, i.e. policy and financial considerations, as well as technical requirements to manage programs in such areas as equipment control and maintenance; technology planning, acquisition and replacement; establishing equipment maintenance schedules; and supervising repair services as well as service contracts. It discusses in significant detail the costs associated with providing in-house equipment repair and maintenance services. In addition, the role of the clinical engineering department in training users to properly use medical equipment, risk management, and quality assurance are presented. All of these activities will require clinical engineers to pay additional attention to improving their administrative skills. In order to supervise technology management programs, the director of clinical engineering must be a skilled manager, communicator, educator, and planner. These increased responsibilities, however, also bring opportunities. By virtue of their responsibility for technology management, clinical engineers can participate in all aspects of the health-care industry.

TECHNOLOGY MANAGEMENT PROGRAM

The development and implementation of a comprehensive technology management program requires a systematic approach. Such programs must embrace not only the technical aspects of maintaining medical equipment, but also the development of institutional policy regarding equipment acquisition, use, replacement, and disposition. In essence, the primary goal of any technology management program is to ensure that the most cost-effective methods for the safe and effective operation of medical equipment are utilized. The stimulus for effective technology management comes from several areas, including these (Carver, 1990; Dickey, 1990; Selsky, 1991):

- Pressure from both the general public and regulatory bodies to improve the quality of patient care. This has focused greater attention on quality assurance and risk management activities. Both the fear of litigation and the desire to provide quality care are strong motivators in the health-care community.
- The potential for hospitals to save money. The modern buzz word is **cost effectiveness.** In light of the continually rising costs associated with health-care, many hospital administrators must evaluate the economic utility (i.e., life-cycle costs) of medical devices.
- Pressure to meet the requirements of the **Joint Commission on Accreditation of Healthcare Organizations** has motivated hospital administrators to employ technology management techniques to ensure JCAHO accreditation.

To meet these pressures, many medical institutions need to be reorganized internally. For example, Figure 3.2 illustrates how the responsibility for technology management might be structured in both small (Figure 3.2a) and large (Figure 3.2b) medical facilities. In both situations, the director of clinical engineering reports directly to a vice-president of support services. Such an organizational structure places significant emphasis on the importance of technology management (Baretich, 1987).

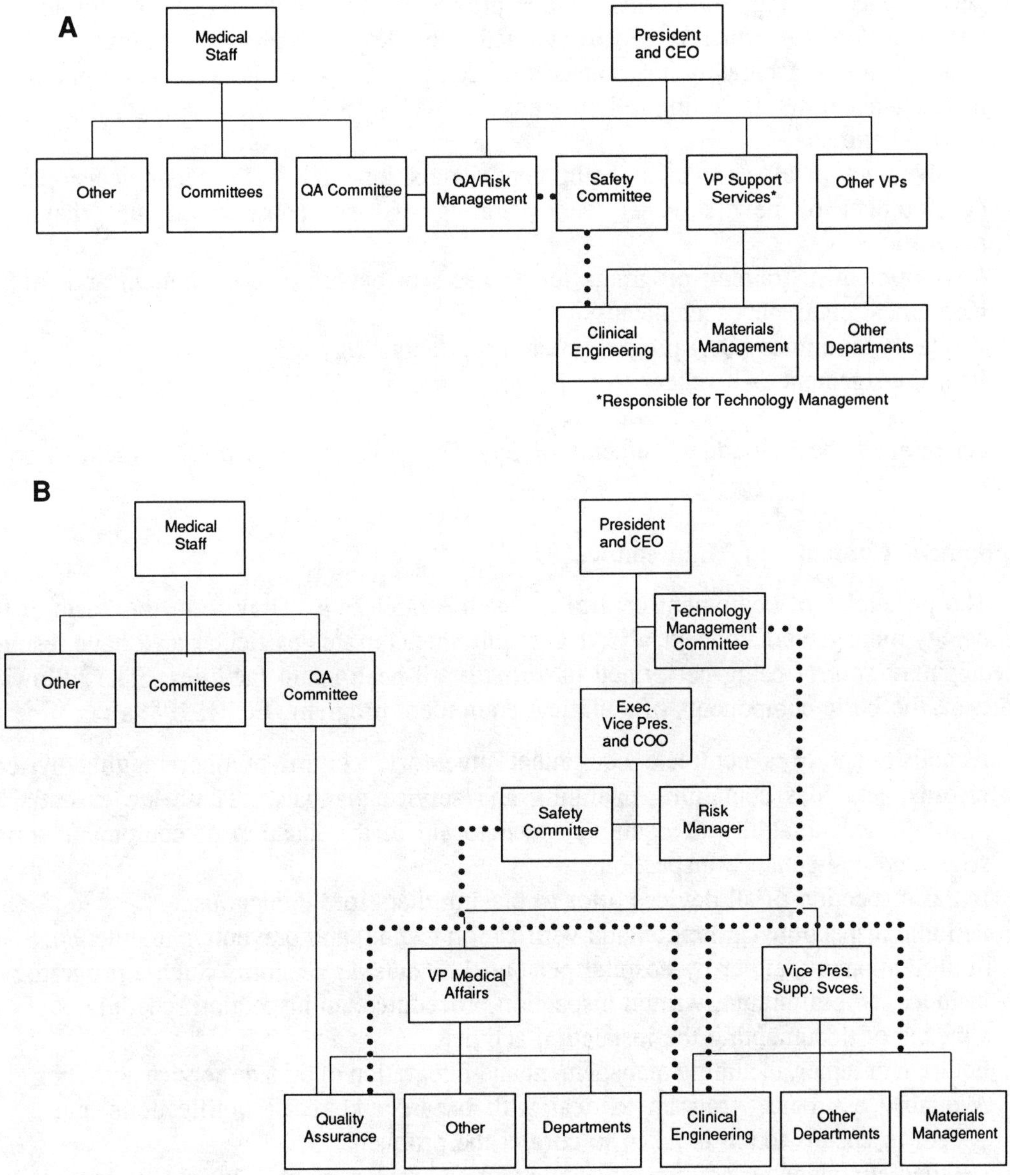

Figure 3.2: Suggested organization chart for small hospitals (A) and large hospitals (B). Solid lines indicate administrative responsibility. Dotted lines indicate committee membership responsibility.

A comprehensive program in technology management (TM) is multidimensional. Although the diversity and complexity of any such program will be dependent on the skills of the clinical engineers assigned to it, it should include the following elements (ECRI, 1989a):

- A program to control and monitor equipment performance, including routine performance testing, initial inspection, preventive maintenance, calibration and verification of performance, repair, and action on device recalls and hazards.
- A program that accurately and consistently computes and monitors total equipment maintenance costs, including in-house costs as well as manufacturer and third-party service contracts.
- Involvement in all aspects of equipment acquisition and replacement decisions, development of new services, and planning of new construction and major renovations.
- Development of training programs for all users of patient care equipment and for biomedical equipment technicians.
- A quality assurance (QA) program relating to technology use.
- Risk management as it relates to technology.

Having defined the individual elements of any TM program, let's discuss them in some detail.

Equipment Control and Maintenance

The principles of equipment control are well established. They form the basis of the technology management concept. JCAHO requirements in this particular area have resulted in equipment control being performed in virtually all health-care facilities. The following represent the basic components of a clinical equipment program (ECRI, 1989a):

- Establishment of a complete equipment inventory, control number tagging system, records, and files containing operating and service manuals. These are essential to maintain accountability of equipment and to aid in the location of equipment during scheduled maintenance inspections.
- Initial inspection of all devices prior to placing them into clinical use.
- Periodic inspection, calibration and verification testing, and preventive maintenance of all equipment, either by hospital personnel or outside vendors. Such a program includes, at a minimum, written inspection procedures, an inspection schedule, and a means of documenting the inspection activity.
- Equipment repair, including management and integration of outside service activities.
- A quality assurance program to deal with hazard and recall notifications and a system to ensure action is taken to correct the problem.
- Detailed strategies for equipment acquisition and replacement. This should include procedures for conducting preprocurement surveys.
- Procedures to dispose of equipment that is no longer needed.
- A method to evaluate the performance and documentation of each of these functions.

Presently, support responsibility for all patient-care equipment is usually assigned to the clinical engineering department. Medical devices used in specific departments, such as clinical laboratory and diagnostic imaging, are often supported by outside vendors or in-house specialists and therefore are not considered the responsibility of the clinical engineering department. However, since JCAHO requires that consistent practices be followed, not only in record keeping, but also in all equipment control functions, it is necessary that each hospital have equipment control policies and procedures that apply hospital-wide and include all organizational segments that support equipment.

Technology Planning, Acquisition, and Replacement

Technology planning is the method by which a hospital plans for the acquisition of new technology. Today, hospitals must plan for the acquisition of new and emerging technologies in order to achieve the best competitive advantage. Experienced clinical engineers, with their unique combination of clinical and technical expertise, must play a major role in hospital technology planning. A detailed discussion of this role for clinical engineers is provided in Chapter 4.

Clinical engineering departments should also be considered essential participants in the planning of new construction and major renovations. They have an important role any time clinical or support services are affected by a new installation of equipment or a renovation of services. Clinical engineers can translate the physical requirements for the optimal operation of clinical equipment into technical specifications. They can serve as advisers to hospital administrators, architects, and engineers to ensure that all requirements to integrate equipment into the hospital are met. A more detailed discussion of the activity of clinical engineers in facility design is provided in Chapter 6.

Technological advances and excessive maintenance costs are the main reasons for equipment replacement. Equipment is replaced as clinical procedures change and when maintaining the device is no longer cost-effective. Although equipment users most often provide the perspective on a medical device's clinical performance, the clinical engineer can provide an equally valuable perspective from the service record of the device. The log of equipment performance, service costs, and availability of repair parts allows a comprehensive review of a device's operating performance and thereby helps in making equipment replacement decisions (Clark and Forsell, 1990).

Training in Equipment Use

Regular training of equipment users is an essential element of any technology-related quality assurance and risk management program. Many experts believe that the vast majority of equipment-related injuries (see Chapter 2) are due to user error, not equipment malfunction (ECRI, 1983). To reduce user error significantly, clinicians must be trained in the proper use of the medical equipment that they operate.

The clinical engineer plays an important role in assisting the hospital staff, not only in the identification of medical equipment that requires special training, but in the actual training process itself. Since training in the use of specific pieces of equipment is often best conducted by someone in the same discipline as those being trained, clinical engineering departments can assist in "training the trainers." Clinical engineers, however, often conduct the training themselves, especially when detailed aspects of highly technical equipment use are to be discussed. Since clinical engineers are familiar with the clinical environment, they can provide the medical staff with the level of understanding necessary to utilize the equipment effectively.

With these factors in mind, hospitals need to develop a training policy regarding medical equipment use that should include the following (Shaffer and Shaffer, 1990):

- Assigning responsibility for the training. In the case of most medical equipment, the clinical engineering department should be involved. However, training should also include sessions provided by manufacturers. These extramural lectures and demonstrations are usually coordinated by the nursing department to fit into the overall training program of the hospital with the least disruption to clinical services.
- Monitoring and assessing equipment-related training for its effectiveness by clinical engineering or by the individual departments.
- Documenting the training program (e.g., when held, who attended, etc.); the evaluations must be available to meet regulatory and accreditation requirements and minimize liability.

Quality Assurance

Quality assurance is an essential activity in all modern hospitals. Due to the demands of third-party payers, hospitals are required to monitor and document systematically all significant aspects of patient-care, analyze the outcome of procedures, and take corrective action when problems are identified. In the past, hospitals have not devoted much attention to the quality of care as it pertains to device-related aspects of patient care. However, by requiring hospitals to analyze their patient care deficiencies systematically and to take corrective measures, the JCAHO has increased the visibility and importance of equipment-related, as well as user-related factors. These new quality assurance requirements provide both a challenge to and an opportunity for clinical engineering departments.

Equipment-Related Risk Management

Risk management is closely related to both technology management and quality assurance. Equipment use, abuse, or nonuse are important factors in many patient incidents. As pointed out in Chapter 2, incident reports from both an equipment and a user perspective are an essential component of a comprehensive technology management program (Bruley, 1988; Alder, 1991).

Clinical engineering personnel should be routinely involved in reviewing all incident and safety reports that involve patient-care equipment. The director of clinical engineering, in concert with the risk manager, should develop criteria for identifying equipment-related incidents involving serious injuries or death and should maintain records of equipment-related incidents. These records can then be used to identify trends with specific types of equipment, specific equipment manufacturers, or groups of equipment users so appropriate action can be taken. Having reviewed the basic components of a comprehensive technology management program, it is important to point out that, at any given facility, the scope of such a plan can vary dramatically based on the skills of the available clinical engineering personnel and the hospital administrators. Technology management programs thus must be tailored to the needs of each particular facility.

MEDICAL EQUIPMENT MANAGEMENT

Each aspect of the technology management program mentioned above is important. In this chapter, however, particular emphasis will be given to equipment control and maintenance activities. With this in mind, let's explore the following tasks in greater detail:

- Initial inspection/acceptance testing.
- Scheduled maintenance services.
- Repair services.
- Scheduled maintenance services.
- Equipment disposition.

Initial Inspection/Acceptance Testing

Although the equipment acquisition process is discussed in detail in Chapter 4, it is important simply to note here that when a new medical device is received, an initial inspection/acceptance test is conducted in order to do the following:

- Verify that all components, accessories, and options listed on the purchase request were received.
- Verify the safety and performance features of the device prior to its initial use for patient care within the facility. Safety and performance should be verified against the manufacturer's specifications.
- Record initial performance and safety values, which can be used for comparison during future inspections if questions arise about the device's performance.
- Satisfy the requirements of the Joint Commission on Accreditation of Healthcare Organizations. As part of their Plant, Technology, and Safety Management (PTSM) standards, JCAHO requires documentation of equipment testing prior to initial use.

There are also a number of administrative considerations during the initial inspection. These include the following:

- Ensuring that the hospital identification tag or unique control number is affixed to the equipment.
- Starting an equipment data file (EDF). This file should include a copy of the original purchase order, the initial performance and safety values, and any warranty/guarantee data.
- Filing the manufacturer's service and operator manuals.
- Entering information about the device (e.g., serial number, purchase price, purchase date, etc.) into the computerized maintenance management system and determining the appropriate scheduled maintenance frequency.
- Stocking appropriate accessories and user supplies, including replacement parts.
- Setting up training programs for users.

MAINTENANCE SCHEDULES

Once the device has been added to the equipment inventory, careful thought must be given to selection of an appropriate maintenance schedule. Inspections that are too frequent may degrade device longevity and may not be cost effective.

Device Category: ____________________

Manufacturer: ____________________ Model: ____________________

1. Equipment function (check all that apply):
   ☐ Life support or resuscitation ☐ Therapeutic ☐ Critical monitor ☐ Diagnostic
2. Application risk – Does failure or misuse of this device have the the potential for serious injury? ☐ Yes ☐ No
   Does the device apply potentially dangerous energies? ☐ Yes ☐ No
3. Review of equipment incident history, experience, and other information sources reveals:
   ☐ No experience available. ☐ No significant findings. ☐ See comments below.
4. Significant problems and special considerations: ☐ See comments below.

General Considerations
- ☐ Backup devices unavailable
- ☐ Component wear
- ☐ Internal cleaning required
- ☐ Internal heating reduces reliability
- ☐ Status of technology
- ☐ Battery failure
- ☐ Mobile or portable
- ☐ Outstanding recalls or hazards
- ☐ Manufacturer-recommended maintenance
- ☐ Device condition

Use Environment
- ☐ Frequent use
- ☐ Incorrect use
- ☐ Poor user maintenance
- ☐ Likely hard use or abuse

Failure Modes
- ☐ Physiologic measurement error
- ☐ Physiologic measurement failure
- ☐ Critical alarm inaccuracy
- ☐ Critical alarm failure
- ☐ Therapeutic output error
- ☐ Therapeutic output failure
- ☐ Backup circuitry failure or error
- ☐ Noncritical indicator failure or error
- ☐ Mechanical safety
- ☐ Electrical safety

5. Risk Level (based on Items 1 through 4):
   ☐ High (life support and resuscitation devices and those devices whose failure or misuse is reasonable likely to result in serious injury)
   ☐ Medium (misuse, failure, or absence will have significant impact, but unlikely to cause serious injury)
   ☐ Low (misuse or failure unlikely to have serious consequences)
6. Special requirements for (explain): ☐ No special requirements
   ☐ Cost: ____________________
   ☐ Operational difficulties: ____________________
   ☐ Codes, standards, or regulations: ____________________
7. Scheduled-support program components:

	Not Required	Intervals	Person/Department Responsible
User training	☐	______	____________
User performance verification	☐	______	____________
User maintenance procedure	☐	______	____________
Minor inspection	☐	___ months	____________
Major inspection	☐	___ months	____________
Scheduled maintenance	☐	___ months	____________

8. Include in equipment-management inventory? ☐ Yes ☐ No

Comments: ☐ See separate sheet.

____

____

____

Assessed by: ____________________ Date: __________

Follow-up review by: ____________________ Date: __________

ESSA-0590
0087DL0A

Figure 3.3: Equipment scheduled-support assessment form. © 1990, ECRI. Used with permission.

Inspections that are not frequent enough may adversely affect reliability, accuracy, and safety. A device should be scheduled for periodic inspection, maintenance, or performance verification only if there is good reason to provide such support (Hertz, 1990). Appropriate reasons include (ECRI, 1990):

- Reducing the risk of injury to patients, staff, or visitors.
- Minimizing equipment down time.
- Avoiding excessive repair costs by providing maintenance at appropriate intervals.
- Correcting minor operational problems before they result in major system failures or inaccurate results.
- Complying with codes, standards, and regulations or the strict recommendations of equipment manufacturers.

It is important to note that, regardless of the decision, JCAHO requires each decision to be documented. The standard states, "*Before a piece or type of equipment is used, it is evaluated for inclusion in the program (scheduled maintenance) and the evaluation is documented*" (JCAHO, 1990). The Equipment scheduled-support assessment form (Figure 3.3) developed by ECRI provides a good example of the documentation required. It will be noted that this type of form permits the tracking of significant medical device problems as well as the work level and costs associated with them.

Although risk alone does not define the scheduled maintenance frequency, it is an important factor. Figure 3.4 lists devices that have been designated as being high, medium, or low risk. High-risk devices are those life-support, therapeutic, and diagnostic devices whose failure or misuse is reasonably likely to cause injury to patient or staff or whose absence or failure could have an immediate or serious impact on patient care. Medium-risk devices are those devices whose failure, misuse, or absence is not likely to cause serious injury to patients or staff but may have an impact on patient care. Low-risk devices are those devices whose failure, misuse, or absence is unlikely to result in injury to patient or staff and will have minimal impact on patient care.

Other major factors that bear on the scheduled maintenance frequency include (1) clinical application, (2) maintenance requirements, (3) manufacturer's recommendations, (4) incident history, including device recalls and hazard alerts, (5) revenue lost due to equipment downtime, and (6) cost of service (either in-house or by contract). All these factors should be evaluated in order to make an appropriate decision regarding which devices will be supported, the type of support, and at what intervals.

A simple scoring system can be established to determine whether scheduled maintenance should be performed and at what frequency. Three factors are considered in order to arrive at an equipment management (EM) number, which is used to make this determination. These three factors are (1) equipment function, (2) physical risk, and (3) required maintenance. This can be expressed mathematically as follows:

$$EM = Function + Risk + Required\ Maintenance$$

Equipment function usually falls into one of the following categories: therapeutic, diagnostic, analytical, and miscellaneous (Figure 3.5). Therapeutic equipment applies some form of energy to the patient and hence has the highest risk score, i.e., 8–10. The risk scores for diagnostic, (6–7), analytical, (3–5) and miscellaneous equipment are provided in Figure 3.5.

Physical risk considers what the possible consequences might be to the patient or operator if the equipment fails or malfunctions. Figure 3.6 illustrates some of the possible outcomes (e.g., patient death, injury, and misdiagnosis) and provides the risk score associated with each outcome.

These levels are based on the risks of injury as a result of device failure or user error; they take into account both outcome probability and severity.

High-risk devices are life-support devices, key resuscitation devices, and other devices whose failure or misuse is reasonably likely to seriously injure patient or staff.

Anesthesia units and vaporizers
Anesthesia ventilators
Apnea monitors (neonatal)
Aspirators (emergency and tracheal)
Autotransfusion units
Defibrillators
Diagnostic radiologic imaging/nuclear medicine systems (all types)
Electrosurgical units
Fetal monitors
Heart-lung bypass units
Hemodialysis units
Humidifiers (heated)
Hypo/hyperthermia units
Incubators (infant, including transport units)
Infusion controllers/pumps
Intra-aortic balloon pumps
Lasers (surgical)
Oximeters (pulse)
Oxygen monitors and analyzers
Pacemakers (external)
Peritoneal dialysis units
Phacoemulsification units
Physiologic monitors and monitoring systems
Radiant warmers (infant)
Radiographic dye injectors
Resuscitators (cardiac)
Resuscitators (pulmonary)
Sterilizers (e.g., steam, EtO)
Regulators (tracheal suction)
Tourniquets (pneumatic)
Transcutaneous O_2 and CO_2 monitors
Ventilators

Medium-risk devices are those whose misuse, failure, absence (e.g., out of service and no replacement available) would have significant impact on patient care, but would not be likely to cause direct serious injury. Many diagnostic devices are in this category.

Ambulatory ECG recorders and scanners
Aspirators (surgical, thoracic, and uterine)
Blood bank refrigerators
Blood gas/pH analyzers
Blood pressure units (noninvasive electronic units used in critical monitoring applications)
Blood warmers
Capnographs
Cardiac output units
Centrifuges
Clinical laboratory equipment (all types)
Cryosurgical units
Electrocardiographs
Electroconvulsive therapy units
Electroencephalographs
Electromyographs
Endoscopes
Evoked potential units
Lithotripters
Oxygen-air proportioners
Phonocardiographs
Phototherapy units
Pneumatic antishock trousers
Pressure transducers (all types)
Pulmonary function analyzers
Radiant warmers (adult)
Regulators (air, O_2, suction [except tracheal])
Scales for critical applications (e.g., hemodialysis and neonatal care units)
Smoke evacuators (laser)
Special care beds (e.g., rocking, circle, flotation)
Surgical drills and saws (powered)
Temperature monitors
Traction units
Treadmills
Ultrasound imaging units/systems
Vectorcardiographs

Low-risk devices are those devices whose failure or misuse is unlikely to result in serious consequences.

Alternating pressure pads
Aspirators (low volume)
Cast cutters
Circulating fluid pumps
Diathermy units (physical therapy)
Duplex receptacles
Electric beds
Electronic scales (used for general patient care)
Electronic thermometers
Examining lights
Fiberoptic light sources
Isolated power systems
Paraffin baths
Pumps (breast)
Sphygmomanometers
Stimulators (low- and high-voltage physical therapy units)
Surgical lights
Surgical microscopes
Surgical tables
Ultrasonic nebulizers
Ultrasonic therapy (physical therapy)
Whirlpool baths

Figure 3.4: Typical device risk levels. © 1990 ECRI. Used with permission.

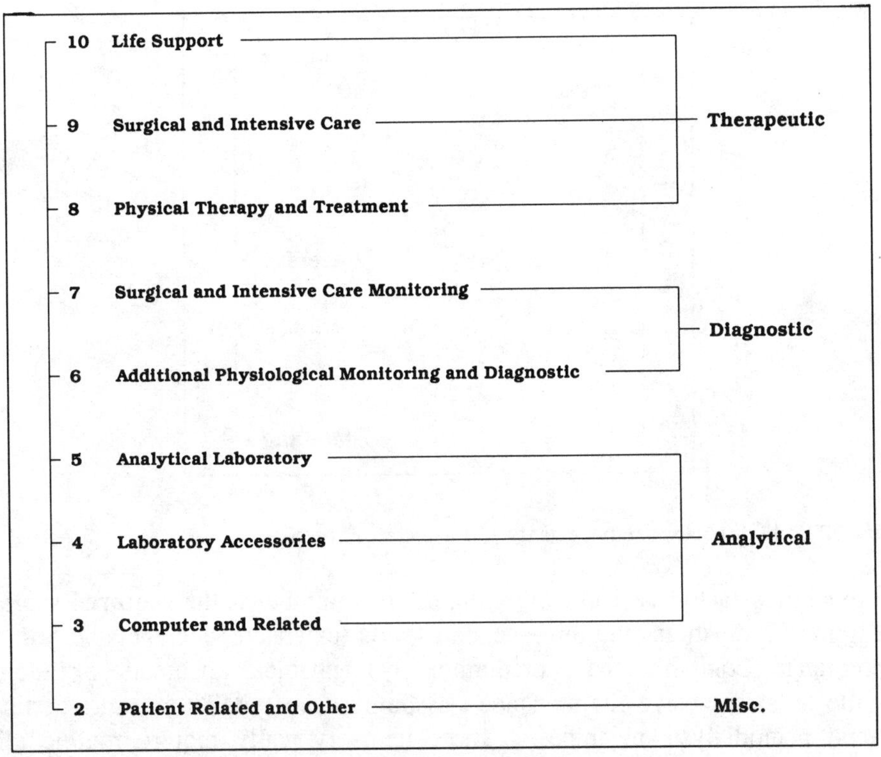

Figure 3.5: Equipment function categories and associated risk scores.

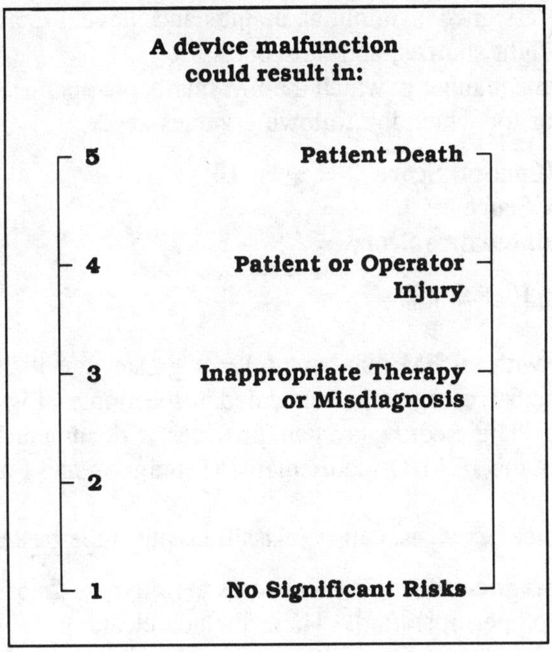

Figure 3.6: Physical risks scores associated with device malfunctions.

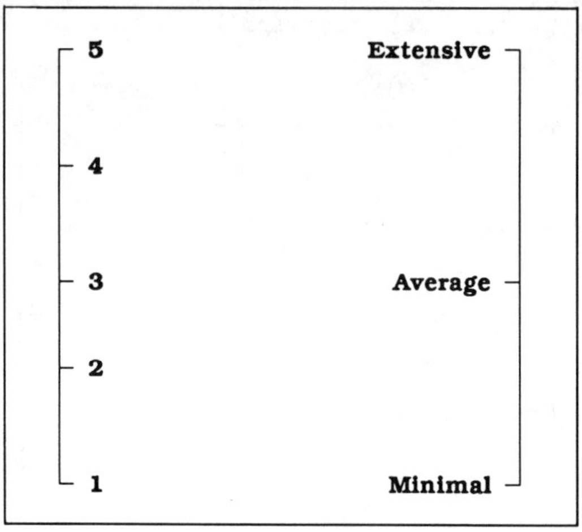

Figure 3.7: Maintenance requirements and associated scores.

The remaining factor used in computing the EM number is the **required maintenance** score. Figure 3.7 illustrates the three general levels (extensive, average, and minimal) and the scoring range. Equipment that is predominantly mechanical, pneumatic, or fluidic usually requires the most extensive maintenance. Examples are ventilators, intra-aortic balloon pumps, and hemodialysis machines. These items typically require routine alignment, calibration, or extensive parts replacement. Devices requiring only performance verification and safety testing are classified as average maintenance level. Included in this category are devices such as physiological monitors and infusion pumps. Devices that require only a visual inspection are assigned a minimal maintenance level. Examples of such devices includes water baths, light sources, and otoscopes.

Having reviewed the manner in which the EM number is obtained, let's compute the EM number for a ventilator for which the following values apply:

Equipment Function Score	=	10
Physical Risk Score	=	5
Required Maintenance Score	=	<u>5</u>
Therefore **EM = 10 + 5 + 5**	=	20

Only those items with an EM number of 12 or greater are included in the equipment control program and receive regularly scheduled inspections. Figure 3.8 provides some typical EM numbers. This scoring system provides a documentable equipment control program that will meet the JCAHO requirements (Fennigkoh and Smith, 1989).

Scheduled Maintenance Services: can be classified into three basic categories:

- **Preventive maintenance:** Periodic procedures to minimize the risk of failure and to ensure continued proper operation. These include cleaning, lubricating, adjusting, and replacing certain parts, but exclude operational maintenance normally carried out by the user (e.g., cleaning defibrillator paddles) (ECRI, 1990).

- **Functional testing, performance verification, and calibration:** To verify that the equipment is fully operational and performing within reasonable, previously specified limits (AHA, 1988).
- **Safety inspection:** Leakage current and ground integrity should be tested in accordance with NFPA 99, Standard for Health Care Facilities. A visual inspection for mechanical safety (e.g., cables, casters, handles) should also be conducted to ensure both the patient and operator are safe from possible harm.

The appropriate scheduled maintenance frequency is important to ensure longevity, reliability, accuracy, and safety of the device. In addition, specific maintenance procedures must be developed for each device to ensure that all critical, mandatory, and necessary tests are performed during the inspection. The JCAHO requires that "each piece or type of equipment listed in the inventory has written equipment testing procedures and user training programs designed to manage the clinical and physical risks." (JCAHO, 1991). Maintenance procedures may cover a number of different models of equipment, requiring only minor modifications to become device specific. *The Health Devices Inspection and Preventive Maintenance System*, published by ECRI, and *Maintenance Management for Medical Equipment*, published by the American Hospital Association, are good resources for general maintenance procedures on a wide variety of devices. Figure 3.9 provides a good example of a basic preventive maintenance check list.

Records of inspections must be kept for accreditation organizations and also for use in any equipment-related lawsuit. The JCAHO and the College of American Pathologists (CAP) are the most noteworthy of the accreditation bodies. The equipment data file should also contain useful information, such as any unusual findings or calibration results, that might be required at a later date.

Device	Function	Risk	Maintenance	EM #	Class	PM Interval
Balloon Pump	10	5	5	20	I	6
BP Amp	7	3	3	13	I	12
Centrifuge	4	3	5	12	I	6
CPR Manikin	2	1	1	3	N	12
Defibrillator	10	5	4	19	I	6
Diathermy	8	4	4	16	I	6
Electrocardiograph	6	3	4	13	I	6
Exam light	2	1	1	3	N	12
Fetal monitor	6	3	3	12	I	12
Hypo/Hyperthermia	9	4	5	18	I	6
Infant incubator	10	5	4	19	I	6
Infusion pump	9	3	2	14	I	12
Pacemaker	10	5	4	19	I	6
Physio monitor	7	3	3	13	I	12
Scale	2	3	2	7	N	12
Terminal	3	1	1	5	N	12
Treadmill	8	4	5	17	I	6
Ultrasound, Doppler	6	3	1	10	N	12
Ventilator	10	5	5	20	I	6
Water bath	4	1	2	7	N	12

Figure 3.8: Equipment maintenance numbers computed for included (I) and nonincluded (N) devices. Preventive maintenance intervals are given in terms of months.

UNIVERSAL INSPECTION FORM

CONTROL NO. ________ LOCATION ________
DEVICE TYPE ________
MANUFACTURER ________
MODEL NO. ________ SERIAL NO. ________
INSPECTOR ________ DATE ________ CHECKLIST NO. ________
[ ] MINOR [ ] MAJOR [ ] ACCEPTANCE

System Components	
Control #	Description

Status	
Passed	[ ]
Service Required	[ ]
Removed From Use	[ ]
WO #	

1	Pass	Fail	QUALITATIVE TESTS	COMMENTS
1.1			CHASSIS / HOUSING	
1.2			MOUNT / FASTENERS	
1.3			CASTERS / BRAKES	
1.4			AC PLUG / RECEPTACLES	
1.5			LINE CORD	
1.6			STRAIN RELIEFS	
1.7			CIRCUIT BREAKER / FUSE	
1.8			TUBES / HOSES	
1.9			CABLES	
1.10			FITTINGS / CONNECTORS	
1.11			ELECTRODES / TRANSDUCERS	
1.12			FILTERS	
1.13			CONTROLS / SWITCHES	
1.14			HEATER	
1.15			MOTOR / PUMP / FAN / COMP.	
1.16			FLUID LEVELS	
1.17			BATTERY / CHARGER	
1.18			INDICATORS / DISPLAYS	
1.19			USER CAL / SELF TEST	
1.20			ALARMS / INTERLOCKS	
1.21			AUDIBLE SIGNALS	
1.22			LABELING	
1.23			ACCESSORIES	
1.24				
1.25				

COMMENTS: ________

TIME REQUIRED ____ . ____ HOURS

2	Pass	Fail	QUANTITATIVE TESTS			COMMENTS
2.1			GROUNDING RES.:			
2.2			LEAKAGE CURRENT Ω			
			Chassis: ____ μA Leads: ____ μA			
2.3						
2.4						
2.5						
2.6						
2.7						
2.8						
2.9						
2.10						
			Set	In	Actual	
	Units					
2.11						
	Units					
2.12						
	Units					

3	CHECK IF DONE	P.M.	DESCRIPTION & COMMENTS
3.1		CLEAN	
3.2		LUBRICATE	
3.3		CAL / ADJUST	
3.4		REPLACE	

Figure 3.9: Example of a universal inspection form.

Scheduled maintenance inspections are usually spread evenly throughout the year. The historical workload, other departmental responsibilities, and the patient occupancy level should be considered during the scheduling review. Seasonal variations in patient occupancy levels may make it difficult to gain access to the equipment, and productivity will suffer. If the workload is not balanced over the year, the department may not be able to handle all scheduled maintenance inspections while also fulfilling other areas of responsibility (Betts, 1989). An alternative approach is to have a group of seasonal workers (i.e., college students who will work under supervision during school vacation times) do a majority of the routine scheduled maintenance procedures.

Hospital departments should be notified as far in advance as possible of scheduled maintenance so that the equipment can be available with minimal disruption to patient services. In areas with high patient throughput, such as radiology and clinical laboratory, proper scheduling may be more difficult. Not only is patient care affected, but hospital reimbursements from these revenue-generating departments may be reduced.

Many devices pose little or no risk to patients and may not be included in the hospital inspection program. While these devices may not require a high degree of maintenance support, they should be periodically checked. Detailed individual maintenance instructions and equipment records are not required for these devices.

Maintenance technicians must be provided with proper equipment to carry out a successful scheduled maintenance program. Some basic items that are required, no matter what the extent of the program, include a multimeter, an ECG simulator, a leakage current meter, a portable vacuum cleaner, adapters for piped gas outlets and operating room electrical outlets, hoses and adapters, a stopwatch or watch with a second hand, accessories for devices to be tested, and a tool kit (ECRI, 1990). There are also a wide range of device-specific testers that may be required, depending on the level of service to be provided. These include analyzers for defibrillators, electrosurgical units, infusion pumps, and ventilators. Some analyzers currently available can test several types of devices and produce a printed report of the results. This may provide a cost-effective method for consolidation of test equipment requirements and automation of report generation.

Walk-through inspections, sometimes called "rounds," should be conducted to supplement the formal scheduled maintenance program. These inspections should be conducted at frequencies based on the department's mission. For example, a walk-through inspection in the ICU or emergency room would be conducted more frequently than in non-patient care areas or areas of limited equipment usage. Figure 3.10 provides some examples of devices and equipment that could be included in a walk-through inspection program.

In conducting a walk-through inspection, clinical engineers should try to ensure that the equipment is functioning properly and being correctly used. During the walk-through, abuse or damage, general safety, and problems with non-patient-care and patient-owned equipment can also be identified. Resolving problems in this way helps to develop and maintain a good relationship between the users and the clinical engineering staff. In turn, the improved communications and cooperative spirit facilitate the equipment management process.

User maintenance is a critical part of any scheduled maintenance program. Equipment operators work with the equipment day in and day out and are most familiar with the operation and peculiarities of their equipment. Thus, they are more apt to notice subtle changes in operation than someone who only sees the equipment occasionally.

The equipment operator also plays a vital role in performing routine user maintenance, as usually described in the equipment operator's manual. Properly performed, user maintenance can significantly reduce equipment downtime and extend useful life. A quick visual inspection provides a good indication of how much attention is being given to user maintenance. If the item looks well cared for, the operators are probably doing a good job of user maintenance. Chances are there has not been much unscheduled maintenance in that section. On the other hand, if the item looks like it's been abused, user maintenance is probably lacking. Poorly maintained equipment may be distinguished by dirty, sticky tape residue, felt-tip marker notes scribbled on the case, or a yellow label with instructions to **"STRIKE HERE IF MACHINE DOESN'T WORK."** Unscheduled maintenance is probably high in these sections.

If the user maintenance program is to be successful, operators must be aware of their responsibilities. Training and feedback should be given to equipment operators during regular scheduled inspections. It is good advice to praise the positive actions taken and offer assistance in areas that need improvement.

Appropriate equipment service, whether performed by hospital personnel, equipment manufacturers, or other outside service organizations, is essential to high-quality, cost effective patient care. Ensuring cost-effective service of medical instrumentation may be simple in principle, but it is complex in execution. There are five elements to responsive, cost-effective equipment service:

- Competent technicians.
- Repair parts.
- Service manuals and documentation.
- Experience with factory back-up.
- Diagnostic software.

In summary, a scheduled maintenance service program helps to increase equipment safety and reliability, reduce unscheduled repairs and equipment downtime, and prolong the useful life of a device. Additionally, it can reduce costs and improve the quality of patient care. The benefits of a properly conducted and administered scheduled maintenance program far outweigh the costs.

Repair Services

Repair services have always been the bread and butter of every clinical engineering program. Customers see the fruits of these efforts, unlike the scheduled maintenance services whose results are less discernible to the user. For this reason, a successful clinical engineering program must have a successful repair program.

Repair can be defined as trouble shooting to isolate the cause of device malfunction and then replacement or adjustment of components or subsystems to restore normal function, safety, performance, and reliability (ECRI, 1990). Repair services are offered by manufacturers, shared-service organizations, third-party service organizations, and in-house departments, with the extent of the repairs varying from circuit board exchange to component-level repairs (Betts, 1987). Depending on the device complexity, component level repairs may be the most cost-effective and desirable method of repair for a given device. Many companies offer exchange prices on circuit boards, which significantly reduces the cost of board replacement.

Audiovisual Equipment
Autopsy Saw
Baby Cribs
Bassinets
Bed Lamps
Buffers
Business Machines
Calculators
Ceilings
Circulating Bath
Coffee Makers
Computer
Conductive Floor Testing
Convection Oven
Deep Fryer
Diluter
Door Latch Tensions
Doors (Manually Operated)
Drinking Fountains
Electric Thermometers
Electrical Beds
Electrocautery Units
Enzyme Treatment Drains
Exam Tables
Exit Lighting
Eye Washers
Floor Coverings
Floor Drains
Floor Machines
General Lighting
Gurneys
Heaters
Heat Sealing Units
Holter Tape Recorder
Hotplates
I.D. Printers
Immersion Heaters/Humidifiers
Insect Controllers
Isolated Power Systems
Laboratory Oven
Laminar Air Flow Hoods
Laundry Chute Doors
Lawn Sprinkler System
Line Integrity Isolation Monitor
Master Clocks
Mechanical Beds
Medical Gas Outlets
Medical Vacuum Outlets
Motorized Tables
Morgue Table
Nonelectrical Food Carts
O.R. Lamps
Ophthalmoscope/Otoscope Wall Sets
Ovens
Oxygen Blender
Paraffin Baths
Parallel Bars
Patient Lifts
Patient Scales
Pipet Shaker
Pipet Washer/Dryer
Portable Exam Lamp
Portable Fan
Portable Heat Lamps
Refrigerator (Non-Med Storage)
Room Furniture
Room Grounding
Rotator
Scrub Sinks
Sewers
Shaker
Showers
Signs and Lighting
Sinks
Slide Dryer/Warmer
Stenographic Equipment
Stirplates
Televisions
Temperature Block
Test Equipment
Time Clocks
Time/Date Stamp Unit
Tissue Float
Toilet Exhausters
Toasters
Transformers
Trash Chute Doors
Typewriters
Ultrasonic Cleaners (Small)
Vacuum Cleaners
Video Equipment
Walls
Warming Cabinets
Water Temperatures
Wheel Chairs
Window Screens
Whirlpool Unit
X-Ray Viewboxes

Figure 3.10: Example of items generally included in a walk-through inspection.

Current technologies using surface-mounted components make it very difficult to trouble shoot at the component level. Each repair must be evaluated to determine the most cost-effective and expeditious way to return the device to service. Many high-technology systems, such as computerized tomography, magnetic resonance imaging, and automated laboratory analyzers, may be better handled by outside service organizations because of the complexity, training and test equipment costs, and replacement part inventory required for their maintenance. Requests for repair services typically come from the equipment operator in written form or verbally. The request should do the following:

- Identify the device requiring repair, usually by use of the hospital identification number or equipment control number.
- Provide as much information as possible regarding the problem.
- Identify the operator of the device at the time of malfunction.
- Give the time and date of the malfunction.
- Provide the equipment location, the department, a point of contact, and a phone number.

Repair work orders should be scheduled on the basis of equipment need, availability of back-up equipment, effect of downtime, and effect on patient care. Prior to making major repairs, the equipment history should be reviewed for previous repair actions and the amount of money already spent on maintenance. Repair -versus- replacement decisions should be made based on equipment age, dollars already spent on repair, frequency of failure, technological obsolescence, cost of repair, and cost of replacement.

All too often when equipment is being examined after a reported failure, no problems are found. Two assumptions may be drawn from this result: (1) there is an intermittent problem, or (2) the operator made an error that led to the conclusion that there was a malfunction. In practice, genuine intermittent equipment problems do occur, but not too frequently. When checking an instrument for a possible intermittent problem, it should be run under all operating conditions for a considerable length of time. However, the majority of intermittent problems occur due to operator error or misuse. In its 1991 *Accreditation Manual for Hospitals*, the JCAHO requires that operator errors be identified, documented, and reviewed by the safety committee. Since these operator error reports cause an unneeded expenditure of technician time and cost to the hospital (Fennigkoh, 1990), the clinical engineer should take an active role in eliminating operator error by providing in-service training; ensuring that instruction manuals are clear, concise, and available; evaluating new equipment; and identifying potential problems before the device is purchased.

Documentation of repairs should be as detailed as practical. A complete description of the malfunction and the corrective action taken should be noted, along with all repair parts used. This information should be placed in the equipment data file for future reference. This information may be useful the next time the device fails and can be used to determine if a trend exists with a particular class of devices.

Managers should be aware that even though in-house service is generally the most cost-effective way to repair most devices, extended amounts of time spent on trouble shooting a problem may be an inefficient use of resources. The time thus spent may be better used performing more pressing tasks. Therefore, it is important to establish guidelines to evaluate technical abilities, local service availability, and backlog of equipment to determine at what point alternate service possibilities should be used.

In order to determine the capabilities of outside providers of service support, considerable information is needed; some of this information is also needed from manufacturers in order to evaluate the ability to service the equipment in-house:

- location of service personnel
- for manufacturer service, whether personnel are employed by it or by an independent dealer
- number of personnel at the local service office who routinely service this type of device; their names, training, experience, or other credentials; and the total number of the device in question that they currently service
- location of backup service
- guaranteed response times (both by telephone and on-site) and penalty for nonperformance; for a manufacturer, to be specified separately for the warranty period and for postwarranty service
- availability of parts (for in-house and third-party service)
- primary location of parts; the range at that location
- location of backup parts; how quickly they are shipped
- for manufacturer service, current parts price lists for all categories of customers
- service manual and diagnostic software availability (for in-house and third-party service)
- hourly labor rate and standard service hours it covers
- hours during which service will be provided at additional cost and overtime labor rate(s)
- how travel time is charged
- attitude toward first-call troubleshooting or screening by hospital personnel (e.g., will a price reduction be offered, or does the organization oppose involvement of in-house staff?)
- for manufacturers, whether a service hot line is provided
- number of IPMs provided and copies of applicable IPM protocols
- number of repair visits provided, if there is a limit
- whether loaner equipment is provided and, if so, how quickly; how conflicting needs for loaners are resolved
- availability of training courses and materials for training of service techs and cost, if any
- years in business
- liability insurance coverage (including types of coverage and policy limits)
- uptime guarantee (including definition of uptime) and penalty for nonperformance
- names and addresses of 10 closest service clients, indicating which of them have the type of device being considered

Figure 3.11: List of information needed concerning sources of service support.

Types of Maintenance Services

There are three traditional methods of servicing medical instrumentation: in-house equipment service, manufacturer service, and third-party or shared service. A fourth option has emerged over the last several years. Maintenance insurance is an option that combines the use of any of the above service methods with financial protection against unusually high service costs. There has always been a debate over which type of service is best. Since the overall goal is to provide high-quality, cost-effective medical care, a mix of all types of service may be the answer. Figure 3.11 provides a list of information required in order to determine which type of service might be best applied to a given situation. Optimizing the service mix means maximizing the use of low-cost service alternatives (e.g., in-house, shared service, parts only) and minimizing the use of high-cost, full-service contracts. There is no magic formula to determine the proper mix, especially since the mix that works now may require change later. Let's discuss the basic advantages and disadvantages of the three major types of service.

In-House Equipment Service. The prime advantages of in-house servicing are immediate availability of service technicians to trouble shoot and repair equipment, facilitation of other aspects of equipment operation, and provision of prompt, ongoing support for clinical personnel. Disadvantages focus on the relative costs associated with operating an in-house clinical engineering service.

Hospitals must make a continuing institutional commitment to support the clinical engineering department. That commitment includes training, equipment, space, tools, management, and parts inventory. These expenses could be considered a disadvantage to the hospital, and unlike service contracts, in-house service offers no financial protection or "insurance" against the cost of catastrophic equipment failure. However, the savings from in-house service can be used to create, either formally or informally, a fund that is used to pay for some extraordinary repairs (ECRI, 1989b).

Manufacturer Service. Manufacturers usually provide service through (1) a full-service contract, which generally includes all labor-related costs, and may include all or certain parts-related costs, (2) a demand service agreement in which the hospital pays on a time-and-materials basis for each service call, as needed, and (3) a combination of the two basic methods. Manufacturer service for some devices may be the only service that is practical. High-tech items like MRI, CAT, and digital imaging equipment require such extensive training and investment in repair parts that it is often not practical to maintain these items in-house. The quality and timeliness of repairs, and the reliability of repair work are usually higher when done by the manufacturer, because the manufacturer is more familiar with the devices, and has greater accessibility to repair parts. [Manufacturer service may be required to obtain an uptime guarantee and may include penalties for nonperformance (that is part of new equipment acquisition).] There are also a number of actual and potential disadvantages to this type of service:

- Cost may be greater.
- Response time is dependent on the location of the manufacturer's service center.
- Technician experience and qualifications may be suspect if subcontractors or dealers are used.
- Clinical engineers must closely monitor the contractors to ensure acceptable

performance and to ensure that the terms of the contract are met. Appropriate records needed by the hospital for quality assurance, accreditation, and future service decisions must also be received.

There are various programs that entail shared responsibility between the hospital and manufacturer. These programs usually involve the performance by hospital personnel of an initial screening of each repair call in exchange for a discount on the contract price. The hospital may be provided with some consigned spare modules and parts or may be required to purchase a parts kit. Other parts can be supplied on a next-day emergency basis. Preventive maintenance may be done by the vendor or by the hospital. Discounts as high as 55 percent can be realized with this type of contract (Brinkman, 1989). Telephone consultations with experienced manufacturer's technicians are an important feature of this type of service.

Third-Party Service. A hospital may elect to obtain service from an independent, third-party service organization. These organizations may be small and specialize in only a few types of equipment, or they may be large enough to provide service on any equipment in the hospital. Hospitals in a region can join in a cooperative arrangement to share amongst themselves services provided by a nonprofit clinical engineering organization, or they may contract with one large hospital to provide services to all. Some third-party service organizations are well established and receive good support from equipment manufacturers. Third-party service, however, requires at least as much management oversight as does manufacturer service. A service organization may have particular difficulty in fulfilling the hospital's needs for support functions beyond narrowly defined equipment repair, and it may be at a serious disadvantage, especially for servicing high-tech equipment, if the manufacturer is unwilling to provide needed parts and diagnostic equipment.

Cost Analysis for In-House Service

The cost of the in-house service program must be known in order to compare it with other service options. One way to determine costs is to set a price or value on services provided to users. Whether this charge is actually collected by the clinical engineering department or if it is just noted for reference, it provides a management tool to establish the value of services provided. Profit or loss is acutely sensitive to pricing. Many of the benefits associated with a clinical engineering profit center could be compromised if the pricing of its services is not carefully established. To establish the price of clinical engineering services, it is necessary to do the following:

- Determine actual hourly labor costs.
- Evaluate cost–volume–profit relationships.
- Establish pricing options and service contract rates.

Hourly Labor Costs. While there are a variety of methods that could be used, those based on an actual hourly labor cost are the most effective and applicable. This cost represents the total effective hourly cost of doing business and becomes the hourly labor rate at which the department's services are billed.

Generally, the hourly labor cost method is easiest to compute, understand, and explain to others. It is also the most popular pricing method used by technical service providers.

It is particularly well suited for use by clinical engineering departments for several reasons:

- It permits direct comparisons between the costs of the clinical engineering department and those of equipment manufacturers, other clinical engineering departments, or third-party service providers.
- It represents the single best aggregate measure of overall department efficiency by acknowledging all department costs and the effects of staff productivity.
- It becomes a useful measure of clinical-engineering management effectiveness.
- It serves as the basis for all service cost estimates or contracts.

Despite institutional variations in financial reporting systems, available data, and terminology, the hourly labor cost method is based on standard (yet simple) cost accounting principles. In using this method, every effort should be made to do the following:

- Identify accurately and use all of the applicable cost factors associated with the hourly labor rate equation (as incurred over a reasonable time period).
- Minimize the use of unsubstantiated estimates or assumptions.

A useful practice to determine all of the factors necessary to derive the hourly labor rate is to imagine that the entire department has just been evicted from the hospital and is now forced to either become financially self-sufficient or be dissolved. The hourly labor rate is determined by the following equation:

Hourly Labor Rate ($/Hr.) = (Variable Costs + Fixed Costs)/Chargeable Hrs.

Variable Costs, sometimes referred to as "direct," "incremental," or "marginal" costs, are the costs that are assumed to vary (linearly) with production volume or service output. Variable costs can also be viewed as those costs that would not exist if there were no labor force. Typically, these costs include:

- The salary and wages (including any overtime, on-call pay, bonuses, or shift premiums) of the active service staff, i.e., personnel whose time is chargeable.
- Employee benefits (often expressed as a percentage of total salaries and wages).
- Continuing education expenses, e.g., service schools, technical meetings, short courses, and journal subscriptions.
- Office supplies and forms.
- Liability insurance costs.
- All nonfixed telephone charges.
- Repair parts and service supplies. (As it is assumed these will be charged back to the customer, these are typically not included in computing the hourly labor rate.)
- Any other costs that would vary with department workload, e.g., travel and fuel costs.

Fixed costs, often referred to as "overhead" or "burden," are typically those costs that do not fluctuate with the level of activity. They include

- Effective cost of hospital floor space and associated utilities.
- Capital depreciation (e.g., test equipment and machines).
- Fixed telephone charges.
- Administrative and clerical labor costs.

- Repair parts inventory carrying costs. While this figure is likely to elude most departments, inventory carrying costs can represent a significant yet hidden cost, especially to those departments stocking an abundance of circuit boards or X-ray tubes.

Typical carrying costs for the manufacturing industry range from 20–40 percent of total inventory costs. The inventory represents a fixed cost for several reasons:

- It takes up space, and space costs money.
- Parts must be put into and taken out of storage (by paid labor).
- The inventory must be managed, counted, and recorded.
- It must be protected from pilferage.
- It can be taxed as property within for-profit organizations.
- It may deteriorate or become obsolete with age.

Optimally, inventory carrying costs must be evaluated against the effective cost of not having the parts available.

Table 3.1 contains a summary of the annual variable and fixed costs incurred by an actual clinical engineering department. Generally accepted cost accounting practices dictate that the production or revenue-producing departments (i.e., profit centers) within an organization recover not only all of their costs, but also all or a portion of those costs incurred by the nonrevenue-generating departments. Within any organization, it is the profit centers that effectively subsidize the cost centers. As applied to a clinical engineering profit center, it is administrative, clerical, and possibly engineering overhead that must be paid for by the revenue-generating service force. Depending on the department's organizational structure, it may be necessary to allocate all or only a portion of its administrative overhead to the revenue-generating divisions. The amount of this allocation is included in the fixed-cost component of the hourly labor rate equation.

Table 3.1: Summary of annual varied and fixed costs

Dept. Division	Number of Technicians	Percent of Total Time	Allocated Overhead
Electronics	7	41.2	$ 52,879
Imaging	2	11.8	$ 15,145
Communication	8	47.0	$ 60,323
TOTALS	**17**	**100.0**	**$ 128,347**

For this particular department, the total administrative overhead of $128,347 is allocated proportionately to each of the department's three divisions based upon the number of technicians in each division.

While other allocation methods could be used (e.g., by processed work orders, equipment volume, or division budgets), the employee-based method is simple and representative.

Chargeable hours, represent the maximum number of labor hours the department can realistically expect to charge, or bill out, in the fiscal year. Total chargeable hours (TCH) is defined as follows:

TCH = **(Number of Employees)** x **(Available Labor Hrs./Employee)** x **(Productivity)**

where:

- **Number of employees**, or full-time equivalents (FTEs) is the combined number of full- and part-time staff whose time will be charged out. This includes all technicians and may or may not include engineering personnel.
- **Available labor hrs./employee** includes only regular and overtime hours. It does not include sick time, breaks, vacations, and holidays. Actual figures can be taken directly from department payroll reports (if available), or they can be estimated by the following equation:

Annual Available Labor Hrs./Employee

= 2080 hrs – (vacation hrs.) – (holiday hrs.) – (sick hrs.)
= 2080 – 80 – 64 – 40 = 1896 **Available Hrs.**

This estimate should be adjusted for institutional variations in vacation, sick time, or holiday availability. However, because there is often considerable variation, actual payroll figures should be used whenever possible.

- **Productivity**, as used here, is simply the number of chargeable hours divided by the number of available work hours for a given fiscal period. It is a "reality factor." Throughout the service industry, real productivity rarely exceeds 75–80 percent. Since productivity effectively reduces the number of chargeable labor hours, its impact must be factored into the department's hourly labor costs. Nonproductivity is not all wasted time. Internal housekeeping, education, and general departmental activities perhaps should be charged as internal overhead. (Mahachek, 1987)

Clinical engineering managers may be shocked to learn just how low their department's productivity really is. A sample two-year productivity history is shown in Figure 3.12. While its 58 percent average seems far from commendable, its consistency and relatively low variability (standard deviation = 6.7 percent) does provide a useful reference on which to improve. In the calculations that follow, however, the optimistic figure and realistic goal of 70 percent is used.

While there are a variety of factors that contribute to overall productivity, these all eventually translate into creating a finite number of chargeable hours per day. The ongoing challenge is to determine how to maximize chargeable hours without doing the following:

- Compromising work quality (by encouraging fast, careless work).
- Overcharging the customer (through exaggerated time reporting).
- Creating an antiservice, uncooperative environment.
- Acquiring the image of a customer-insensitive, profit-only department.

For the entrenched, cost-centered manager who changes to a profit-centered mode, these issues are particularly significant.

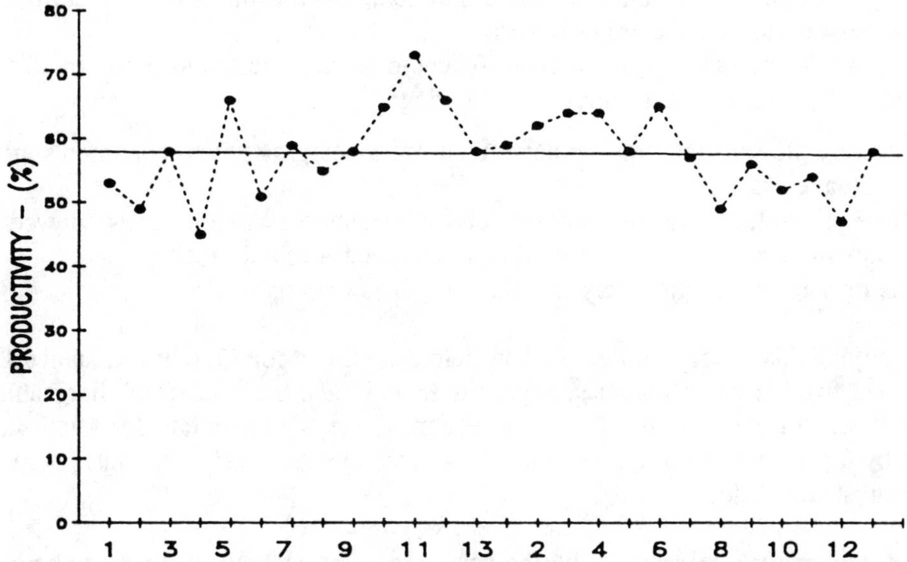

Figure 3.12: Graph illustrating productivity history of the medical electronics division over a two-year period. Average productivity over the entire period was 58 percent.

Once all of the known costs associated with the labor rate equation have been identified, calculating the hourly labor rate can proceed.

Hourly Labor Rate ($/Hr.) = (Variable Costs + Fixed Costs)/Chargeable Hrs.

= **[(Variable Costs – Parts) + (Dept. Fixed Costs) + (Admin. Fixed Costs)/ (FTEs) x (Available Labor Hrs.) x (Productivity)**

= [($348,221 – 115,367) ($55,729)] + ($52,879)/(12,600 hrs.) (0.70)

= ($341,462)/(8820 hrs.)

= $38.71/hr.

= $39.00/hr.

This figure represents an actual total obtained from a 1986 year-end payroll report.

Based on the chargeable number of labor hours (8820), $39/hour represents the absolute minimum labor rate the department should have used during 1986 in order to break even. The profound effect of staff productivity on the required hourly labor rate is illustrated in

Figure 3.13. It is the dramatic effect of this relationship on costs (and hence profits) that makes productivity improvement such an important issue.

Once the break-even hourly rate is known, it is then appropriately increased to produce a desired profit margin. For the in-house department, profit could simply be defined as the additional cost of doing business next year.

Not only would such a profit policy be sufficient to cover projected increases in all variable and fixed costs, it also accomplishes the following:

- Effectively prevents an in-house department from charging other departments more than actual costs.
- Is more psychologically palatable for service customers in that it can be viewed as a minimum-necessary profit rather than a maximum-desired profit.
- Is the only profit margin likely to gain administrative approval.

In applying this concept to the $39/hour rate determined for 1986, it is assumed that the variable and fixed costs will increase 6 percent in 1987 and the number of chargeable labor hours will remain constant at 8820. Consequently, the $39/hour rate for 1986 will also increase by 6 percent to $41/hour for 1987. For convenience, hourly labor rates are rounded to the nearest whole dollar.

Cost–volume–profit analysis. Using the cost accounting technique of cost–volume–profit (CVP) analysis, the relationships between revenue, service volume (i.e., chargeable hours), and variable and fixed costs become apparent. Such an analysis assumes that linear relationships exist between revenues, volume, and variable costs.

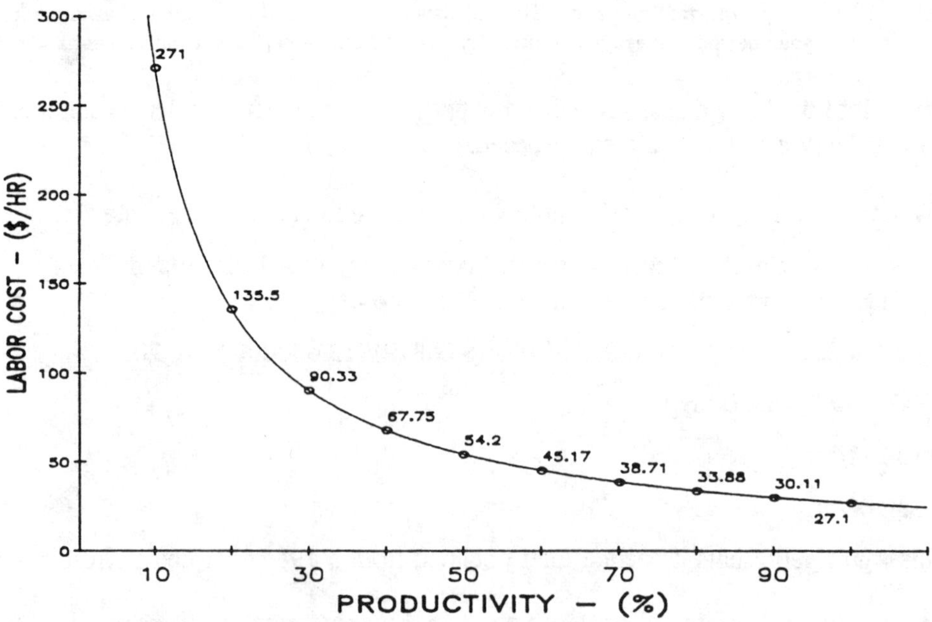

Figure 3.13: Graph illustrating the impact of productivity on hourly labor costs.

To complete the CVP analysis, the following data are required. As derived or presented earlier, they include:

Hourly Labor Rate = \$41/hour
Total Fixed Costs = (department + administrative) + 6 percent
= (\$55,729 + \$52,879)(1.06)
= \$115,124
Chargeable Hours = 8820
Variable Costs/Hour =
Profits = Revenue – Expenses

However, since **Profits** = 0 at break even,

Revenues = Expenses
Revenues = Fixed Costs + Variable Costs

Of the above, only Variable Costs/Hour has yet to be derived.

Variable Costs = Revenue – Fixed Costs
Variable Costs/Hr. = **[(Labor Rate) (Chargeable Hrs.)] – (Fixed Costs/Hr.)**
= **(Labor Rate) – (Fixed Costs)/Chargeable Hrs.**
= \$41/hr. – (115,124)/(8820 hrs.)
= \$41/hr. – \$13.05/hr.
= \$27.95/hr.

Figure 3.14 shows the resultant CVP, or break-even, chart. It should be noted that, as expected, the department will operate at a loss until 8820 hours of service have been charged. Also evident is the effect of changes in fixed costs, revenues, and variable costs on the break-even point.

The results of any financial analysis, of course, will be only as accurate as the data used to produce it. Because accurate data are not always available, it is frequently necessary to use assumptions. While the use of assumptions should be limited, their use is tolerated as long as the effect of their limitations and uncertainty is understood.

The accountant's measure of this uncertainty is called "sensitivity." As applied here, the assumptions used in deriving the hourly labor rate, i.e., productivity and the omission of some unknown fixed costs, should be tested for their effect on department profits. Specifically, profits are evaluated for changes in productivity (with fixed costs constant) and fixed costs (with productivity constant).

All changes are referenced to the break-even point, the point at which income equals expenses. Mathematically, profit sensitivity can be determined as follows:

For changes in productivity:

Profits = Revenues – Expenses
= **(Labor Rate)**(1 + n*)(hrs.) – **Expenses**

For changes in fixed costs:

Profits = Revenue – [**(Fixed Costs)**(1 – n*) + **Variable Costs**]

[* where -0.4 ≤ **n** ≤ 0.4, thus representing a 40 percent variation in the estimates used.]

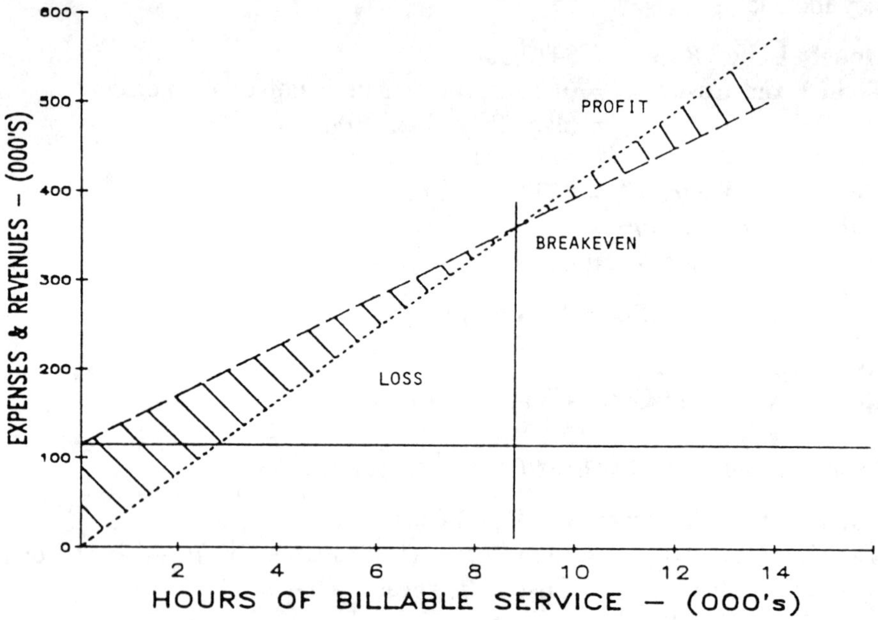

Figure 3.14: Graph of projected cost–volume–profit relationships. Solid line represents fixed costs level, dashed line represents variable costs level, dotted line represents revenue level.

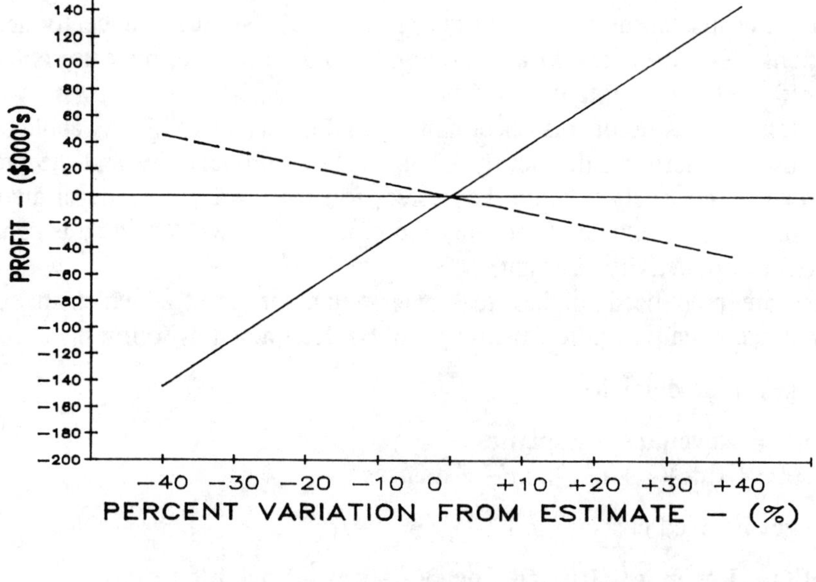

Figure 3.15: Graph illustrating the sensitivity of profits to productivity (solid line) and fixed costs (dashed lines).

These relationships are also illustrated in Figure 3.15. Note, for example, that a 10 percent increase in productivity translates to approximately a $35,000 increase in profits and that a 20 percent reduction in fixed costs results in a $23,000 increase in profits. Figure 3.15 also demonstrates the profound impact of staff productivity on profits (Fennigkoh, 1987).

With the rapid advancement of medical technology over the past 20 years, even the best in-house maintenance program cannot always maintain every piece of equipment in today's hospitals. Items such as CT scanners, and other high-technology systems are often difficult to maintain with in-house resources. Lengthy training courses, expensive test equipment, and the high cost of stocking repair parts make it difficult to maintain these systems in a cost-effective manner. Only if there is a sufficiently large amount of equipment on-site is an in-house specialist justified.

Service Contracts

Level of Service. One of the big functions of clinical engineering departments is to manage service contracts. Since this activity is so important, it is necessary to discuss it in some detail. In selecting service to be provided, the level of service required for a particular device must first be determined. Is 24-hour-per-day, seven-day-per-week coverage needed, or is eight hours per day, five days per week acceptable? Is two-hour response or 48-hour response required? Is equipment uptime of 99 percent or 90 percent needed? There are many other questions, based on the hospital's location and particular needs, that must be considered as well. Service contractors will attempt to meet the most stringent requirements specified by the hospital, but the tighter the requirements, the more the contract will cost. Even with in-house services, overtime and on-call costs can mount quickly. The hospital must determine exactly what its requirements are for each device. Remember, requirements drive costs. An understanding of the following terms is essential when dealing with service contracts.

- **Full service** includes a specified number of preventive maintenance (PM) calls at regular intervals, unlimited repair calls, all parts except consumable supplies, all labor and travel charges, and availability 24 hours per day, seven days per week, 365 days per year.
- **Limited-hour service** includes a specified number of PM calls at regular intervals, unlimited repair calls, all parts except consumable supplies, and all labor and travel charges during a specified work week (normally Monday to Friday, 8:00 A.M. to 4:00 P.M.).
- **Limited service** includes a specified number of PM calls at regular intervals, all parts except consumable supplies, and all labor and travel up to a maximum number of service calls specified in the contract.
- **Demand Service** includes PM and repair service provided upon request by the customer and paid on a time-and-materials basis (Anderson, 1989).
- **Depot Service** includes all parts, all labor for repairs, some freight charges, and sometimes a loaner instrument, and a specified number of PM inspections at regular intervals. All work on defective equipment must be performed at the factory or a regional depot.

After determining the level of service required, the costs for each type of service need to be considered. Figure 3.16 is a work sheet used to determine the costs of service types.

Service Analysis Work Sheet. After total costs and nonfinancial considerations have been identified for each service option, the final selection can be made in a variety of ways. A detailed matrix comparing all relevant factors will be helpful, especially for service involving costly equipment, many devices of one or more types, or a hospital's entire equipment inventory. Figures 3.17a and 3.17b provide a good service analysis matrix to aid in decision making. Unfortunately, there is no formula that will automatically generate the best choice when the information is inserted into the matrix. The selection will depend on the devices involved, the geographical area, the level of service, the response time required, and the characteristics of the hospital. If no choice is obvious and the costs are similar, the hospital should first attempt to identify the most important criteria. The selection can be based on weighing each criteria to determine the best option. If costs and other considerations are similar, basing a decision on the preference of those closely involved may be appropriate (ECRI, 1989b). In the following example, vendors were requested to provide quotes to service three CT scanners, covering the following service options:

- **Full service,** which included parts and labor for all necessary corrective maintenance and weekly preventive maintenance inspections.
- **Hospital participation,** in which routine inspection and initial problem screening would be performed by technicians from the clinical engineering department, with major corrective maintenance (parts and labor) being performed by the service provider.
- **Parts only,** for which all corrective and preventive maintenance labor would be provided by in-house technicians.
- **Tubes,** which would either be supplied on the basis of a fixed-fee contract or purchased individually as needed for a fixed price.

Vendors submitted quotes based on a three-year contract. The annual costs for services provided appear in Table 3.2. Scanning these figures it seems as though Provider A offers the greatest savings. However, the cost differences do not represent the net cost savings (Table 3.3). Additional assumptions included the following:

- The full-service option from Provider A will be used for the first six months while the in-house staff is being trained. The hospital participation option will be used for the next 18 months, and the parts-only option will be used during the last 12 months of the contract.
- An existing, unrelated service contract with Provider B will increase 10 percent per year if Provider B is not awarded the new contract.
- A 6 percent cost-of-money factor is used to compute the cost saving net-present-value.

In Table 3.4, the three-year projected savings obtained earlier is recomputed for each likely variation in tube use. For example, as shown in Table 3.4, if five 8800 tubes and only two 9800 tubes are used, the total savings increases to $299,671. However, if only three 8800 tubes but four 9800 tubes are used, the total savings decreases to $260,003. In Table 3.2, we assumed an annual tube usage of four 8800 and three 9800 tubes. This assumption was made based on previous usage and may be subject to change. Given the relatively high cost of these tubes, slight variations in actual tube use can have a major effect on the actual net savings. A measure of this effect can be demonstrated through sensitivity analysis.

Service Cost Work Sheet

Cost Category	In-House Service	Manufacturer Service: Contract	Manufacturer Service: Demand	Third-Party Service: Contract	Third-Party Service: Demand	Maintenance Insurance with Outside IPM
Direct-Service Labor Cost	$________	N/A	$________	N/A	$________	$________[1,2]
Contract Price	________[3]	$________	N/A	$________	N/A	________[1,2]
Cost of Exclusions	N/A	________	N/A	________	N/A	N/A
Spare Parts	________	________[2]	________	________[2]	________	________[1,2]
Inventory Stocking Cost	________	N/A	N/A	N/A	N/A	N/A
Training Costs	________	N/A	N/A	N/A	N/A	N/A
Depreciation of Test Equipment	________	N/A	N/A	N/A	N/A	N/A
Diagnostic Software Costs	________	N/A	N/A	________[2]	________[2]	________[1,2]
Software Update Cost	________	N/A	N/A	N/A	N/A	N/A
Travel Time Cost	N/A	________[2]	________[2]	________[2]	________[2]	________[1,2]
Cost of Maintenance Insurance	N/A	N/A	N/A	N/A	N/A	________
Maintenance Insurance Claim Cost & Disallowed Claims	N/A	N/A	N/A	N/A	N/A	________
Misc. Costs (e.g., down-time, overtime)[2]	________	________	________	________	________	________[1]
Management Costs	________	________	________	________	________	________
Overhead Costs	________	________	________	________	________	________
Total Costs	$________	$________	$________	$________	$________	$________

Notes:
IPM = Inspection and preventive maintenance
N/A = Not applicable
(1) = For IPM only
(2) = Depends on contractual provisions
(3) = Estimated cost of special outside needs (e.g., calibration)

Figure 3.16: Example of a service cost work sheet used to determine the relative cost of various types of service.

CHARACTERISTIC	IN-HOUSE SERVICE	MANUFACTURER SERVICE	THIRD-PARTY SERVICE	MAINTENANCE INSURANCE (service by mfg)
Estimated Total Cost	$3,200	$8,000	$4,500	$6,500
Type of Service	Full support	Service contract	Demand	Demand + Insurance
Location of Primary Service Personnel	Within the hospital (Bluetown, PA)	Bluetown, PA	Bluetown, PA	Bluetown, PA
Number of Primary Service Personnel	Three BMETs, one clinical engineer	Four service engineers	Four BMETs	Four service engineers
Service Personnel Qualifications	With additional manufacturer training	Yes	Yes, completed manufacturer training course	Yes
Location of Backup Service Personnel	In the hospital	New York, NY	Hilltown, PA	New York, NY
Guaranteed Response Time:				
On-site	20 minutes	2 hours	2 hours	2 hours
By Phone	N/A	30 minutes	30 minutes	30 minutes
Penalty	N/A	10% discount on labor charge for each late response	10% discount on labor charge for each late response	None
Nearest Location of Parts	Bluetown, PA (not complete inventory)	Bluetown, PA (not complete inventory)	Hilltown, PA (complete inventory)	Bluetown, PA (not complete inventory)
Location of Backup Parts	Redtown, PA	Redtown, PA	Must receive from manufacturer	Redtown, PA
Parts Availability	Generally good, within 24 hours	Good, within 24 hours	Fair	Good, within 24 hours
Software Diagnostics Availability	Will be available	N/A	Unclear, apparently not	N/A
Service Manual Availability	Available	N/A	Yes	N/A
Service Hours Covered by Cost Estimate	8:00 a.m.-6:00 p.m.	8:00 a.m.-5:00 p.m.	8:00 a.m.-5:00 p.m.	8:00 a.m.-5:00 p.m.
Hours Outside Cost Estimate That Service Will Be Provided	On-call	5:00 p.m.-Midnight	5:00 p.m.-Midnight	5:00 p.m.-Midnight
Uptime Guarantee	90%	95%	90%	95%
Uptime Definition	% of normal workweek	% of normal workweek	% of normal workweek	% of normal workweek
Penalty for Uptime Failure	N/A	2% credit on next year's contract for 90%-94.9% and 10% credit for below 90%	5% rebate on total labor charge for that year's service	Below 95%, a 5% discount on a future insurance premium

Figure 3.17(a): Sample of a service analysis matrix used to evaluate various types of service.

CHARACTERISTIC	IN-HOUSE SERVICE	MANUFACTURER SERVICE	THIRD-PARTY SERVICE	MAINTENANCE INSURANCE (service by mfg)
In-service Training of Clinical Personnel	N/A; personnel already trained	Same	Same	Same
Number of Repair Calls Provided Per Year	Unlimited	Unlimited	Unlimited	Unlimited
Loaner Equipment Available	No	Yes	No	No
Service Hotline Available	Yes	Yes	No	Yes
Organizational Stability	N/A	Excellent	Very good	Service – excellent Insurer – good
Number of Years in Business	N/A	29	11	Service – 29 Insurer – 8
Adequately Insured	Yes	Yes	Yes	Yes
Manufacturer Supportive	Yes	N/A	No	Yes
Quality of Service:				
Response Time	Excellent	Good	Excellent	Good
Parts Available	Good	Excellent	Fair-Good	Excellent
Repairs Made Correctly the First Time	Yes	Yes	Yes	Yes
Repairs Made Timely	Yes	Yes	Yes	Yes
Overall Satisfaction	Good	Excellent	Excellent	Excellent; ins. carrier references generally pleased; 50% felt it saved $
Other Equipment Support Functions	N/A (single device)	N/A (single device)	N/A (single device)	N/A (single device)
Miscellaneous Factors	Will involve learning curve until fully trained.			Will require extra time and effort filing claims. Some risk of claim disallowances.

Figure 3.17(b): Continuation of the service analysis matrix.

Table 3.2: Annual cost of service options.

Service Options	*Provider A*	*Provider B*	
Full Service	196,535	282,956	
Tubes	115,500[1]	128,875[2]	
Total	312,035	411,831	
Difference			$99,796
Shared Service	161,525	249,055	
Tubes	115,500[1]	128,875[2]	
Total	277,025	377,930	
Difference			$100,905
Parts Only	132,250	not available	
Tubes	115,500[1]	not available	
Total	247,750	337,930	
Difference			$90,180

1 Assumes an annual tube usage of four 8800 tubes @ $13,500 each, and three 9800 tubes @ 20,500 each.

2 Represents a fixed-fee tube contract regardless of usage.

Table 3.3: Calculation of net contract savings.

	Year 1	Year 2	Year 3	3-Year Total
Service Options Savings				
Full Service (6 mo.)	$43,211	--	--	43,211
Shared Service	$43,765	87,530	--	131,295
Parts Only	--	--	116,805	116,805
Tubes	$13,375	13,375	13,375	40,125
Total	$100,351	100,905	130,180	331,436
In-House Cost Increases				
Training, 3 Technicians*	?	?	?	?
Airfare (est.), 3 @ $300	$900	--	--	900
Room and Board (21 days @ $73/day x 3)	$4,599	--	--	4,500
Total	$5,499	--	--	5,499
Increase in Other Contract	$8,370	9,207	10,128	27,705
Total Cost Increases	$13,869	9,207	10,128	33,204
NET SAVINGS	$86,482	91,698	120,052	298,232
Net Present Value**	$86,482	$86,508	$106,846	279,836

*Readers are encouraged to compute the effective cost of in-house training.
**This represents the present worth of some future amount. It acknowledges the time value of money and is computed from the formula P = F(P/F, i%, n), where F is the future amount (in this case, the net savings), P/F is the present worth factor, obtained from a table of interest factors, i is the interest rate, and n is the number of periods. For example, at the end of year 2: P = $91,698(15,723 x 6% x 1) = $91,698(.9434) = $86,508.

Table 3.4: Illustration of the effect of tube usage on projected savings.

8800 tubes → / 9800 tubes ↓	1	2	3	4	5	6
1	$510,759	$472,508	$434,257	$396,006	$357,755	$319,504
2	$452,674	376,127	337,921	337,921	299,671	261,420
3	$394,589	356,339	318,088	279,836	241,586	203,335
4	$336,505	298,254	260,003	221,752	183,501	145,250
5	$278,420	240,169	201,918	163,667	125,416	87,166
6	$220,335	182,084	143,834	105,583	67,332	29,081

Based on this analysis, the following recommendations were made (Fennigkoh, 1988):

- Select the service options offered by Provider A, being sure to include a cancellation clause in case their quality of service is lower than expected.
- Enroll the in-house clinical engineering staff in the training program offered by Provider A as soon as possible.

Negotiating a Contract. The best means the hospital has to obtain favorable terms and conditions and an attractive price is to be sure that it does not lock itself into a situation where there is only one alternative, i.e., buying a contract from a single vendor. Alternatives should include other ways to obtain the service (time and materials or maintenance insurance) and other vendors (manufacturer, distributor, shared service, and independent). Without this leverage, the hospital will be at a disadvantage during negotiations and will usually be unable to gain any concessions.

Based on the hospital's evaluation of its own requirements, it should have some idea of what service should cost. The next step is to generate a list of qualified vendors. If each vendor understands that it is bidding against other service companies or manufacturers, the hospital will maintain maximum leverage during the negotiations (Brinkman, 1989). Vendors can be qualified by analyzing their answers in the service analysis matrix (Figures 3.17a and 3.17b).

Monitoring Outside Vendor Service. The award of the service contract is not the end of the process. The vendor's performance must then be monitored to ensure that the hospital receives the services for which it has contracted. There is only one effective way to do this. Each time a service call or PM visit occurs, the vendor must be required to check in and out of the clinical engineering department. A detailed service report must be provided, listing the problem, corrective action, labor hours, travel hours, and repair parts used, with the price for each item. The hospital can use these reports to determine the actual costs of service.

Repair Parts Management

Effective management of repair parts is essential to the operation of the clinical engineering department. Management effort is required to prevent overstocking or accumulation of rarely needed or unusable repair parts. Only those repair parts required on a continuing basis should be maintained in bench stock within the department. If scheduled maintenance inspections are conducted properly, most repair part requirements, especially for high cost items, can be anticipated and procured on an as-required basis. Limited exceptions may be justified to ensure adequate maintenance support for items with long supply time or to enable immediate repair of selected items of equipment judged essential to life support, emergency resuscitation, or continuity of operations.

Repair parts maintained in the clinical engineering section should be classified as bench stock. Exceptions are common bulk hardware items, such as nuts, bolts, washers, resistors, capacitors, general-purpose semiconductor devices, etc., and repair parts ordered for immediate use.

Clinical engineers should consider the following factors when determining what parts and quantities to place in bench stock:

- **Critical nature of equipment.** If the hospital can function safely without the equipment for a short period of time, minimize or eliminate bench stock levels for repair parts.
- **Cost of downtime.** If the item is out of service, will patient appointments be canceled and hospital revenue significantly affected? The loss of revenue may be more than the cost of maintaining repair parts in inventory.
- **Number of units on hand.** The greater the number of units on hand, the greater the probability that repair parts will be required and should be in bench stock. However in some cases, the urgency of repair may be lessened since there may be sufficient items for exchange.
- **Consumption rate.** If a repair part is being used on a recurring basis, it should be considered for inclusion in bench stock.
- **Lead time.** If the time from when the repair part is ordered until it is received is excessive, some should be kept in stock.
- **Cost of the repair parts.** There are three factors that determine the overall cost of a repair part: the dollar value of the part, the administrative cost of processing the purchase order, and the minimum order level of the vendor. When ordering low-cost items, it is reasonable to stock a one-year supply. This is usually less costly than ordering the item several times during the year.
- **Shelf life.** Low levels should be kept on items that deteriorate while in storage to ensure that they are used before they deteriorate.
- **Age of the equipment.** As equipment gets older, breakdowns normally increase, resulting in greater demand for repair parts. Increasing bench stock to meet these demands can result in large dollar losses if new equipment is purchased.

Since the use of repair parts is typically very sporadic, investment of excessive capital in stock parts should be avoided. The location of the hospital from sources of repair parts, equipment importance, and potential for lost revenue will probably be the most significant determining factors in the decision on whether to stock a repair part.

Equipment Disposition

Equipment seems to come in and out of a hospital as frequently as patients. Clinical engineers must stay abreast of technological changes that bring about this rapid turnover of medical equipment. There are several reasons for disposing of old devices:

- Changes in the standard of care. New clinical procedures may cause a device to become obsolete. Technological changes in performance criteria or accuracy necessitate the purchase of state-of-the-art equipment.
- Safety factors resulting in increased risk of injury to patients, staff, or visitors.
- Maintenance problems that cause frequent or expensive repairs and excessive downtime.
- Nonavailability of repair parts or service.
- Operational costs. Newer equipment may require less technician time, use less costly consumable supplies, be more economical to lease than to buy, or be more reliable.
- Newly purchased equipment may incorporate a number of different functions in a single device.

Upon identification of a device for disposal, the clinical engineering department should take certain actions. First, the section responsible for ordering consumable and spare parts unique to that device should be notified so that additional money isn't spent. The device may then be placed in storage and held as a back-up unit. This is the least desirable option because it requires continued support with repair parts as expendable supplies. Other possibilities include offering the item as a trade-in on new equipment, cannibalizing parts to support other similar equipment, transferring the equipment to a research laboratory, or donating it to a charitable organization or a third-world country. The last resort is to make the item unserviceable and sell it as scrap metal.

COMPUTERIZED MAINTENANCE MANAGEMENT AND INFORMATION SYSTEMS

The equipment control function of technology management requires extensive records to comply with regulatory and accreditation requirements. These records and files must be converted into meaningful information used to schedule and track work orders, follow up on repair part requests, forecast equipment replacement, and locate recalled devices. Computerized systems are available to support the clinical engineer and hospital (see Chapter 9 for a detailed discussion of these systems) in the following ways:

- Produce maintenance work schedules and track inspection and work order requests.
- Produce reports to determine personnel productivity, notify departments with higher than average equipment repair costs, identify repeat repairs on the same device, and document potential user errors or equipment abuse.
- Provide documentation for malpractice suits involving medical equipment.
- Demonstrate to accreditation inspectors that equipment is being properly maintained.
- Support repair–versus–replacement decisions with historical data.
- Forecast equipment replacement requirements.
- Determine if and where recalled devices are located in the hospital.

- Determine charges to user departments and prepare operating budgets.

Any clinical engineering department can manage its work more effectively and make better management decisions with computerized equipment control records. With such a system, department supervisors can manage workloads, monitor productivity and work order completion, and obtain end-of-month summaries of labor and parts costs. In addition, computerization can provide data for quality assurance indicators of equipment performance (e.g., data on downtime or mean time between repairs) as well as information that aids the hospital-wide QA and utilization review efforts (e.g., how discharges can be increased as a result of fewer diagnostic decisions delayed by equipment downtime).

Standard informational items that should be included in any clinical engineering computerized database for equipment control include the following:

- **Equipment control number**: A unique number identifying a specific equipment item; individual equipment modules may also be given specific control numbers.
- **Manufacturer**: The name of the company that manufactured the equipment.
- **Model number**: An equipment type identifier assigned by the manufacturer and labeled on the equipment.
- **Serial number**: An identifier assigned by the manufacturer for a specific piece of equipment.
- **Manufacturer code**: A unique code identifying the company that manufactured the equipment.
- **Device Code**: A code indicating the type or class of the device.
- **Device code description**: An industry-accepted standard nomenclature for the device.
- **Vendor**: The name of the company that sold the device.
- **Vendor code**: A unique code indicating the company that sold the device.
- **Department code**: The department to which the equipment was assigned.
- **Location**: The building or room where the device is normally located.
- **Contractor code**: The equipment contractor if the item is under a maintenance contract or warranty.
- **Risk code**: The relative risk to a patient in the event of equipment failure or misuse.
- **Purchase date**: The date the item was ordered.
- **Received date**: The date the item was received.
- **Installation date**: The date the hospital accepted the equipment for use.
- **Warranty/contract expiration date**: The date the device is no longer under warranty or contract.
- **Purchase price**: The total amount paid for the device.

Additional data elements required for service include the following:

- **Work order number**: A unique number to identify a particular maintenance request. It should include date and time of request.
- **Requestor**: The name and department of the individual placing the service request.
- **Requestor's telephone number**: A phone number for contacting the requestor.
- **Service required**: A narrative description of the perceived problem or the service that is required.
- **Service source**: The provider of the service.

- **Service response time/date**: The time and date that the technician responded to the work order.
- **Service complete time/date**: The time and date that the work order was completed.
- **Work order action code**: A code indicating the status or completion of the work order.
- **Equipment status code**: A code that indicates if the device was still serviceable upon initiation of the work order.
- **Priority**: The relative urgency of the work order.
- **Service time**: The actual labor time expended.
- **Repair parts cost**: The total cost of repair parts used.
- **Contract costs**: The labor/travel costs of contract maintenance.
- **Technician code**: A unique code identifying a specific technician.

These elements provide some idea of the data most likely used by the clinical engineer. With the relative ease of with which the data may be collected and processed, the clinical engineer must be prudent in the selection of data so as not to become overloaded. For example, a bar code system can help automate data entry and also reduce errors due to manual entry.

With thousands of individual equipment control records to maintain, computer use substantially improves the clinical engineering department's efficiency (see chapter 9 for details) as well as the overall effectiveness of the technology management program and the quality of patient care throughout the hospital. A computerized equipment/service database provides unique opportunities for managing and documenting the department's activities. For example, consider the following:

- **Computation of downtime**: Downtime can be expressed as (**service completed**, time and date) – (**work order opened**, time and date). This provides a gross indicator of the time the equipment is not available for patient treatment or diagnosis. Factors affecting downtime are technician response time (either in-house or contractor), service time, and the time waiting for repair parts to arrive. With the current emphasis on reducing average-length-of-stay by patients, equipment downtime is an important factor.
- **Average time to repair**: This is computed as (**total service time**) (**total service calls**) and can be broken down by device code to determine devices that exceed the expected repair times, by manufacturer to identify poor-quality products, or by technician to determine the need for training.
- **Response time**: Response time is defined as (**service response**, time and date)– (**work order opened**, time and date). Customer satisfaction is directly linked to responsiveness of service.
- **Operator error/no defect actions**: Use work order action codes to identify problems. The **JCAHO** requires that these work order outcomes be reviewed and analyzed to determine if user training is required.
- **Repeat repair**: In these cases, historical data are used to identify repeat repairs. Excessive repeats can indicate that a technician may need training, the operators may be abusing the equipment, or the equipment has become unreliable. For example, alerts might be indicated for items with two work orders in seven days, or three work orders in 90 days.

A clinical engineer with a good imagination can devise any number of additional uses for these data. Productivity, budgeting, and forecasting are areas that could be aided by the proper use of these data. Finally, such a data base will enable the clinical engineer to meet the documentation requirements of accreditation and regulatory agencies (Minsent, 1990).

Some features of an appropriately established database will include ease of record updates and suppression of unneeded data elements. Such a database will meet the documentation requirements of accreditation and regulatory agencies and will also provide the flexibility required by clinical engineers (Minsent, 1990).

SUMMARY

Comprehensive technology management plays an important role in a hospital's ability to provide high-quality, cost-effective medical care. Moving from equipment control to technology management may not be easy for some hospitals or for some clinical engineers. For those clinical engineers who accept this challenge, the rewards can be substantial, not only for themselves, but also for the hospital and society at large. The long-range opportunities for clinical engineers lie in the development of executive-level business skills that lead to positions such as assistant administrator for hospital technology, assistant administrator for support services, or vice-president of technology (Gordon, 1990).

With this in mind, this chapter reviewed those aspects of technology management that are the responsibility of clinical engineering departments. Because of its relative importance, equipment control and maintenance procedures, including the establishment of program guidelines and the determination of costs for in-house repair and maintenance services were presented in significant detail. Activities of clinical engineering departments related to negotiating and monitoring service contracts; performing technology planning, acquisition and replacement; and establishing a computerized equipment data base have also been discussed.

EXERCISES

1. The basic components of a clinical equipment program include

   (a) a complete equipment inventory.
   (b) periodic inspections of all equipment.
   (c) a complete inventory of expendable supplies.
   (d) equipment disposition procedures.

2. The majority of equipment-related injuries are caused by

   (a) equipment malfunctions.
   (b) manufacturer's defects.
   (c) inappropriate maintenance procedures.
   (d) user errors.

3. A typical training policy for medical equipment should include

   (a) assigning responsibility for training.
   (b) allowing manufacturers to present portions of the training.
   (c) documenting and assessing the training provided.
   (d) all of the above.

4. The scope of a technology management program

   (a) is the same at all facilities.
   (b) varies based on the skills of the clinical engineer.
   (c) changes based on geographic area.
   (d) is determined by the educational background of the clinical engineer.

5. A device should be scheduled for periodic inspection, maintenance, or performance verification only if

   (a) the manufacturer suggests it.
   (b) there is a good reason to provide such support.
   (c) it always breaks.
   (d) the clinical engineering department needs to increase its chargeable workload.

6. Determine the scheduled maintenance frequency for the following items. Provide the rationale for your decisions.

   (a) Defibrillator/monitor used in the emergency room as a primary unit for ambulance dispatches. There is one back-up system. The manufacturer has had three recalls on this particular model in the last 18 months.
   (b) Electric bed used in the general ward area. There are 250 other beds identical beds in the facility. The average daily census is 178 patients.
   (c) Infusion pump used in ICU. There are thirty other similar pumps within the section. You have had an increased number of repair calls in the last six months. Eighty percent of these maintenance calls resulted in no equipment defects being found. What appears to be the underlying cause of the increase in repair calls?
   (d) Computed tomography scanner, one of only two in the region. Your hospital has a trauma unit. This is a major revenue-producing item for the hospital. It is maintained by a full-service contract by the manufacturer.

7. The most cost-effective and desirable method to repair a device is

   (a) manufacturer repair.
   (b) board swapping.
   (c) component level repair.
   (d) to buy a new device.
   (e) dependent on the particular situation.

8. The following items require repair. List them in priority sequence, and explain your rationale.

   (a) Ventilator from ICU, four back-up items, normally only two in use at any one time.
   (b) Clinical chemistry analyzer, manual back-up, major revenue producer.
   (c) Cardiac monitor in ICU, 12 other monitors available for back-up, average daily patient load is eight. The charge nurse is very demanding.
   (d) Infant incubator, six back-up items, average daily patient load is four. Your bosses wife is pregnant and has a history of delivering early.
   (e) Surgical drill, two back-up items. The surgeon is a prima donna with the hospital administration and this is his favorite drill.

9. Using figures 3-17a and 3-17b, determine the best maintenance option for the devices described below, justify your answer.
   (a) The device is a treadmill system. Your hospital is willing to train one of your technicians. The cost of training is $1000. Seven procedures are done each day with the equipment. You need no additional test equipment.
   (b) There has been a request for six steam sterilizers. Reliability of the sterilizers is poor and adequate back-up capability exists. The cost of training is $5000 for your technician. You have a constant backlog of work within your section and limited administrative support.
10. Discuss the three types of services that hospitals can elect to maintain their medical devices and systems.
11. Identify the major factors affecting the cost of in-house service provided by a clinical engineering department.
12. If a department had 8 employees, compute the annual available labor hours per employee and the total chargeable hours that the department can bill out in the fiscal year.
13. For a relatively small department of 5, a clinical engineering director and 4 BMETs conduct a cost-volume-profit analysis. To proceed, make appropriate assumptions explaining your rationale.
14. Identify the different levels of service contracts. What are the major factors determining which level is appropriate?

REFERENCES

American Hospital Assoc. "Maintenance Management for Medical Equipment," AHA, 840 North Lake Shore Drive, Chicago, IL, 1988.

Alder, H.C. "Safe Medical Device Act: What You Need to Know Now to Comply with the New Law," *Health Facilities Management*, 14–22, November 1991.

Anderson, J.T. "Evaluating Medical Equipment Service Options," *Biomed. Instr. Technol.*, 23:195–198, 1989.

Baretich, M.F. "Clinical Engineering Effectiveness from the Hospital Administrator's Perspective," American Society for Hospital Engineering, Technical Document Series, Number 055888, February 1987.

Betts, W. F. "Using Productivity Measures in Clinical Engineering Departments," *Biomed. Instr. Technol.*, 23:120–127, 1989.

Betts, W. F. "Cost-Effective Clinical Engineering Programs: An Expanding Role In Hospitals," *J. Clin. Engin.*, 12:119–125, 1987.

Brinkman, M.O. "Managing Equipment Service Contracts," *Biomed. Instr. Technol.*, 23:445–447, 1989.

Bruley, M.E. "Medical Device Accidents: Causes, Prevention, Liability, and Investigation," Emergency Care Research Institute, Plymouth Meeting, PA, 1988.

Carver, M.E. "Technology Management in the Health Care Environment--Yesterday, Today, Tomorrow: Part 1," *Biomed. Instr. Technol.*, 24:320–326, 1990.

Clark, J.T., and Forsell, R. "Clinical Equipment Replacement Planning," *Biomed Instr. Technol.*, 24:271–276, 1990.

Dickey, D.M. "Surviving and Growing in the '90s: Managerial Methods for the Hospital-Based BME/CE Department," *Biomed. Instr. Technol.*, 24:345–354, 1990.

Emergency Care Research Institute, "Equipment Related Injury: Design Defect vs. User Error," *Health Devices*, 12(9-10):253-256, 1983.

Emergency Care Research Institute, "Technology Management: Preparing Your Hospital for the 1990s," *Health Technology*, 3(1), 1989a.

Emergency Care Research Institute, "Special Report on Managing Service Contracts," *Health Technology*, 3(4), Winter 1989b.

Emergency Care Research Institute, "Health Devices Inspection and Preventive Maintenance System," Plymouth Meeting, PA, 1990.

Emergency Care Research Institute, "Safe Medical Device Act Requires User Reporting," *Health Technology Management*, Legal and Regulatory 4, February, 1991a.

Emergency Care Research Institute, "An Action Plan: Handling Medical Device Hazards and Recalls," *Health Device Alerts*, 1991b.

Fennigkoh, L. "How to Convert a Cost Center into a Profit Center," in *Management of the Clinical Engineering Department*, Quest Publishing Co., Brea, CA, 1987.

Fennigkoh, L. "CT Scanner Maintenance: A Financial Comparison of Alternatives," *Clinical Engineering Section*, May–June 1988.

Fennigkoh, L. "Clinical Engineering and the Management of Operator Error", *American Society for Hospital Engineering Technical Document Series*, Number 055930, April 1990.

Fennigkoh, L., and Smith B. "Clinical Equipment Management," *Plant, Technology, and Safety Management Series*, 2:5–14, 1989.

Gordon, G.J. "Hospital Technology Management: The Tao of Clinical Engineering," *J. Clin. Engin.*, 15(2):111–117, 1990.

Hertz, E., "Establishing the Priority of Equipment Inspections," *Biomed Instr. Technol.*, 24(6):410–416, 1990.

JCAHO. *The 1991 Joint Commission Accreditation Manual for Hospitals*, JCAHO, Oak Brook, IL, 1990.

Mahachek, A.R. "Management and Control of Clinical Engineering Productivity: A Case Study," *J. Clin. Engin.*, 12(2):127–132, 1987.

Minsent, D.R. "USAF Medical Logistics System Medical Equipment Maintenance Module," *Proc. of 12th Ann. Int. Conf. IEEE/EMBS*, 12(5):1985–1986, 1990.

Selsky, D.B., et al. "Biomedical Equipment Information Management for the Next Generation," *Biomed. Instr. Technol.*, 25(1):24–32, 1991.

Shaffer, M.J. and Shaffer, M.D. "Strategies for Improving Clinical Engineering In-Service Instruction," *Biomed. Instr. Technol.*, 24(5):336–342, 1990.

CHAPTER 4

MEDICAL TECHNOLOGY: ASSESSMENT AND ACQUISITION

The deployment of medical technologies in the American health-care system is now on a relatively fast track. New devices, diagnostic procedures, equipment, and systems of health-care delivery are continually being produced and flow rapidly into the nation's medical mainstream. This process has created additional burdens for the hospital administrators, clinical engineers, and medical staff who are responsible for the assessment and acquisition of new medical technology. As a result, there is a pressing need for clinical engineering departments to assume more responsibilities in these two areas. Prepurchase evaluation has been a traditional and well-accepted function of most clinical engineering departments. On the other hand, technology assessment is in its infancy, but it is essential if obsolete health-care technology is to be replaced and new technology is to be properly infused into the health-care system.

This chapter focuses on basic concepts associated with technology assessment, highlighting the processes of innovation, development, and diffusion of medical technology in the modern health-care system. The various organizations and agencies, both public and private, that play important roles in technology assessment are provided, and how technology assessment may be incorporated into the mainstream of an individual hospital's activities is discussed. The chapter then moves on to the equipment acquisition process and describes the sequence of steps necessary to implement a successful acquisition program and illustrates the role of the clinical engineer in this process.

TECHNOLOGY ASSESSMENT

Any discussion regarding the management of medical technologies must include an evaluation of safety, efficacy, and cost-effectiveness as well as a consideration of the social, legal, and ethical effects of these devices. Unfortunately, these considerations have significantly lagged behind the procurement and use of new medical technologies in the clinical environment. For health-care institutions to remain cost-effective and competitive, it is absolutely essential that any new medical technology be chosen or selected based on the "knowledge" gathered about its performance, value, and availability (Institute of Medicine, 1985). Therefore, one would hope that such a selection process would be guided by an orderly, well-conceived, unified system of assessing and testing the new, comparing the new with the existing technology, and making decisions based on valid, reliable information. At present, however, this hope is only partly fulfilled.

Today, hospital administrators are under continuous pressure to understand and react to regulation and competition, to deal with various forms of "government rationing" (e.g., limited reimbursement and franchise control), and to function within increasing financial constraints. Given these pressures, the following list illustrates the challenges facing those responsible for technology management:

- To ensure that hospitals effectively assess the impact of technology on all health-care services.

- To make effective adjustments in planning to ensure that any new technologies will better serve the organization's mission.
- To compare technology-based options.
- To gain knowledge from post-deployment experiences .

To meet these needs, advocates of technology assessment have become very vocal. Exactly what is "technology assessment?" According to the National Institutes of Health (NIH), the term refers to assessing the results of clinical trials and creating state-of-the-art reports on specific medical technologies. Consider the following: *"Technology assessment ... consists of synthesizing complex scientific information in such a way that the reports are useful for decision making by practitioners or policymakers,"* (NIH, 1985). More simply, technology assessment is the analysis of the effects of the introduction or widespread use of a technological innovation. Assessment of medical technology is only a small part of the technology assessment universe. The former process has its own distinctive methods, purposes, and consequences. Yet, on a smaller scale, it replicates all the characteristics of the larger universe of technology assessment in general. When the term "technology assessment" is used in this book, it is the technology of health-care that is of concern (Tomasik, 1992; McConnell, 1992).

The assessment of medical technology occurs in essentially a sequential order, ultimately leading to the deployment of the technology. The first stage is to establish the **feasibility** of a technique, i.e., to determine if it is safe and can produce technically acceptable results. This information, however, provides little data about the utility of a particular medical technology. Therefore, the next step is to establish the **efficacy**, i.e., the performance of the technology under ideal conditions using selected patients. If the technology under consideration does not work effectively under the most favorable of circumstances, it certainly cannot be expected to be effective under less than favorable circumstances. Next comes the test of **effectiveness**. Even if a particular technology does perform well when guided by its innovator or medical champion, it may still prove insufficiently robust to produce substantial benefit when used routinely in a less controlled environment. Success here often depends on how readily the skills associated with the technical procedure are learned and how successful the procedure is in improving the health status of patients in the general population. The final step in assessment is the **economic appraisal**. This step is concerned with the value of the technology, i.e., its contribution to quality care in terms of both **cost effectiveness** and **cost benefit**.

All of these steps are important, and must be completed in order to assess properly the benefits and costs associated with a particular medical technology. To do anything less may be expedient, but it is not correct.

Innovation, Development, and Diffusion of Medical Technology

The process by which medical technology is developed for and distributed throughout the health-care system is illustrated in Figure 4.1. It should be noted that the process begins with basic research, which may lead to a new technological innovation. Once a device is created, it then moves through the various stages of development, evaluation to ensure compliance with federal regulatory requirements, adaptation for market use, use, and finally obsolescence.

The stage, at which a medical technology enters and becomes a part of the health-care system can be referred to as "diffusion." The diffusion curve of an innovation is typically described by an S-shaped curve (Figure 4.2a). The diffusion process usually begins with a slow initial introduction, has a takeoff phase characterized by an increasing rate of adoption, then slowly levels off to a mature phase, and eventually decreases as obsolescence approaches. It is important to note that the rate of adoption of new medical technologies at hospitals affiliated with medical schools is usually higher than that of nonaffiliated hospitals (Mantil et al., 1991).

The results of several empirical studies have shown that specific medical technologies have followed such a course (OTA, 1978; Russell, 1979). For example, consider the adoption and use of the computed tomography (CT) scanner in the United States (Figure 4.2b). The CT scanner was introduced into the United States in the early 1970s. By 1974, there were four scanners in operation. Only two years later there were 475 operational scanners, i.e., a ten-fold increase. By 1977, CT scanners were being bought and installed at a rate of about 40 per month. A year later, although total volume continued to increase, the rate of increase was cut in half and this rate has continued to decline ever since. During the mid- to late 1970s, there was a great deal of public debate over control of capital expenditures for health-care. As a result, Congress enacted the Health Planning and Resources Development Act of 1974, which quickly instituted a system of local health planning agencies. These regional agencies promptly halted wide spread proliferation of many high-cost medical technologies. If any single technology was specially targeted for regulatory control with the intentions of creating a more orderly process of diffusion, it was the CT scanner.

In the 1980s, a similarly expensive and dramatic diagnostic technology, magnetic resonance imaging (MRI), reached the diffusion stage in the American health-care system. By 1985, MRI was reported in the takeoff phase of the diffusion curve. However, certificate-of-need (CON) regulations enacted during the mid-1980s significantly retarded the diffusion rate of MRI in the United States (Steinberg et al., 1985).

It should be emphasized that the life cycle of many medical technologies, such as CT and MRI scanners have occurred essentially in the absence of any assessment process. A case study commonly cited to illustrate the problems encountered when assessment is not performed prior to diffusion is that of gastric freezing, i.e., the use of a special cryogenic probe to cure ulcers (Fineberg, 1979). Introduced in 1962, 2500 of these probes were sold in the United States, and an estimated 25,000 operations were performed before the technique was properly evaluated. All this was due to the erroneous results of a few uncontrolled case studies that were purported to have shown dramatic benefits in curing ulcers without medication or surgery. However, controlled randomized trials performed several years later showed that gastric freezing to be of no benefit whatsoever.

When should technology assessment occur? Referring once again to Figure 4.1, it has been suggested that technology assessment should occur at the point of crossover from the innovation phase to the diffusion phase. The basis for this suggestion lies in the need to address concerns (safety, efficacy, cost effectiveness, and even social and ethical issues) that might first be raised by those organizations and institutional committees that must approve human research.

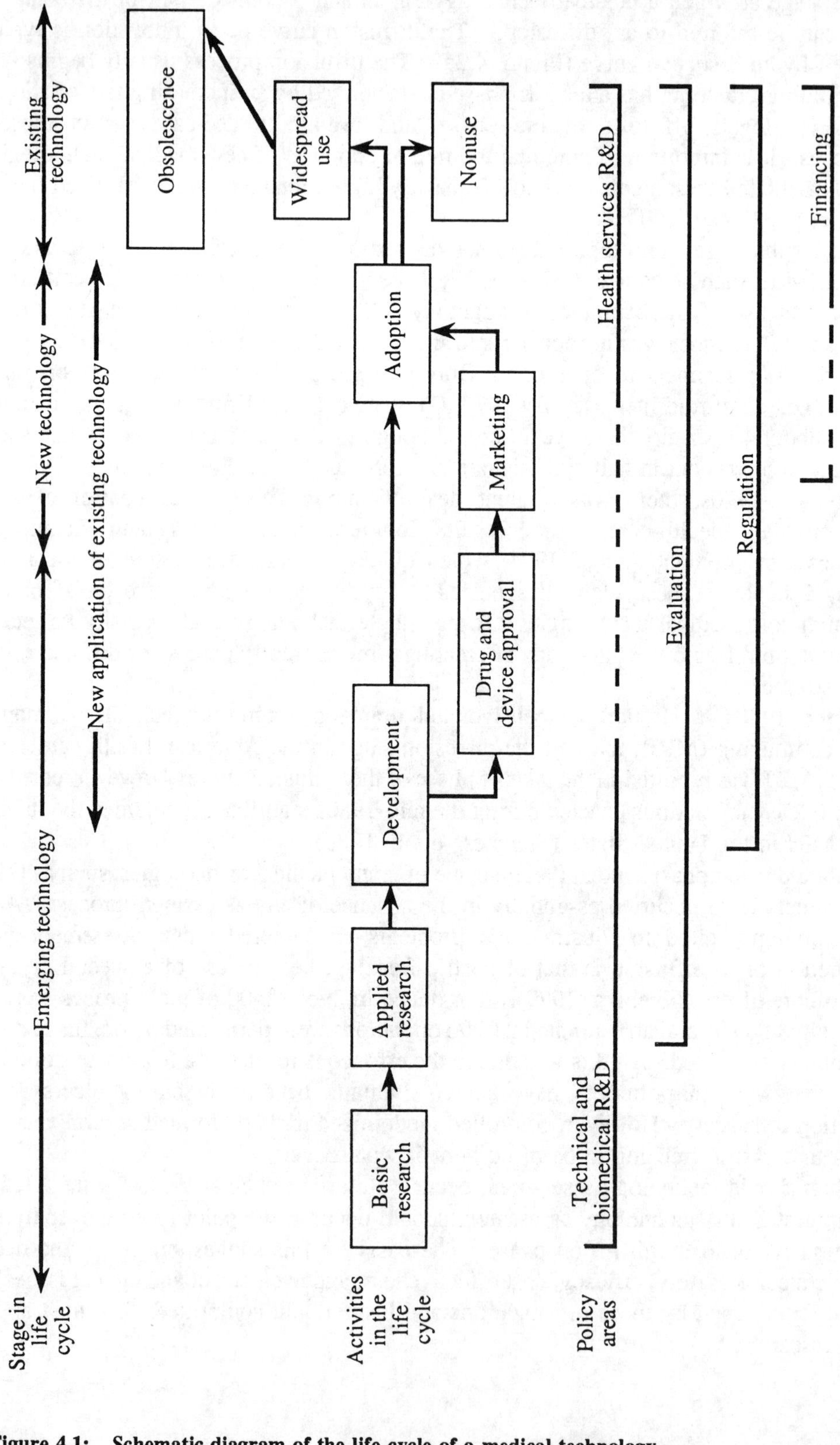

Figure 4.1: Schematic diagram of the life cycle of a medical technology.

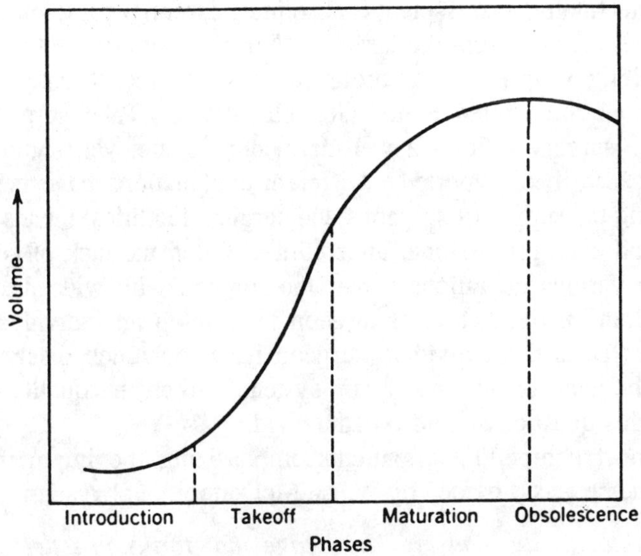

Figure 4.2a: Diffusion curve for medical technology innovations.

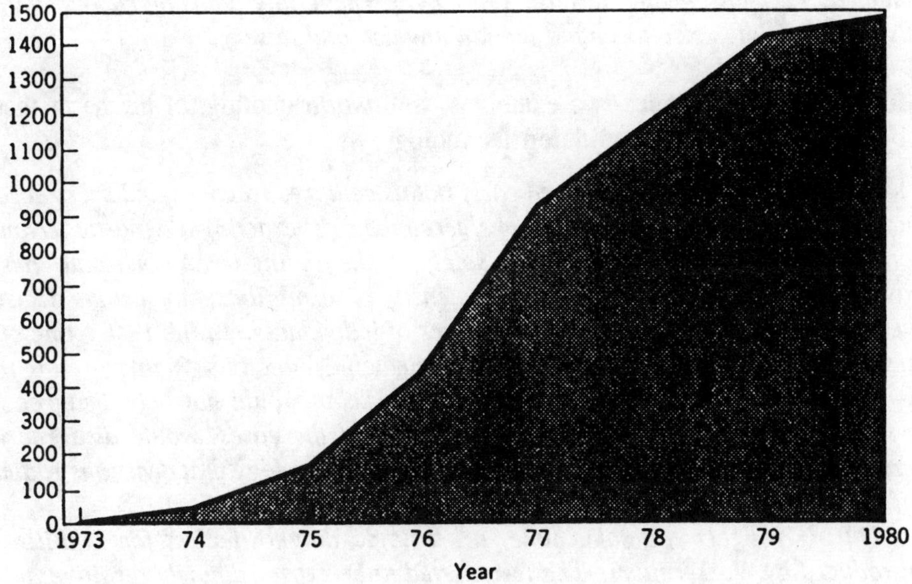

Figure 4.2b: Graph illustrating the number of CT scanners installed in the U.S. between 1973 and 1980.

Evidence that technology assessment is absolutely essential comes not only from the case studies given above, but also from the large number of papers (more than 150) published in the last decade citing significant variations in many of the so-called "standard clinical practices" throughout the United States (Jennett, 1988). Take surgical procedures, for example. Usually, surgery follows a well-defined rationale; yet, significant variations in surgical outcomes have been reported. Different explanations have been given for these variations, including the supply of surgeons and surgical facilities, means of reimbursement, patient demand, and even professional uncertainty. Often the lack of consensus regarding the indications for various operations leaves the surgeon with wide discretion (Weinberg, 1984). This freedom encourages each surgeon to develop an individual practice style or surgical signature. Does the individual surgeon have too much discretion? Maybe yes, maybe no, but if the goal for our health-care system is to ensure quality of care throughout the country, then this question should be addressed.

One of the most compelling arguments emphasizing the importance of technology assessment in medicine was provided by Walsh McDermott, a physician (McDermott, 1977).

> *"At any one time ... the body of knowledge that forms practice, especially the therapeutic practice, of medicine is a curious mixture of a highly effective technology interspersed with islands of dogma, empiricism, conventional wisdom, and at times, superstition. With the exponential growth of "interventions," however, this situation can no longer be tolerated. The persistence of unvalidated technologies leads not only to serious diagnostic error but to waste of skilled services and of money; it also contributes to the increasing load of medically induced, i.e., iatrogenic, disease and, by perpetuating untruths about chronic diseases, can give rise to untold human anguish and misery."*

McDermott also provides two examples, well worth quoting, of the harm that can be done by the utilization of **unvalidated technology**:

> *"Chest X-rays were introduced early in this century, became standard procedure in the 1920's, and had come to be considered the most exacting diagnostic technique for tuberculosis by the early 1930s. Solely on the finding of an abnormal chest X-ray or a change in the appearance of a density in serial films, momentous decisions were made that profoundly altered the lives of individuals. In the 1940s, one of the first attempts at validating a technology in medicine found that, in interpreting these X-ray films, in one out of three cases, the physician would not only disagree with a second or third "reader", but in 20 percent of the cases, would disagree with himself. Yet it was on this supposedly "decisive" technology that decisions radically affecting the lives of people were made.*
>
> *During roughly the same time, a serologic diagnostic test for syphilis was introduced by Wassermann. The test proved to be extraordinarily sensitive, in that few patients with untreated active disease yielded negative reactions. What was not realized was that the test was overly sensitive. Of all those people yielding positive reactions, only about one-half were syphilitic. But this "validation," so to speak, of the test, this characterization of its inadequacies, was performed decades after large-scale public health campaigns (including laws governing premarital examinations) had brought thousands of people under treatment."*

Although the Food and Drug Administration ensures that prescription drugs and certain medical devices are safe and efficacious when applied under prescribed conditions, no agency exists to ensure that medical or surgical procedures pass an initial safety and efficacy test prior to diffusion into general practice. Once any technology is available, whether it is a drug, device, or a medical or surgical procedure, physicians are constrained in their use by training, ethics, economic considerations, their estimate of patient benefit, and the threat of malpractice suits. Thus, the appropriate use of all available medical technologies has, in the main, been left solely to physician and patient discretion. Does this freedom need to be corrected? All of these factors clearly point to the need for more and better technology assessment throughout the U.S. health-care system. Some institutions have begun to lead the way and their example must be emulated.

Organizations for Technology Assessment

Since the assessment of medical technologies has assumed such an important role, there are a number of organizations in government and the private sector that have assumed responsibilities in this area. Some of the more important organizations in this area are described in this section.

The Food and Drug Administration. The FDA, a division of the Public Heath Service, is the primary U.S. government agency that is responsible for medical technology assessment. It regulates entry into the U.S. market of all drugs and medical devices, requiring manufacturers to demonstrate that their products are safe and efficacious. Thus, the FDA requires rather than conducts assessments. It is charged with the protection of the public health in the U.S. by establishing and developing product standards although none yet have been promulgated, regulating the testing of products, developing or approving clinical protocols, evaluating technical and clinical evidence provided to it by manufacturers, and regulating product labeling. The FDA does no actual clinical testing itself. It generally requires that companies demonstrate safety and efficacy only as claimed in their labeling, but not relative to other products or procedures.

Drug Regulation. In order for drugs to enter the U.S. market, the manufacturer must proceed through two major steps established by the FDA: (1) the investigational new drug (IND) application process, and (2) the new drug application (NDA) process. The IND process normally precedes testing in humans in the United States and requires that the firm describe the proposed clinical studies, the qualifications of the investigators, the chemical properties of the drugs, and the results of all pharmacologic and toxicity testing gained from laboratory animals, and the results from any available human studies, usually from other countries. If the FDA approves the IND application, the firm may proceed with the NDA step, which normally consists of a three-phase clinical testing program in humans, culminating in a relatively large (usually 700–3000 patients) multisite, randomized, controlled trial. The results of these studies are then presented to the FDA for market approval. In some instances, additional "Phase 4" postmarketing surveillance studies are required. The entire drug development process takes as long as seven to 12 years and is extremely expensive (FDA, 1977).

Device Regulation. The 1976 Medical Device Amendment to the Federal Food, Drug, and Cosmetic Act and its successor, the Safe Medical Devices Act of 1990 (see Chapter 5 for a detailed discussion of this act), provide the FDA with the authority to regulate medical devices during their development, testing, production, distribution, and use. These new laws require that all medical devices be classified into one of three risk-based categories: Class I, general controls; Class II, performance standards; and Class III, market approval. The laws require any device-related patient death or injury to be reported immediately.

In general, the approval process for medical devices is less onerous than that for drugs. Class I devices (e.g., medical and surgical supplies) are the least stringently regulated, essentially requiring only FDA notification of intention to market; Class II devices (e.g., noninvasive diagnostic test equipment) must pass general performance standards; however, Class III devices (e.g. pacemakers, total hip prostheses) are regulated for safety and efficacy and must pass through a clinical testing phase similar to that mandated for drugs (although much less demanding).

A manufacturer of a Class III device is required to file an investigational device exemption (IDE) application (which is similar to the IND drug process). The IDE permits the firm to test the device on humans in controlled settings in order to establish its safety and efficacy. The resulting evidence is then submitted to the FDA in the form of a premarket approval application (PMAA).

The National Institutes of Health. The NIH contributes to medical technology assessment in two major ways. The first is by sponsoring clinical trials and conducting consensus development conferences on specific medical practice issues. Although the NIH's principal mission is to support basic and applied biomedical research in the United States, it does spend a portion of its budget, approximately 5 percent in 1985, on clinical trials. Most trials are investigator-initiated by research clinicians from medical centers all over the United States.

Another major technology assessment activity of the NIH is the consensus development program organized by the Office of Medical Application of Research (OMAR). Whereas NIH-sponsored clinical trials are typically conducted on medical and surgical procedures in a very early phase of development, the consensus development conferences typically concern medical practice that is in a much more advanced stage of diffusion. Some topics (e.g., CT scanner) are chosen because they are important or controversial new technologies; others (e.g., screening for cervical cancer) are chosen because they are widespread and controversial issues.

Consensus development occurs at meetings of experts who discuss the appropriate use of a given medical technology. These experts review evidence of safety and efficacy/effectiveness of the technology under study. The panel then reaches a consensus on a statement of what is known about application of that technology. The results of these conferences are disseminated, first by holding a news conference, by publishing results in the *Journal of the American Medical Association* (JAMA), and through the wide distribution of booklets summarizing the findings.

The Office of Technology Assessment. The Office of Technology Assessment (OTA) is an arm of Congress that acts as its technology research and advisory source. Established by Congress in the early 1970s it assists in understanding complex technological issues. The OTA has a number of programs, including the Health Program within the Health and Life

Sciences Division. Since the main thrust of the OTA Health Program is to assist Congress in developing policies concerning medical technologies, its reports draw conclusions from evidence and expert opinion rather than from its own assessment of specific technologies. For example, following a specific request from a congressional committee, the OTA normally conducts its studies by forming an advisory panel for each major topic, gathering evidence from the literature and expert opinion, writing a report on its findings, and circulating drafts of the report to a wide audience for comment. A final report is then released to the requesting committee (OTA, 1982).

The Health Care Financing Administration. The Health Care Financing Administration (HCFA) is responsible for administering Medicare and federal aspects of state Medicaid programs. Its medical technology activities are mainly associated with coverage and reimbursement policies and, to a lesser extent, research and demonstrations.

New procedures are first evaluated at the local level to determine if they should be included in the reimbursement schedule. If coverage cannot be resolved at the local or regional level, the HCFA's central office initiates a more formal process, first by referring the issue to its internal physician panel and then, if still unresolved, to the Office of Health Technology Assessment (OHTA) within the Public Health Service (PHS) for a more structured review and recommendation.

Although the HCFA Office of Research and Demonstrations (ORD) does conduct and sponsor some studies associated with medical technology and its assessment, these studies are generally aimed more at general delivery and reimbursement of services than at individual technologies. An exception was the National Heart Transplant Program in which the HCFA sponsored a study to help to establish a reimbursement coverage policy.

The National Center for Health Services Research and Health Care Technology Assessment. The National Center for Health Services Research and Health Care Technology Assessment is involved in technology assessment by sponsoring extramural studies of technologies and by conducting intramural assessments, mainly through the OHTA. Located within the HCFA National Center, the OHTA is primarily responsible for advising on coverage policy. As stated earlier, when the HCFA cannot resolve a coverage issue within its own system, it formally requests the Public Health Service for advice. The PHS refers that request to the OHTA, which then publishes a notice to that effect in the Federal Register, requesting information and advice from interested and knowledgeable parties.

OHTA assessments are normally concerned with safety and efficacy/effectiveness, not cost effectiveness, and generally address the acceptability and appropriateness of a procedure. In the past, the OHTA advice was to either cover or not cover a procedure, with explicit guidance as to the appropriate conditions of use. More recently, however, the OHTA has been addressed the conditions under which a technology should be covered. For instance, in 1986, the OHTA recommended to the HCFA that heart transplants be covered, but only for persons age 55 and under and only when performed in facilities meeting certain criteria (e.g., high volume, high success rate).

The Prospective Payment Assessment Commission. As part of the 1983 Amendments to the Social Security Act, Congress established the Prospective Payment Assessment Commission (ProPAC) to advise and assist both Congress and the Secretary of Health and Human Services in maintaining and updating Medicare's Prospective Payment System (PPS).

Appointed by OTA, ProPAC has two primary responsibilities: (1) recommending to the secretary the annual economic update factor for the entire system, which includes an adjustment for changes in technology, and (2) recommending changes in the relative weights to the diagnostic-related guidelines (DRGs). The latter responsibility empowers ProPAC to study individual technologies as they apply to hospital in-patient care.

When a new technology starts to diffuse into the hospital environment, it must be included within some DRG that has been calibrated on the basis of previous practice methods. If the new technology changes the cost of providing care, the DRG may no longer accurately reflect the relative resource intensity required and thus may inappropriately compensate the hospital for that case. ProPAC's responsibility is to assist in determining when a DRG needs to be created or recalibrated and what that change should be.

Two examples illustrate the issues involved as well as the potential effect of the diffusion of new technologies. The first is magnetic resonance imaging, which, as mentioned previously, was assessed in the 1980s. MRI is an expensive technology that can be applied to a growing number of hospital cases (i.e., DRGs). The question becomes whether the Medicare prospective payment system should be modified to reflect the additional costs of providing MRI care and if so, how. If no change is made, hospitals that adopt MRI will lose money on cases for which it is used (Chu and Cotter, 1986). If all relevant DRGs are increased to reflect the additional costs to the entire system, hospitals that are slow to adopt MRI will be overcompensated, and hospitals that adopt MRI will be undercompensated (since the additional payment is spread across all cases). If an additional DRG "add-on" is made only for those hospitals that adopt MRI or for only those cases where MRI is used, payment may be more equitable on a case-by-case basis. However, such a method begins to resemble the previous inflationary cost-based system that the PPS was designed to reform. In 1987, ProPAC's recommendation was to pay an add-on to the DRG for each scan. However, the HCFA has been reluctant to adopt such a policy.

Extracorporeal shock wave lithotripsy (ESWL) provides another example of the new technology-related DRG dilemma. Prior to lithotripsy technology, the treatment of kidney stones in a hospital could be managed either medically or surgically, depending on clinical indications, with the surgical DRG being roughly three times more expensive than the medical DRG. Although the lithotripster is an expensive machine to buy and install (costing approximately $2 million), it destroys kidney stones noninvasively. Its use tends to be more expensive per case than medical management, but considerably less expensive than surgery. Fitting lithotripsy into either category could either under- or overpay a hospital for adopting the technology. After studying hospital cost data, ProPAC recommended that the HCFA temporarily use the higher of two medical DRGs, which it calculated would just cover costs if the machine were used efficiently. The HCFA decided to simply pay ESWL within the existing medical DRGs (OTA, 1986).

Both MRI and ESWL illustrate the importance of ProPAC's role and the potential far-reaching effects of reimbursement policies on the adoption, diffusion, and ultimately innovation and development of new technologies.

Private Sector Technology Assessment Activities. Although public policies and agencies tend to dominate medical technology assessment issues, the private sector is also very active in this area. Consider the following:

Pharmaceutical and Device Industries. The pharmaceutical industry devotes enormous resources to the assessment of its products. This investment includes all the preclinical and clinical trial research required for FDA premarket approval. The medical device industry also spends large amounts of money on assessments of its products, although on a much smaller scale.

Due to increased pressures from a competitive marketplace and a price sensitivity to costly new technologies, both drug and medical device firms are beginning to invest in cost-effectiveness analyses (CEA) of their products. Rather than being compared to a placebo, new technologies are being examined for cost effectiveness compared to competing choices of therapy. For example, coronary artery bypass surgery is compared to percutaneous transluminal coronary arteriography (PTCA), a procedure that uses a balloon catheter to increase the inner diameter of restricted coronary arteries.

Insurance Health-Care Associations and Providers. Other technology assessment activities sponsored by private-sector organizations rely on analyzing existing information to assist technology policy making. Very seldom are new data collected.

All health-care insurance organizations must have some system to determine coverage policies, although many private insurers often take a "follow-the-leader" approach. The leader may be the HCFA (for Medicare) or possibly the Blue Cross and Blue Shield Association. In other cases, such as in organ transplantation issues, the HCFA has been slower than commercial insurers in making coverage decisions. Just as the HCFA relies on the Public Health Service, many private insurers rely on the appropriate medical societies for guidance in addition to their own internal medical advisory panels.

A prominent and well-defined private insurer assessment activity is the Blue Cross and Blue Shield (BCBS) Association's Medical Necessity Program (MNP). Established in 1977, the MNP attempts to assist in formulating coverage policy by selectively reviewing existing technologies in order to eliminate or reduce coverage for outmoded, ineffectual, and/or misused medical and surgical procedures. The MNP uses BCBS's Medical Advisory Panel and requests cooperation from such medical societies as the American College of Radiology to guide its assessments.

The American College of Physicians (ACP) sponsors the Clinical Efficacy Assessment Project (CEAP), an expansion of the MNP. This program relies on literature review and expert opinion from its membership to review the appropriate application of new technology used in the practice of internal medicine.

The American Medical Association (AMA) sponsors the Diagnostic and Therapeutic Technology Assessment (DATTA) program, which is designed to educate its members to the values and appropriate use of technologies. The DATTA program tends to concentrate more on new and emerging diagnostic and therapeutic technologies. For each topic, the DATTA program reviews existing evidence, formulates relevant questions, and surveys a panel of experts within the AMA's membership ranks.

The American Hospital Association's (AHA) Hospital Technology Series is a program that focuses on hospital devices and equipment from the hospital administrator's point of view. The evaluations are concerned primarily with the cost and service implications of technologies that are entering clinical practice. Evaluations are based on analysis of technical reports and the professional literature and on selected and focused interviews with technical and hospital experts.

The Emergency Care Research Institute (ECRI) focuses on consultation services and the evaluation of specific medical devices.

The International Society for Technology Assessment in Health-care (ISTAHC) through its publications and conferences, promotes academic, research, and policy-making activities that relate to health-care technology.

The Institute of Medicine. The latest entrant into the field of medical technology assessment in the United States is the Institute of Medicine's (IOM) Council on Health Care Technology. Since Congress earmarked matching funds through the auspices of the National Center for Health Services Research and Health Care Technology Assessment, the IOM was given a charter to establish an organization cosponsored by both private and public monies, to help guide and coordinate technology assessment policy. The council is made up of leaders from private industry and the academic community and has set an agenda to develop a clearinghouse for technology assessment literature and reports, to assist in guiding the development of methods for assessment, to promote education and training, to the available identify information and data, and to develop guidelines for evaluation. The new council is mandated to sponsor, coordinate, and commission assessments (IOM, 1989).

Improving the Use of Medical Technology

While recognizing the limitations of technology assessment as a method of improving medical practice, there seems little prospect of moving toward more rational, more effective, and more humane uses of medical technologies without a strategy based on reliable data. Such a strategy needs to identify effective technologies, to determine the limits of appropriate use based on the sliding scale of benefits and burdens, and then, to determine the affordable level of use (Jennett, 1985, 1986, 1988).

The two most important concerns in assessment of medical technology are efficacy and safety (Banta et al., 1981):

> *"Efficacy and safety are the basic starting points in evaluating the overall utility of a medical technology. If a technology is not efficacious, it should not be used, and if its efficacy is unknown, statements about its overall value cannot be made. ... In addition, efficacy and safety data are needed to evaluate the cost effectiveness of a technology. Neither the need for a technology nor its appropriate use in medical care can be established without reliable and valid information on efficacy and safety. Federal programs to regulate and provide medical care and medical technology depend on efficacy and safety information to assure wise decisions. Information obtained from assessment of the efficacy and safety of new and existing medical technologies might help to ensure that new technologies demonstrated to have potential benefits with acceptable risks are made available rapidly, might constrain the diffusion and use of technologies which either lack efficacy or cause excessive harm, and might guide the appropriate use of all technologies."* A useful definition has also been provided by Banta et al. (1981):

Efficacy: The probability of benefit to individuals in a defined population from a medical technology applied for a given medical problem under ideal conditions of use.

Over the years, several factors have been identified as especially important to a medical technology's efficacy:

- The benefit to be achieved.
- The medical problem giving rise to the technology.
- The population affected.
- The conditions under which the technology is applied.

The most complex factor is the first, i.e., the benefit to be achieved.

Benefit to be Achieved — Diagnostic Technology. One might think that a diagnostic technology is beneficial to the extent that it facilitates the clinician's ability to distinguish diseased from nondiseased persons or to assess the severity of disease. Assessment of diagnostic technology, however, is not this simple. To determine the diagnostic benefit, several important factors must be considered:

- Technical capacity: Does the device or procedure perform reliably and deliver accurate information?
- Diagnostic accuracy: Does the test contribute to making an accurate diagnosis?
- Diagnostic impact: Does the test result influence the pattern of subsequent diagnostic testing? Does it replace other diagnostic tests or procedures?
- Therapeutic impact: Does the test result influence the selection and delivery of therapy? Is more appropriate therapy used after application of the diagnostic test than would be used if the test was not available?
- Patient outcome: Does the performance of the test contribute to the improved health of the patient?

If a diagnostic technology fails completely at any stage of this hierarchy, then it must fail at all later stages. If it succeeds at some stage, this presupposes success at prior stages but leaves undetermined whether success may occur at later stages. Thus a test may be accurate without leading to a more accurate diagnosis, or it may lead to an accurate diagnosis without leading to better therapy, etc.

The example of the syphilis test used in the first three decades of this century, described above, illustrates the harm inflicted on thousands of patients by a diagnostic technology that was overly sensitive. Poor performance in any of these aspects of diagnostic accuracy could result in unnecessary exposure of well patients to the risks associated with specific medical procedures or in the failure to treat patients who would benefit from therapy.

One of the major difficulties in determining the performance characteristics of diagnostic tests, however, is the lack of appropriate reference standards (gold standards) against which to judge the test. The true state of nature is generally not known in clinical medicine. For the majority of diseases, even the best diagnostic test has some error rate associated with it. In practice, the clinician is forced to accept the best available, albeit imperfect, diagnostic test as a pseudo reference standard. The evaluation of a diagnostic test against an imperfect standard obviously results in an inaccurate measurement of test performance.

If this is correct, then it is not possible to make perfect discrimination between patients with a given disease and those without. Therefore, assessment of diagnostic technologies will always be somewhat less than perfect. A new diagnostic technology can only be measured against existing technologies designed to differentiate between those who have a given disease and those who do not. However, the unavoidable susceptibility of these technologies to some degree of error makes them a less than perfect basis upon which to evaluate a new technology.

Benefit to be Achieved — Therapeutic Technology. The benefits to achieved in the case of therapeutic technology include improvements in morbidity, mortality, and life expectancy as consequences of a particular technology's ability to correct physiology and control pathology. In other words, therapeutic technologies are developed with the aim of relieving illness, saving lives, and increasing life spans. These relatively quantifiable aspects of a technology's performance can be referred to as its "medical benefit." Although medical benefit is extremely important, it is not all that should be considered when assessing a therapeutic technology. As Laurence Tancredi (1982) has noted, the scientific training of clinicians often disposes them to emphasize the measurable aspects of the disease process and to think solely in terms of what is relatively amenable to measurement. Yet, to recognize only the medical benefit of a technology is to omit aspects of therapeutic benefit that are especially important to patients.

This leads to the second element of the benefit sought by using therapeutic technologies, improvement of the patient's quality of life, which can be referred to as the personal benefit of the technology. Five dimensions of this element of therapeutic benefit have been identified (Tancredi, 1982).

The first consideration regarding the quality of life is whether the patient will be able to return to a baseline of functioning, particularly in cases requiring dramatic therapeutic technologies such as renal dialysis or the proposed nuclear-powered heart. The medical treatment may be effective in keeping the patient alive and in correcting the biochemical and physiological abnormalities of disease or defect, but it may at the same time create significant difficulties that change the quality of the patient's life.

Although a technology may rate highly in terms of medical benefit because it relieves illness or saves life, it may leave the patient unable to return to work, unable to pursue favorite avocations, unable to have a normal sexual life, or otherwise unable to engage in activities that are central to the quality of the patient's life. A technology can have a high measure of medical benefit without having an equally high measure of personal benefit or even much personal benefit at all.

The second consideration involving the quality of the patient's life would be the degree of relief from expected symptoms. The patient would be most concerned with personal freedom from pain or discomfort, including those induced by the treatment itself. A therapeutic technology may be very effective at preventing a patient's death, yet may fail to provide any measure of relief from the pain or other unpleasant effects of the disease. In some cases, the technology itself may cause the patient much suffering. In either situation, the technology may rank very poorly with respect to personal benefit even if it is an excellent source of medical benefit.

The third consideration, the requirements of the treatment, would also be particularly important to patients suffering from chronic illness such as end-stage renal disease. The hemodialysis patient, for example, may have to spend as much as six hours, three times a week, attached to an artificial kidney machine in an institutional setting. A technology may excel at keeping a patient alive and at relieving the symptoms of a particular illness yet so tax the patient's time, energy, and other personal resources as to undermine significantly the quality of life. This is especially important where the ailment is chronic and requires long-term use of a necessary technology. In this kind of circumstance, the medical benefit of a technology may be overcome by the personal burdens it imposes on the patient.

The fourth consideration would be the psychological effects of the technology: the short-term as well as the more permanent long-term changes that may ensue. In the case of patients on hemodialysis, studies have demonstrated a significant increase in suicide rate, estimated in one study to be one-hundred times higher than the normal rate, which is about ten in 100,000 individuals in the United States. A therapeutic technology can rate very highly with respect to medical benefit yet be a source of intense psychological distress to the patient—distress great enough to discourage the patient from even short-term use of the technology. In some patients, a technology worth great medical benefit may cause relatively permanent psychological dysfunction and thereby undermine the quality of life. Again, it is clear that while often closely linked, medical benefit and personal benefit do not always go hand in hand.

The fifth consideration in understanding quality of life issues is the effect of the new technology on self-image. This issue has particular relevance to mutilative surgery such as radical mastectomies, jaw resections, and other extreme surgery procedures for seriously ill cancer patients. Although radical procedures are generally employed only when dictated by severe necessity, and although they entail the potential of curing the disease, they can create immense difficulties for patients by causing distortions in body images and self-evaluation. Therapeutic technologies that mutilate the patient's body, even when such mutilations save the patient's life or permanently relieve the illness, may see their medical benefits outweighed by the personal cost they force the patient to endure.

Both medical benefit and personal benefit must be taken into account when assessing the benefit of a given therapeutic technology. The former consists of the technology's ability to relieve illness, avert premature death, and extend the life expectancy as a result of its ability to correct physiology and control pathology. The latter consists of the technology's effect on the patient's quality of life. Because medical benefit is relatively amenable to quantification and so to measurement, it may therefore seem more "real" to scientifically minded medical practitioners. Yet how a technology affects a patient's quality of life is no less real and no less important to the patient because it is resistant to precise measurement. For very many patients, the medical benefit of a therapeutic technology is meaningful only insofar as it leads to an acceptable quality of life and an acceptable level of personal benefit. Accordingly, attention must be paid to both of these dimensions when assessing a new therapeutic technology.

Medical Conditions Giving Rise to Use of the Technology. *"A technology's efficacy can be evaluated only in relation to the disease or medical conditions for which it is applied,"* (Banta et al., 1981). The range of medical conditions for which a particular technology is beneficial must be established empirically. That a technology offers benefits for one type of ailment may mean nothing for its efficacy for other conditions. Although highly efficacious when applied to a particular condition, a technology may not merit support because this condition is exceedingly rare or not particularly urgent. In any case, use of a technology in ways that maximize benefits to patients and minimize their risk of harm requires knowing as precisely as possible the ailment for which it is best applicable.

Population Affected. The effect of a medical technology varies, depending on the individual treated. Sometimes, however, enough uniformity exists to permit careful generalizations that apply to a specific population. For example, in the late 1960s the Veteran's Administration conducted a multi-institutional controlled clinical trial of treatment for hypertension, using the drugs hydrochlorothiazide, reserpine, and hydralazine. The treatment was shown to be efficacious for patients with diastolic blood pressures above 105 mm of mercury. However, all the patients in the trial were males. Thus, the treatment could be considered to be efficacious, based on that trial and other evidence, for the population studied — males — but no automatic assumptions can be made concerning its efficacy for females (Banta et al., 1981).

Even after the efficacy of a technology has been established for a given condition or range of conditions, it is important to determine whether its efficacy is stable for all populations who suffer that condition or range of conditions. A technology may be highly efficacious for some populations and far less so for others even for the same ailment. Accordingly, knowing how a technology's efficacy varies across different patient populations is central to avoiding harmful use and maximizing benefits to patients.

Conditions under which the Technology is Applied. The outcome of the application of a medical technology is partially determined by the skills, knowledge, and abilities of physicians, nurses, and other health-care personnel; by the quality of the drugs, equipment, and institutional settings; and by support systems used by those personnel during the application. Cardiac surgery, for example, may result in better outcomes when conducted by skillful, well-trained surgeons who frequently perform such operations than when conducted by surgeons who rarely use that technology. A situation in which the physician is skillful and experienced, medication is administered carefully, and the patient receives the best care possible must be described as ideal. By definition, not all physicians are the most skillful, and not all conditions of use are of the highest quality (Banta et al., 1981).

A distinction should be noted between the efficacy and effectiveness of a technology. **Efficacy** concerns the benefit likely to be generated by a technology under ideal conditions of use. As Jennett (1986) has noted, " ... It is natural that early exercises in evaluation [of new medical technologies] are carried out in centers of excellence where the technical performance is unusually high, resulting in maximum benefit and minimal iatrogenic mishaps." Yet, although such centers of excellence are natural sites for first assessments of a new technology, they are not likely to be the sites where most patients will come into contact with the technology when it is integrated into the health-care system. These latter sites are likely to fall short of the more optimal conditions of Jennett's centers of excellence. Consequently, evaluation must continue beyond those optimal conditions to the less ideal conditions under which many, perhaps most, patients receive health-care. A technology's **effectiveness** is its likelihood of benefit under these conditions. Complete evaluation of a technology must determine effectiveness as well as efficacy. A technology that is not efficacious does not merit dissemination. If it is efficacious yet cannot be made effective, i.e., cannot be made to offer reasonable benefits under "typical" conditions of use, its dissemination should be severely limited. In particular, its use should be limited to the more optimal conditions of Jennett's centers of excellence. Such limitation might make supporting a technology unwise even though it has been shown to be genuinely efficacious.

Safety. *"Safety, like efficacy, is a relative concept: no technology is every completely safe or completely efficacious,"* (Banta et al., 1981). Every medical technology poses some degree of risk with its use. Accordingly, a safe technology is not and cannot be entirely risk-free.

surgery. Although done in the past, contemporary medical professionals and medical ethicists would surely condemn the performance of sham surgery. Such operations would subject patients to risk of harm with no possibility of benefit that could not have been achieved at lower risk. In recent years, American society has become very reluctant to accept such conduct even when it promises significant benefits for society as a whole. Accordingly, when the control group in an RCT cannot be provided with a suitable placebo, efforts of some sort must be made to determine to what degree the placebo effect is at work and to prevent the ultimate assessment of a technology from being contaminated by it.

Using randomization to determine which patients are assigned to the control and experimental groups is important for at least two reasons. First, it protects treatment comparisons from being rendered invalid by biased assignment of individuals to the two groups. Failure to make unbiased selections can occur with even the most conscientious efforts to be fully objective. Such bias may go undetected until the harm is done. Random assignment of patients between the experimental and control groups ensures the elimination of bias. Second, randomization ensures that the two groups are identical with respect to all relevant factors except treatment, even when some of those factors are unknown. Randomization renders the two groups genuinely comparable.

The main difficulty with randomization is ethical in nature. The traditional concept of the physician's relation to the patient is one of unqualified fidelity to the patient's health. The conduct of a patient's doctor in an RCT appears to conflict with these traditional norms. In the RCT, a physician (or a group of physicians) determines each individual's precise therapy by considering not only the patient's needs, but also the needs of the experimental design, and the needs of the society that will benefit from a randomizing scheme. This certainly poses a moral dilemma for the physicians. This dilemma cannot be solved here. However, rigorous and objective assessment of medical technology is critical if patients are to be provided with the best possible care and if undue harm is to be avoided.

TECHNOLOGY ASSESSMENT IN HOSPITALS: AN EXAMPLE

Overview

To illustrate how technology assessment may be implemented within a medium-size hospital, let's use a specific example (David, 1990). Realizing that the proper use of technology assessment could facilitate strategic planning and enhance competitiveness, our model facility instituted a technology assessment plan that permitted the establishment of organizational priorities to reflect appropriate capital budgeting and resource allocation.

Upon conducting a review of the health-care market, it became clear that because of the intense competition for patients and physicians and the demand for centers of excellence (i.e., increased quality of care) this facility could benefit significantly from the implementation of an appropriate technology assessment plan. The need for such a program became evident when the following problems were continually encountered:

- The lack of a central clearinghouse to collect, index, and monitor all technology information for future planning.
- The absence of procedures for identifying emerging technologies for potential acquisition.
- The lack of a systematic plan for conducting technology assessment, which prevented maximization of the benefits from deployment of available technology.

- The inability to benefit from the organization's previous experience with a particular type of technology.
- The random replacement of medical technologies, rather than a systematic plan based on a set of well-developed criteria.
- The lack of integration of technology acquisition into the strategic planning of the hospital.

To address these issues, efforts to develop a technology assessment plan were initiated with the following objectives: (1) to accumulate information on medical equipment, (2) to monitor the replacement of outdated technology, (3) to facilitate systematic planning, (4) to create a standard assessment methodology, and (5) to improve the capital budget process by focusing on long-term needs relative to the acquisition of medical equipment.

In order to achieve these goals, our model hospital developed specific standards and criteria to evaluate each piece of medical equipment. For example, it was decided that each piece of equipment must do the following:

- Have high technical and diagnostic accuracy, specificity, and reliability.
- Aid in influencing subsequent diagnostic tests or replace existing diagnostic tests or procedures.
- Aid in determining the most appropriate form of therapy, i.e., enable the clinical staff to determine whether a more appropriate therapy would be used after the diagnostic test than would be used if this test were not available.
- Provide new knowledge that would increase the level and quality of care for patients.
- Assist in reducing or eliminating the use of outdated or inappropriate technology.
- Contribute to reducing the number of employees required to obtain the same information or results using other approaches.

Adherence to these standards was viewed as essential.

Getting Started

To implement this technology assessment plan, the first phase required the establishment of a hospital-wide Medical Technology Evaluation Committee (MTEC), charged with three major functions: (1) assess new and emerging technology to identify potential acquisitions; (2) review existing technology; and (3) monitor and set priorities for new technologies. To perform these functions, the committee essentially became responsible for assessment of all medical equipment within the hospital. Given this charge, the committee had to determine: (1) what any new technologies fit the mission of the hospital; (2) how that technology compared with alternative technologies; (3) what stage of the product life cycle the technology was in; and (4) what effect the technology would have on patient care, payment, demand for services, and physician interest.

Technology Assessment Criteria and Tests

The MTEC also assumed responsibility for obtaining performance standards for various pieces of medical equipment, for reviewing specifications for equipment, and facilities needed to support that equipment, and for defining the life-cycle cost parameters.

As it was necessary that medical equipment be assessed prior to acquisition, attention had to be paid to each of the following:

- **Safety**: Analysis of the risk involved in using an item in a specified situation.
- **Homogeneity**: Determination of whether the technology would perform a required function and corresponded to the nature and goals of the hospital, and whether it would be used. That is, would the technology "fit" appropriately into the facility as a whole?
- **Efficacy**: The benefit of using a particular technology for a given medical problem under expected conditions of use.
- **Cost/benefit analysis**: The actual costs of acquiring and operating a technology relative to the actual benefits derived. Cost effectiveness here refers to the cost of a technology relative to alternative solutions to the medical problem. The latter is usually expressed in terms of lives saved, disability avoided, quality of life, and cultural issues (Doessel, 1986).
- **Monitoring and reassessment**: Consideration that after acquisition decisions are made, periodic postdeployment determinations would follow to determine the success achieved and identification of specific factors to be corrected in the future.

In our model facility, the clinical engineering department played a major role in assisting the committee. For example, periodic hospital-wide surveys of the location, cost, and condition of existing equipment, were conducted to provide the necessary information for the department to prepare an equipment replacement and relocation plan for review by the committee. In addition, the clinical engineering department designated a coordinator to assist the committee in prioritizing and reviewing the requests for assessment and acquisition, which was ultimately reviewed by the committee.

After assessing the condition of existing equipment, an evaluation of specific medical devices, including a comparison of the capabilities of the different equipment vendors, was made. To accomplish this evaluation, the following tests were conducted:

- Engineering laboratory testing to determine equipment or system performance.
- Randomized clinical trials designed to test the safety, efficacy, and effectiveness of a medical technology. Patients are assigned to experimental or control groups and outcomes are compared. This type of trial is usually considered the most effective method of comparing the relative benefits of two or more treatments.
- The application of epidemiological and observational methods, such as case studies and longitudinal studies, to determine the benefits derived by patients from a particular medical technology.
- Cost analyses, including cost/benefit and cost effectiveness studies to quantify and compare benefits and costs.
- Simulation/modeling techniques to determine which factors produce the most tangible effects.
- Solicitation and comparison of experiences from peers at other hospitals who have used the same technology on a similar patient population and comparison with experiences within the hospital.
- Operational impact analyses to determine how the new technology will affect protocols, delineation of responsibilities, supplies, stock levels, and operator training.
- Solicitation of expert opinions from outside sources, such as technology assessment organizations, consultants, or information services.

- Literature searches, integration, and summary of reported research findings.
- Group judgments and consensus by experienced personnel to integrate the above findings.

MTEC also had to then agree upon acquisition and replacement criteria for all new pieces of medical equipment. These criteria developed included the following:

- Technical capacity: Does the device or procedure perform reliably and deliver accurate information?
- Diagnostic accuracy: Does the information provided by the medical device contribute to making an accurate diagnosis?
- Diagnostic impact: To what degree do the test results influence the pattern of subsequent diagnostic testing or replace other diagnostic tests or procedures?
- Therapeutic impact: To what degree do the test results influence the selection and delivery of therapy? Is the selection of a particular therapy more definitive as a result of the diagnostic test than if this test were not performed?
- Patient outcome: Does the performance of the test contribute to the health of the patient?
- Reputation of vendor: Do the financial strength and support capabilities of the vendor make the equipment a viable acquisition?
- Research: Does the technology provide a source for new knowledge and increase the potential level of care for patients?
- Utility: Does the technology assist in eliminating outdated or old equipment? Does it contribute to reduction of personnel by eliminating nonnecessary medical protocols or procedures?

In reviewing these steps, it should be clear that our model facility has attempted to make the acquisition and replacement of technology a proactive, rather than a reactive, process. By asking the questions posed above, gathering the information indicated, and monitoring the state of existing equipment, it is possible for decisions related to specific medical technologies to be made on a more timely basis, as opposed to an emergency or *ad hoc* basis.

Having outlined some of the operational procedures to be followed in developing a technology assessment (TA) plan, let's now discuss how TA is actually conducted in our model hospital.

Operational Aspects of Technology Assessment in a Hospital Setting

Figure 4.3 illustrates the technology assessment process at our model hospital. It begins with a department or individual filling out two forms: (1) a Request for Review (RV) form, and (2) a Capital Asset Request (CAR) form (Figures 4.4a and 4.4b). These forms are submitted to the hospital's Medical Technology Evaluation Committee, which conducts the review. Both forms must be sent to the MTEC if the requested item is not currently used by the hospital or does not conform to previously adopted hospital standards. On the RV form, the originator delineates the rationale for acquiring the medical device, e.g., how the item will improve patient care, generate cost savings, support the quality of service, and provide ease of use, and who will be the primary user. On the CAR form, the originator describes the item, estimates its cost, and offers some justification for why it should be purchased. The CAR is then routed to the capital budget office for review.

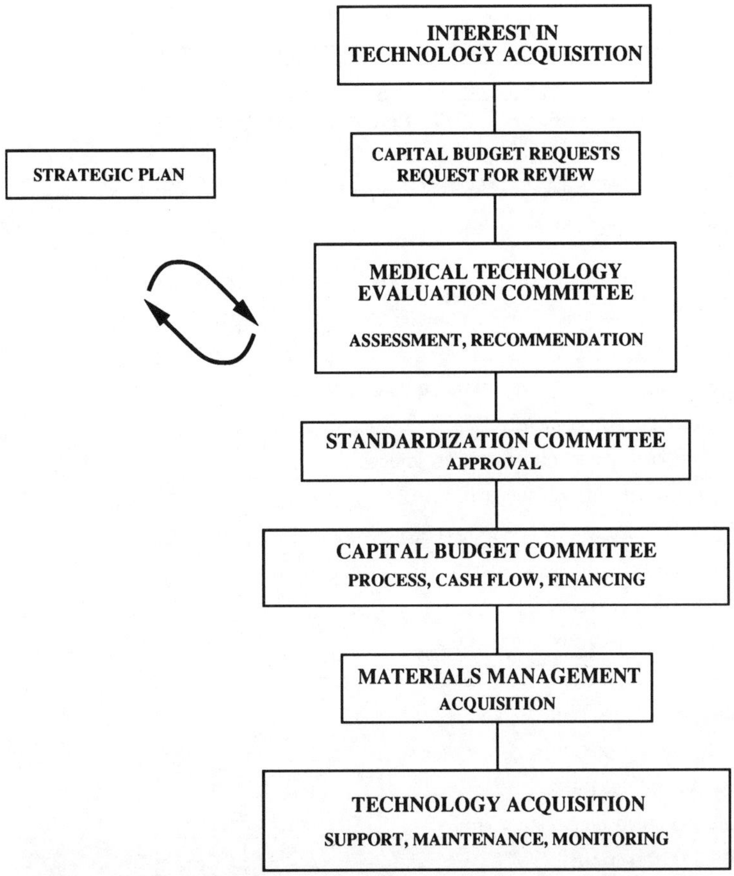

Figure 4.3: Flow chart of the technology assessment process.

Both forms must be sent to the MTEC if the item requested is not currently used by the hospital or if it does not conform to previously adopted hospital standards. During this process, the optimal financing method for acquisition is determined. If funding is secured, the CAR is routed to material management where, together with the RV, it is processed.

The rationale for having the RV accompany the CAR is to ensure that pricing information is included as part of the assessment process. The CAR is the device by which the purchasing department sends product requests out for bid. Any request for evaluation that is received without a CAR, or any CAR involving medical equipment that is received without a request for evaluation, is returned to the originator without action. Both forms are then sent to the clinical engineering department, where a full-time employee designated as a coordinator reviews and prioritizes the various requests submitted to the committee. The committee then has the authority to recommend either acceptance or rejection of any request, based on a consensus of its members.

If the request is approved by the MTEC, then the requested technology or equipment is evaluated using technical and performance standards. Upon completion of the review, a recommendation is sent to the hospital's Products Standardization and Review Committee (PSRC), which reviews the results of the technology assessment, determines whether the particular product is suitable as a hospital standard, and decides if it should be purchased.

REQUEST FOR REVIEW BY THE

MEDICAL TECHNOLOGY EVALUATION COMMITTEE
(COMPLETE ALL PERTINENT INFORMATION)

☐ NEW PRODUCT ☐ NEW EQUIPMENT ☐ REPLACEMENT ITEM ☐ SINGLE USER ☐ OTHER ______

SUBMITTED BY ______ (Name) TO ______ (Name) DATE ______

YOUR POSITION (TITLE) ______ DEPARTMENT NAME & NUMBER ______

BRIEF DESCRIPTION OF THE ITEM (MANUFACTURER & CATALOG NO.) ______

ITEM USED FOR ______

ITEM UNIT COST______ ANTICIPATED ANNUAL USAGE ______

CURRENT ITEM BEING REPLACED (IF APPLICABLE) ______

WHAT IS THE ANNUAL USAGE OF THE ITEM CURRENTLY BEING USED?______

UNIT COST OF THE ITEM CURRENTLY BEING USED (IF NOT STOCK) ______

MANUFACTURER & CATALOG NO. ______

PLEASE GIVE YOUR ASSESSMENT OF THE PROPOSED ITEM OVER THE CURRENT ITEM:

☐ BETTER PATIENT CARE EXPLAIN: ______

☐ COST SAVINGS EXPLAIN: ______

☐ BETTER QUALITY EXPLAIN: ______

☐ EASIER TO USE EXPLAIN: ______

☐ OTHER EXPLAIN: ______

WHO WILL BE THE MAIN USER OF THIS ITEM? ______

WHAT OTHER FACILITIES ARE USING THIS ITEM? (IF ANY)______

LIST CURRENT USER OF THIS ITEM (IF ANY) ______

ANY OTHER PERTINENT INFORMATION (ATTACH ITEMS/LITERATURE)______

______

AUTHORIZED SIGNATURE ______ DATE ______

Medical Technology Evaluation Committee Use Only

REQUEST RECEIVED BY ______ DATE ______

DOES THIS ITEM COMPLY WITH STANDARDS REGULATIONS? (IF APPLICABLE)______

ADDITIONAL ACTION TAKEN ______

PRESENTED TO PRODUCT STANDARDS COMMITTEE ON ______

WAS NOT PRESENTED TO THE PRODUCT STANDARDS COMMITTEE DUE TO ______

ACTION TAKEN ______

FROM: CHAIRMAN OF THE PRODUCT STANDARDS COMMITTEE TO:______

PLEASE ACCEPT OUR APPRECIATION FOR YOUR RECOMMENDATION. THE ITEM YOU SUGGESTED WAS:

☐ CONSIDERED AND APPROVED FOR EVALUATION ☐ CONSIDERED AND NOT APPROVED

☐ REFERRED FOR FURTHER EVALUATION ☐ PENDING CONSIDERATION DUE TO LACK OF INFORMATION

☐ OTHER, ______

Figure 4.4a: Example of a Request for Review form.

CAPITAL ASSET REQUEST
(C.A.R.)

This Form Is Required For All Fixed Asset Purchases With A Cost Of $500 Or More.
Please Type and Complete All Requested Information.

I. Originator

Date | Department | Cost Center | Requested By | Extension

(Includes Model #, Mfg., Name, Accessories, Color, Size, Style, Etc. Attach Any Brochures, Pamphlets, Spec. Sheets, Etc.)

Item Description

Estimated Unit Cost	Quantity	Total Cost	Date Required
$		$	

Is Item In The Approved Capital Budget? ☐ Yes ☐ No If Yes, What Is The Budget Number?

Suggested Vendor(s)

Are Building Modifications Needed? | If Yes, Have You Contacted Facilities Management?

Is Installation Required?

Will There Be A Maintenance Contract? If Yes, Have You Contacted BIOMED?

☐ Inhouse

☐ Vendor Estimated Annual Cost $

Comments

Signature Of Department Manager Date

II. Purchasing

Quotes Obtained From:

Vendor #1 ______ Terms: ______ F.O.B. ______
☐ Recommended ______ Contact: ______ Delivery ______
Phone: ______ Total Price $ ______
C.O.S. Status ______

Quotes Obtained From:

Vendor #2 ______ Terms: ______ F.O.B. ______
☐ Recommended ______ Contact: ______ Delivery ______
Phone: ______ Total Price $ ______
C.O.S. Status ______

Quotes Obtained From:

Vendor #3 ______ Terms: ______ F.O.B. ______
☐ Recommended ______ Contact: ______ Delivery ______
Phone: ______ Total Price $ ______
C.O.S. Status ______

Signature Of Purchasing Manager Date

III. General Instructions

Routing	Initial	Date Rec'd.	Initial	Date Fwd.
1. Facilities (Furniture Only)				
2. HIS (Computer Only)				
3. Biomed (All Items Except Furniture)				
4. Purchasing				
5. Originating Department				
6. Accounting				

Step 1: Department Completes Section 1
Step 2: Furniture Only Forwarded To Facilities
Step 3: Computers Only Forward To HIS
Step 4: All Items Excluding Furniture Forward To Biomed
Step 5: Forward To Purchasing
Step 6: Purchasing Complete Section 2
Step 7: Return To Department
Step 8: Forward Requisition To Accounting
Step 9: Secure Proper Approvals
Step 10: Forward Requisition To Purchasing

PUR-737 1/90

Figure 4.4b: Example of a Capital Asset Request form.

If approved by the PSRC, the request to purchase is reviewed by the Capital Budget Committee (CBC) to determine if the required expenditure meets with available financial resources of the institution and if or when it will be feasible to make the purchase. To ensure coordination of the TA plan, the chairman of the MTEC also serves as a permanent member of the hospital's CBC. In this way, technology assessment is accorded a priority status in budget decisions.

The final recommendation to purchase is thus an evaluation based on strategic, financial, and clinical elements, which directs action toward the selection of a particular vendor by the material management or purchasing department. The overall results of such a program include development of a more structured capital equipment asset management system that provides a mechanism for keeping pace with required equipment replacement, improvement of employee and physician morale, and a diminishment in the frequency of unbudgeted equipment requests. In this way, the TA process can increase operational efficiency and enable the hospital to remain competitive. Fortunately, these efforts are underway at other institutions (Gordon and Tan, 1992) and need to be expanded.

The Role of the Clinical Engineer in Technology Assessment

Technology assessment is one of the five major functions of a modern clinical engineering department (Figure 4.5). Therefore, it is important that clinical engineers be well prepared for the challenge. They must have a full understanding of the mission of their particular hospital, a familiarity with the health-care delivery system, and the support of both the hospital administration and the medical staff. To aid in the process, clinical engineers need access to database services and libraries, the ability to visit scientific and clinical exhibits, and the capability to establish an industrial network and a relationship with peers throughout the country. The final product will be reports that will be read by a variety of clinical and administrative professionals (Shaffer and Shaffer, 1991).

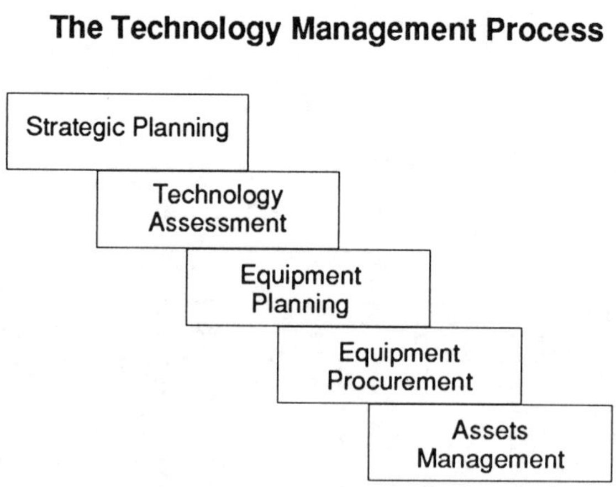

Figure 4.5: The major functions of the clinical engineering department related to the technology assessment process.

Note that while the MTEC is chaired by the director of clinical engineering, another clinical engineer serves as the committee's designated technical coordinator. After accepting a request, the committee identifies other users with an interest in the item and authorizes the technical coordinator to assemble a task force. This task force then serves as an *ad hoc* committee responsible for assessing the equipment described on the RV form. During any specific period, there may be multiple task forces, each focusing on a specific equipment protocol. After the establishment of a task force, the clinical engineer/technical coordinator analyzes the evaluation objectives and devises appropriate technical tests as recommended by the task force. Only equipment that has successfully passed technical tests will proceed to clinical trial. A clinical coordinator collects and reports the summary of experiences gained during the clinical trials to the task force. The technical coordinator puts these results into a summary report, and prepares recommendations for MTEC approval. In this role, the clinical engineer/technical coordinator serves as a multidisciplinary professional, bridging the gap between the clinical and technical needs of the hospital.

ACQUISITION OF NEW EQUIPMENT

Successful management of technological assets requires that an institution adopt policies and procedures based on clear objectives. The prepurchase evaluation of medical instrumentation is one of the most important functions of any clinical engineering department. This process can take just a few hours for simple devices or up to several months for more complex instrumentation. Regardless of the type of device or the time required to perform an evaluation, the required skills and the sequence of steps to follow remains essentially the same. Figure 4.6 presents a flow chart of the prepurchase evaluation process. Note that the first three steps involve assurance that the clinical engineering department has:

- Acquired the proper clinical requirements from the medical and nursing staff.
- Assessed the safety, user interfaces, environmental impact, and conditions under which the equipment must operate.
- Conducted an appropriate survey of the state of the technology and the commercially available equipment.

Only after this data gathering has been completed and the needs of the medical staff have been converted into detailed and quantitative engineering requirements, will the decision-making phase begin. At this point, the choice is usually either to purchase the desired equipment or to have it constructed by the clinical engineering staff or an outside vendor.

If the decision is made to purchase the equipment, a purchase order is issued. Custom construction takes place if the desired system requires specially designed features. In this case, the steps taken include generation of system specifications, solicitation of proposals, proposal evaluation, vendor selection, and contractual acquisition. After this decision has been made, the procedures for equipment acceptance must be prepared. Once the device has been received and accepted, the device is listed in the equipment inventory and maintained in accordance with the technology management policies and procedures outlined in Chapter 3.

Based upon the particular needs of their specialty, physicians and nurses may request a specific medical device or indicate objectives that a device should achieve. Physicians or hospital staff personnel generally do not have the technical resources or direct knowledge or information to select medical equipment on a rational and impartial basis.

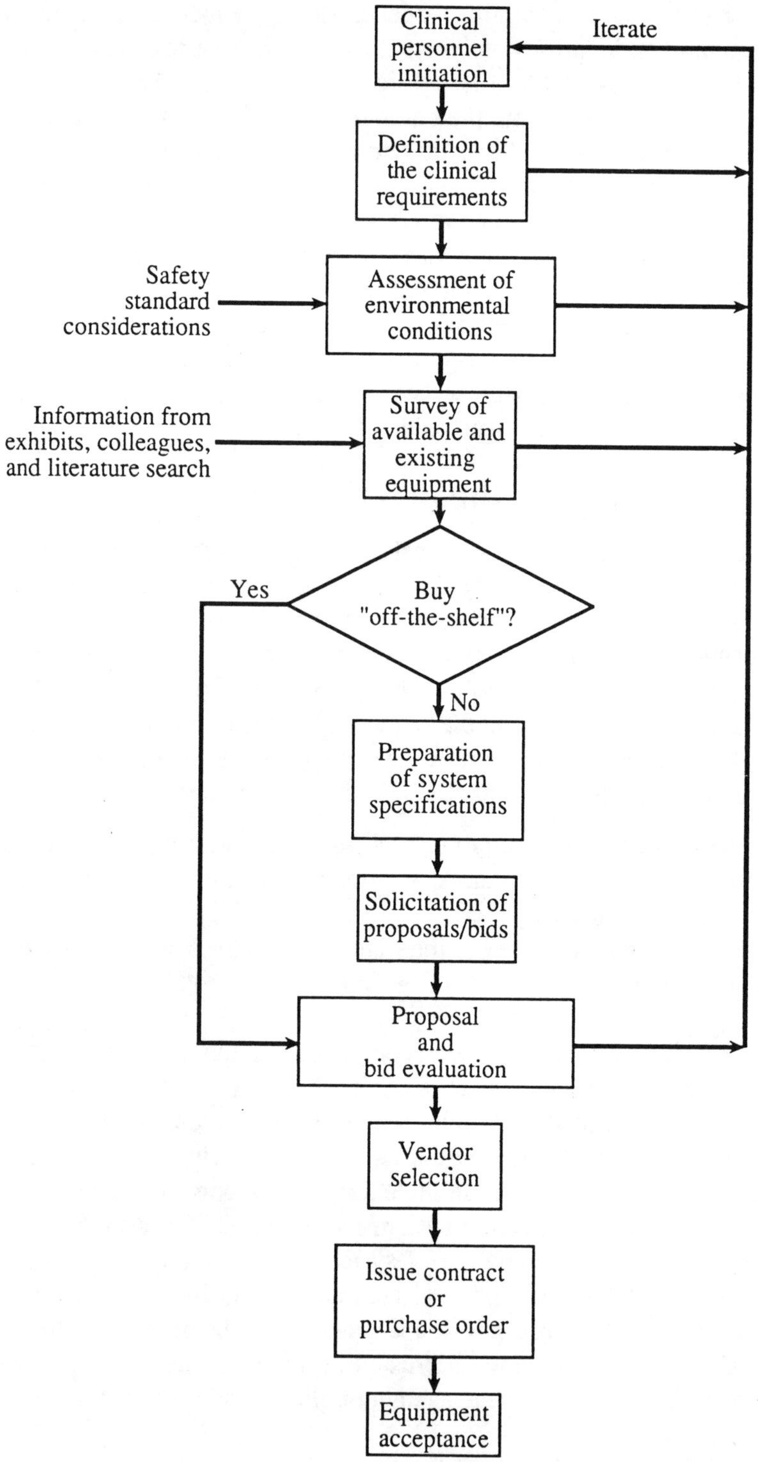

Figure 4.6: Flow chart diagramming the steps in the equipment acquisition process.

Definition of Clinical Requirements

However, it should be pointed out that medical specialists, i.e., physicians or technicians, often have a technical background and extensive experience in the field. The clinical engineer must be capable of interacting with the clinical staff to accomplish the following:

- Define the general clinical goals. The development of a clear, concise statement of the relevant clinical objectives is essential because it serves as a basis for choosing, evaluating, and ultimately accepting the equipment.
- Quantify the type and range of the physiological variables being measured, recorded, or analyzed. The establishment of a list of desired physiological parameters and the degree of accuracy required for each parameter will make it easier to develop engineering specifications for vendors and to determine the criteria for evaluation of competing manufacturers.
- Monitor technology life cycle, research innovations, and determine their clinical utility.

Assessment of Environmental Conditions

In addition to the definition of clinical requirements, the environment in which the equipment will operate is also significant. The clinical engineer must be aware of any potential restrictions that the environment places on the use of the equipment (e.g., heat and electric power) as well as restrictions placed on the environment by the equipment (e.g., the magnet of an MRI unit). Some of the restrictions to consider are reviewed below (Oakes and Gordon, 1974):

- Space: Space is generally considered a restriction applying only to large systems. However, the question of space should be raised for all equipment to be acquired, even if it is then disregarded for small systems. Thus, any potential problems related to physical device size or its use are recognized early. This concern is especially essential in institutions where negotiations for additional space may take many months and involve the highest echelons of the organization.
- Utilities and facilities required: The initial environment survey should also include a study of the available electric power in the proposed area, including details of the feed system, voltage, number of phases, current capacity, and the presence and type of emergency power. The availability of compressed air to power some equipment should also be noted, along with access to central air, oxygen, and vacuum systems. Additionally, for an anesthetizing location, nitrous oxide and gas evacuation are required. All areas should be surveyed for water, light, heating, and air conditioning, radiation protection, and waste disposal services. There must also be sufficient space for storage of routine supplies, housekeeping activities, and, most importantly, the staff's patient-related activities.
- Applicable standards: A detailed review of codes, standards, and regulations applying to health-care activities is the subject of Chapter 5. It will be particularly useful for the clinical engineer to make a list of the specific standards that apply to the equipment being acquired. For example, if the equipment is to be used in an area where there is a magnetic field (the MRI suite), special equipment design and power methods may be required to eliminate the danger of interaction. High-voltage systems, such as those used in imaging rooms, require additional fire-

protection measures.

- Special environmental conditions: Most medical devices are designed to function under normal operating conditions, which include temperature, humidity, vibration and shock, and electric and magnetic fields. If, however, the medical equipment will be subjected to any abnormal environmental conditions, it must be so indicated.

Market Survey

With the clinical requirements defined and the environmental conditions known, the next step in the acquisition process is a search for specific information on available equipment that meets these needs. In carrying out this survey, it will be helpful to have a check list of the most significant characteristics of the desired equipment for ready reference. The survey is important and should be carried out thoroughly regardless of the level of experience of the clinical engineer or the level of complexity of the tool to be acquired.

In many cases, it is reasonable to expect that the system requirements can be met, more or less fully, by commercially available equipment. In this case, advertisements serve as initial sources of information about what is available. If, however, the search proves to be unsuccessful or only partially successful, it may mean that some special design is required or that a different approach to system implementation may be necessary. In this case, a more comprehensive search into the technical literature is appropriate. The purpose of this search is to determine where there is development being carried out in the particular area of interest and what instrumentation is being used in this effort. One of the quickest ways of accessing this literature is through use of one of the medical indexing systems available in most medical libraries and many public library systems.

An effective method of obtaining technical information is to use a prepurchase questionnaire (Figure 4.7). This comprehensive questionnaire can provide a wealth of data, including technical, liability, and business information about the product and manufacturer under consideration. It is important that the form be completed and signed by the manufacturer's manager. The acquisition of the signature provides greater confidence in the validity of the technical information contained than if it is filled out by sales or customer service department representatives (Bronzino and Hayes, 1988).

During this data collection, it is also useful to establish some idea of the cost of the equipment. A useful approach is that of developing a "running cost estimate," which is accumulated and modified as one gathers technical information about the equipment. As the equipment needs change, based on requirements and restrictions, approximate costs can be assigned and a running total established.

Once the vendor has responded to your informal request or formal request for proposal information, the clinical engineering department is usually responsible for evaluating the technical responses, and the purchasing department evaluates the financial responses. One common approach to conduct this evaluation is a structured Matrix. This system consists of two phases—a technical evaluation and a clinical evaluation—which produce a conclusion that can be easily understood and justified.

In the Matrix method, key features or "must-have" attributes of the desired device are identified. Any device not offering these features is automatically rejected. For example, in the selection of a software package to interpret ECG waveforms, a key feature may be its ability to operate in real time. In this case, then, any product that does not provide this capability will not be considered.

New Equipment Pre-purchase Evaluation Form

This form is to be completed by the manufacturer and returned to the Director of Materials Management with manuals and attachments as indicated below. This form must be completed by an employee of the manufacturer with sufficient technical information or knowledge to provide answers to the items below. If the manufacturer is uncertain about specific portions, it is suggested he send available materials promptly so further communication, if needed, will not be delayed. Refer questions to the Director of Materials Management or ______________________. Information detailing specific hospital requirements is outlined in the Saint Francis Hospital and Medical Center Electric/Electronic Equipment Specification pamphlet. Copies of this form are available on request from the Director of Materials Management.

1. TO:

DATE:

ITEM: PROJECT #

2. LISTINGS:
   Is the unit listed with U.L.? Yes ☐ No ☐ If yes, please specify UL Listing # ______________
   Is it listed with other certifying agencies? If so, please give specific standards/listing number.

3. LINE-OPERATED EQUIPMENT, INCLUDING BATTERY CHARGERS:
   Line voltage limits for stable operation: Frequency Limits:
   From To VAC From To Hz
   Phase: Normal Operating Current: __________ Amp. Surge Current: __________ Amp.
   How will safety and/or operation be affected if the voltage goes outside the range of 100–130 volts: _____

   ____

4. BATTERY-OPERATED EQUIPMENT:
   Type of Batteries or Packs: Number per Unit: Recharge Time:
   ______________ ______________ (where applicable) __________
   Discharge Time:
   (under specified load)
   ____
   Can unit be line-operated when batteries are fully discharged? Yes ☐ No ☐
   Willl batteries charge while unit is line operated? Yes ☐ No ☐

5. POWER CORD:
   Required minimum is an 18 gauge, 3 conductor industrial or hospital grade cord at least 10′ long with a Hubbell lock or Hospital grade U ground type plug.
   Does your power cord meet these requirements? Yes ☐ No ☐
   If not, specify differences and indicate cost of modification in Section 13.

   ____

6. POWER SWITCH AND OVERCURRENT INTERRUPTERS:
   Type of power
   Switch (i.e., toggle, slide, etc.):
   ______________ Single Pole
   ______________ Double pole
   Is power switch clearly labeled? Yes ☐ No ☐
   Is power switch in line of sight from operator position? Yes ☐ No ☐
   Type of Overcurrent Protection:
   Ampacity:

   ____

   Must protect all line (hot conductors) to all parts of unit. Must be easily accessible. If fuse, the size must be marked beside the holder and a clearly marked space provided. *If overcurrent protection does not conform to these specifications, see Section 13.*

7. MECHANICAL DESIGN FOR PHYSICAL PROTECTION:
   Unprotected openings on exposed horizontal surfaces not allowed.
   Other openings must be guarded against spillage.
   Small appliances used in patient's bed must be immersible in conductive fluid without macroshock hazard.
   If design does not conform to these specifications, see Section 13.

8. ENVIRONMENTAL AND INTERFACE CHARACTERISTICS:
   Temperature / Humidity Limits
   For Operation: From To °F From To %R
   For Storage: From To °F From To %R
   Maximum allowable storage time: ______________
   Sensitive to RF interference? Yes ☐ No ☐
   Known to generate RF interference? Yes ☐ No ☐
   Sensitive to power line transient? Yes ☐ No ☐
   Known to generate power line transient? Yes ☐ No ☐
   Known to require other utilities? Yes ☐ No ☐

Figure 4.7: Sample Pre-Purchase Evaluation form.

Are exposed to metal surfaces underground? Yes ☐ No ☐

If answer is "yes" to any of these questions, give details on separate page.

Specific sterilizing procedures to be used? ______

Type of labeling for O_2 & Flammable location:

Quality of radiation emission:

Type of shielding: ______

9. PROVIDE THE FOLLOWING MANUALS AND TECHNICAL INFORMATION:
   - Operator's Manual
   - Wiring Diagrams
   - Schematic Circuit Diag.
   - Parts List
   - Statement of known potential hazards
   - Block Diagrams
   - Preventive Maint. Prog.
   - Operational Tests
   - Performance Specifications
   - Service Manual

10. WARRANTY/GUARANTY

    Warranty will start after delivery and initial installation (if applicable).

    If modifications are made to conform to our specifications, will warranty be violated? Yes ☐ No ☐

    Length of warranty: ______

11. SERVICE AND TRAINING INFORMATION

    Estimated response time for service calls from time of notice: ______ hours

    Is local service available? Yes ☐ No ☐

    Give location and working hours of nearest service facility ______

    ______

    A replacement unit is available in ______ hours.

    Are training programs for service personnel available? Yes ☐ No ☐

    Are training programs for users available? Yes ☐ No ☐

    Give location, schedule, cost and instructor's qualifications for both types of training programs on a separate sheet.

12. LEAKAGE/RISK CURRENTS

	ACCEPTABLE LIMITS			
Measurement Site	Device for patients with Intra Cardiac Leads	General Patient Devices	Non-Patient Devices	TYPICAL DEVICE VALUES Indicate Worst leakage current
Patients leads or attachments to gnd.	10 microamperes	50 microamperes	Not applicable	
With 120V applied to patient leads	20 microamperes	Not applicable	Not applicable	
Worst case to ground	100 micro-amperes	500 micro-amperes	500 micro-amperes	

13. MODIFICATIONS/COMMENTS:

    Please list description and cost quotations for any modifications, accessories, or other items necessary to fulfill the requirements stated. *Cost of upgrading unit will weigh heavily on our decision to purchase.*

    1. ______
    2. ______
    3. ______
    4. ______

14. This form is to be completed and signed by the manufacturer's product manager or his equivalent.

    COMPLETED BY:

    Name ______ Title ______

    Address ______ Date ______

    ______

    Signature ______ Telephone ______

Figure 4.7: Continuation of the sample Pre-Purchase Evaluation form.

Equipment Evaluation

Once the "must-have" attributes have been satisfied, the remaining "candidate" devices are evaluated technically. This is accomplished by assigning a weighing factor (which is usually 0 to 10) to denote the relative importance of each of the desired attributes. Once the weighing factors have been assigned, often in collaboration with the clinical users, the clinical engineering department (again in collaboration with the users, if necessary) determines how well each device meets each attribute. A score (once again 0 to 10) is assigned and then multiplied by the weighing factor to determine a weighted score for each attribute for each device. These weighted scores are then totaled to determine the overall rating for each device. These ratings determine the relative ability of each device to meet the user requirements. For example, consider the following attributes:

Accuracy	**Reliability**
Serviceability	**Performance**
Interchangeability	**Repeatability**
Safety	**Cost**

Each of these attributes is important, but some are more important than others. In assigning the weighing factors used in Figure 4.8, the clinical engineer must take into account the relative importance of each of these attributes:

- **Accuracy** is a measure of the device's ability to provide measured values within an acceptable range of some known standard. Since many clinical decisions are based on physiological or clinical chemistry measures, it is extremely important that the accuracy of a device be evaluated and tolerances established.
- **Reliability** of an instrument can be discussed quantitatively in terms of the instrument's "mean time between failures." It is possible to estimate mathematically or to test statistically the MTBF of a device. However, for most patient-care devices, this information is not available for the total system. One can, however, develop some quantitative feel for the probable engineering reliability by examining component quality, evidence of sound manufacturing, heat dissipation, and evidence of mechanical resistance to shock, impact, and vibration. Another valuable resource in reliability estimates is consultation with clinical engineers in other hospitals that use this equipment. Information is also available in private databases such as *Health Devices*, a publication that reports comparative data on medical devices.

- **Safety** issues relating to patients, the clinical staff, and visitors are covered in detail in Chapter 2. The clinical engineering department must ensure that each vendor adheres to some certain performance specifications insofar as leakage current and power interruption are concerned. Furthermore, it is important to check the provisions each vendor has made for various types of safety (mechanical, thermal, electrical, chemical, radiation, etc.).
- **Serviceability** is an important consideration because all patient-care equipment degrades or fails with time. Here, statisticians refer to "mean time to repair" (MTTR) of equipment. Minimization of MTTR requires attention to the availability of quality maintenance documentation, the spacing and ease of removal of components when they do fail, the rapid availability of any manufacturer-specific

components in the equipment, the availability of a local or central manufacturer-supported maintenance facility, and the availability of specialized training for the hospital's technicians at the vendor's plant or within the hospital.

Having determined the weighing factors and constructed the matrix, the next step is to evaluate how well each vendor meets the objectives (attributes). In Figure 4.8, the left side of the box under each vendor shows the actual score, and the right side shows the weighted score. When the weighted scores for all these attributes are totaled, Vendor #3 has the highest score. Using this approach, the clinical engineer has a quantified method for justifying any recommendation made.

Following phase 1, qualified vendors are invited to submit their equipment to the clinical evaluation phase. Once user feedback and clinical experiences are documented and tabulated and the prepurchase evaluation has been carried out, the clinical engineer is in a position to provide a fact-based recommendation to the MTEC, the clinical staff, and the hospital administrator. Based upon this recommendation, which can be justified in a quantified manner, the decision is then made.

ATTRIBUTE CATEGORIES

	Reliability	Accuracy	Repeatability	Safety	Serviceability	Interchangeability	Performance	Cost	TOTAL SCORE
Weighting Factor	9	9	8	10	9	5	9	7	
Vendor # 1	2 / 18	5 / 45	4 / 32	8 / 80	7 / 63	8 / 40	3 / 27	8 / 54	359
Vendor # 2	7 / 63	8 / 72	8 / 64	10 / 100	10 / 90	8 / 40	7 / 63	8 / 56	548
Vendor # 3	9 / 81	9 / 81	9 / 72	10 / 100	10 / 90	8 / 40	9 / 81	5 / 35	580

Figure 4.8: Matrix system used to evaluate device and vendor choices.

ITEM	CONDITION-OF-SALE NO.	DATE

VENDOR	MANUFACTURER

Part I - RADIOLOGY EQUIPMENT

In accepting this purchase order, the manufacturer or his licensed representative shall assume the responsibility of complying with the "Regulations for the Administration and Enforcement of Radiation Control for Health and Safety Act of 1968". In the event of noncompatibility, the manufacturer or his licensed representative shall petition for a variance to the FDA Center for Devices and Radiological Health and make available to this institution a copy of this variance, whether the variance is accepted or not.

Part II - GENERAL PATIENT-RELATED DIAGNOSTIC AND THERAPEUTIC ELECTRICAL EQUIPMENT

The electrical equipment in this purchase order must meet the standards set forth by the Biomedical Instrumentation Department. No payment shall be made to the manufacturer or his licensed representative unless the following standards are met:

Applicable	Not Applicable	See Comments		
			1.	Equipment shall pass the appropriate electrical leakage current tests at 115 volts, 60 cycle power in the grounded, and ungrounded correct and reverse polarities. All measurements are referenced to ground:
			a.	**Patient Contact Equipment** - 50 ua from leads and 100 ua from chassis.
			b.	**Patient Contact Equipment, Isolated Patient Connection** - 10 ua from the leads and 100 ua from the chassis.
			c.	**Nonpatient Equipment** - 500 ua from the chassis.
			d.	**Battery Operated Equipment.**
			2.	Equipment will be supplied with a 3-wire power cord & Hospital Grade Plug.
			3.	Equipment shall pass an initial inspection of all the performance specifications advertised by the manufacturer of the equipment. All tests will be performed at this institution by the manufacturer, his licensed representative, or the Biomedical Instrumentation Department. Test results documentation will be filed with the Biomedical Instrumentation Department.
			4.	Upon successful completion of the initial inspection, a 30-day operational trial period will be required. If at the end of the 30-day evaluation period the equipment does not perform as advertised, the equipment will be returned at the manufacturer's expense and this purchase order shall be voided.
			5.	Upon being placed in operation, inservice training as determined by the hospital will be provided to the hospital staff free of charge by the manufacturer or his licensed representative prior to the expiration of the warranty period.
			a.	Authorized technical service training will be made available to in-house service personnel tuition-free.
			b.	Technical service training to be held in the Houston area.
			6.	Two complete sets of operating instructions, schematics, and maintenance manuals for each separate identifiable item of equipment shall be provided.
			7.	The manufacturer will guarantee the direct sale to this institution of test fixtures and spare parts that are needed to maintain the equipment in proper condition during its life expectancy. Copies of all engineering change orders, field modifications, etc., that affect the operation of any equipment purchased under this sale, must be provided to this institution for as long as the equipment is manufactured. Parts, fixtures, etc., that are part of the above modifications will be made available for sale to this institution for installation into the equipment purchased under this order.
			8.	The manufacturer will supply to this institution, as they are published, all service bulletins, device alerts, and field modifications that pertain to the above equipment.
			9.	Compliance with all applicable local and national codes and standards is required. Including the standards of organization such as NFPA, JCAH, AAMI, EPA, ANSI, and UL.
			10.	The vendor warrants that the equipment shall be free from defects under normal use and service for a period of ____ months after the date of installation.

COMMENTS:

CONDITIONS OF SALE ISSUED BY:	DIRECTOR, BIOMEDICAL INSTRU. DEPT.	DATE
CONDITIONS OF SALE ACCEPTED BY:	MANUFACTURER'S REPRESENTATIVE	DATE

CONDITIONS OF SALE MET — APPROVED FOR PAYMENT

PURCHASE ORDER NO.		DIRECTOR, BIOMEDICAL INSTRU. DEPT.	DATE

WHITE — BIOMED COPY CANARY — VENDOR COPY PINK — ACCOUNTING COPY GOLD — PURCHASING COPY

Figure 4.9: Sample Condition of Sale form.

INSTRUMENT			CONTROL NUMBER
MANUFACTURER		MODEL	
SERIAL NUMBER	ACQUISITION COST	DATE PLACED IN SERVICE	WARRANTY EXP.
VENDOR OR SOURCE			PURCHASE ORDER NO.
DEPARTMENT		SERVICED BY	
NORMAL LOCATION(S)		LOCATION OF OPERATOR'S MANUAL	

DOCUMENTATION RECEIVED:	OPERATOR'S MANUAL	ELECTRICAL SCHEMATIC	SERVICE MANUAL
Yes			
No			

SPECIALIZED TEST EQUIPMENT REQUIRED: ____________________

ADDITIONAL TRAINING REQUIRED: ____________________

SERVICE SCHOOLS AVAILABLE: ____________________

OPERATIONAL IN ACCORDANCE WITH MANUFACTURER'S MANUAL: __________

☐ Yes

☐ No

COMMENTS: ____________________

PRECAUTIONS REQUIRED: ____________________

RELEASED TO DEPARTMENT: ________________ (DATE)

TECHNICIAN:	DATE:

Figure 4.10: Sample Incoming Inspection form.

CONTROL NO.	INSTRUMENT/MODEL	SERIAL NO.	LOCATION

After a close evaluation of the subject equipment, the following disposition is suggested:

- [ ] Obsolete
- [ ] Inadequate for intended use
- [ ] Safety Hazard to patient and/or operator
- [ ] Lack of replacement parts availability
- [ ] Requires extensive maintenance
- [ ] Requires extensive repairs
- [ ] No longer meets performance specifications
- [ ] Excess

Recommendations:

- [ ] Remove from service
- [ ] Destroy
- [ ] Sell
- [ ] Store as emergency back-up equipment

Remarks:

TECHNICIAN:	DATE:

Figure 4.11: Sample Equipment Disposition form.

EXERCISES

1. Technology assessment

   (a) concerns only the assessment of the technical performance of a medical device.
   (b) is a systematic approach to evaluating the impact of using a specific piece of medical equipment.
   (c) analyzes the impact made by the diffusion of a medical technology.
   (d) is solely concerned with the cost effectiveness of a medical technology.

2. List the various stages of technology assessment.

3. Select a specific medical technology (e.g., the excimer laser used in corneal sculpting) and discuss its relative position on its own diffusion curve.

4. The federal agency most involved in performing technology assessment for reimbursement policy is the

   (a) FDA.
   (b) OTA.
   (c) OHTA.
   (d) OMAR.

5. Propose a signal flow graph for a technology assessment process to be implemented at a medium-size hospital, as seen from the perspective of the director of clinical engineering.

6. List the steps involved in the equipment acquisition process.

7. What equipment considerations are most important to the physician? To the nurse? To the clinical engineer? To the administrator?

8. List the major steps carried out in an environmental survey regarding medical equipment procurement.

9. What is a "running cost estimate," and how is it used in equipment acquisition?

10. Discuss the matrix approach in evaluating a specific medical device (e.g., a defibrillator).

11. What four factors are especially important in assessing the efficacy of a specific medical technology?

12. List the four factors that are crucial to a diagnostic technology's accuracy.

13. Explain the differences between the medical benefit and personal benefit of a therapeutic technology.

14. Explain the difference between the efficacy and the effectiveness of a medical technology. Use a specific medical device to illustrate the distinction.

15. What are the most important differences between randomized clinical trials and the method of natural history as means of assessing a medical technology?

16. List several quality assurance related reasons for implementing a technology assessment program.

17. Does TA serve a strategic planning role? Discuss the interrelationship between TA and strategic planning.
18. What types of standards should be used in evaluating medical equipment and how would you verify compliance with such standards?
19. What key factors should be addressed by a TA program? Select a medical device and discuss its relative performance using these factors.
20. Outline the technology assessment process, as illustrated in Figure 4.3, for a specific piece of equipment such as a magnetic resonance imager.
21. What are the three priorities of a Medical Technology Evaluation Committee and how should a clinical engineer be prepared to support the MTEC?

REFERENCES

Banta, H.D., Clyde J.B., and J.S. Williams, *Toward Rational Technology in Medicine: Considerations for Health Policy*, Springer Verlag, New York, 1981.

Bronzino, J.D. and Hayes, T.P. "Hospital-Based Clinical Engineering Programs," in *Handbook on Biomedical Engineering* (J. Kline, ed.), Academic Press, New York, pp. 565–595, 1988.

Chu, F. and Cotter, D. "PPS Policies Should Reflect Payment Adjustments for New Technologies," *Business and Health*, 4:60, 1986.

Committee on Technology and Health Care Assembly of Engineering, National Research Council and Institute of Medicine. *Medical Technology and the Health Care System: A Study of the Diffusion of Equipment-Embodied Technology*, Office of Publications, National Academy of Sciences, Washington, D.C., 1979.

Council on Health Care Technology, Institute of Medicine. *Improving Consensus Development for Health Technology Assessment: An International Perspective*, (C. Goodman and S. Baratz, eds.), National Academy Press, Washington D.C., 1990.

David, Y. "Technology Evaluation at the Hospital Level," *Proc. 6th Ann. Meeting of the International Society of Technology Assessment in Health Care*, Cambridge University Press, Cambridge, 1990.

Doessel, D. "Medical Technology and Expenditure: An Economic Review and Proposal," *International Journal of Health Planning and Management*, 1:253–273, 1986.

Fineberg, H.V. "Gastric Freezing: A Study of Diffusion of a Medical Technology," in *Medical Technology and the Health Care System: A Study of the Diffusion of Equipment-Embodied Technology*, National Academy of Sciences, Washington D.C., 1979.

Food and Drug Administration, U.S. Department of Health and Human Services. *General Considerations for the Clinical Evaluation of Drugs*, U.S. Government Printing Office, Washington, D.C., 1977.

Gordon, G.J. and Tan, K.M. "Technology Assessment and Equipment Planning in Kaiser Permenente, Northern California Region," *J. Clin. Engin.*, 17(3), pp. 209–213, 1992.

Institute of Medicine. *Assessing Medical Technologies*, National Academy Press, Washington, D.C., 1985.

Institute of Medicine. *Assessment of Diagnostic Technology in Health Care*, National Academy Press, Washington, D.C., 1989.

Jennett, B. "Benefits and Burdens of Surgery," *Brit. J. Surg.*, 72:939–941, 1985.

Jennett, B. *High Technology Medicine, Benefits and Burdens*, Oxford University Press, Oxford, 1986.

Jennett, B. "Assessment of clinical technologies," *Internat. J. Technol. Assessment in Health Care*, 4:435–445, 1988.

Mantil, J., Willett, R., and Sawyer, W. "Medical High-Technology Assessment and Implementation in a Community Hospital: Nuclear Magnetic Resonance," *Biomed. Instr. Technol.*, 25(4):289–296, 1991.

McConnell, E.A. "Technology Assessment in Health Care," in *Plant, Technology, and Safety Management*, Series No. 1, JCAHO, Oakbrook Terrace, Il, pp. 7–12, 1992.

McDermott, W. "Evaluating the Physician and his Technology," *Daedelus*, 10:135–157, 1977.

National Institutes of Health. *Draft Research Plan, FY:1985*, NIH, Bethesda, MD, 1985.

Oakes, J.B., and Gordon, D.H. "Equipment acquisition," in *Clinical Engineering: Principles and Practices*, (J. Webster and A. Cook, eds.), Prentice Hall, Englewood Cliffs, NJ, pp. 195–234, 1974.

Office of Technology Assessment, U.S. Congress. *Policy Implications of the Computed Tomography (CT) Scanner: An Update*, U.S. Government Printing Office, Washington, D.C., 1978.

Office of Technology Assessment, U.S. Congress. *Strategies for Medical Technology and Assessment*, U.S. Government Printing Office, Washington, D.C. 1982.

Office of Technology Assessment, U.S. Congress. *Health Technology Case Study 36: Effects of Federal Policies on Extracorporeal Shock Wave Lithotripsy*, U.S. Government Printing Office, Washington, D.C. 1986.

Russell, L.B. *Technology in Hospitals: Medical Advances and Their Diffusion*, The Brookings Institution, Washington, D.C., 1979.

Shaffer, M.D., and Shaffer, M.J. "Clinical Engineering Participation in Hospital Technology Assessment," *Biomedical Instrumentation and Technology*, 25(4):282–286, 1991.

Simmons, D.A., and Wear, J.O. *Clinical Engineering Manual*: 3rd ed., Scientific Enterprises, North Little Rock, AR, 1988.

Steinberg, E.P., Sisk, J.E., and Locke K.E. "The Diffusion of Magnetic Resonance Imagers in the United States and the World," *Internat. J. Technol. Assessment in Health Care*, 1:537–545, 1985.

Tancredi, L.R. "Social and Ethical Implications in Technology Assessment," in *Critical Issues in Medical Technology*, (D.J. McNeil and E.J. Cravalho, eds.), Auburn House, 1982.

Tomasik, K.M. "Assessing and Acquiring New Technologies: An Introduction," in *Plant, Technology, and Safety Management*, Series No. 1, JCAHO, Oakbrook Terrace, Il, pp. 5–6, 1992.

Weinberg, J.H. "Dealing with Medical Practice Variations: A Proposal for Action," *Health Affairs*, 3:6–32, 1984.

CHAPTER 5

CODES, STANDARDS, AND REGULATIONS

The subject of codes, standards, and regulations is often considered to be a rather dry and tiresome topic. But this need not always be the case, especially in light of the dynamics associated with modern health-care, i.e., the concerns regarding cost and quality assurance. Since most individuals, including health-care professionals, consider it an affront to be told what to do and how to do it, one look at the current version of the Code of Federal Regulations would be enough to make most members of the medical staff cringe at the prospect of knowing and understanding every applicable requirement. For practicing clinical engineers, the best approach is to acquire a solid overview of the standards that apply to the various applications falling within their domain and to develop or have access to a comprehensive library of reference materials.

There are many advocates for the development, publication, and use (both mandatory and voluntary) of standards. One well-known proponent declares: "*One general statement can be applied to all (technical) standards. Standards consolidate scientific and technical knowledge, making possible a mechanism that brings the benefits of scientific research into widespread application. Standards are mankind's best communication medium for broadcasting technical progress*" (Batik, 1989).

To justify the existence of standards, one need look no further than the foundation upon which the United States form of government is based. The Founding Fathers included as a basic tenet in the Preamble of the Constitution of the United States the need "to promote the general welfare." Since it is reasonable to characterize the health-care industry as intimately tied to the general welfare of the nation's citizens, codes and standards are required to ensure safe and effective health-care services. Clinical engineering, as a distinct professional discipline, owes its existence to the desire to ensure the safe and beneficial use of modern technology in the provision of health-care.

Another positive aspect of the promulgation of and adherence to standards is the avoidance of "reinventing the wheel." As discussed in Chapter 1, it is unlikely that any single clinical engineer can acquire expert knowledge that encompasses the entire discipline. Although it is theoretically possible that through education and experience each clinical engineer can develop and implement criteria for the evaluation, acquisition, and safe use of technology in the modern hospital, the availability of codes and standards makes this task more efficient and manageable.

A third motivating factor associated with the need to be familiar with applicable codes, standards, and regulations is liability. Failure to adhere to established norms for performance of services in the public sector may result in consequences that range from personal disciplinary action through nonaccreditation of a hospital and include civil prosecution, fines, and even imprisonment. Since ignorance of requirements is not an excuse that holds up in court, it is essential that every effort be made to establish and document compliance with appropriate standards.

Finally, in reviewing the Canon of Ethics for engineers, it is clear that the efforts and activities of all engineering professionals are subject to certain standards. As discussed in more detail in Chapter 10, professional engineering ethics requires that engineers *"strive to increase the competence and prestige of the engineering profession."* Furthermore, they are encouraged to exchange information and experience with other engineers. Since professional engineers are licensed according to rules and regulations established by the state in which they practice, consider the following: **The Connecticut Department of Consumer Protection**, Board of Registration for Professional Engineers and Land Surveyors, Rules and Regulations, Section 20-200-12, Code of Ethics, Part I, states that *"(1) The engineer shall at all times recognize his (her) primary obligation to protect the safety, health and welfare of the public in the performance of his (her) professional duties,"* and *"(2) The rules of professional conduct as promulgated herein are an exercise of the police powers invested in the Board by virtue of the Acts of the Legislature, and as such, the Board is authorized to establish conduct, policy, and practices in accordance with the powers herein above stated."* Thus, when employed in combination with technical knowledge and competence, codes, standards, and regulations provide necessary guidelines through which this obligation may be achieved.

The purpose of this chapter is to present some of the more relevant codes, standards and regulations that affect the practicing clinical engineer. Also provided is a historical perspective on the regulatory influences in our society and definitions that will assist in understanding the differences between codes, standards, and regulations. Highlights of some documents and document-producing agencies that most affect clinical engineers are discussed.

Before considering the world of codes, standards, and regulations, it is important to note that it is one steeped in acronyms. Thus, **OSHA** is used instead of **the Occupational Safety and Health Administration** and **FDA** is used instead of **The Food and Drug Administration**. In the spirit of simplification, "codes, standards, and regulations" will be referred to as "CS&Rs," and similar acronyms will be used at every opportunity.

HISTORY

Even in antiquity, certain measures were present for the protection of the uninformed layperson. For example, more than four thousand years ago, the **Code of Laws** of Hammurabi, a king in the region now known as Iraq, contained the following regulations dealing with builders: *"If a builder erect a house for a man and do not make its construction firm, and the house which he built collapse and cause the death of the owner of the house, that builder shall be put to death."*

Even in the Bible, one finds the presence of standards. In Genesis, for example, the Lord instructs Noah: *"Make thee an ark from resinous wood, sealing it with pitch."* Today, such instructions would be called a standard specification for ark building.

Advances in technology have often been the primary stimulant for the development of standards and regulations. Often, stimulated by certain disasters, the use of new technologies has led to the creation of standards or regulations that control their safe use. Consider the following examples:

- **Steam power**. Although a major factor in the industrialization of modern society, the misuse of steam power was initially very destructive. In 1884, at the height of the American Industrial Revolution, approximately 10,000 boiler explosions and failures occurred in the United States alone. The property damage, fatalities, and injuries were staggering. However, with the development of the **American Society of Mechanical Engineers (ASME) Boiler and Pressure Vessel Code**, these horrible statistics were significantly improved. In recent times, e.g., for the period 1974–1984, there was not a single boiler failure in the United States.

- **Electricity**. The initial use of electricity in the latter part of the nineteenth century also produced a significant number of accidents, thereby motivating the development of a safety code for its use. What is now the **Institute of Electrical and Electronics Engineers** (IEEE) National Electrical Safety Code (not to be confused with the NFPA National Electrical Code) evolved from concerns regarding the safe use of electrical energy.
- **Fire Protection**. In 1895, a small group of men representing sprinkler and fire insurance interests gathered in Boston to discuss the inconsistencies in existing automatic sprinkler systems. For example, nine radically different standards for piping sizes and head spacing were being used within a one hundred mile radius of the city. As a result of their efforts, a standard for the uniform installation of sprinklers was developed. The descendants of this standard can be found today among some 280 specific fire safety standards maintained by the **National Fire Protection Association (NFPA)**. Consider the following two examples:

1. Baltimore was the site of an early twentieth-century fire that went out of control and spread throughout the city. Fire companies from as far away as one hundred miles rushed to the aid of the stricken city, but to no avail. It was found that their hose couplings could not attach to the hydrants, nor to other hoses—there were no standard couplings. As a result, the firemen watched helplessly as Baltimore burned. This disaster stimulated the establishment of standard hose couplings by the NFPA and standard screw threads by the ASME.
2. In 1911, the Triangle Shirtwaist Company, a sweat shop in the lower part of Manhattan in New York where women's blouses were made, was the scene of a tragic fire. Situated in a loft building that had no fire escapes, fire extinguishers, or sprinklers, hundreds of seamstresses were laboring over their sewing machines when a fire broke out. With its piles of cloth and oily machinery, the loft was quickly ablaze. Trapped, many women leaped to their deaths from the sixth floor, their long hair and full skirts ablaze. Photographs of this horror were published in newspapers and shocked the nation, stimulating the development of the NFPA National Fire Code and significant New York State safety legislation.

- **Ship Safety**. In 1912 the "unsinkable" Titanic went down in the North Atlantic with an estimated 2200 people aboard, of whom only 705 were saved. Given her tonnage, the British Board of Trade regulations of the day required lifeboat space for only 962 people. As a result of this tragedy, these regulations were reviewed and modified.

Throughout the twentieth-century, rapidly changing economic and social conditions also played a major role in the evolution of regulatory activity. The Progressive Era, the years between the turn of the century and World War I, ushered in a number of reforms relating to labor and working conditions, partly in reaction to the power of the reigning captains of industry.

The 1920s were the Golden Age of Standards. The influence of technology was profound. The secretary of the Department of Commerce was an engineer, and many of the great corporations were headed by technical people. There was a significant appreciation of industrialization, mass production manufacturing, and the need for standardization. As a result, it was the heyday of trade associations, and even of the federal government became involved and started to develop commodity and commercial standards through the **National Institute of Standards and Technology**.

The financial crisis triggered by the stock market crash of 1929 paved the way for the introduction of socially motivated legislation aimed at alleviating the plight of the people during the Great Depression. Franklin Roosevelt's New Deal initiatives included major laws regarding social security, food and drug regulation, child labor, and public health services. Roosevelt's insistence that there was a national interest superior to and separate from the business interest justified an enormous growth in the prestige and power of the federal government. This growth may have been the single most important phenomenon of the 1930s.

Whereas the years leading up to World War II can best be characterized by industrial development, the last 50 years have been nothing short of a technological revolution. Advances in nuclear science, electronics, communications, molecular biology, lasers, computers, robotics, and a host of other science-based technologies have been overwhelming. Not surprisingly, there has been a high level of activity in developing standards and regulations aimed at controlling these powerful instruments of progress. An additional factor propelling the growth of CS&R effort has been the reawakening of a social awareness. Protecting the health and safety of the worker and consumer has become a concern to all. To illustrate the power of social awareness, two examples of media-induced standards development come to mind. The first is the article published in March 1971 in which Ralph Nader claimed that more than 1,200 hospital patients were being electrocuted each year by faulty medical devices. Drastic changes in code requirements for equipment and facilities resulted almost overnight. In the second example, a former anesthesia resident wrote an article describing his experiences working in an operating room. Within two years, the **National Institute of Occupational Safety and Health** issued guidelines for anesthetic gas waste scavenging systems and work practices in operating rooms.

Clearly, events, and especially tragic ones, have shaped our views in regulating technology. With these historical perspectives in mind, the specific CS&Rs that affect the practice of clinical engineering can now be discussed.

DEFINITIONS

The terms "codes," "standards," and "regulations" are often used interchangeably and thus can cause a great deal of interpretive confusion. The compact edition of the *Oxford English Dictionary* (there ought to be a standard for minimum print size!) cites no less than 30 different definitions of the word "standard." Perhaps the most appropriate definition here is the one that states: *"A definite level of excellence, attainment, wealth, or the like, or a definite degree of any quality, viewed as a prescribed object of endeavor or as a measure of what is adequate for some purpose."* In effect, the term "standard" is the starting point or foundation of a legal hierarchy. The following definitions will be used throughout the remainder of this chapter:

Standard: Documents that are perceived to establish a minimum level of performance or to standardize such items as test methods, specifications, properties, definitions, or practices. These documents do not have the force of law.

Code: A system of standards relating to the same topic (e.g., fire code, electrical code). The code may be adopted by government or private entities in whole or in part. Enforcement of the provisions of the code lies with the government (local, state, or federal), turning the standards into regulatory documents, or with the private entity (NFPA National Electric Code), by weight of its standing in the community.

Regulation: A document that is issued originally by a government or private entity. It may include in whole or in part a standard or, in lieu of inclusion, reference to a standard. A regulation has the force of law from the start.

"Regulation," in a more narrow interpretation, means setting restraints on individuals and groups, directly compelling them to take, or not to take, certain actions.

An important subgroup of standards are the "voluntary consensus standards." The term "voluntary" applies to both the preparation and use of this type of standard. In its preparation, those involved, freely and without coercion, gave of their time, effort, and knowledge to develop the standard. In its use, the standard is applied or not applied with full knowledge that lack of conformity to the standard will be subject to judgment by those who promulgated the standard, by consumers of services, and possibly by the courts. The term "consensus" is not synonymous with compromise, but rather implies an agreement arrived at by those concerned. "Compromise," on the other hand, is a position arrived at by mutual concessions. The two terms are not mutually exclusive. Many of the most important hospital clinical engineering standards were developed as voluntary consensus standards.

"Proprietary" standards are those developed either by a company for its own internal use or by a trade association for use by its members. These standards can serve as a basis for voluntary standards or regulations if appropriate exposure is provided and if consensus is reached among all parties.

ROLE OF THE UNITED STATES GOVERNMENT

As highlighted in the discussion about the historical development of standards, the role of the federal government as "regulator" is essentially a twentieth-century phenomenon. An analysis of the structure of government as it relates to regulatory affairs, especially from a political perspective, would go far beyond the scope or intent of this chapter. Suffice it to say that the underlying motivation of the regulatory activities of the federal government is the protection and welfare of its citizens.

At the federal level, laws originate as acts that have been passed by both the House of Representatives and the Senate and have been signed by the president. They are numbered according to the number of the congressional session in which they were approved, followed by a number designating the consecutive number in which each measure (bill or resolution) was passed. Thus, Public Law 94-295 was the 295th measure passed by the 94th Congress.

Texts of measures which become statutory laws may be found in *Public Laws, Statutes at Large*, and the *United States Code* (USC). The USC groups all laws according to titles (e.g., Food and Drugs, Labor, Public Buildings, Property, and Works), the broad topics with which the laws deal. Revised every six years and kept up to date with supplements between revisions, the most recent edition is the eleventh USC, which was revised in 1988.

Officials and agencies of the U.S. government that have the responsibility of carrying out the laws enacted by Congress issue regulations to put them into effect. Although they are not called laws, the regulations issued by the executive departments and agencies of the federal government generally have the force of law. U.S. government regulations are published in the **Code of Federal Regulations** (CFR), a codification of the general and permanent rules published in the Federal Register. The CFR groups the regulations under 50 titles. The numbers are frequently consistent with the USC.

Keeping informed about these regulations or even locating one is no easy task because so many are issued or changed each year. Each volume of the CFR is revised at least once each year and is issued on a quarterly basis in a staggered fashion. The CFR is kept up to date by individual issues of the Federal Register, which is published five days a week and is often a hundred pages or more in length. The CFR and the Federal Register must be used together to determine the latest version of any given rule. The task is made somewhat less formidable by the monthly publication of the *Cumulative List of CFR Sections Affected.*

The Office of Management and Budget

Circular A-119, dated 17 January 1980 and titled "Federal Participation in the Development and Use of Voluntary Standards," announced the intention of the federal government to save money by obviating the development of in-house federal standards for use in the procurement process. The memorandum established the following criteria for acceptance of voluntary standards: the process must include open meetings, representation of all concerned parties, consensus decisions, mechanisms in place to handle complaints and appeals, adequate public notice, and periodic review. This policy has been very effective and has avoided the development of conflicting standards and unnecessary duplication of effort and cost.

The Food and Drug Administration

The origins of the FDA can be traced to one individual, Harvey W. Wiley, Chief chemist of the Agriculture Department's Bureau of Chemistry during the early twentieth-century. Soon after joining the bureau in 1883, he began experimenting with food and drug adulteration. His most famous experiments took the form of feeding small doses of poisons to a group of human volunteers. The substances fed to the volunteers were similar or identical to those found in then-common food preservatives. Dubbed the "Poison Squad," the volunteers generated publicity for Wiley's experiments and created a public awareness of the dangers of eating adulterated foods. This publicity led Congress to enact the Food and Drug Act of 1906, which called for the protection of the public from the potential health hazards presented by adulterated and mislabeled foods and drugs. That law since has been extended by the Food, Drug, and Cosmetics Act of 1938 and various amendments to it, the Public Health Service Act of 1944, the Fair Packaging and Labeling Act of 1966, the Radiation Control for Health and Safety Act of 1968, and the Drug Price Competition and Patent Competition Act of 1984.

The FDA was given additional powers in 1976 when Congress passed legislation requiring regulation of medical devices and diagnostic products. The 1976 Medical Device Amendments (MDAs) provide the following definition of products subject to regulation 201(H): The term device means an instrument, apparatus, implement, machine, contrivance, implant, in-vitro reagent, or other similar or related article including any component, part, or accessory which is:

1. Recognized in the official National Formulary, or the United States Pharmacopoeia, or any supplement to them.

2. Intended for use in the diagnosis of disease, or other conditions, or in the cure, mitigation, treatment or prevention of disease, in man or other animals.
3. Intended to affect the structure or any function of the body of man or other animals, and which does not achieve any of its principal intended purposes through chemical action within or on the body of man or other animals and which is not dependent upon being metabolized for the achievement of any of its principal intended purposes.

The MDAs establish a device classification scheme that subjects products to three levels of scrutiny:

Class I: General controls: A device that is found to be adequate, as specified in Sections 501, 502, 510 (registration), 516 (banned device), 518 (notification), and 520 (device controls), to provide a reasonable assurance of safety and effectiveness. These controls include

- Adulteration.
- Mislabeling.
- Classification change.
- Records and reporting.
- Good manufacturing practices.
- Traceability.
- Custom devices
- Restricted devices.
- Administrative restraint.

Class II: Performance standards: A finding must be made that general controls are insufficient to provide reasonable assurance of safety and effectiveness, that standards would be sufficient, and that there is sufficient information available about the device to establish a standard.

Class III: Premarket approval: Devices in this classification will be required to undergo premarket approval according to requirements of the Amendments and implementing regulations. Devices in this class will be those for which not enough is known to determine if general controls would provide a reasonable assurance of safe and effective performance and not enough is known to establish a performance standard. Further, a device will not be assigned to Class III unless

1. It is intended for a use in supporting or sustaining human life or is of substantial importance in preventing impairment of human health.
2. It presents a potential unreasonable risk of illness or injury. New devices will be automatically placed in a premarket clearance category unless and until a petition to reclassify the device is approved.

Additional MDA provisions allow for the granting of Investigational Device Exemptions (IDEs), protection of trade secrets, device manufacturing facility inspections, state and local requirements, and exportation. IDEs preserve a mechanism for clinical research on new devices, but in return, the FDA requires an application, the maintenance of records, ongoing progress reports, filing of clinical testing protocols, Institutional Review Board oversight, and the obtaining of informed consent from test subjects.

Once a product has been approved for release to the market, it is then subject to the reporting and recall provisions of the MDAs. Medical device problems are more often than not discovered by users in the field, and they usually consist of such deficiencies as improper labeling, defective components, performance failure, inadequate instructions, erroneous information, or improper use. Upon notification of a problem, the FDA may require the manufacturer to remove the device from the marketplace or correct distributed products. There are three recall classifications. Note that the order of importance or degree of consequence is exactly the reverse of approval classes:

Class I: URGENT — LIFE THREATENING

A situation in which there is a reasonable probability that the use of or exposure to a violative product will cause serious, adverse health consequences or death.

Class II: SERIOUS — CORRECTIVE ACTION REQUIRED

A situation in which the use of or exposure to a violative product may cause temporary or medically reversible health consequences or where the probability of serious, adverse health consequences is remote.

Class III: ADVISORY

A situation in which the use of or exposure to a violative product is not likely to cause adverse health consequences.

Manufacturers must report problems directly to the FDA. In those instances in which a problem is detected in the field, a reporting mechanism has been available for many years through the United States Pharmacopoeia and its Voluntary Medical Device and Laboratory Problem Reporting Program (Figure 5.1). The **Emergency Care Research Institute (ECRI)** also supports a User Experience Network and publishes forms for reporting a problem or hazard related to equipment (Figure 5.2). Upon receipt of a report, the FDA may then publish its findings and actions in the Device Enforcement Notifications (DENs).

In 1983, the FDA initiated a reorganization that combined the **Bureau of Medical Devices** and the **Bureau of Radiological Health** into the **Center for Devices and Radiological Health (CDRH)**. It also combined the **Bureau of Drugs** and the **Bureau of Biologics** into the **Center for Drugs and Biologics (CDB)**.

In 1990, Congress passed the Safe Medical Devices Act (Public Law 101–629), which granted the FDA additional authority to obtain information concerning serious device problems, to remove defective devices from use more quickly than previously, and to provide enhanced assurance of the safety and effectiveness of new medical devices (see Chapter 2). This new law places significant emphasis on postmarket surveillance and regulatory controls. Under the new law, device user facilities—i.e., hospitals, ambulatory surgical units, outpatient treatment and diagnostic facilities, and nursing homes—are required to report incidents in which a medical device caused or contributed to the serious injury, illness, or death of a patient or to the potential thereof. Furthermore, the new law required that device distributors be included in the reporting requirements that already applied to device manufacturers. Manufacturers of certain types of devices (implants, life-support or life-sustaining devices) must fulfill additional requirements, such as tracking devices and conducting postmarket surveillance of their own products.

Form Approved; OMB No. 0910-0143

DATE RECEIVED

ACCESS NO

Medical Device & Laboratory Product Problem Reporting Program

SMDA

1. PRODUCT IDENTIFICATION:

Name of Product and Type of Device
(Include sizes or other identifying characteristics and attach labeling, if available)

Manufacturer's Name __________

Manufacturer's City, State, Zip Code __________

Is this a disposable item? YES ☐ NO ☐

Lot Number(s) and Expiration Date(s) (if applicable)

Serial Number(s)

Manufacturer's Product Number and/or Model Number

2. REPORTER INFORMATION:

Your Name __________ Today's Date __________

Title and Department __________

Facility's Name __________

Street Address __________

City __________ State ______ Zip ______ Phone ( ) ______ Ext: ______

3. PROBLEM INFORMATION:

Date event occurred __________

Please indicate how you want your identity publicly disclosed:

No public disclosure ☐

To the manufacturer/distributor ☐

To the manufacturer/distributor and to anyone who requests a copy of the report from the FDA ☐

This event has been reported to: Manufacturer ☐ FDA ☐

Other __________

If requested, will the actual product involved in the event be available for evaluation by the manufacturer or FDA? YES ☐ NO ☐

Problem noted or suspected (Describe the event in as much detail as necessary. Attach additional pages if required. Include how and where the product was used. Include other equipment or products that were involved. Sketches may be helpful in describing problem areas.)

Figure 5.1: Example of a Product Problem Reporting Program form of the type supported by the ECRI.

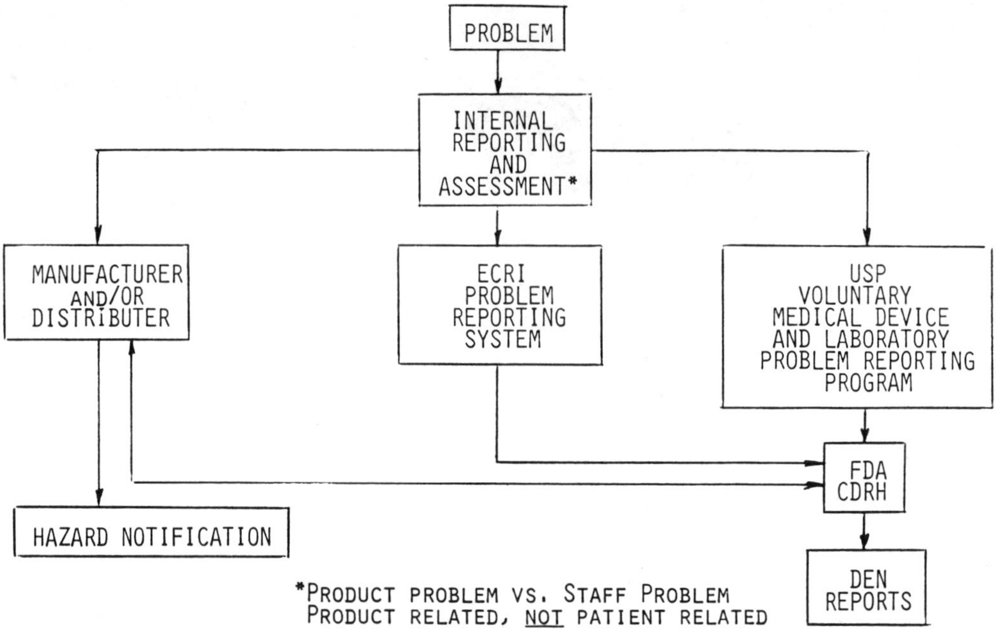

Figure 5.2: Reporting procedures supported by the ECRI for medical device problems.

The new law also gave the FDA additional enforcement powers. The FDA can now order manufacturers to immediately stop distribution of a medical device and to notify health professionals and users to stop its use. The new law also establishes civil penalties for violations of these new provisions, with fines of up to $15,000 for each violation and up to $1 million for all violations in a single suit. The FDA can issue subpoenas for evidence and testimony in civil proceedings.

Under the new law, mandatory performance standards are no longer required for each Class II device. Instead, standards are one of several "special controls" the FDA may use to regulate Class II products. Other provisions of the new law provide for reclassification of transitional devices, humanitarian exemptions for life-saving devices used to treat conditions affecting fewer than 4000 patients, the regulation of combination products, and preproduction quality assurance.

The Occupational Safety and Health Administration

The Occupational Safety and Health Administration (**OSHA**) was established as an agency within the **Department of Labor** by the Occupational Safety and Health Act of 1970. One of OSHA's major tasks is to develop standards to protect individuals in the work place. The agency's standards fall into four major categories: general industry, maritime, construction, and agriculture. When it first started, OSHA adopted many of the consensus standards that had been developed over the years by the **American National Standards Institute** and the **National Fire Protection Association**. These standards, however, frequently represented minimum rather than ideal degrees of protection. OSHA has worked to update, revise, and add to these standards to cover as many potential workplace hazards as possible.

OSHA can begin standards-setting procedures on its own initiative or on petition from other parties, including the secretary of the **Department of Health and Human Services (HHS)**, the **National Institute of Occupational Safety and Health (NIOSH)**, state and local governments, nationally recognized standards-producing organizations, employers, labor representatives, or any other interested person.

In order to enforce its standards and regulations, OSHA is authorized to conduct workplace inspections and investigations. With very few exceptions, inspections are conducted without advance notice. Before 1978, OSHA compliance officers were allowed to enter a workplace without a search warrant. However in May 1978, the Supreme Court ruled in *Marshall versus Barlow's Inc.* that an employer has the right to refuse admission to an OSHA inspector who does not have a search warrant. The ruling has not had a dramatic effect on the agency, however, since employers have usually been willing to admit the compliance officers without a warrant.

The general industry standards (29 CFR Part 1910) that are most applicable to hospitals cover the following areas relating to occupational safety and health:

- Walking–working surfaces.
- Means of egress.
- Powered platforms, manlifts, and vehicle-mounted work platforms.
- Occupational health and environmental control.
- Hazardous materials.
- Personal protective equipment.
- General environmental controls.
- Medical and first aid.
- Fire protection.
- Compressed gases and compressed air equipment.
- Materials handling and storage.
- Machinery and machine guarding.
- Hand and portable tools and other hand held equipment.
- Welding, cutting, and brazing.
- Special industries.
- Electrical.

Effective November 1985, OSHA promulgated 29 CFR Part 1910.1200, the Hazard Communication Standard (HCS), the purpose of which was *"to ensure that the hazards of all chemicals produced or imported by chemical manufacturers or importers are evaluated, and that information concerning their hazards is transmitted to affected employers and employees. This transmittal of information is to be accomplished by means of comprehensive hazard communication programs, which are to include container labeling and other forms of warning, material safety data sheets (MSDSs), and employee training."*

This HCS initially covered 14 million workers in more than 300,000 manufacturing establishments. The ink was barely dry on the HCS, however, when labor organizations and citizens groups began to protest the standard's limited coverage. In August 1987, after two years of deliberation, OSHA completed an expansion of the HCS. The coverage now extends to more than 32 million workers at some 3.8 million firms, including hospitals, determined simply by whether the company, firm or institution uses hazardous chemicals. The HCS outlines several steps required for compliance:

1. Hazard Evaluation. Chemical manufacturers and importers are required to evaluate the chemicals produced or imported to determine if they are hazardous. Any substance that presents a physical or health hazard, as defined by OSHA, is considered regulated under the HCS. OSHA has designated four separate lists of chemicals that make up a baseline for regulated chemicals:

- 29 CFR Part 1910 Subpart Z: Toxic and Hazardous Chemicals (OSHA)
- National Toxicology Program (NTP), Annual Report on Carcinogens (latest edition)
- **International Agency for Research on Cancer** (**IARC**), Monographs (latest edition)
- Threshold Limit Values for Chemical Substances and Physical Agents in the Workplace Environment, American Conference of Governmental Industrial Hygienists (ACGIH)

There are about 1200 chemicals specifically listed as regulated. However, it is important to note that a substance may be regulated even though it is not on any list. These regulations also address substances that are exempt from the standard, such as those already regulated by other government agencies or where exposure is minimal:

2. Labels and Other Forms of Warning. The purpose of labels on hazardous chemicals or on products containing them is to warn about potential danger or significant risk. They serve as an immediate warning on containers and as a reminder for more detailed information provided in other formats (posters, MSDSs, written programs). The HCS covers two types of hazard: physical and health. Table 5.1 illustrates these categories.

Beyond the general requirements for substances in the four lists given above, OSHA has developed specific health standards for more than 20 substances. Of particular concern within the hospital environment are asbestos (found in building materials), benzene (sometimes used in clinical chemistry and research reagents), formaldehyde (used in anatomic pathology as a tissue preservative), and ethylene oxide (used as a gas sterilant).

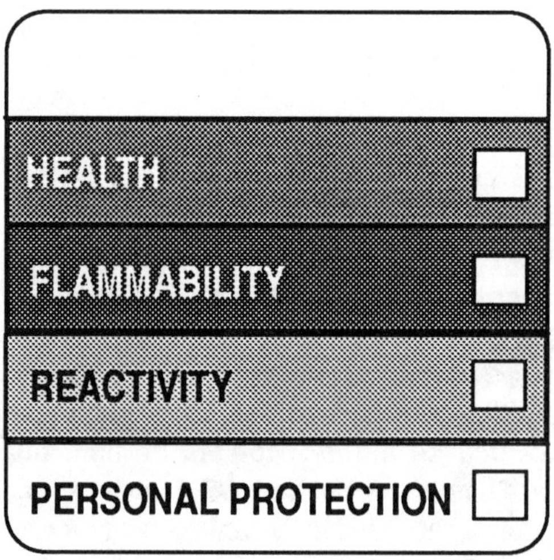

Figure 5.3: The NCPA hazardous materials identification labeling system.

Table 5.1: Hazards Associated with Chemicals

Health Hazards	Physical Hazards
Carcinogenic	Combustible liquid
Acutely toxic	Compressed gas
Chronically toxic	Explosive
Reproductive toxin	Flammable
Irritant	Organic peroxide
Corrosive	Corrosive
Sensitizer	Oxidizer
Hepatotoxin	Pyrophoric
Nephrotoxin	Unstable (reactive)
Neurotoxin	Water-reactive
Agents damaging to the lungs, skin, eyes, or mucous membranes	
Agents which act on the hematopoietic system	

Two of the most common labeling systems in use today are those developed by the NFPA and the **National Paint and Coating Association.** Figure 5.3 illustrates an example of the NPCA *Hazardous Materials Identification System* (HMIS) label. In label, poster, or sign form, the HMIS provides information on:

- Chemical identity.
- Degree of acute health, flammability, and reactivity hazards. Each label contains three colored horizontal bars: blue for health, red for flammability, and yellow for reactivity, each has a separate numerical code on a scale of 0 to 4; 0 denotes a minimal hazard, 4 denotes a severe hazard.
- Proper personal protective equipment (often designated by symbols or coded letters).

The NFPA labeling system is very similar to the HMIS. When known, the specific target organ effect must be part of the hazard warning.

Material Safety Data Sheets. Chemical manufacturers and importers must obtain or develop an MSDS for each hazardous chemical they produce or import. The appropriate MSDS must be provided to all distributors and employers with the initial shipment of the chemical, and with the first shipment after an MSDS is updated. Certain information, at a minimum, must appear on every MSDS:

- Identity (chemical and common names).
- If a mixture, hazardous ingredients and concentrations.
- Physical and chemical characteristics.
- Physical hazards.
- Health hazards (including if it is a carcinogen).
- Primary routes of entry.
- Symptoms of overexposure.
- Permissible exposure limits.
- Emergency/first aid procedures.

- Precautions for safe handling.
- Recommended engineering controls.
- Date of preparation.
- Name, address, and telephone number of manufacturer.

Employers must maintain copies of MSDSs for each hazardous chemical in use at their workplaces and ensure that they are available during each work shift to employees at their workplaces.

OSHA developed a data sheet in the 1970s primarily for the shipbuilding industry. Designated as Form 20, it is now obsolete. In 1986, responding to many industry requests, OSHA released a new form that complied with the requirements of the HCS; Form 174. The use of this form is not mandatory, but the minimum information content given above is

4. **Employee Training.** Under the HCS, employers must establish a training and information program for all employees routinely exposed to hazardous chemicals in their workplace. This training must be provided at the time of initial assignment and whenever a new hazard is introduced. The standard is performance-oriented, specifying the results but not mandating the methods to be used. At a minimum, the following topics must be thoroughly covered:

- The Health Communication Standard: Employees must be informed of the existence of the HCS, what it requires, and what it will do for them.
- Terminology: Must be understandable.
- MSDSs: Availability and content.
- Labels.
- The written HCS program.
- Specific chemicals used by each employee.
- Appropriate personal protective equipment.
- First aid and emergency procedures.

It is advisable to document which employees have been trained and when they received the training. If any Subpart Z substances with specific health standards are used, their specific requirements for safe use must be incorporated into the training program.

5. **Written Hazard Communication Program.** This program is the written record of what your institution has done to comply with the HCS. The written record should include

- An inventory of all hazardous chemicals on-site.
- The corresponding MSDS files.
- The labeling program.
- Training policies, procedures, and attendance records.
- Evidence that employees have been informed about the hazards of nonroutine tasks.

Effective January 1991, OSHA promulgated 29 CFR 1910.1450, *Occupational Exposure to Hazardous Chemicals in Laboratories*, also known as the Chemical Hygiene Plan (CHP), a more stringent standard that targets laboratories.

A citation is issued if violations are discovered during an OSHA inspection. This document describes the violation and allows a reasonable amount of time for its correction. Review of contested inspections is the responsibility of the **Occupational Safety and Health Review Commission (OSHRC)**, an independent agency not connected with OSHA. OSHA only proposes penalties; the final orders imposing them are issued by the OSHRC. The law requires the commission to consider four factors when determining civil penalties: (1) the size of the business involved; (2) the gravity of the violation; (3) the good faith of the employer; and (4) the employer's history of previous violations.

The Environmental Protection Agency

Created by executive order in December 1970, **the Environmental Protection Agency (EPA)** is an independent agency in the executive branch of the federal government. The EPA took over the various air pollution, water pollution, solid waste, and radiation programs then scattered throughout the federal bureaucracy. Established at a time when the nation was becoming increasingly concerned about declining air and water quality and a general deterioration of the environment, enthusiasm for environmental legislation was sustained throughout the 1970s:

1970: Water Quality Improvement Act Amendments
Clean Air Act Amendments
1972: Federal Environmental Pesticide Control Act
Noise Control Act
Marine Protection, Research, and Sanctuaries Act
Water Pollution Control Act
1974: Safe Drinking Water Act
1976: Toxic Substances Control Act
Resource Conservation and Recovery Act (RCRA)
1980: Comprehensive Environmental Response, Compensation, and Liability Act (CERCLA)

Most of the environmental protection regulations can be found in CFR Title 40. Like OSHA regulations, they are kept up-to-date by individual issues of the Federal Register. The RCRA is the most comprehensive legislation to cover solid waste management, particularly chemically hazardous waste. Its regulations establish requirements regarding identification, labeling, packaging, transportation, and storage limitations. The hazardous waste manifest system tracks these wastes and documents "cradle-to-grave" responsibility and liability in the event that they are mishandled and damage the environment. The actual monitoring and enforcement of RCRA regulations has been delegated primarily to state environmental protection agencies. The CERCLA, also known as the Superfund act is a complicated regulation that sets up procedures for reporting and controlling hazardous substances, regulates their release into the environment, and designates waste sites targeted for federally funded clean-up. A $1.6 billion emergency fund was started, 86 percent of which was obtained from the chemical and oil industries, and 14 percent from general revenues.

The Superfund Amendments and Reauthorization Act of 1986 (SARA) established emergency planning and community right-to-know requirements. The SARA encourages and supports emergency planning efforts at the state and local levels and requires businesses to provide the authorities with information concerning toxic chemical releases and other potential chemical hazards in the community. The EPA is required to publish a list of hazardous substances and to establish a threshold planning quantity for each substance on the list. Facilities across the country are required to disclose to state and local governments information on use and storage of these hazardous substances that meet or exceed the threshold planning quantities so that emergency response plans can be developed.

The use of chlorofluorocarbons (CFCs) has been recognized as a potentially serious environmental hazard, and much discussion and activity is afoot regarding this issue. The effect on hospitals is primarily in the use of chillers, ethylene oxide sterilizers (utilizing a standard 12 percent ETO/88 percent Freon mixture that is directly exhausted into the atmosphere), and common air conditioner/refrigerator/freezer refrigerants. In 1987, the original Montreal Protocol on Substances That Deplete the Ozone Layer called for an assessment and review of control measures beginning in 1990 and occurring at a rate of one review at least every four years thereafter. The second review took place in June 1992. At that time, the phase-out schedules for CFCs, halons, carbon tetrachloride, and methyl chloroform were reviewed on the basis of available scientific, environmental, technical, and economic information. Three assessment panels have assembled this information into reports. Under the technical and economic assessment panel, six committees have completed reports on aerosols and miscellaneous uses, economic options, solvent options, halon options, refrigeration options, and foam options. Summaries from each committee were submitted to the United Nations Environment Program in October of 1991.

A great deal of the technical information gathered to date is from operations that have been successful in finding alternatives for these substances. Little information has been forthcoming on applications that are having difficulties with finding alternatives. At least one manufacturer of these chemicals (Dow/Corning) is offering consumers an opportunity to provide input to the standards development process. This opportunity is another example of a mechanism available to allow widespread participation in an activity that affects society as a whole.

As a result of significant media coverage during the summer of 1988 regarding medical waste, especially syringes and needles washing ashore on public beaches in the Northeast, The Medical Waste Tracking Act (MWTA) was enacted by Congress in the fall of 1988. It amended the RCRA by the addition of Subtitle J and directed the EPA to establish a two-year demonstration program for tracking medical wastes. Under this new law, the EPA issued regulations entitled "Standards for the Tracking and Management of Medical Waste," 40 CFR Part 259, as an interim final rule (i.e., in effect only until the MWTA is made permanent, revised, extended, or repealed). Required participants in the program included the states of Connecticut, New York, New Jersey, and Rhode Island, and the Commonwealth of Puerto Rico (the Great Lakes states respectfully declined the invitation to participate). Participating states are authorized to enforce the program. The regulations detail the following definitions and procedures:

1. **Definition of regulated medical wastes:**

   - Cultures and stocks of infectious agents.
   - Human blood and blood products.
   - Human pathological wastes, including those from surgery and autopsy.
   - Contaminated animal carcasses from medical research.
   - Wastes from patients isolated with highly communicable diseases.
   - All used sharp (e.g.,needles and scalpels) and certain unused sharp implements.

2. **Definition of generators:**
   - Physicians, dentists, veterinarians, hospitals, laboratories, etc.
   - Institutions that generate 50 pounds or more of regulated medical waste per month on- site.
   - Generators with special requirements or exemption.

3. **Pretransportation procedures:**
   - Waste segregation and separation.
   - Packaging.
   - Labeling.
   - Indelible marking.
   - Storage.

4. **Transportation requirements.**

5. **Treatment, destruction, and disposal facility requirements.**

6. **Tracking Requirements:**
   - The tracking form.
   - Exception and discrepancy reporting.
   - Exportation.

7. **Recordkeeping.**

8. **Enforcement.**

The results of the demonstration program are to be reported to Congress and are intended to help determine whether such a program should be extended nationwide. The current prevailing opinion is that even if the federal mandate does not materialize nationally, most or all states will eventually enact their own programs. The primary advantage of a federal program, discounting any disagreements about the specifics, would be its uniformity from state to state. This is a significant issue because existing permitted disposal facilities often require interstate delivery. If medical waste control becomes a permanent federal program, it will probably be incorporated into the RCRA regulations.

In addition to waste regulation under RCRA, EPA encourages the minimization of all wastes that pose a risk to human health and the environment. Minimization techniques focus on source reduction or on recycling activities that reduce either the volume or toxicity of hazardous wastes.

The Nuclear Regulatory Commission

The **Nuclear Regulatory Commission** (NRC) was created by the Energy Reorganization Act of 1974 and took over the nuclear regulatory and licensing functions of the Atomic Energy Commission, which was then abolished. The NRC is specifically charged, under authority of the Atomic Energy Act of 1954, to do the following:

- License construction and operation of nuclear reactors.
- License possession, use, transportation, handling, packaging for and disposal of nuclear materials.
- Conduct public hearings on radiological safety.
- Develop and implement rules and regulations governing licensed nuclear activities.

This charge includes certain work practices and the control of potential workplace exposures. These rules also apply, to some extent, to X-ray sources, accelerator sources, and to all radioisotope sources. Radioisotope sources are often found in the hospital environment for to cancer services (isotope "seeds" or implants), nuclear medicine imaging, blood irradiation, and research. NRC rules are found in the CFR Title 10. There is an advisory committee on the medical use of isotopes within the structure of the agency.

Most hospitals use health or medical physicists for the application and safe handling of nuclear materials. Radiation safety is more of an exact science than a management function. Usually, clinical engineers do not have responsibility for radiation safety (see Chapter 2 for a discussion).

In many states, the regulation of non-ionizing and ionizing radiation is the responsibility of the state health department. The state accepts the regulatory responsibility under the conditions of an "agreement state." Those states that participate have regulations that are at least as restrictive as those of the NRC.

The Federal Communications Commission

The **Federal Communications Commission (FCC)** is an independent regulatory agency established under the authority of the Communications Act of 1934. The first federal regulation of interstate electrical communication began with the Post Roads Act of 1866, authorizing the postmaster general to fix rates annually for government telegrams. The Radio Act of 1912 was the first law for the domestic regulation of radio communications in general. The 1934 Act set up the FCC as an agency to regulate all interstate and foreign communication by wire, radio, telephone, telegraph, and broadcasting.

The FCC regulates the offering for sale and use of devices that radiate RF energy (non-ionizing radiation). In the hospital, these may include X-ray sources, diathermy units, ultrasound systems, biomedical telemetry, and various forms of radio voice communication. For obvious reasons, there is a need for control over the frequencies of both signals and any spurious radiation (noise) generated by these devices, in terms of both preventing interference with other forms of communication and by establishing safe distances from signal sources.

BUILDING CODES

In order to design and construct a health-care facility properly, certain minimum construction standards must be followed. Typically, authority for enforcement of building standards lies at the state level, although local, city, and county authority often exists as well. Most states have in their regulations specific construction standards that are required for plan review and building permit authority. These state standards are often developed within state government with input from various groups of the design and construction industry and from user groups within the state. Quite often, however, state authorities will reference one of the three model building codes:

1. The Building Officials and Code Administrators (BOCA) International Inc. National Building Code.
2. The Southern Building Code Congress International (SBCCI) Standard Building Code.
3. The International Conference of Building Officials (ICBO) Uniform Building Code.

These model codes were developed principally by building officials charged with regulating construction activity within their areas of jurisdiction. Although each of the three model building code–writing organizations are structured independently, many of their rules and code change procedures are similar. In general, the only voting power lies with the building officials; other industry representatives are only permitted to advise during deliberations.

The three model building codes are used in different parts of the country are not referenced by the Joint Commission or Medicare, and have had very little input from the health-care industry. Quite often, however, state authorities will references the three model building codes (BOCA, SBCCI, or UBC) during hospital construction. Consequently, it is easy for a building official who might not clearly understand the function or purpose of a particular health-care service to hold to requirements that could create conflicts in the operation of the facility after it has been built. These conflicts could be related to construction, design, hardware, or function.

The Life Safety Code (LSC), published by the **National Fire Protection Association,** is the most widely referenced standard in the U.S. affecting health facility planning, design, construction, and operation. The LSC is recognized by the JCAHO and by the federal Health Care Financing Administration (Medicare). The American Society for Hospital Engineering has published a technical document that cross-references the LSC and the model building codes to help health-care facility designers and facility managers identify the similarities and conflicts. An overview of the provisions of a typical building code (BOCA) should be compared with the NFPA Life Safety Code given later in this chapter:

- Plans and specifications.
- Use classifications (e.g., Group I—Institutional).
- Type of construction.
- Siting.
- Height and area limitations.
- Interior environment and design requirements.
- Fire performance.
- Structural performance (including materials and tests).
- Exterior envelope.
- Building service systems.
- Precautions during construction (see also 29 CFR 1926).
- Energy conservation.

The BOCA Building Code references 42 other standards organizations.

Another document often referred to in the design and construction of health-care facilities is "Guidelines for Construction and Equipment of Hospital and Medical Facilities," which is published by the **American Institute of Architects** (**AIA**) in cooperation with the **U.S. Department of Health and Human Services.** The original general standards appeared in the Federal Register of February 1947 as part of the implementation regulations of the Hill–Burton program. Sections 603(b) and 1620(2) of the Public Health Service Act require the secretary of HHS to prescribe by regulation, general standards for construction, modernization, and equipment of projects assisted under Title VI and Title XVI of the act. Since the grant and loan authorities of Title VI and Title XVI have expired, there was no need to retain these standards in regulation. In 1984, HHS removed from regulation the requirements relating to minimum standards of construction, modernization, and equipment (having retitled the standard in 1974 to emphasize that the requirements were generally minimum rather than recommendations of the ideal).

The AIA guidelines contain information intended as a model standard for constructing general hospitals, skilled nursing care facilities, outpatient facilities, and rehabilitation facilities:

- Medical/surgical/postpartum nursing units.
- Intensive care units.
- Newborn nurseries.
- Pediatric and adolescent units.
- Psychiatric nursing units.
- Surgical suites.
- Obstetrical (birthing) facilities.
- Emergency service.
- Radiology suites.
- Nuclear medicine units.
- Laboratory suites.
- Rehabilitation departments.
- Respiratory therapy service.
- Morgue.
- Pharmacy.
- Dietary facilities.
- Administration and public areas.
- Medical records.
- Central services.
- General stores.
- Linen services.
- Housekeeping services.
- Employee facilities.
- Engineering service and equipment areas.
- Waste processing services.
- General standards for details and finishes.
- Design and construction, including fire-resistive standards.
- Elevators.
- Mechanical standards.
- Electrical standards.

There are extensive details, including such criteria as HVAC filter efficiencies; proper number and type of medical gas outlets for different patient-care applications; appropriate ventilation air exchange rates and temperature and humidity ranges; sound transmission limitations; hot water use; flame spread and smoke-production limitations on interior finishes; and energy management control systems. The guidelines are not intended to restrict innovations and improvements in design or construction techniques, but they do assume that appropriate architectural and engineering practice and compliance with applicable codes will be observed. This document references 18 other standards organizations and regulatory agencies.

VOLUNTARY CONSENSUS STANDARDS ORGANIZATIONS

As defined previously, a voluntary consensus standard is one that is developed by a group of individuals who give freely of their time and knowledge and who reach an agreement on the best achievable measure of performance. There are more than four hundred standards-developing organizations in the United States and more than 32,000 voluntary consensus standards. Although they are not regulatory agencies, these organizations play an important role in today's regulation activities. Many government regulations are adopted from or based upon their standards. Some of these organizations also play a prominent role in establishing standards specifically for the health-care industry. An overview of the structure and operational characteristics of some of these organizations will be helpful in gaining an understanding of how this process works.

National Fire Protection Association (NFPA)

The purpose of NFPA, (One Batterymarch Park, P.O. Box 9101, Quincy, MA 02269-9101), as stated in Article 2 of its bylaws, is to *"promote the science and improve the methods of fire protection and prevention, electrical safety and other related safety goals; to obtain and circulate information on these subjects; and to secure the cooperation of its members and the public in establishing safeguards against loss of life and property."* The primary thrust toward meeting those goals is in developing and updating standards covering all areas of fire safety. The goal of the NFPA standards program is the *"development, publication, and dissemination of timely consensus standards which are responsive to the needs of society, which are produced through a democratic, dynamic, expeditious system, and which so far as practicable, are based on performance criteria."*

The NFPA Board of Directors has general charge of all NFPA activities and it adopts the Regulations Governing Committee Projects under which all committees involved in standards-making operate. The board also appoints a 13-member standards council to administer the association's standards-development activities and regulations. Members of the council are familiar with the technical and standards-development functions and have selected from a broad range of appropriate interests.

Anyone can submit a request for a new safety standards project. The NFPA publishes an announcement in the membership newsletter, acknowledging the receipt of the request and soliciting comments on the need for the project, organizations that may be active in the subject matter, resource material that is available, and an indication of who would be willing to participate in the project if it is approved by the standards council.

If the council determines the need for the proposed project, it either assigns the project to an existing technical committee (TC) or establishes a new committee whose membership reflects a fair balance of concerned interests. All NFPA standards are developed and periodically revised by TCs. Members of the TCs are appointed by the standards council and include volunteer experts representing the government, educational institutions, business, insurance companies, industry, and consumers. Some 4,500 people with diverse interests and knowledge of fire safety make up the two hundred committees within the system. Each committee member is classified by interest:

M	Manufacturer
U	User
I/M	Installer/maintainer
L	Labor
R/T	Applied research/testing laboratory
E	Enforcing authority
I	Insurance
SE	Special expert
C	Consumer

Each committee is structured so that no more than one-third of the membership is from a single interest group. The standards council assigns a scope of activity to each committee to avoid duplication of effort or conflict.

Once a TC has been established, the NFPA issues public notices announcing the Committee's next meeting date and calling for specific proposals from interested persons. Anyone may submit a proposal to be included in the new document or, in the case of an existing committee, to amend an existing document. This public notice appears in the NFPA *Fire News*, the American National Standards Institute *Reporter*, the Federal Register, and relevant trade journals.

The TC meets to consider all proposals received and then drafts a proposed document or an amendment to an existing document, which takes the form of a committee proposals (CP). The submitter of a public proposal may address the TC on his or her proposal at the meetings. Letter ballot approval by at least two-thirds of all TC members eligible to vote is required for approval.

If the standards council determines that a project is of sufficient magnitude that it spans the scope of more than one TC, the council may appoint a correlating committee (CC) to direct the activities of all the TCs that have primary responsibility in areas of concern. It is the responsibility of the CC to coordinate and supervise the work of the TCs under its charge to ensure that no conflicts arise and that the TC activities have been conducted in accordance with the regulations and operating procedures of the NFPA.

All proposals, together with the TC's action on each proposal and proposed new documents appear as a report in the NFPA's "Technical Committee Reports" (TCR). A two-thirds letter ballot approval vote is required for TC approval on action on the proposals. Should the committee revise or reject a proposal, in whole or in part, it must include in its report the reasons for this change or rejection. These TCRs are sent automatically to each proposer and to all affected TC members and are available to anyone else on request. They are widely distributed. The NFPA provides at least a 60-day comment period for all proposals in the TCRs.

Anyone can submit a public comment to the proposed changes published in the TCR. At the conclusion of the comment period, the TC reconvenes to discuss the public comments and to decide its action on each comment. The submitter of a public comment may address the TC on his or her comment at the meeting. A two-thirds letter ballot approval vote of committee members is required for approval of actions taken on comments. All comments, and TC action on comments, and reasons for revising or not accepting them are published as a supplementary report in the NFPA's "Technical Committee Documentation" (TCD). The TCD is supplied automatically to each commenter and committee member and is available to anyone on request.

The TCR and TCD are then presented for open debate at the NFPA's annual meeting in May or the fall meeting in November, which are held in various cities throughout the United States and Canada. Anyone, regardless of membership in NFPA, may present views at these meetings. However, only NFPA members of record for at least 180 days may vote on the adoption of the TCRs (to prevent packing a meeting with adherents to a particular point of view). The only amendments that may be proposed from the floor at an NFPA meeting are those that have been previously published as proposals in the TCR or as comments in the TCD. Such amendments may be proposed only by the submitter of the original proposal or comment or by his or her duly authorized representative. Anyone, however, may propose that an entire TCR be returned to the committee for further study, and anyone may propose that a portion of a report be returned to the wording published in the TCR or be returned to the committee for further study, that is, returned to the wording in the previous edition of the document, but only if there has been a change in that portion of the document between the TCR and TCD. After the debate, an informed NFPA membership votes to approve, amend, or return a portion of or the entire report to the Committee.

The final step for a standard is the issuance of the document by the standards council. The decision is based on all of the information presented, including the vote of the membership and the disposition of any complaints filed with the council. Anyone who is dissatisfied with action taken within the system may file a complaint with the council. Complaints may cover (1) the council's decision on whether a certain document should be developed; (2) the association's action on a proposed committee report at an NFPA meeting; (3) the technical validity or fairness of a document or part of a document; or (4) the council's decision on the appointment of a nominee to a committee. Appeals on the action of the standards council may be made to the board of directors.

An excellent example of this process occurred at the annual meeting in 1978. At that time, the regularly scheduled revision of NFPA 56A, Standard for Use of Inhalation Anesthetics, was up for membership vote. A number of significant proposals and amendments had been received by the technical committee, including the removal of the requirement for isolation distribution transformers in nonflammable anesthetizing locations. The committee had rejected these proposals, but they were reintroduced from the floor according to the rules and were overwhelmingly approved by voice vote. Because the committee rejected the amendments again, the document reverted back to the 1975 edition until the appeals process was completed. The revised document did not go into effect until 1981.

NFPA 101: The Life Safety Code. The Life Safety Code (LSC) originated in the work of the Committee on Safety to Life, which was appointed in 1913. For the first few years of its existence, this committee devoted its attention to a study of the notable fires of the time involving the significant loss of life (recall the Triangle Shirtwaist Company fire mentioned earlier in this chapter) and to an analysis of the causes of this loss of life. This work led to the preparation of standards for the construction of stairways, fire escapes, for fire drills in various occupancies, and for the construction and arrangement of exit facilities for factories, schools, etc. These standards form the basis of the present LSC. In 1921, the committee was enlarged to include representatives from groups not previously participating. Work was started on the further development and integration of previous committee publications to provide a comprehensive guide to exits and related features of life safety from fire in all classes of occupancy. Various drafts of the Building Exits Code were published, circulated, and discussed over a period of years. The first edition was published by the NFPA in 1927.

A number of disastrous fires in the 1940s (including the Coconut Grove Night Club fire in Boston in 1942 which left 492 dead) focused national attention upon the importance of adequate exits and related fire safety features. However, the code of 1927 was not suitable for adoption into law, as it had been drafted as a reference document containing many advisory provisions that were useful to designers of buildings but were not appropriate for legal use. This situation led the committee to revise the entire code, limiting the body of the text to requirements suitable for mandatory application and placing advisory and explanatory material in notes. The revision also involved adding provisions on many features in order to produce a complete document. Editions published from 1948 to 1963 were substantially revised. In 1963 the committee was restructured, and the title of the document was changed from "Fire in Buildings and Structures" to "Code for Safety to Life." In 1977, the committee was reorganized into a technical committee, with an executive committee and standing subcommittees responsible for various chapters and sections. The code is on a three-year revision cycle. The 1991 edition contains numerous new requirements for mandatory sprinklers in new health-care facilities, hotels, apartment buildings, lodging and rooming houses, and board and care facilities as well as mandatory sprinkler requirements for existing high-rise hotels and apartment buildings. The LSC consists of five major parts. Part 1 contains Chapters 1 through 7, which cover the following:

- Administrative responsibilities.
- Fundamental requirements.
- Definitions.
- Classification of occupancies and hazard of content.
- Features of fire protection:
    - Construction.
    - Compartmentalization.
    - Smoke barriers.
    - Special hazard protection.
    - Interior finishes.
- Building service and fire protection equipment:
    - Utilities.
    - HVAC systems.
    - Smoke control.
    - Vertical and horizontal transport systems.
    - Chutes.
    - Incinerators.
    - Fire detection, alarm, and communication.
    - Automatic sprinklers.
    - Other extinguishing equipment.

Part 2 consists of Chapters 8 through 30, which address specific types of occupancies, including new and existing health-care facilities. Parts 3 and 4 consist of Chapter 31, on operating features and Chapter 32 on mandatory referenced publications. Finally, Part 5 consists of Appendices A and B, which contain useful additional information.

NFPA 70: The National Electrical Code. The NFPA National Electrical Code (NEC) is one of the most widely adopted standards in the world. In 1881, the **National Association of Fire Engineers** met in Richmond, Virginia and produced a proposal that served as the basis for the first national electrical code. It covered such topics as the use of insulated conduit and single disconnect devices. The first nationally recommended electrical code was published by the National Board of Fire Underwriters (now the American Insurance Association) in 1895. In 1897, the NEC was drafted; it was the product of the combined labors of architectural, electrical, insurance, and allied interests. The National Conference of Standard Electrical Rules, composed of delegates from various national associations, unanimously voted to recommend this draft to their respective associations for approval and adoption. In 1911, the NFPA assumed sponsorship and control of the NEC, and since 1920, this code has been officially endorsed by the **American National Standards Institute**.

Article 90 of the NEC states its purpose as *"the practical safeguarding of persons and property from hazards arising from the use of electricity,"* and notes that the code *"contains provisions necessary for safety,"* and the proviso that *"compliance therewith and proper maintenance will result in an installation essentially free from hazard, but not necessarily efficient, convenient, or adequate for good service or future expansion of electrical use. This Code is not intended as a design specification nor an instruction manual for untrained persons."*

The format of the NEC is similar to that of the Life Safety Code in that some chapters are dedicated to basic or fundamental requirements, while other chapters address specific or "special" occupancies and equipment. Chapter 2 addresses branch circuits, feeders, service equipment, overcurrent protection, grounding, and surge arresters. Chapter 3 specifies wiring methods and materials, including conductors, cable, conduit, raceways, busways, boxes, switches, switchboards, and panelboards. Chapter 4, "Equipment for General Use," covers flexible cords and cables, lighting fixtures, appliances, fixed space heating, outdoor de-icing and pipeline electric heating equipment, motors, air conditioning and refrigeration equipment, generators, transformers and vaults, capacitors, resistors, reactors, and storage batteries. Article 517 of Chapter 5, "Special Occupancies," is dedicated to health-care facilities and details the requirements of such applications as essential electrical systems, inhalational anesthetizing locations, X-ray installations, communications, and isolated power.

NFPA 99: Standard for Health-care Facilities. This document's genesis can be traced to a series of explosions in operating rooms during surgery in the 1930s. The problem was traced to static discharges of sufficient energy to ignite the flammable anesthetic agents being used at the time. A series of recommendations to mitigate the hazard were then promulgated. In addition, the Committee on Hospitals was established with responsibility to review and revise these recommendations periodically. Since then, the concerns of this committee have grown to encompass many other fire and fire-related hazards associated with health-care services. The committee was allowed to enlarge its scope to include all health-care facilities.

Whereas both the Life Safety Code and the National Electrical Code have sections that apply specifically to health-care facilities, NFPA 99 is the one document that is devoted exclusively to this type of occupancy. The idea for the document arose as the number of documents under the original NFPA Committee on Hospitals expanded. By the end of 1980, 13 documents existed on a variety of subjects:

NFPA 3M	Manual on Health Care Emergency Preparedness
NFPA 56A	Standard on the Use of Inhalation Anesthetics
NFPA 56B	Standard on Respiratory Therapy
NFPA 56C	Standard on Laboratories in Health Related Institutions
NFPA 56D	Standard on Hyperbaric Facilities
NFPA 56E	Standard on Hypobaric Facilities
NFPA 56F	Standard on Nonflammable Piped Medical Gas Systems
NFPA 56G	Standard on Inhalation Anesthetics in Ambulatory Care Facilities
NFPA 56HM	Manual on Home Use of Respiratory Therapy
NFPA 56K	Recommended Practice on Medical Surgical Vacuum Systems in Hospitals
NFPA 76A	Standard on Essential Electrical Systems in Health Care Facilities
NFPA 76B:	Standard on Safe Use of Electricity in Patient Care Areas of Health Care Facilities
NFPA 76C:	Recommended Practice on Safe Use of High Frequency Electricity in Health Care Facilities

The Health Care Facilities Correlating Committee concluded that combining all the documents under its jurisdiction would be beneficial for the following reasons:

- The referenced documents were being revised independently of each other.
- Combination into one document would place all of them on the same revision cycle.
- It would place, in one volume, many documents that referenced each other.
- It would be an easier and more complete reference for users and enforcers.

A request for public comments on this proposal in the spring of 1981 drew a 75 percent positive response, with the support of 90 percent of health-care facilities and organizations. In January 1982, a compilation of the latest edition of each of the 13 documents under the jurisdiction of the Correlating Committee was published. It was designated NFPA 99, Health Care Facilities Code, because it was, and still is, the intention of the committee to develop this document into a Code. The committee also entered the document into the revision cycle, reporting to the 1983 fall meeting for the purpose of formal adoption.

The primary focus of this document is to alleviate the hazards associated with operating a health-care facility, treating patients, and operating laboratories. Each general chapter (3 through 11) has been organized into the following sections:

Section 1 Scope
Section 2 Nature of Hazards
Section 3 Source
Section 4 Distribution
Section 5 Performance Criteria and Testing
Section 6 Administration

Chapters 12 through 18 are "facility" chapters, listing requirements from Chapters 3 to 11 that are applicable to special facilities.

The major topics considered in each facility chapter are arranged in the following order:

- Electrical systems.
- Gas and vacuum systems.
- Environmental systems.
- Materials.
- Electrical equipment.
- Gas equipment.

Of special interest are the electrical requirements for anesthetizing locations, patient-care areas, and emergency generators in Chapter 3; the requirements for oxygen, medical air, and medical vacuum supply and distribution systems in Chapter 4; the ventilation requirements in Chapter 5; the requirements for performance testing and maintenance of patient-care equipment in Chapter 7; respiratory therapy equipment requirements in Chapter 8; manufacturer requirements in Chapter 9; and laboratory requirements in Chapter 10. Appendix A provides useful explanatory notes, and Appendix B lists referenced publications. Annex 1 addresses disaster planning, and Annex 2 contains guidelines for the safe use of high frequency electricity.

Many other NFPA documents also have application in the design, construction, equipping, and operation of health-care facilities.

The American National Standards Institute (ANSI)

ANSI (1430 Broadway, New York, N.Y. 10018) is the clearinghouse and coordinating body for the voluntary consensus standards system in the United States. Approval has been granted to more than ten-thousand standards as American National Standards, of which approximately 1,500 have been published by ANSI on behalf of constituent bodies. ANSI is a federation of trade associations, technical societies, professional groups, and consumer organizations. Some one thousand companies are affiliated with the institute as company members.

ANSI also represents the interests of the United States in international standards development through its membership in the International Electrotechnical Commission (IEC) and the International Standardization Organization (ISO), both of which are based in Switzerland. The range of standards activities is extremely broad, although a major area is safety. Within ANSI, the Medical Devices Standards Board is responsible for medical product standards. A review of the list of ANSI standards reveals many of particular interest to the clinical engineer:

ANSI C2-1990	National Electrical Safety Code (IEEE)
ANSI N449.1	Procedures for Periodic Inspection and Maintenance of Cobalt-60 and Cesium-137 Teletherapy Equipment
ANSI S3.6	Specifications for Audiometers
ANSI Z88.2	Practices for Respiratory Protection
ANSI Z136.3	Safe Use of Lasers in Health Care Facilities
ANSI/ADA 26	Dental X-Ray Equipment and Accessory Devices
ANSI/CGA G7.1	Commodity Specification for Air
ANSI/NFPA 70	National Electrical Code
ANSI/UL 187	X-Ray Equipment

American Society for Testing and Materials (ASTM)

By far the largest single source of voluntary consensus standards in the U.S., the ASTM (1916 Race Street, Philadelphia, PA 19103) has promulgated more than eight thousand standards in its 90-year history. It came into being at the turn of the century because railways were having problems with the nonuniform quality of steel rails they obtained from the steel companies. The ASTM Committee F-4 on Medical and Surgical Materials and Devices was organized in 1962. Volume 13.01 of the *Annual Book* of ASTM Standards is titled *Medical Devices* and contains standard specifications, test methods, practices, guides, and terminology on medical and surgical devices; orthotics, external prosthetics, and mobility aids; anesthetic and respiratory equipment; emergency medical services; and forensic services. Additional subcommittees have been formed in the areas of orthopaedics, cardiovascular, neurosurgical, plastic and reconstructive surgery, and urological materials and devices and the reprocessing of medical devices. Standards range from the Specification for Rubber Contraceptives (D 3492-90) through the Specification for Direct-Reading Liquid Crystal Forehead Thermometers (E 1061-85) to the Specification for Wrought Cobalt-Nickel-Chrome-Molybdenum-Tungsten-Iron Alloy for Surgical Implant Applications (F 563-88). The largest source of income for the ASTM is the sale of its standards, as is to be expected.

Association for the Advancement of Medical Instrumentation (AMI)

The AAMI (3330 Washington Blvd., Suite 400, Arlington, VA 22201-4598), founded in 1967, is an alliance of medical and nursing professionals, engineers, and government and industry representatives with an interest in increasing the understanding and beneficial use of medical devices and instruments. The AAMI offers a variety of programs that assist these groups in developing, evaluating, using, and maintaining this instrumentation. These programs include continuing education, conferences, and the publication of standards and recommended practices, periodicals, and other technical documents.

Through its 38 technical committees, subcommittees, and working groups, the AAMI produces two types of consensus documents: medical device standards and recommended practices. It is the AAMI's view that these documents can contribute significantly to the advancement of medical instrumentation provided that they are drafted with the objectives of increasing the safe and effective application of technology to patient care and of encouraging new technologies and provided that arbitrary and restrictive uses are avoided.

The AAMI medical device standards include recommendations (1) to the device manufacturer of the information that should be provided with or on the product, (2) of the basic safety and performance criteria that should be considered in qualifying the device for clinical use, (3) the measurement techniques that should be used to determine if the device conforms with the safety and performance criteria, and sometimes, comparison data on the performance of similar products. AAMI-recommended practices contain guidelines for the use, care, and processing of a medical device or system. Without addressing device performance *per se*, a recommended practice describes procedures that will help ensure that a device is used safely and effectively and that its performance is maintained. A recommended practice may also address the protection of the environment in which the device is used. The AAMI device standards and recommended practices are grouped into six categories:

- Cardiovascular monitoring and surgery (e.g., blood pressure transducers, defibrillators).
- Equipment maintenance and electrical safety (Guideline for Establishing Medical Instrumentation Maintenance Programs; Safe Current Limits for Electromedical Apparatus).
- General surgical devices (e.g., autotransfusion, electrosurgical devices).
- Nephrology (e.g., hemodialysis systems).
- Neurosurgery (e.g., implantable spinal cord stimulators).
- Sterilization (e.g., Ethylene Oxide Gas Vessels, Steam Vessels).

VOLUNTARY ACCREDITATION ORGANIZATIONS

Although not regulatory agencies or standards-producing organizations in the sense of the descriptions given thus far, voluntary accreditation organizations play an important role in establishing and maintaining quality in the health-care field. These organizations can be very helpful to the hospital. They can provide assistance with standards interpretation, technical databases, continuing education, and resource materials. Many organizations provide on-site survey programs. These programs help the hospital ensure minimum regulatory compliance and advance the cause of patient care. As we shall see, sometimes compliance with accreditation is somewhat less than voluntary.

The Joint Commission on Accreditation of Healthcare Organizations (JCAHO)

The JCAHO (One Renaissance Blvd., Oakbrook Terrace, IL 60181) is an outgrowth of the Hospital Standardization Program established by the American College of Surgeons (ACS) in 1918. The aim of this program was to encourage the adoption of a uniform medical record format that would facilitate the accurate recording of a patient's clinical course. The ACS appreciated the need for a system of standardization that would provide the means of identifying those institutions devoted to the highest ideals of medicine.

Although the ACS's standardization program was successful, it grew to be a financial burden on the college, and participation by other national professional organizations was solicited to continue the program. In 1951, an event occurred that was unique in the history of medicine: five major associations of North American medical groups and hospitals jointly created an organization whose sole purpose was to encourage the voluntary attainment of uniformly high standards of institutional medical care. The founding members of the **Joint Commission on Accreditation of Hospitals (JCAH)** were the American College of Surgeons, the American College of Physicians, the **American Hospital Association**, the **American Medical Association**, and the **Canadian Medical Association (CMA)**. The CMA continued its participation in JCAH until 1959, when the **Canadian Council on Hospital Accreditation** activated its own program. The **American Dental Association** became a corporate member of JCAH in 1979.

The standards developed over a period of 35 years by the ACS were adopted by JCAH, and the hospitals listed by the Hospital Standardization Program were accepted as accredited. On January 1, 1952, the JCAH officially began the task of reviewing hospital survey reports, of granting accreditation based upon these reports, and of carefully reviewing the standards. After the first year's experience, these standards were amended in a few details. The standards were revised six times between 1953 and 1965.

In 1965, Public Law 89-97 (Medicare) was enacted. Reference to JCAH in this law represented the confidence of Congress in the ability of the private health-care sector to voluntarily assess the quality of care being provided. Written into the Medicare Act was the provision that hospitals participating in the Medicare program were to maintain a level of patient care that had come to be recognized as the norm. The JCAH standards were specifically referred to in the law, and the Medicare Conditions of Participation for Hospitals, subsequently promulgated and published by the **Social Security Administration**, reflected the 1965 JCAH standards.

One result of the 1965 Medicare legislation was that hospitals accredited by the JCAH were "deemed" to be in compliance with most of the federal Medicare Conditions of Participation for Hospitals and, thus, met the eligibility requirements for participation in Medicare. The 1972 Amendments to the Social Security Act, Public Law 92-603, provided for "validation" surveys of JCAH-accredited hospitals. Although accredited hospitals continue to be deemed to meet eligibility requirements, this provision meant that the Secretary of Health and Human Services was authorized to validate JCAH findings on the basis of either a selective sample or a substantial complaint.

In August 1966, the JCAH Board of Commissioners voted to review, reevaluate, and rewrite accreditation standards so as to encourage hospitals to further strive for excellence in patient care. Consequently, the standards underwent extensive revision, resulting in the 1970 edition, which, for the first time was called, the *Accreditation Manual for Hospitals* (AMH). Since then, the AMH has undergone continual review and revision.

In 1981, JCAH began revising the AMH to develop less prescriptive, more goal-oriented standards that focused on essential elements of quality care. At that time, the section of the AMH relating to engineering activities and responsibilities was entitled "Functional Safety and Sanitation" (FS&S). The accent was on having written policies and procedures to specify what was to be done to maintain functional safety and how it was to be accomplished and on written records to certify that the procedures were in fact, followed. The FS&S standard specified clinical engineering responsibility for participation in the hospital safety committee and program; inspection of new equipment before use; regular, documented equipment maintenance records and inspection frequency data; a hazard surveillance program; participation in staff orientation and continuing education regarding the use of medical technology; and provision of technical advice.

In April 1984, the JCAH Board of Commissioners adopted a new set of standards. These standards were designed to be an intermediate step in an evolution from the previous standards, which were highly prescriptive, to new standards, which would be oriented to a management system designed to ensure the quality and safety of the patient-care environment. The relevant section of the AMH was retitled "Plant, Technology, and Safety Management" (PT&SM) and consisted of 19 sections:

I Buildings (Life Safety 101, Statement of Construction).
II Grounds.
III Safety system/committee.
IV Safety education.
V Emergency preparedness.
VI Hazardous substances and wastes.
VII Fire safety.
VIII Communications systems.

IX Clinical equipment.
X Nonpatient care equipment.
XI Electrical distribution systems.
XII Emergency power.
XIII Vertical/horizontal transport systems.
XIV HVAC systems.
XV Plumbing systems.
XVI Boilers.
XVII Compressed medical gases.
XVIII Medical/surgical vacuum.
XIX Safety devices and safe operation practices.

The third and most recent revisions to the PT&SM standards went into effect in January, 1989, under what is now called the Joint Commission on Accreditation of Healthcare Organizations. This new version condensed the previous 19 sections into four: Safety Management, Life Safety, Equipment Management, and Utilities Management. These four standards reflect the key functions that are considered to be essential for the effective management of the quality and safety of the physical environment in which patient care is provided.

A significant concept that has matured along with the evolution of the PT&SM is the "quality assurance loop." For each standard, required characteristics focus on the collection of information, problem identification, problem resolution, and monitoring of results. Now, instead of merely documenting that policies and procedures have been followed to the letter, data must be collected and analyzed to show evidence that whatever the policies and procedures are, they work well. If not, evidence must be shown that they have been evaluated and, if necessary, revised. This process is an ongoing one, with the goal of continually improving quality. In other words, the quality assurance loop is to be closed.

College of American Pathologists (CAP)

The College of American Pathologists (325 Waukegan Rd., Northfield, IL 60093-2750) is a voluntary organization that accredits hospital laboratories. The CAP evaluates the quality of pathology services (clinical chemistry, transfusion services, hematology, microbiology, anatomic pathology, etc.). A laboratory safety program is also required. Laboratories have long been recognized as one of the more hazardous locations in the hospital from both a chemical and a biological viewpoint. The CAP helps clinical laboratories and pathology areas ensure that the working environment is safe from recognized safety hazards.

TRADE ASSOCIATIONS

Trade associations are generally composed of companies in the same business serving a specific industry. Trade associations have many functions, including collecting economic, marketing, and production statistics and developing standards. They are often active politically, protecting the interests of their constituent members on matters such as tariffs, trade regulations, and environmental issues. Not all trade associations have programs to develop standards. Those that do have a variety of motivations, such as to assist the industry in increasing production, lowering costs, increasing quality, and making the products of the industry competitive with alternatives. Trade association standards often help in marketing by making the products easier and safer to use, and ensuring a certain level of quality. Some trade associations maintain a certification program for products that they write standards for. Organizations that may be of interest to clinical engineers include the following:

Compressed Gas Association (CGA)
Crystal Gateway #1, Suite 501
1235 Jefferson Davis Hwy
Arlington, VA 22202

Health Industry Manufacturers
Association (HIMA)
1030 15th St. N.W., Suite 1100
Washington, D.C. 20005

National Electrical Manufacturers
Association (NEMA)
2101 L St. N.W.
Washington, D.C. 20037

Pharmaceutical Manufacturers
Association (PMA)
1100 15th St. N.W.
Washington, D.C. 20005

Scientific Apparatus Manufacturers
Association (SAMA)
225 Reinekers, Suite 625
Alexandria, VA 23314

PROFESSIONAL SOCIETIES

Some of the larger developers of standards are professional organizations, such as organizations of mechanical, electrical, or chemical engineers, architects, physicians, and dentists that existed prior to major standards-development efforts. The technology-of-the-times often creates safety concerns, and the only organizations that can help are the professional societies. It was these organizations that started to write standards for their particular disciplines as a professional obligation. Professional societies that produce standards of interest to clinical engineers include the following:

American Dental Association (ADA)
211 E. Chicago Ave.
Chicago, IL 60611

Illuminating Engineering Society (IES)
Delta House
222 Balham High Rd.
London SW12 9BS, England

Instrument Society of America (ISA)
P.O. Box 12277
67 Alexander Dr.
Research Triangle Park, NC 27709

American Society of Heating,
Refrigerating, and Air Conditioning
Engineers (ASHRAE)
1791 Tullie Circle N.E.
Atlanta, GA 30329

American Heart Association
7320 Greenville Ave.
Dallas, TX 75231

Institute of Electrical and Electronics
Engineers (IEEE)
345 E. 47th St.
New York, NY 10017

LISTING ORGANIZATIONS

Another type of standards-preparing organization is the "listing" agency. Years ago, insurance companies began paying claims for fires, personal injury, and property losses caused by faulty mechanical and electrical devices. It became clear that if the quality of these products was improved, the necessity for payments would be lessened. But one cannot just look at a fire extinguisher and know if it will put out a fire—it has to be tested. Tests must be uniform and relevant to the objective. Thus, the need for standard test methods arose.

Underwriters Laboratories (UL) (333 Pfingsten Rd., Northbrook, IL 60062) is perhaps the most recognized name in listing organizations. It is a nonprofit organization that maintains laboratories to evaluate the safety of products. Nearly 1,300 electrical, fire, and mechanical safety evaluation standards have been prepared by UL. Products that have been evaluated and have passed the requirements of these standards are listed in published directories. Although UL does derive revenue from the sale of its standards, the vast proportion of its revenue comes from the actual test work done in its several laboratories. Products passing the appropriate tests are allowed to carry the distinctive UL label. Among the many UL standards, several are of particular interest to clinical engineers:

187	X-Ray Equipment	544	Electric Medical and Dental Equipment
1022	Line Isolation Monitors	1047	Isolated Power Systems Equipment
1069	Hospital Signalling and Nurse Call Equipment	1262	Laboratory Equipment

Other listing agencies include the cities of Los Angeles and Detroit, the Factory Mutual Engineering and Research Group, and the Canadian Standards Association. In other parts of the world matters are somewhat simplified. Typically, there is a single national standards body, such as the British Standards Institution (BSI), which derives some income from dues, some from standards sales, and some, from its national government. The existence of such a national organization does not preclude some standards being developed by a trade association, such as the Society of British Aerospace Companies, or a professional organization, such as Verband Deutscher Elektrotechniker (German Electrical Engineers).

INTERNATIONAL STANDARDS

The object of international standards and related activities is to facilitate the exchange of goods and services, and to promote cooperation in scientific and economic activities. International standards should not act as nontariff barriers. There exist four types of standards bodies whose documents cross national boundaries: international nongovernment, international intergovernment, regional nongovernment, and regional intergovernment bodies. Of the many standards organizations in existence, the two most concerned with medical devices are the International Electrotechnical Commission and the International Organization for Standardization.

SUMMARY

The pervasiveness of codes, standards, and regulations presented in this chapter illustrates the need for clinical engineers to become familiar with the documents that affect their responsibilities and activities. Equipment selection and acquisition, performance assurance, in-service education, maintenance and repair, documentation, design and fabrication, and, as we shall see in the next chapter, facilities design and operation are all clinical engineering functions that are enhanced through the guidance provided by standards. These standards are the results of a great deal of work, knowledge, experience, and lessons learned from mistakes. They should be viewed as helpful resources for meeting the responsibilities of the clinical engineer in managing health-care technology.

EXERCISES

1. Describe the circumstances under which adherence to a standard becomes mandatory.
2. What are the ramifications for a health-care facility of noncompliance with "voluntary" JCAHO accreditation standards?
3. Investigate and compare the requirements of NFPA 70 and NFPA 99 for equipment grounding in a general patient-care area.
4. Locate and report on the latest revision of, amendment to, or proposal for rulemaking under 29 CFR 1910.1200. Cite your reference.
5. What are the advantages and disadvantages of adopting international standards?
6. Describe at least two mechanisms through which a practicing clinical engineer can contribute to the standards-making process.

REFERENCES

AAMI, "Standards and Recommended Practices," Association for the Advancement of Medical Instrumentation, Arlington, VA, 1987.

ANSI. Z136.3, "Safe Use of Lasers in Health Care Facilities," American National Standards Institute, New York, 1986.

ASHE. "Electrical Safety Compendium," American Society for Hospital Engineering of the American Hospital Assocation, Chicago, 1990.

Ballard, R.D. "The Discovery of the Titanic," Madison Press, Toronto, 1987.

Batik, A.L. "A Guide to Standards," Parker, CO, 1989.

Hospital and Medical Facilities, American Institute of Architects Press, Washington, D.C., 1987.

JCAHO, "Accreditation Manual for Hospitals," Joint Commission on Accreditation of Healthcare Organizations, Chicago, IL, 1991.

NFPA No. 70, "National Electrical Code," National Fire Protection Association, Quincy, MA, 1990a.

NFPA No. 99, "Standard for Health Care Facilities," National Fire Protection Association, Quincy, MA, 1990b.

NFPA No. 101, "Life Safety Code," National Fire Protection Association, Quincy, MA, 1991.

Nunes, B.A., et al. "The Guide to Biomedical Standards," Quest Publishing Co., Brea, CA, 1991.

State of Connecticut, Department of Consumer Protection, State Board of Registration for Professional Engineers and Land Surveyors. "Rules and Regulations," Hartford, CT, 1978.

"United States Code of Federal Regulations," Title 21, Food and Drugs. U.S. Government Printing Office, Washington, D.C.

"United States Code of Federal Regulations," Title 29, Labor. U.S. Government Printing Office, Washington, D.C.

"United States Code of Federal Regulations," Title 40, Protection of the Environment. U.S. Government Printing Office, Washington, D.C.

CHAPTER 6

FACILITIES MANAGEMENT AND DESIGN

Since clinical engineering departments often provide support functions that maintain or enhance the ability of a medical facility to deliver quality health-care, it is essential that clinical engineers be cognizant of all operational aspects of the facility in which they perform their wide range of functions. To be effective, therefore, it is important that clinical engineers understand the wide range of activities associated with facilities management, which includes housekeeping, grounds maintenance, design, construction and renovation, engineering services (e.g., heating, ventilation, and air conditioning), and operations (e.g., policy, organization, budget, personnel, and financial activities). The level of involvement of the clinical engineer in facilities management or facilities design activities is determined by a number of factors, including the expertise and willingness of the hospital's engineering personnel. In any event, collaboration between facilities and clinical engineers is critical in today's cost-conscious health-care environment. With this in mind, this chapter initially presents an overview of a facilities management (FM) program and then describes, in detail, those FM functions in which clinical engineers may become involved. The chapter is divided into two sections. "Facilities Management" examines those functions that pertain to the day-to-day management of a health-care delivery facility, and "Facilities Design" emphasizes the planning, design, and construction or renovation of new or existing facilities.

FACILITIES MANAGEMENT

The effective management of a modern medical facility represents a significant challenge. The range of responsibilities encompassed by the **facilities manager**, the **director of clinical engineering**, and their respective departments has grown larger and become more complex as a result of the continuous infusion of new technologies and state and federal regulations (AHA, 1990; Sloane and Sloane, 1992). This fact and the realization by hospital administrators that effective facilities management translates to cost-effective health-care delivery have served to redefine and expand the role of both clinical and hospital engineers. Given the importance of the medical facility in the overall delivery of health-care, this section presents the fundamental activities of a facilities management department and examines several areas — including utilities, medical gases, regulated medical waste, and safety — that are of specific concern to clinical engineers.

Functions of a Facilities Management Department

At the onset, it is important to emphasize that the primary objective of any facilities management support program is to provide and maintain the proper environment for the delivery of health-care services. Therefore, FM programs ensure that medical buildings and associated utilities, transport, and communication systems are acquired, operated, and maintained in a manner that promotes the most efficacious and productive environment for normal hospital operations and the delivery of quality medical care (AHA, 1980).

Figure 6.1 presents the organizational chart of the FM department for a major academic medical center that includes medical and dental schools, and a 240-bed teaching hospital. The major positions within this organization can be noted from this figure:

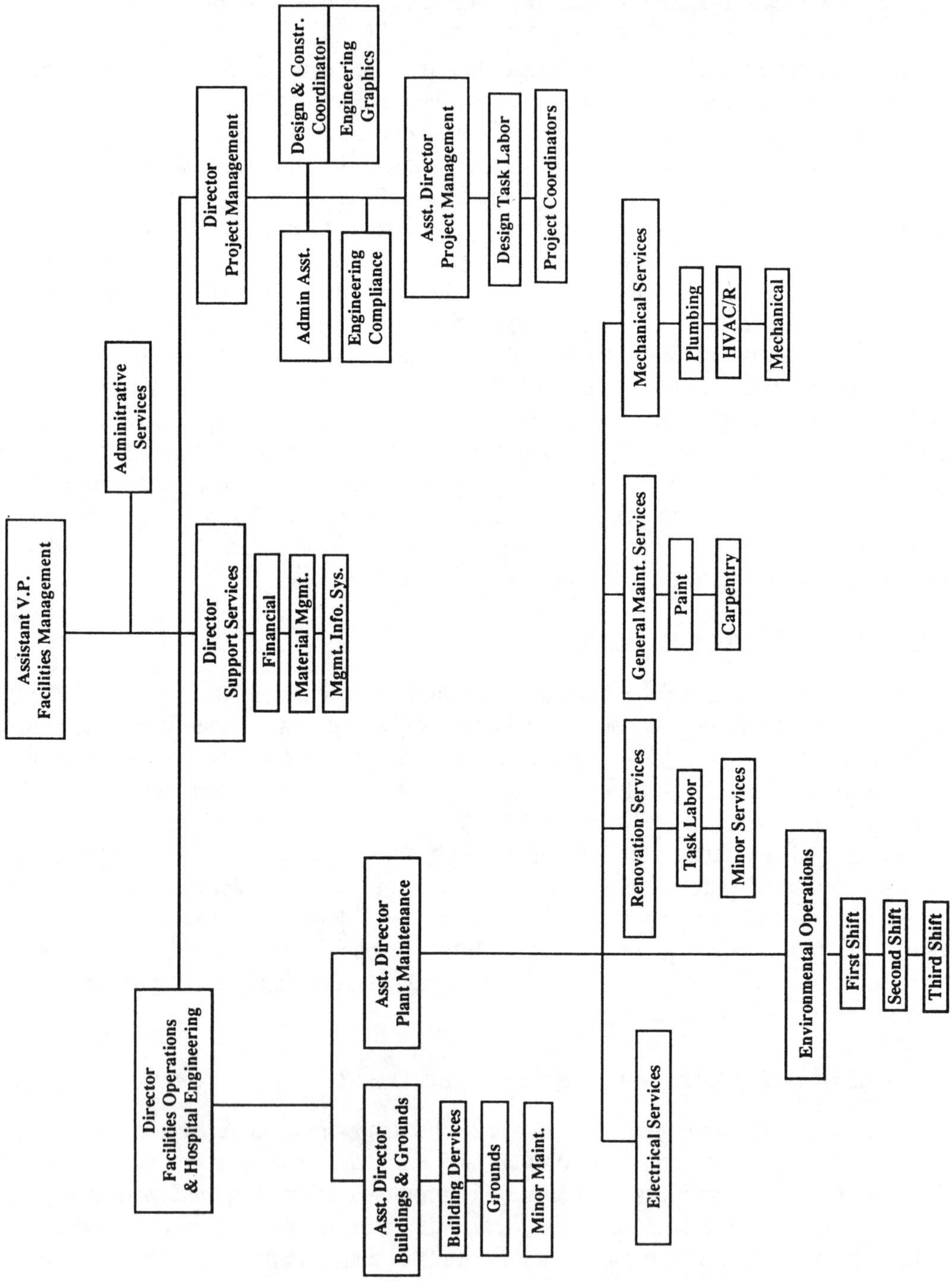

Figure 6.1: Facilities Management organizational chart.

- Assistant vice-president of facilities management.
- Director of facilities operations and hospital engineering.
- Director of support services.
- Director of project management.
- Assistant director for buildings and grounds.
- Assistant director for plant maintenance.

Since each of these positions entails responsibility for a major function of the FM program, a brief discussion of the primary responsibilities of each position should provide insights into the overall activities of FM within such an academic health-care center.

Assistant Vice-President of Facilities Management. The assistant vice-president of facilities management is usually responsible for the management of effective projects, buildings maintenance, and plant maintenance organizations, and for the administration of policy, organization, budget, personnel, and financial activities within the department. Specific responsibilities include the following:

- Define, establish, implement and maintain the facilities management organization to meet effectively the programmatic needs of the health-care facility.
- Ensure that quality assurance and control programs are developed, adhered to, and reported on.
- Ensure the timely delivery of quality facility-related services to the health-care center. These services include building operations and maintenance, project design and construction, housekeeping services, and grounds maintenance.
- Develop and maintain effective communication between the facilities department and user/customer departments.
- Define, acquire, and control budget allocations sufficient to support all facilities management and operations functions.
- Interact with federal, state and local agencies and regulatory boards.
- Keep current with the development of new technologies and management concepts in the facilities field by active participation in professional organizations and groups.

Director of Facilities Operations and Hospital Engineering. The director of facilities operations and hospital engineering is responsible to the vice-president of facilities management. The duties of this position include assuming the duties of the vice-president in that individual's absence and directing the plant maintenance and buildings and grounds functions of the facilities management department. The director also serves as the hospital safety officer, providing the daily administrative direction necessary to coordinate all hospital-related plant maintenance and buildings and grounds activities. Specific duties include the following:

- As the hospital safety officer, report at least once a month to the safety committee on findings, recommendations, actions, and monitoring. Complete semi-annual loss review report. Develop safety policies and procedures. Aassist with safety training.
- Review and prepare personnel, equipment, and other expense budgets.
- Establish and approve preventive maintenance procedures.
- Review plans and specifications for code compliance and accreditation standards. Institute corrective action and follow-up documentation.

- Establish training programs in all areas.
- Establish and supervise quality assurance, training, and continuing education programs.
- Prepare service contracts.
- Supervise computerized plant maintenance/facilities management reporting system.
- Maintain service requests and preventive maintenance schedules.
- Maintain facilities management policy and procedure manuals for all divisions.
- Coordinate labor relations and affirmative action activities for facilities management and operation.
- Maintain performance standards and compare to actual performance.
- Evaluate or approve evaluation of employee performance and abilities.
- Set department standards and reporting procedures.
- Represent the department on various committees, such as animal care, risk management, disaster planning, etc.
- Evaluate department efficiency, organization, and performance. Institute changes where needed.
- Provide administrative direction and coordination of services relative to facilities operation and hospital engineering.

Director of Support Services. The director of support services is responsible for all aspects of departmental budgets and financial accounting and control and is directly responsible to the assistant vice-president of facilities management. The director of support services also works closely with the institution's budget officer, hospital fiscal officer, and the fiscal officers of the medical and dental Schools. Examples of the duties of this position include the following:

- Direct the preparation, submission, and management of all departmental budgets, including budget analysis, and report to the assistant vice-president for facilities management.
- Monitor and report on all fiscal trends. Oversee all activities related to purchase requisitions, contracts, and other expenses.
- Have administrative responsibility for maintenance of financial records, accounts, ledgers, etc.
- Coordinate efficient and effective resolution of all fiscal matters.
- Supervise information systems division.
- Establish and maintain communication links between facilities management and purchasing department.
- Supervise materials management to ensure timely procurement and effective control of materials flow.
- Develop, implement, and maintain departmental auditing systems.
- Monitor all activities related to departmental billing and cost accounting.
- Oversee office automation systems such as, word processing, work order, inventory, and preventive maintenance systems.
- Provide fiscal direction on the budget process, including minor capital and capital budget requests.
- Define and communicate specific goals of each department subdivision based on user needs.

Director of Project Design and Management. The director of project design and management is responsible for administering the project design and management functions and is directly responsible to the assistant vice-president of facilities management (Grattendick, 1990). The duties of this position include the following:

- Review and prepare personnel, equipment, and other expense budgets.
- Establish policies, procedures, and guidelines for scheduling, cost estimation, bidding processes, building standards, design, project staffing, change order processing, and materials control.
- Establish and approve design standards and procedures.
- Review plans and specifications related to renovation projects prepared by in-house staff, outside architects, and engineers.
- Evaluate or approve evaluation of employee performance and abilities.
- Prepare reports, forms, surveys, etc., as required.
- Serve as a technical resource for the facility.
- Establish training programs.
- Prepare and approve purchase requests.
- Prepare service contracts and specifications.
- Attend prebid meetings with contractors; prepare and review bid forms.
- Represent the department on various committees, such as animal care, risk management, disaster planning, etc.
- Evaluate department efficiency, organization, and performance. Institute changes where needed.
- Serve as the general contractor, utilize material purchased through vendors and labor provided through personal service contracts.

Assistant Director for Buildings and Grounds Maintenance. The assistant director for buildings and grounds maintenance is responsible to the director of facilities operations for housekeeping, general maintenance, and groundskeeping for the entire facility, including the hospital, medical and dental schools, research laboratories, animal care facilities, administration, and other buildings. The duties of this position include the following:

- Develop, implement, and maintain regulated medical waste and recycling programs.
- Review and prepare personal services, capital equipment, and other expense budgets.
- Coordinate snow and ice removal in the winter.
- Review plans and specifications for interior design compliance and accreditation standards within the hospital.
- Evaluate or approve evaluation of employee performance and abilities.
- Prepare service contracts and specifications.
- Approve and prepare purchase requests and orders.

Assistant Director for Plant Maintenance. The assistant director for plant maintenance is responsible to the director of facilities operations and hospital engineering. The duties include managing, supervising, and coordinating the operations, renovations and general maintenance functions of the facility. Specific duties include the following:

- Establish and supervise facilities operations, maintenance, repair, and renovation procedures.

- Establish and supervise scheduling procedures to ensure compliance with regulatory requirements, etc., and budgetary allocations.
- Establish and supervise personnel services necessary to operate, maintain, and repair the facilities efficiently and effectively.
- Establish and maintain inventories of materials, spare parts, tools, and equipment needed to support all aspects of facilities operation and maintenance.
- Prepare and manage operations, maintenance, repair, and renovation budgets.
- Coordinate all operations, maintenance, repair, and renovation projects.
- Prepare monthly and annual reports such as, personnel time records, service requests, and status of ongoing projects and renovations.
- Establish and supervise a quality assurance program for all levels of the operating and maintenance functions.

Functions of the FM Department

In reviewing the responsibilities of the major positions in a large FM program it should be clear that the activities of any FM program are extensive and touch all aspects of the operation of the health-care facility (Magee, 1988). Certainly, the extent and complexity of the organizational chart and the personnel positions associated with this chart can be reduced or modified when it is applied to medical facilities comprised only of hospitals or to smaller facilities. However, the broad base of FM activities remains constant regardless of the size of the institution; only the degree of complexity of the activities and the management of these activities changes.

The responsibilities of the facilities manager are summarized in Table 6.1, which divides these responsibilities into four categories: engineering, management, supervision, and liaison functions (AIPE 1990; Kaiser, 1989). Having introduced the various responsibilities of a facilities manager, let us now take a closer look at some of the major functions of the FM department that are of particular interest to clinical engineers. The responsibilities include the following:

Engineering. The physical plant must be properly maintained. It must also be operated to minimize the consumption of resources and to prevent contamination of the surrounding environment.

Life Safety. Building systems must function reliably and safely. They must meet current codes and standards applicable to the occupancy classification of each part of the facility. Patients, staff, and visitors must be protected against undue risk of fire or other hazards.

Hospital Safety. Facilities personnel, patients and visitors must be protected from both physical and biological hazards. Proper management and disposal of medical waste is but one example of the type of programs required to ensure that facilities and personnel are protected.

Security and Resource Protection. The facility must be maintained to provide a secure environment for patients, visitors, and staff. Adequate provisions must also be made for the protection (security) of facilities, property and personnel.

Professional Environment. The interior and exterior appearance of the facility must be conducive to the delivery of high-quality medical care. The term "professional environment" encompasses the entire facility and includes air quality, heating, cooling, lighting, etc.

Medical Functionality. Adequate space that can be efficiently used to accommodate people and equipment with physical access for all patients, including the handicapped, must be provided.

Table 6.1 FACILITIES MANAGEMENT RESPONSIBILITIES

Engineering	Management	Supervision	Liaison
Ensuring that maintenance and testing procedures are performed on critical utility systems at appropriate intervals and documented per JCAHO requirements. Ensuring reliable and adequate emergency power in the event of service interruption. Ensuring compliance with JCAHO, NFPA, OSHA and EPA standards to the maximum extent possible.	Managing "in-house" housekeeping functions. Developing and maintaining long-range facility master plan. Preparing budget and financial plans to support facilities management functions. Managing the facility resource protection program. Managing, tracking, disposal and documentation of regulated medical waste. Managing facilities and grounds maintenance programs.	Monitor work requests involving facilities systems, e.g., utilities, HVAC, communications. Review contracts of external service vendors, e.g., elevator, refuse removal, hood and duct cleaning, etc. to ensure compliance with all relevant codes. Develop and monitor energy efficiency programs.	Interact with outside support groups, including contractors, vendors and police, fire and disaster relief agencies such as the Red Cross, etc. Serve as a member of the Safety Committee.

Although each area of responsibility has its own set of considerations, all must occur synergistically to promote the continuously smooth operation demanded of a health-care delivery facility. Because each of these areas is critical to the proper functioning of a medical facility, let us discuss them in greater detail.

Engineering

The physical plant is a complex network of building-related subsystems that provides the services necessary for day-to-day operations. To be effective, this system must be operated in an efficient and cost-effective manner. Often, operation of the physical plant is transparent to the staff and patients until a problem exists. Water, electricity, heating, cooling, and ventilation are all clearly essential to the proper operation of medical technology, thus, the absence of any one of these basic utilities would have a serious impact on the delivery of health-care. Are there other major engineering systems that facilities managers must control?

To answer this question, let us examine the following eight systems:

Medical Air. Medical air is defined as air intended for human respiration, which may also be mixed with oxygen to treat patients. This is particularly significant in dealing with neonates on respirators. The **Compressed Gas Association** has established quality standards, which must be met before air can be classified as medical air. For example, included in these standards are requirements that the central compressor systems must be equipped with dry-type intake filter-mufflers (after coolers and/or air dryers), line filters appropriate for the specific compressor type and the intake air conditions, and pressure regulators to ensure the delivery of medical compressed air (Slack, 1989; NFPA 99, 1990).

Medical/Surgical Vacuum Systems. These systems are required to provide vacuum pressure for drainage, aspiration, and suction during medical procedures. Generally, these systems are centrally piped and consist of two or more vacuum pumps that operate alternately or simultaneously, according to the demand. Each pump should be capable of maintaining a minimum required vacuum equal to 75 percent of peak calculated demand.

Piped Medical Gas Systems. These systems provide oxygen, nitrous oxide, nitrogen, carbon dioxide, helium, and air to specifically identified outlets within procedural rooms throughout the facility. Figure 6.2 illustrates a typical medical gas distribution system. These gases are generally piped to areas of use from central manifolds. Because there have been several reports of incorrectly connected gas lines resulting in patient death, each line must be properly marked to eliminate the possibility of cross-connection. Because all of these gases are used in surgical procedures, their availability is critical. Faults occurring within any of these gas systems can have catastrophic consequences. As a result, emergency alarms are present throughout the system to alert users of low pressure, and system outlets are routinely tested for leaks to protect against fire, gas loss, and low system pressure.

Heating, Ventilation and Air Conditioning. The HVAC systems maintain the ambient hospital environment. Many areas of the hospital have specific environmental requirements. As an example, temperature control in surgical suites is often set automatically, depending upon the requirements of the surgical procedure. Relative humidity in such suites must be maintained at a level no lower than 35 percent. Smoke originating within surgical suites (e.g., resulting from laser surgery) must be eliminated without recirculation and positive pressure must be maintained in such surgical suites to ensure that contaminants are not drawn into the room from adjacent rooms during a procedure.

Electrical Systems. All hospitals are dependent upon electrical power, e.g., power for HVAC ventilators, electrical motors and equipment, and lighting. Figure 6.3 illustrates a typical electrical power distribution system for a large hospital (Martin, 1987). Complex medical procedures, such as those requiring artificial circulation of blood, mechanical respiration, and aspiration, are examples of situations that have critical electrical power requirements. Because interruption of electrical service during such procedures would represent a life-threatening situation, contingency plans in the event of power loss and the periodic inspection and testing of the electrical distribution system are required (IEEE, 1986).

Guidance in the planning and execution of inspections of the electrical power system is provided in NFPA 99, Standard for Health-care Facilities (NFPA 99, 1990).

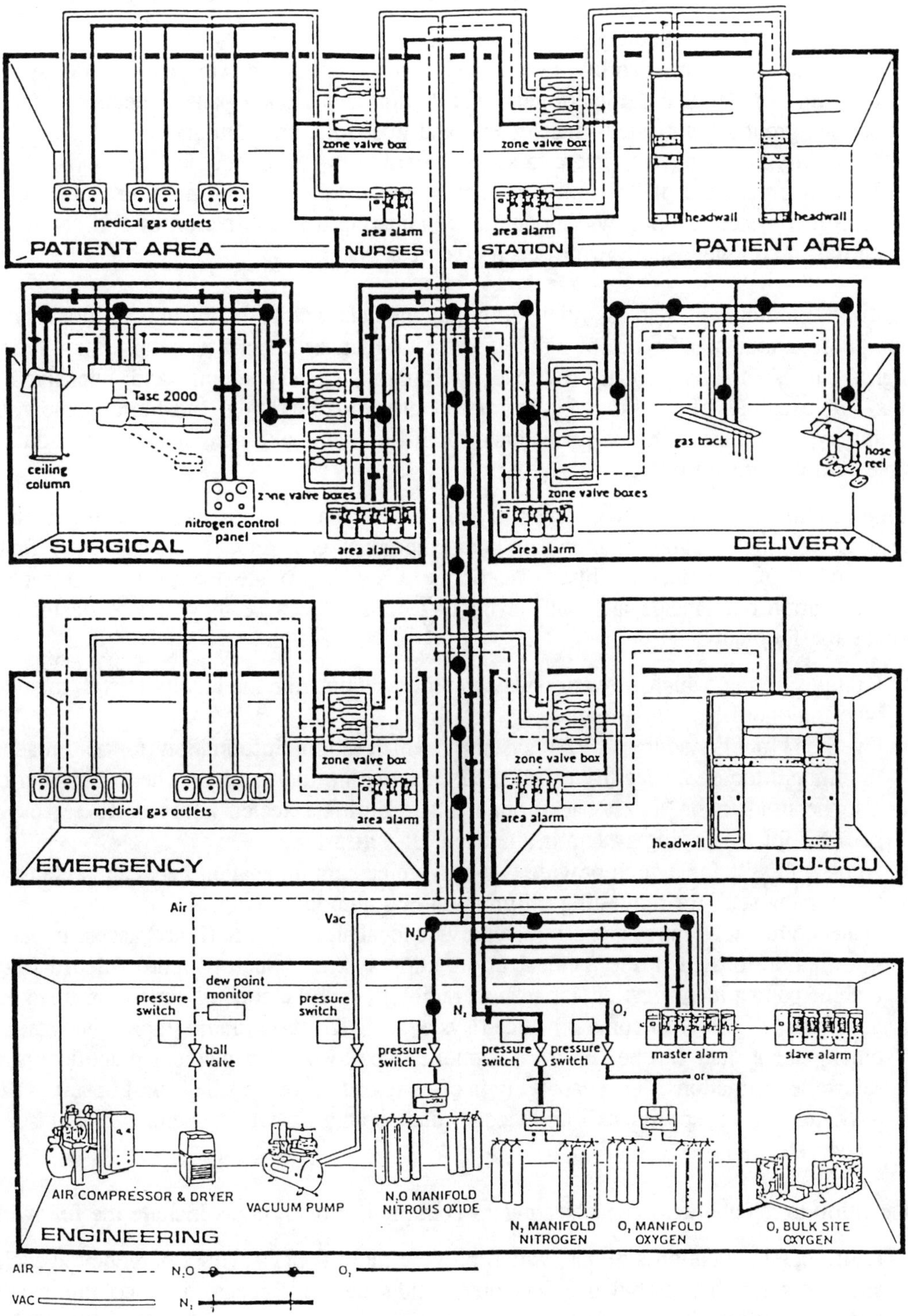

Figure 6.2: Diagram of a typical medical gas distribution system.

At a minimum, such inspections should include assessment of the following:

- Testing of alternate sources, i.e., generators.
- Condition and serviceability of all components of the power distribution system, including switch gears, transformers, distribution and breaker panels, electrical feeders, outlets, ground fault circuit interrupters, and line-isolation monitors.
- Capability of the power system to safely meet the in-house electrical demands.
- Written procedures that specify the action to be taken during a failure of essential electrical systems, along with documents indicating the distribution of and control for partial or complete shutdown of each electrical system.

Lighting. Illumination is an essential part of any medical facility. Clinical practitioners need appropriate amounts and types of lighting to treat patients. Special hospital units—such as surgical suites, delivery rooms, cystoscopy rooms, recovery rooms, and intensive-care units—are examples of areas that require special attention to lighting. In addition, emergency lighting systems must be properly designed to ensure that health-care delivery can continue in the case of a power outage.

Communication Systems. The capability to communicate, access data, locate personnel, broadcast information, and summon help in an emergency is essential to the safe and efficient operation of any medical facility. Telephone systems provide the principal means of communication both inside and outside many facilities, because they can be designed to provide the following:

- Paging systems, which allow one-way communication from the facility to staff members who may not be on the premises.
- Overhead public address (PA) systems, which allow information to be broadcast throughout the entire facility or selected areas within the facility. The PA system can also be used to broadcast background music during selected hours or to serve as a back-up for the paging system in the event of a disaster.
- Nurse call systems, which provide two-way voice communication between patients and the nursing staff for requesting information or summoning help.
- Data communications systems, which provide local area network (LAN) access to patient information located in the medical information system. Such patient-related data can include patient identification, lab results, radiology reports, doctors' orders for treatment, and nursing notes. In some advanced systems, ECG traces, radiographic images, and other patient data can be sent by telephone lines to outside medical practitioners for referral consultations. This capability is often used to provide small rural hospitals with easy access to specialists' knowledge and opinions, which would otherwise be unavailable.

In addition to telephone systems, secondary communication systems include the following:

- Radio communication systems, which provide radio contact with emergency agencies, such as police, fire, ambulance, helicopter, and security. Because these communication links are critical for conveying information to and from the site of an emergency and for coordinating emergency response in the event of a disaster, the FCC has set aside special radio frequencies for the health-care industry.

- Television systems, which provide patient recreation and staff training. Because educational tapes or programming on a number of medical topics are now available, such systems can be used to provide required staff training. In conjunction with satellite transceivers, these systems can also be used for teleconferencing and satellite symposia, thereby providing immediate access to medical techniques and information that serve to enhance the quality of health-care delivery within the facility.

Fire protection systems. These systems consist of alarm boxes, smoke detectors, automatic fire door closures, and sprinkler systems. Because the ratio of nonambulatory patients to staff personnel makes it difficult to evacuate a medical facility safely in the event of fire, fire emergencies must be quickly contained and controlled to avoid the necessity of evacuating the entire facility. This consideration requires that testing, inspection, and maintenance of fire protection systems be a priority concern of the FM department.

The basic service components of a medical facility presented above combine to form a complex system requiring extensive engineering and management expertise. Most of these systems have a direct impact on the medical equipment and instrumentation used for the daily delivery of health-care, and without them, medical care would be severely impaired. Therefore, the facilities manager–clinical engineer interface is critical to ensuring that treatment and diagnosis of patients can continue without interruption.

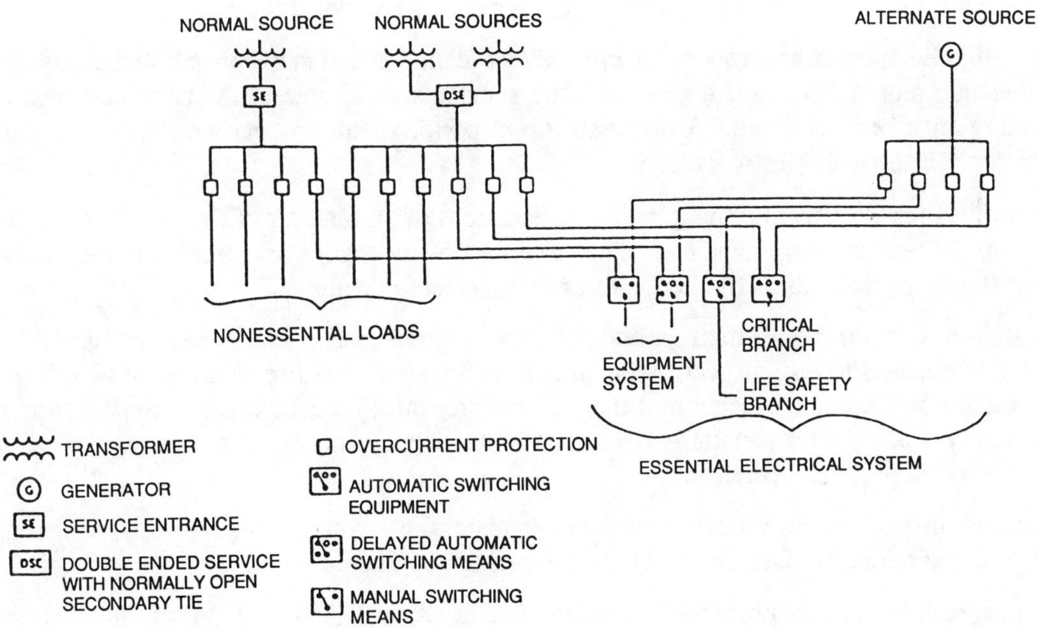

Figure 6.3: Diagram of a typical electrical system in a large hospital.

Life Safety

The objective of life safety is to reduce the probability of injury and loss of life from the effects of fire and other emergencies or hazards. The level of safety is defined by the combination of prevention, protection, facility exit routes, and other features enumerated within the individual chapters of NFPA 101: Code for Safety and Life from Fire in Buildings and Structures. These combined chapters are referred to as the Life Safety Code and address the following:

- Life safety from fire and similar emergencies.
- Construction, protection, and occupancy features necessary to minimize danger to life from fire, smoke, fumes, or panic.
- The minimum criteria for the design of exit routes that permit prompt escape of occupants from buildings or, where desirable, into safe areas within the building.

Because life safety is more than a matter of egress, the facilities manager must ensure that the following requirements are met to maintain an effective fire safety program:

Code compliance. Each hospital building that houses patients overnight or in which patients receive treatment must be in compliance with the appropriate provisions of the Life Safety Code.

A comprehensive statement of construction. A statement must be prepared that describes the structural characteristics of fire protection systems for each building that houses patients overnight. If code violations exist, the facilities manager must develop a plan of equivalent protection for the facility and a written plan for the correction of these deficiencies.

An effective inspection process. A process that identifies and maintains all features of fire protection required by the Life Safety Code standards applicable to the particular type of facility must be established. A qualified fire inspector should inspect the facility annually for compliance with NFPA standards.

Drawings (or documents) that provide the locations of all features of fire protection in the facility. These drawings must be updated to reflect every change or alteration to the facility and should be maintained by the facilities management department.

Installation, testing, and maintenance of the fire alarm system in accordance with NFPA 101. Procedures to test, inspect, and maintain all fire alarm and fire detection systems must be established, and the execution of these procedures must be documented. Such testing is generally conducted on a quarterly basis and should include all circuits and annual preventive maintenance of all components.

Annual inspection and testing of all automatic fire extinguishing systems, including sprinkler systems and kitchen dry-chemical discharge systems.

A program to manage portable fire extinguishers. A program that defines hospital policy for extinguisher identification, placement, and use must be developed. Facilities managers should request assistance from the local fire department to help train personnel in the use of portable extinguishers. Portable extinguishers should be inspected quarterly, and this inspection should be documented. The program should also include scheduled preventive maintenance of these devices.

A written fire plan that delineates specific staff responses to a fire emergency. The plan should include the type of fire alarm in the building and its' distinctive sound; hospital staff responsibilities in the event of fire; departmental responses to fire alarms; number and/or sections to call to report a fire; evacuation procedures and evacuation responsibility; use of fire extinguishers; assembly areas; staff member education in all elements of the fire plan; and quarterly fire drills for all hospital personnel on all shifts in all patient-care buildings.

A strict smoking policy that limits smoking to a minimum of designated areas.

Policy statements designed to ensure that interior furnishings, wall coverings, and carpeting that are purchased or installed within the facility are assessed for fire safety code compliance (flame spread, combustibility, etc.).

The facilities manager should review the fire safety management program annually and ensure that a summary of the program is reviewed by the hospital safety committee and executive staff. The facilities manager must ensure that deficiencies identified in the fire safety program and all actions taken to alleviate the problems are properly documented in committee minutes and appropriate program folders.

Hospital Safety Program

The goals of any hospital safety program are to ensure a safe environment for patients, staff, and visitors and to reduce the risk of human injury in the facility or on the grounds. The facilities manager is responsible for overseeing the development, implementation, and monitoring of the hospital safety management program. Therefore, the facilities manager is responsible for managing an ongoing process of collection and evaluation of hazard and safety practice information, which can be used by the safety committee to address safety management issues.

The safety committee should meet at least every other month with appropriate membership as required by the JCAHO. At these meetings, the safety committee analyzes safety discrepancies, develops action recommendations, and monitors the actions taken to determine their effectiveness. The safety committee oversees the following:

- Development of the medical facility's safety policies and standards.
- Review and approval of departmental safety policies.
- Monitoring and investigation of accident and injury situations, including the timely reporting and resolution of situations that pose an immediate threat to life, health, and/or property.
- Identification and elimination of hazards, including, but not limited to, grounds, buildings, internal systems, and remodeling or construction projects. This identification includes a risk assessment program that evaluates the risk posed by equipment, building, grounds, and internal building systems, to patient care and safety.
- Development, review, and evaluation of the safety education program.
- Development, review, and evaluation of the fire prevention program.
- Review of equipment failures or user errors that result in the generation of incident reports; review of relevant equipment hazard reports.
- Development of policies and procedures relating to the operation of the hospital waste management program, including investigation and resolution of identified waste management problems, and evaluation of program effectiveness.

As an example, consider the development of programs for the prevention of biological contamination of the hospital environment. The development, implementation, and management of medical waste tracking and disposal programs represent a key functions of any modern FM department (Lee, 1990).

Regulated medical waste is defined as any solid waste generated in the diagnosis, treatment, or immunization of human beings or animals, in research testing of biologicals, or in the production of biologicals, which is not specifically excluded from the following classes:

Class 1: Cultures and stocks of infectious agents and associated biologicals.
Class 2: Pathological waste from humans, including tissue, organs, body parts, and body fluids that are removed during surgery, autopsy, or other medical procedure.
Class 3: Discarded human blood and blood products that contain free-flowing blood and blood components.
Class 4: Used sharps (i.e., scapel blades, needles, etc.) from animal or human patient care or treatment or from medical, research, or industrial laboratories.
Class 5: Animal waste, containing carcasses, body parts, and bedding of animals that were known to have been exposed to infectious agents during research, production of biologicals, or testing of pharmaceuticals.
Class 6: Waste from patients with highly virulent diseases contaminated with blood, excretion, exudates, or secretions from humans who are isolated to protect others from certain highly virulent organisms.
Class 7: Unused sharps, i.e., hypodermic needles, suture needles, syringes, and scalpel blades.

Every facility must develop a regulated waste tracking system that includes a comprehensive plan outlining the manner of segregation and disposal of waste products. The following procedures should be considered:

- Establishment of a **waste management committee** that includes personnel from Infection Control, Environmental Health, Nursing Services, Hospital Services (covers those who deal with waste, but are not under Nursing Services; i.e., Laboratory, Radiology), Facilities Management, Housekeeping, Safety, and Medical Material. It is important that all parties are included since the proper management of regulated medical waste involves many disciplines within the facility. This committee is responsible for development of the waste management plan.
- Definition by the committee of what constitutes regulated medical waste. This includes defining the categories of waste that must be specifically handled to protect the environment and health-care workers. In this regard, definitions found in the **Medical Waste Tracking Act** (MWTA) can serve as a guide to which any additional state or local requirements may be added.
- Development of a **Facilities operating instruction (FOI)**, which defines the facility-specific procedures for handling regulated medical waste. The instruction should include the facility segregation policy, a description of the disposal method used, a definition of responsibilities, and a copy of the contingency plan.
- Establishment of a segregation policy and standards for packaging waste. Medical waste should be contained in specially colored bags (**red bags**) or marked with the universal

biohazard symbol. Color codes and the types of bags and containers to be used should be determined and implemented throughout the facility. Each department or unit of the facility will require equipment for segregating waste according to the procedures set down by the committee. All housekeeping personnel should receive instruction and regular training in the procedures for regulated waste collection, transport, and disposal. All medical waste should be placed in containers explicitly marked for this purpose and separated from containers used for general refuse.

- Allocation and identification of securable storage space for regulated waste. Such storage areas must maintain the integrity of packaging and provide protection from water, rain, and wind.
- Destruction of medical waste. Regulated medical waste can be disposed of in a number of ways, including incineration, sterilization, and grinding/shredding. Expert advice from a consultant regarding federal, state, and local requirements may be desirable to ensure that the disposal program meets regulations. Each facility must keep a destruction/treatment log and submit copies of incineration destruction reports to the state or federal agencies that require such documentation. Records are usually maintained for three years from the date that the waste was treated or destroyed.
- Development of contingency plans for emergency disposal of regulated medical waste. The plan should include alternative arrangements for the disposal of regulated medical waste in the event of an equipment (incinerator, autoclave, shredder, grinder, etc.) failure or cancellation of a contract.

Security and Resource Protection

Major objectives of the security and resource protection program are to minimize loss, theft, and damage of hospital resources and to maintain order during emergencies. Hospitals are unique facilities that are open 24 hours a day and must be accessible to all patients. Facilities managers, therefore, are responsible for hospital security and resource protection. They must coordinate building security plans with the local police and should request police assistance in determining appropriate security measures. An effective medical facilities security program should include:

- Provision of proper exit and entrance, parking lot, and sidewalk lighting.
- Development of procedures to secure exterior entrances after normal operating hours.
- Protection of individuals during disasters; contingency response planning.
- Evaluation of requirements and adequacy of resource protection measures, such as security alarm systems, vaults, and safes.
- Protection of critical systems (e.g., access to emergency generators, medical gas supply, fuel supply, and primary electrical distribution systems) and control of access to radio base stations, overhead paging systems, and telephone closets.
- Development of a program to track reported thefts and security protection problems and to seek appropriate corrections or elimination.
- Control of facility keys and combinations by establishing and maintaining a key control program. The program should include the safeguarding, issuance, documentation, inventory, and recovery of all keys issued to hospital personnel.

Security and resource protection is everyone's responsibility. With rising crime rates across the nation, security is now more important than ever. With the federal government reducing funding for federal, state, and local law enforcement, greater emphasis will be placed on the hospital security department (Martin, 1991).

Professional Environment

An attractive, professional-looking facility will attract both patients and highly qualified medical providers. It is the responsibility of the facility manager to develop a long-term plan for maintaining and improving the appearance of the facility. The plan should include painting, floor covering renovation (tile or carpeting), wall covering replacement, and maintenance and renovation of any portion of the hospital.

Housekeeping functions must be performed in an effective and timely manner. This is not only important to maintaining the aesthetics of the hospital, but it is also essential essential to providing an aseptic environment, which facilitates medical treatment. The most important tool in the infection control arsenal is the use of appropriate cleaning agents by a qualified cleaning staff. Frequent nosocomial infections are an indicator of problems with cleaning agents or techniques.

Designing a pleasing environment involves more than selecting textures and finishes; Life Safety Code and infection control requirements must be considered. Factors such as wear, soil-hiding capabilities, how well body fluids can be removed, regular maintenance requirements, and ease of equipment transport are some basic considerations. The philosophy that a pleasing environment can support healing and promote well-being has been scientifically tested and documented. The benefits derived from such a notion present some interesting perspectives. There is a definite financial benefit to reducing the length of stay under today's hospital payment system. A clean, well-kept environment can also produce positive results by improving staff productivity (Ruga, 1989).

Medical Functionality

In order to allocate adequate space to accommodate both people and equipment efficiently it is necessary to (1) develop a facilities master plan that provides an overall view of the activities planned for the facility and, (2) establish guidelines for space utilization.

The Facilities Master Plan. The facilities master plan is a long-range planning tool that can be used to prioritize minor and major construction projects necessary for the operation, maintenance, and future development of the hospital. The facility master plan usually is a single document identifying requirements, resources, and priorities for at least a ten-year program of facility projects. The level of detail declines for later years. When developed properly, the master plan facilitates a coordinated, integrated approach to equipment planning, preparation for and compliance with accreditation standards and safety codes, security and resource protection requirements, meeting space utilization objectives and energy goals, adapting to mission changes, cosmetic enhancements, etc. The development of a master plan assists the facilities manager in efforts to manage maintenance and repair as well as minor and major construction projects.

In developing the facilities master plan, input should be solicited from the hospital executive committee and senior staff members. The facilities manager should also attempt to incorporate the hospital strategic plan, facility utilization studies, JCAHO accreditation survey results, resource protection reports, and any other appropriate documentation to develop this plan. To ensure that the master plan remains current, the facilities manager and various administrators should jointly review the priorities on a regular basis.

The following elements of the facility master plan are essential:

- An up-to-date, comprehensive **statement of construction and fire protection** that follows the JCAHO format. This should be a copy of the actual statement sent to the JCAHO.
- A comparison of all building designs to applicable current standards based on the type of occupancy as listed in NFPA 99 and 101.
- A list of all building systems and plant equipment in the hospital showing the age of the equipment, a brief assessment of its condition and the estimated fiscal year and cost for the next replacement or overhaul.
- A schedule of facility projects planned within the next three to five years in priority order, as determined by the executive committee.

Space Utilization. Attempting to integrate new technology into a medical department can be extremely challenging. The addition of one new system can result in a domino effect that requires moving several other departments to accommodate the new technology. As a result, the allocation of space for any project should be carefully examined (DeChant, 1988; see also Chapter 4).

The allocation of hospital space to various clinical users and departments is usually accomplished by a **facilities utilization board**, a hospital-wide committee that evaluates space requests and recommends actions to the hospital executive committee (Mills, 1990). At a minimum, this board should consist of the following:

Director of nursing, who has the knowledge of patient and staff requirements and can give infection control input.

Director of capital planning, who can determine financial feasibility.

Director of facilities management, who has knowledge of code compliance, structural capabilities, utility availability, housekeeping, etc.

Director of clinical engineering, who is familiar with technology integration, installation requirements, clinical applications, and their relation to other functional areas.

A representative from the hospital's board of directors.

The facility utilization board serves several purposes. It assists the hospital's executive committee in determining the adequacy of medical support facilities, ensures that medical facilities are used for medical purposes, and makes recommendations to eliminate inadequacies (adjusting the medical mission within physical plant constraints or pursuing major or minor construction projects to alleviate significant space shortfalls).

In this respect, computer systems can be of tremendous assistance to the facilities manager in determining space utilization. Computer-aided design (CAD) systems offer exceptional flexibility in providing high-quality drawings and in making changes to these drawings during various phases of project management. Various concepts and alternatives discussed with hospital administration can be quickly turned into drawings so the most appropriate solution to a given problem or situation can be determined.

CAD systems also permit standardization of frequently used details and symbols (Peglow, 1987). Floor plans can be overlaid, allowing analysis of structural, mechanical, electrical, or plumbing systems during the design process, thus ensuring that conflicting spatial issues are reconciled. CAD systems interfaced with appropriate database systems have been developed that allow building information to "grow" as the facility changes. Space productivity can be analyzed to ensure the hospital is getting the most for its investment. Accurate square footage measurements can lead to higher Medicare reimbursements of overhead expenses that can be prorated on a square foot basis. Although this is primarily a facilities management tool, the entire facility can benefit from a properly configured and up-to-date graphic computerized space inventory system.

Maintenance Programs. Figure 6.4 illustrates the general work flow of a typical FM system. In this system, requests for specific services are received by letter, telephone, or even over a local area network (LAN) via computer transmission. If the service request pertains to new equipment, testing prior to its use may include safety testing, functional testing, and performance verification as outlined in Chapter 4. Once accepted, the item is placed on the equipment inventory and preventive maintenance schedules are developed in much the same manner as described in Chapter 3 for medical equipment.

Today, identification data, including the item description, identification number, manufacturer, model and serial numbers, acquisition date, life expectancy, location, cost, etc., are entered into an automated maintenance information system, where these data are accessible for a wide variety of purposes including scheduling, work order control, analysis of historical data, productivity evaluation, budgeting, and accreditation documentation.

Corrective maintenance requests are received in the same manner, and the resulting work request is assigned to the appropriate personnel for action. As with the repair of biomedical equipment, response to work requests is usually prioritized by the level of risk to patients, staff, and visitors and the impact on medical care. Utility system failures, for example, would significantly interfere with the ability of the clinical staff to perform necessary medical procedures and, thus, require prompt attention. The fact that the Safe Medical Devices Act of 1990 also applies to plant equipment systems that are connected to medical devices demands that physical plant and utility systems be maintained with the same competence and attention as the medical equipment they support.

FACILITIES DESIGN

The design of clinical facilities is an activity not normally associated with the "traditional" duties of the practicing clinical engineer. Generally, licensed architectural, civil, mechanical, and electrical engineers are hired to design and construct buildings. As discussed in the previous chapters, biomedical and clinical engineers, on the other hand, are primarily involved in the design, development, and proper operation of medical devices and systems. Why, then, is it necessary to involve clinical engineers in the process of designing health-care facilities? The answer to this question lies in the desirability of incorporating the experience of the clinical engineer into the design of medical facilities.

Experienced clinical engineers usually are familiar not only with the specific medical devices, but also with the environment in which they are used. These environments range from the relatively simple surroundings of patient rooms found in general-care nursing units to the more complex units used for surgery, imaging, and critical care. As a result of their capabilities and insights, experienced clinical engineers can make significant contributions to the proper (optimal) design of patient-care facilities. Their participation in this area is, therefore, to be encouraged.

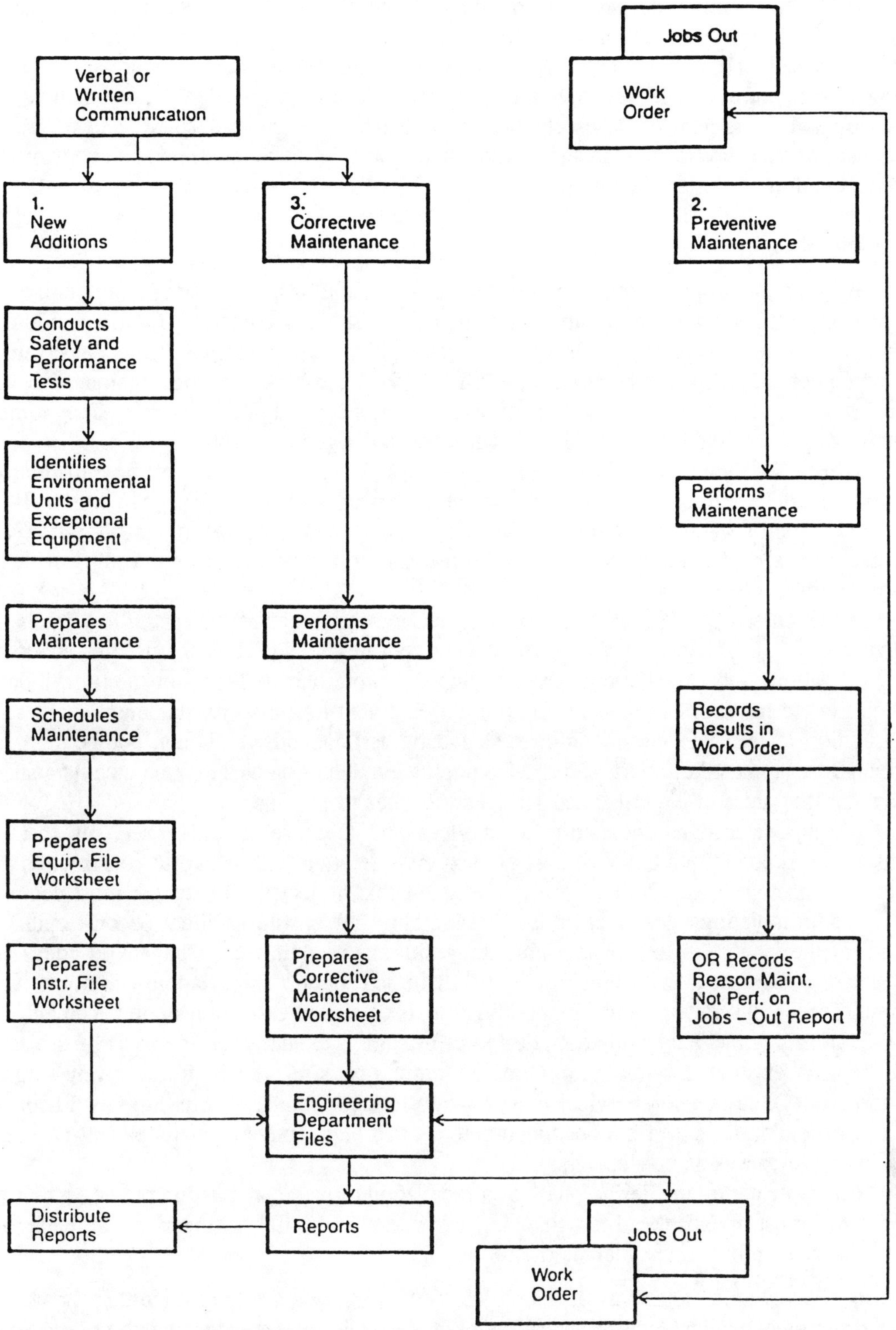

Figure 6.4: Work flow model for a facilities management program.

With this in mind, the aspects of facilities design discussed in this section are limited to clinical facilities. The design of employee cafeterias, laundry rooms or business offices is not discussed. These nonclinical facilities can be more than adequately addressed by other engineering professionals who do not need the more detailed knowledge of how medical care is provided. The goal of this section is to emphasize how most hospitals can utilize the services of an in-house clinical engineer to enhance and facilitate the design and construction or renovation of clinical facilities.

Design Issues

In general, hospitals are complex and costly buildings. The larger community and university-affiliated institutions are essentially miniature cities, containing multiple buildings, roadways and pedestrian walkways, major utility distribution systems, specialized environmental control systems, business offices, food services, laundries, maintenance and repair services, computer networks, and even chapels for religious services. The primary activity of these "cities" is providing health-care to the general public.

As one would imagine, the capital investment in the physical assets of these institutions is significant. Therefore, when it is deemed necessary or desirable to engage in design efforts related to modifying or expanding medical facilities, the task is not taken lightly. When such a decision is made, many factors must be taken into account before proceeding with the design process.

As discussed in Chapter 1, the overall mission statement of the institution drives the activities of the facility. Within the context of present social concerns and economic considerations, most institutions have developed a more narrow focus for the utilization of their limited resources. Consequently, the development of a mission statement enables the institution to take into consideration such factors as financial well-being, competition, the strengths of the medical staff, and service population demographics to announce its goals in terms of the areas of expertise and services it wishes to provide.

Having determined the particular services and the level of these services that the institution is committed to providing, the next consideration with regard to construction and renovation projects is, "Is there really a need for this project?" One of the most common reasons for initiating a design effort is that, ultimately, all existing facilities become outdated, and for the institution to remain viable, they must be modernized. Changes in codes and standards, advances in technology, and increased public expectations combine with obsolescence and deterioration of buildings to necessitate renovation or replacement. In addition to this inevitable situation, design efforts are also started on the basis of decisions to expand existing services (e.g., provide more operating rooms for a given surgical subspecialty), initiate new services (e.g., begin offering secondary- or tertiary-level neonatal care), or reallocate space from one function to another (e.g., convert general patient-care beds to intensive-care beds or vice versa).

Prior to entering the design phase of a renovation or new construction project, a number of factors must be considered for which input from the "in-house" engineering staff can prove to be very helpful. These include the following:

Costs. "What is the total cost of the project?" It is important to recognize that the cost of construction of medical facilities usually runs at least twice that associated with normal office building projects. Total costs, however, include not only actual construction, but also architect and engineer fees, cost estimating, construction management, asbestos abatement (in existing spaces), building permits, insurance, change orders, and contingencies. All of these components of the total cost of the design project must be taken into account.

New construction versus renovation. Factors that affect the decision to build a new facility or to renovate an existing space include a comparison of relative costs for new versus old construction. For inner-city institutions, zoning limitations on any increase in the ratio of total building "footprint" sizes to land plot size must also be taken into account. Whatever the reason, if the decision is to renovate, it is critical to understand that there can be significant limitations on design options. For example, it is highly likely that the ideas that administration or clinical staff may have regarding optimum designs for clinical spaces of various types will not fit exactly into the "footprint" (i.e., perimeter shape) of an existing building.

Space. "How much space is actually needed?" Based on experience, published guidelines, standards, or equipment manufacturers' recommendations, there are well-established minimum space requirements for most hospital services. To what extent a given design goes beyond minimum requirements or implements innovative design techniques is usually a function of available space. In renovation projects, for example, the usual experience is that there is not quite enough space to implement the desired design.

Adjacencies. "How does this project affect other services?" A critical factor to consider in design projects that involve clinical services is that of "adjacencies," i.e., the proximity of medical services that interact directly. Some examples of this interrelationship include the surgical intensive-care unit and the operating room; the helicopter landing pad, the emergency trauma room, and the CAT-scanning facilities in radiology; and the delivery room and the neonatal intensive-care unit. The efficiency and quality of patient care is improved as access to adjacencies is optimized.

Handicap access. The **Americans with Disabilities Act (ADA)**, passed by Congress in 1990, has had a significant impact on all building designs. This legislation mandates that design attention be paid not only to the physically challenged patient, but also to staff members and visitors who may be handicapped. The impact of these requirements has been particularly significant in the design of patient-care areas intended for overnight stays.

Utility Systems. "What are the utility requirements of the project?" Often, the demand for utility services in clinical services area projects is substantial. Therefore, the design process must carefully evaluate the demand level to avoid overtaxing existing service capacities or, if necessary, provide for the expansion of these capacities. Such an analysis should include the following:

- The number of electrical receptacles, lights, systems, and devices connected to the various branches of the essential electrical system (emergency generator and distribution) versus the capacity of that system.
- The cooling load (people, lights, equipment) versus the cubic feet per minute (cfm) ventilating capacity and Btu/h cooling capacity of the HVAC system.
- The number and utilization of medical gas outlets (oxygen, medical or surgical vacuum, compressed medical air, nitrous oxide, nitrogen, etc.) versus bulk, tank manifold, pump, or compressor capacities, pipeline sizes, and distribution distances.
- The number of telephones versus switch and backup capacities.
- Contingency planning for interruption of utility service.

The Design/Development Process

Once the fundamental decision to proceed with a facility design effort has been made, several steps will enhance the likelihood of success. These include the following:

- Determination of and contractual arrangements with the appropriate planning, architectural, and engineering services, such as the architect, the director of FM, representatives of hospital management, etc. Individuals from these areas form the nucleus of the design team. The architect often assumes the lead in directing the initial phases of this effort, starting with preliminary discussions to define the scope of the project, and identifying the goals of the owner/institution. Previous experience in health-care facilities design should be a major factor in selecting an architect for a medical facilities project. The design process is often greatly facilitated by the presence of the chief clinical engineer, who can serve as an effective interface between user, medical equipment, and facility.
- Establishment of a schedule. It is vital for individual and group deadlines to be established to prevent the process from taking an unacceptably long period of time. In the programming phase, the design team usually expands to include specific "user representatives" (e.g., physicians, nurses, clinical and ancillary support personnel). Differences in opinion are likely to increase, causing delays in the project schedule. Because it is a cardinal rule that the longer the process takes, the more expensive it becomes, it is critical to organize meetings to achieve consensus as quickly as possible. During this phase, solicitation of input from users is encouraged. Within any medical facility, there are several different user groups that can provide insight and practical information concerning incorporating the functional program of a particular clinical service within the design space. Specific clinical user groups and the focus of their interests are presented in Table 6.2.
- Identification of the space "footprint." Whether an existing space is to be renovated or a new space is to be built, each clinical function is usually confined to a space defined by a perimeter geometry. This geometry may be a total building shape or a section within that shape. The area must conform to the minimal requirements for the function (operating rooms, ICU, imaging suite, etc.) and must satisfy the requirements of adjacencies associated with that function. Figure 6.5 provides an example of how this geometry may be defined. Note that each clinic is confined to a particular space identified in the footprint. Although most of these shapes are quite regular, some can be rather unusual (e.g., diagnostic X-ray department space).
- Development of a floorplan block diagram based on function. This process is initiated by defining the functional spaces and quantity of individual spaces. For example, it may be decided that an adult cardiac ICU will require 12 beds, based on the characteristics of the hospital's service population, availability of necessary ancillary and support services (cardiac catheterization laboratory, electrophysiology laboratory, cardiac operating rooms, etc.), and competitive goals. Each bed requires a certain amount of space. Beyond this, all of the appropriate support spaces (nursing station, medication room, equipment storage, etc.) must fit into the footprint and be appropriately positioned. This process is often difficult, especially if the project is a renovation and the footprint is less than ideal for the function. However, the design team usually can produce a functional block diagram that meets appropriate design criteria or, in the extreme, can reject the space as unworkable and offer suitable alternatives.

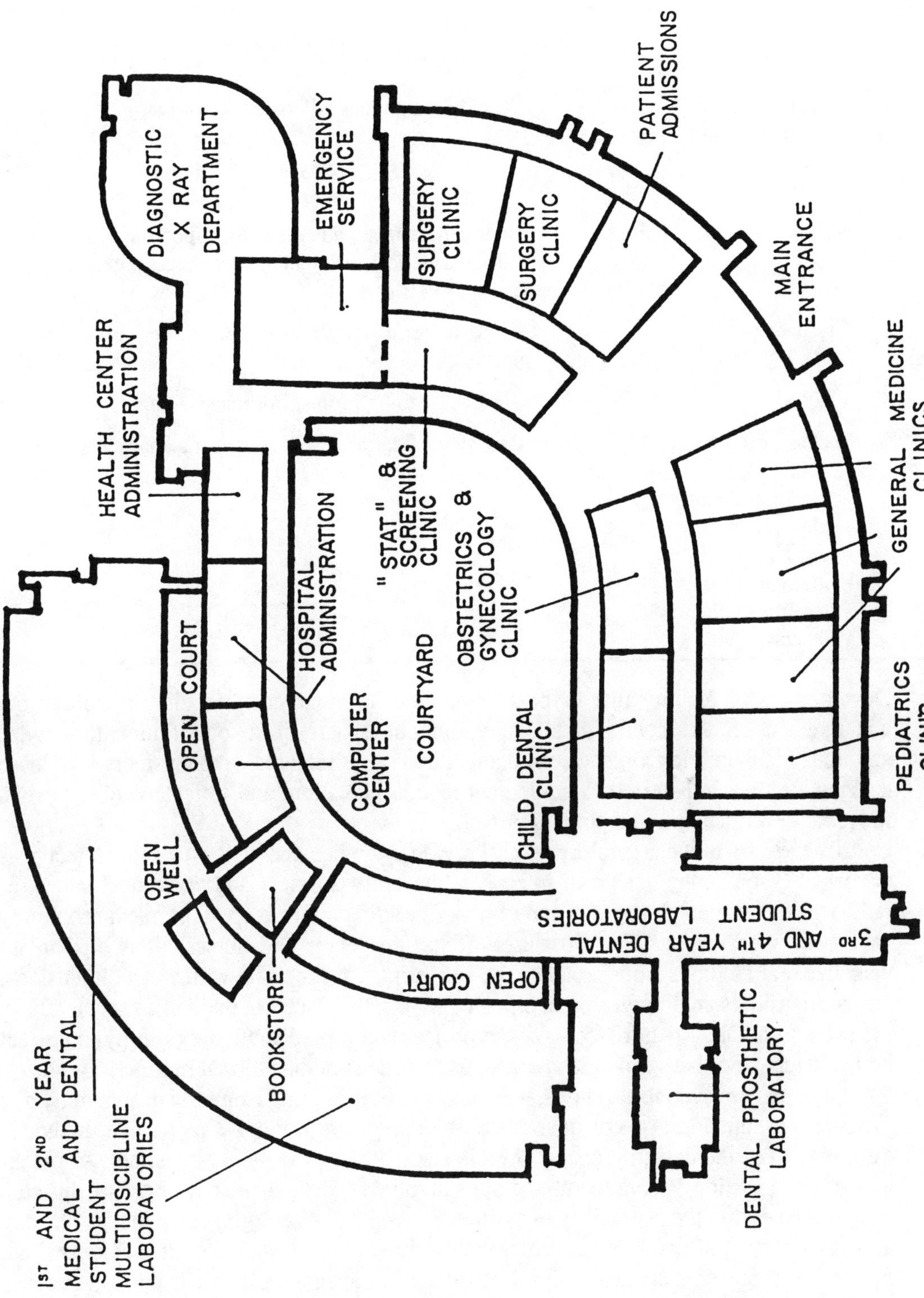

Figure 6.5: Basic plan of the main floor – University of Connecticut Helath Center, Farmington, CT.

Table 6.2 Specific User Input to the Design Process

User Group	Topics of Interest
1. Patients, i.e., - children - adults - the elderly	Windows; lighting; toilets; colors; privacy
2. Nurses	Bedside/treatment-side services; support staff (dietary, clerical, respiratory care, housekeeping, etc.
3. Physicians	Adjacencies; privacy/consulting; charting; education
4. Visitors	Signage; waiting rooms; in-room visiting
5. Technicians, i.e., - radiology - radiation therapy - physical therapy - surgical - medical (laboratory) - respiratory therapy - others	Bedside or treatment area services; adjacencies

- Development of functionality layouts. Once the floorplan configuration is worked out and agreed upon, the specific details of equipment layouts, utility outlet quantities, styles and locations, interior finishes, and any other requirements are considered. These designs are then transferred to equipment layout, elevation, and reflected ceiling prints for review, refinement, and final approval.
- Construction of models (prototypes). Previously, when the scope of the project was extensive (such as the design of intensive-care units, surgical and obstetrical suites, or radiology departments), the cost and effort of building a mock-up of a typical room may have been worthwhile. For most users (e.g., physicians and nurses), it is difficult to visualize real facilities from sketches and blueprints. A mock-up with exact dimensions, drawn-in utilities, and moveable equipment physically placed in the design space allows the users to obtain a better "feel" for the project and provides the opportunity to correct both discrepancies between design drawings and the anticipated final product. However, CAD systems are available today that are capable of providing isometric design drawings to serve this function at a considerable cost savings over model construction methods.
- Termination of the design process. At this stage of the process, it is desirable to obtain agreement, in writing, from the user groups involved. More than anything else, this step provides an end to the possibility of further discussion. Although such a maneuver may seem arbitrary, it offers a few advantages that are extremely valuable. It recognizes that the design represents the best efforts of the entire design team to accomplish specific goals within the limitations of available space and resources. It limits the duration of the design process and precludes the likelihood of change orders occurring during the actual construction, which can be extremely costly.

- Construction documents. After the above steps have been accomplished, all of the detailed design information is taken by the licensed architectural and engineering professionals and transformed into specification books and blueprints that are used by local building authorities to issue building permits, by the hosptital design team for cost estimating and competitive bidding purposes, and by construction contractors to build the facility. Experience suggests that hospital engineering personnel, including the clinical engineer, should review these documents to ensure that the interpretation of design information is correct and has been accurately translated into the final specifications and prints.

With this understanding of the design and development process in mind, let us now discuss how these concepts may be applied to specific clinical areas.

Intensive-Care Areas

At the end of World War II, the concept began to take shape of a nursing unit where concentrated care could be rendered to seriously ill patients under conditions where more continuous monitoring and intensive treatment could be offered than in ordinary or "general" nursing units. Today, the evolution of this approach is reflected in the existence of several types of intensive-care units. These units, which may include adult general surgical, medical, cardiac, neurosurgery, trauma, burn, cardiovascular surgery, pediatric, and neonatal units, are often found within the confines of a single institution, especially if that facility is designated at a "tertiary-care" level for a given geographical area. Each type of unit, however, requires design considerations common to all intensive-care environments as well as special criteria inherent to its medical subspecialty. With this in mind, the common needs of ICUs are covered first, then the special needs, depending on the medical specialty are discussed.

Bed Space. Space allocated to individual patient beds in ICUs varies, according to whether the unit is based on a large open area, cubicle, or individual room design. The open area concept has the advantages of greatest visibility and least amount of space required per bed, but many other considerations, such as ventilation control, privacy, and equipment maneuverability, make this choice less than ideal for most modern applications. The cubicle concept provides for solid partitions with viewing panels between beds, a solid headwall and open space in the direction of the nursing station. It offers a greater degree of privacy while still maintaining substantial visibility and accessibility (Figure 6.6). Control of ventilation and noise abatement, however, remain problematical. The individual room concept, on the other hand, maximizes privacy and ventilation control, but it requires the most space, the greatest investment in floor space, and the highest construction cost. Furthermore, it often impedes visibility. The space required for each bed is directly related to the severity of the patient's illness or injury. By definition, intensive-care units (ICU's) house those patients who require the most care. Therefore, ICUs need the greatest area per bed. The AIA/HHS (1987) guidelines specify a minimum of 120 square feet for an ICU bed. An evaluation of the space required for the bed itself, access to the patient (from three or four sides), provision of utility services, and the placement of various pieces of equipment (e.g., ventilator, infusion pumps, intra-aortic balloon pump, dialysis machine, hyperthermia unit, etc.) needed at the bedside, however, usually increase this minimum. In view of the range and complexity of the medical technology available in today's armamentarium for intensive care, a single-bed ICU room may require upwards of 250 square feet.

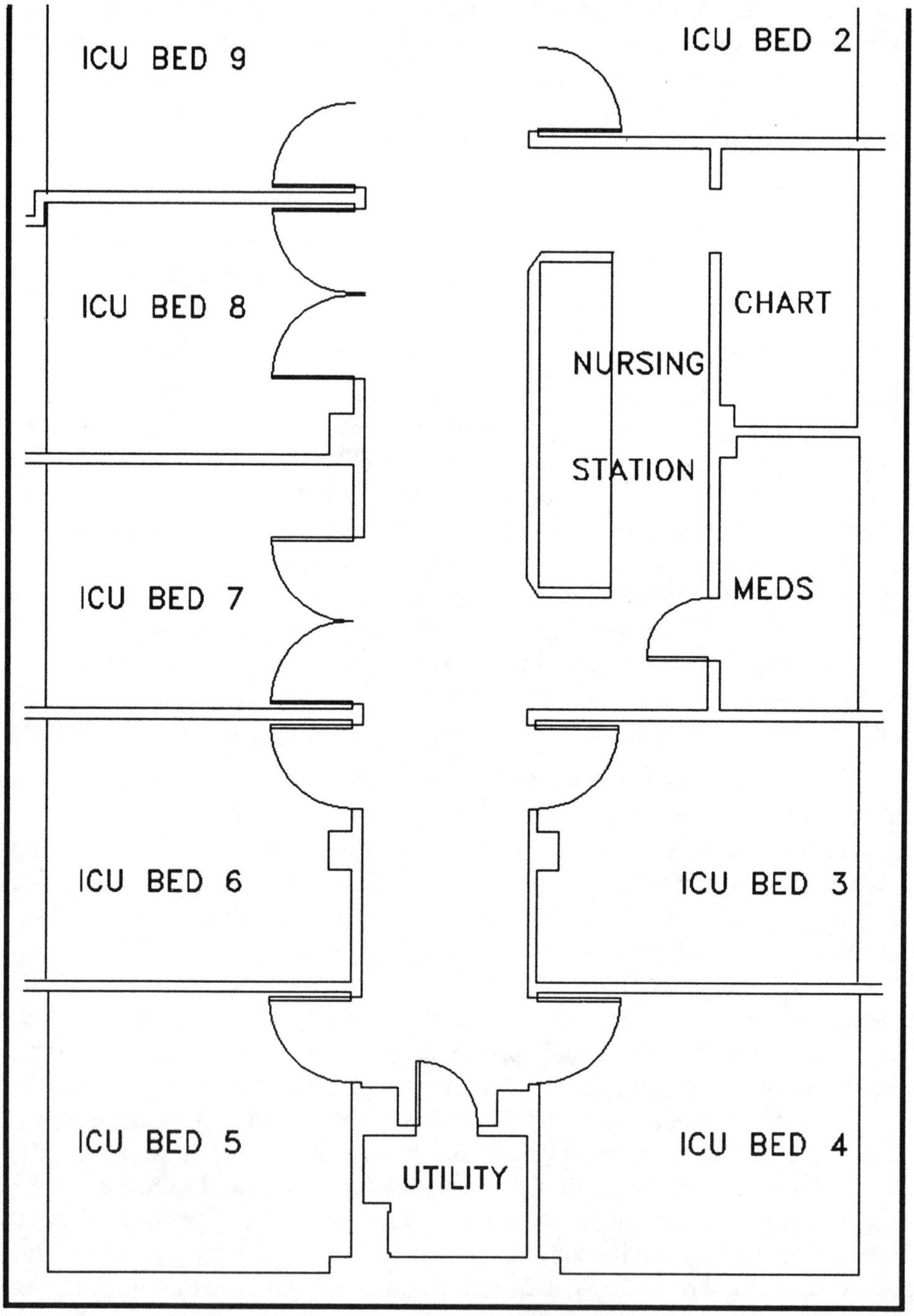

Figure 6.6: Floor plan of a cubicle-type layout used in the ICU.

There are definite limits to the total number of beds accommodated in a given intensive-care unit. The prevailing wisdom—based on nursing staff and support service requirements which include distances from nursing station to beds, the total number of nurses on duty during a given shift (i.e. nurse-patient ratio), and the need for ancillary support spaces, generally supports a unit size of no more than 12 to 16 beds. Thus, in ICUs, the total net square foot requirements for bed space alone may be as high as 4,000 square feet.

Support Functions. The total area of an ICU generally approximates 2.5 to 3 times the area required for bed space alone (Laufman, 1981; Moderow, 1991). Functions that need to be located in close proximity to patient bed spaces include the following:

The Nursing Station. As the command post of the ICU, the nursing station must be sized, configured, equipped and located to accommodate all of the activities situated at and emanating from this hub. These activities include the following:

Communications. Space is needed to accommodate telephones, nurse call consoles, intercoms, data terminals, printers, and also verbal communication with nurses, physicians, visitors and ancillary support staff. A nursing station desk design often incorporates a physical barrier (such as an elbow-height partition with a small counter cap at the top) on the outer side of the desk surface to protect those surfaces from "intrusion" by personnel approaching the desk.

Clerical. Adequate space for the record-keeping requirements of the nursing unit staff is needed. This includes open writing space and filing spaces for forms, records, and references required by current regulatory and accreditation requirements. Desk depth is an important design specification because the presence of numerous consoles and devices could easily eliminate adequate writing space.

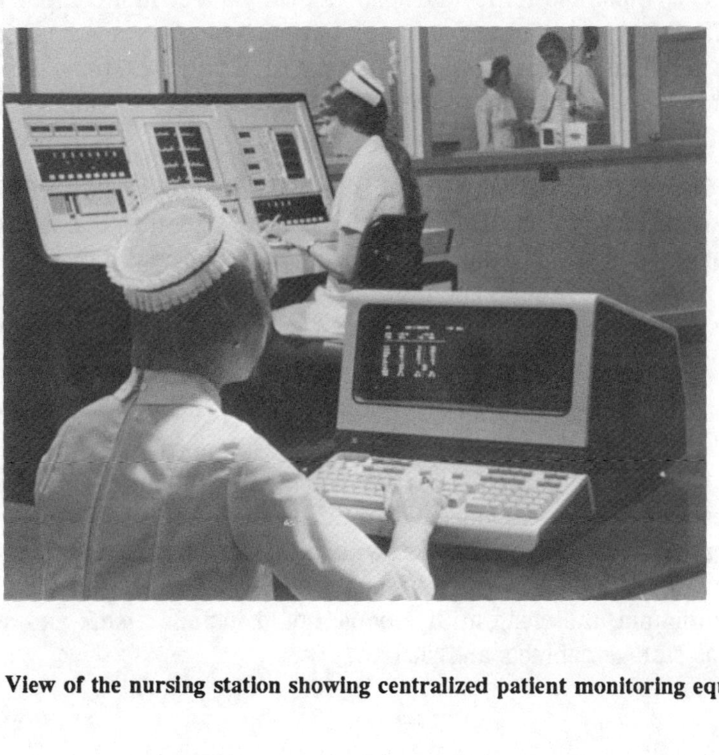

Figure 6.7: View of the nursing station showing centralized patient monitoring equipment.

Central monitoring. Bedside physiologic monitors are included as a standard of the type of care found in ICUs. Most monitoring systems incorporate central station displays and recorders that are normally located at the nursing station and can be placed directly on the desk (again, adequate depth must be provided for these devices without affecting writing space), placed on shelves or suspended from the ceiling (Figure 6.7).
The position of these monitoring displays should always allow for ready access and proper visibility at the nursing station. The issue of constantly viewing monitors to inspect patients is a difficult one for nursing staff. With this in mind, many manufacturers incorporate automatic alarms, recording, and arrhythmia detection capabilities into their equipment.

Visual access to patients. Typically, nursing stations are located in such a way as to provide visual access to all patients within the unit and to be equidistant from all beds. In single-bed room designs, vision panels (glass doors or windows) must be incorporated into partitions separating the nursing station from patients to maintain visual access. Moveable curtains are placed over these vision panels when privacy is needed and appropriate (e.g., when a nurse is tending to the patient).

Charting Activities. The maintenance of patient charts and medical records is a continuous process that is performed by nurses, physicians, and allied health personnel, such as respiratory therapists or dialysis technicians. Because a substantial portion of this activity occurs at the bedside, provision should be made within patient rooms or cubicles for writing space, either at sitting (30") or standing (36") heights. Because charting also occurs at the nursing station (especially by physicians), serious consideration should be given to the concept of a separate charting area that is quiet yet not too far from the nursing station. In addition, if the hospital utilizes electronic access to medical records, laboratory results, etc., a separate charting area should be provided for terminal access. Clearly, the emergence of the "paperless record" is a factor that must be taken into account for modern ICU design (Moderow, 1991). Input and retrieval of patient data via a central computer system (Figure 6.8) is recognized as a powerful tool to help alleviate the common complaint of nurses that they spend too much time on paperwork. For expansion purposes, provision should be made not only for immediate installation of terminals at the bedside, nursing station, and charting areas, but for future installations as well.

Medication Preparation. Usually, a separate area for the stocking and preparation of medications is necessary. In an ICU, this space is often larger than that needed for a general-care nursing unit. An adequate supply of medications, refrigerated storage devices, ancillary supplies (such as syringes, needles and intravenous (I.V.) solutions), and a sink are necessary. As a side note, it should be pointed out that an I.V. hanger or track above the sink is often handy for the preparation of I.V. medications, and can save considerable space.

Clean Utility Activities. In this era of disposables, a storage space specifically dedicated to sterile medical and surgical supplies, additional I.V. solutions, and other "clean" items is a necessity. Although there is a tendency for nursing personnel to ask for massive storage capacity because supplies are often used up quickly, space and budget limitations may often preclude this luxury. Careful coordination with materials management personnel and supply delivery procedures is therefore crucial when the design team focuses on the size of this space. At a minimum, the clean utility room should include a sink and adequate counter space as well as storage cabinets and shelves.

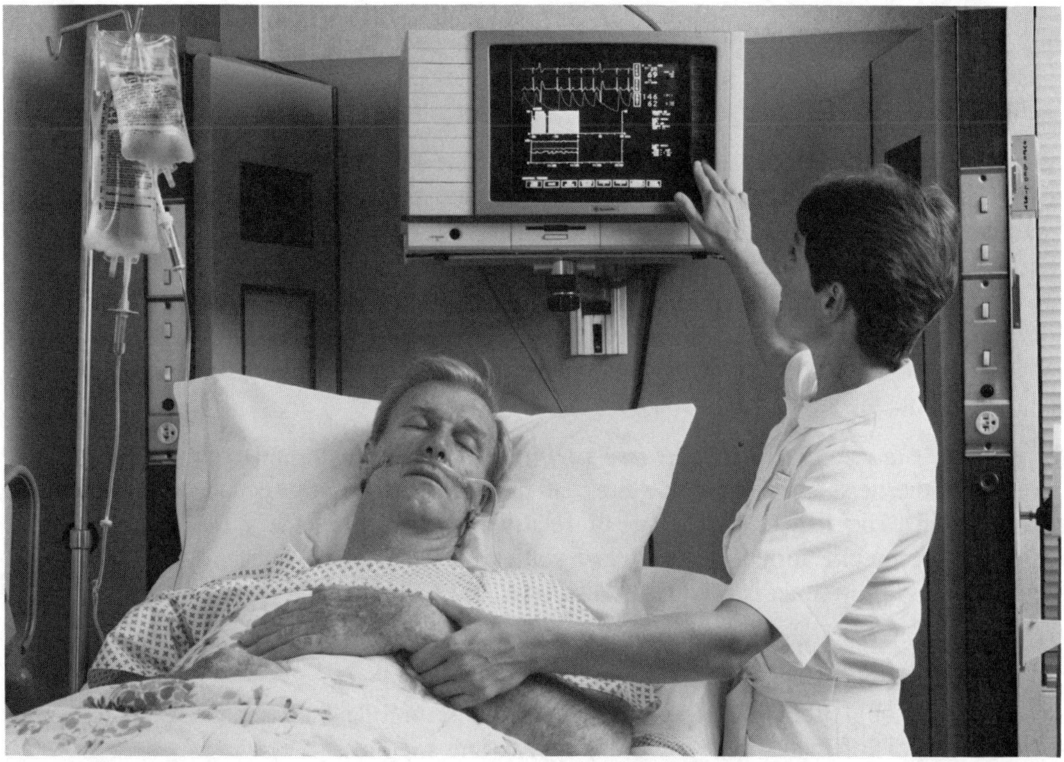

Figure 6.8: Nurse entering patient data to cental computer linked to bedside terminal.

Soiled Utility Activities. A separate, compartmentalized space for holding normal trash, biomedical (red bag) waste, reusable items awaiting return to the central supply department for reprocessing, and bagged, soiled linen is often required. This space should include a utility sink, a clinical sink (rim flushing for liquid wastes), and a bedpan sanitizer.

Nourishment Station. Although the dietary needs of patients are met primarily by intravenous nutrition or dietary tray services, a small pantry is desirable for special needs, such as reheating food for patients who were undergoing tests or treatment when trays were delivered. Provision should be made for a refrigerator, a small heating or microwave oven, an ice machine, a handwashing sink, and minimal storage cabinets.

Linen Storage. Space is needed for the storage of clean linen. An attractive alternative to a space with fixed storage shelves is the exchange cart system. Using this approach, a day's supply of clean linen is delivered to the unit on a cart, and the previous day's supply cart is removed for restocking. With this system, a linen supply can be accommodated in a corridor alcove (if the cart has a cover) rather than a separate room.

Equipment Storage. For equipment that is dedicated to the unit (rather than supplied on an as-needed basis from a central location), storage is required. Space is determined by the amount and type of equipment to be stored, either on shelves or floor space for rolling devices. If battery charging is necessary, an adequate number of electrical receptacles should be provided. If the support of clinical engineering services requires on-site trouble shooting, repair, and provision for other biomedical equipment, appropriate space and facilities for this function should also be incorporated into the design.

Staff Lounge/Lockers. A space for staff to take breaks, write shift change reports, and conduct in-service education sessions is desirable, as are changing areas, lockers, and lavatory facilities.

Visitor Waiting Space. Because visiting times for the families of seriously ill patients are necessarily restricted, a pleasant and comfortable area outside of the ICU for visitor use while waiting is a major consideration. The decor and layout of the area should avoid the classic "bus station" environment through compartmentalization and noise abatement. Communication should be provided (e.g., a restricted telephone; an intercom may not provide enough privacy or confidentiality) between this room and the nursing station, so that visitors can inquire about appropriate times to enter the unit and the nursing staff can communicate status or events to family members.

Head Nurse's and Assistant Head Nurse's Offices. The administration of the ICU is usually the task of the head nurse, who requires, at times, privacy or the isolation necessary for concentration. The office should be in relative proximity to the nursing station with appropriate communication links (such as a station on the nurse call system) so that the head nurse may respond immediately to the desk or to individual rooms.

Housekeeping Functions. The equipment and supplies required by housekeeping personnel to keep the unit clean must be accommodated. The unit design should include a janitorial closet large enough for a floor sink, mops, brooms, mobile buckets and carts, cleaning solutions and disinfectants, and any other appropriate supplies.

Utility Services. Once all required functional spaces, their sizes, and adjacencies have been identified and an architectural solution is achieved through an acceptable floor plan, the next major design step is the specification and detailing of utility services. These services include electrical power, lighting, plumbing and fixtures, heating, ventilation, air conditioning, piped medical gases, and communications. Requirements for each vary, according to the functional space under consideration. The most crucial space is, appropriately, the patient space.

The environment immediately surrounding an intensive-care patient bed must be able to support and accommodate a multitude of skilled professionals focusing their attention on the well-being of the patient while utilizing a variety of devices to administer to the needs of the patient. To accomplish this, a number of utility services are required in appropriate configurations, capacities, locations, and specifications.

Electrical Power

Receptacles. It is important to provide an adequate number of receptacles. As the utilization of medical technologies increases, so does the need for power. Therefore, it is critical to analyze the probable locations of devices (e.g., physiologic monitor located near the head of the bed; ventilator to the side or behind the head; infusion pumps at the sides; intra-aortic balloon pump or hyperthermia unit at the foot) and to distribute receptacles accordingly. In addition, it is appropriate to specify receptacle types: hospital grade 3 prong, twist lock for life-support devices, etc.

Circuits. Because the number and distribution of electrical circuits is important, an analysis of total loads (present and future) must be made. In this study, it is critical that circuits have a rated capacity and protection of 20 amps or more. In addition, the use of emergency versus normal power and the consequences of circuit failure must be determined. For example, a quad receptacle (two duplex receptacles) could be fed by two different circuits that may share other receptacles in the room so that if one fails, quickly replugging the device into an adjacent receptacle will restore power.

Emergency power. Life-support devices, which are now almost always found in the intensive-care environment, must be powered from the critical branch of a hospital's essential electrical system, as specified in NFPA 70 and 99. However, a combination of both emergency and normal power receptacles should be considered on the basis of (1) the capacity of the alternate power source (e.g., diesel generator) and (2) the likelihood of a total external power outage versus an internal distribution failure.

Isolated power. During the 1970s, ICUs were required to be constructed with isolation transformers and line-isolation monitors. This type of electrical distribution is no longer required in ICUs, although it is still a design option, albeit expensive. As discussed in Chapter 2, isolated power does not protect against microshock hazard; however, it does provide the users with a warning of equipment faulting and enhanced protection against macroshock.

Equipotential grounding. The need to protect the patient from microshock hazard in the ICU is critical because of the common use of "externalized cardiac conductors" (e.g., Swan-Ganz catheters, temporary pacemaker leads, etc.), which can provide a pathway for very small electrical currents to cause cardiac fibrillation. In addition to the performance of equipment preventive maintenance procedures and leakage current testing, the installation and testing of equipotential grounding in the ICU patient environment ensures no that there will be no potential difference between grounded surfaces and equipment in the room. Physically, all receptacles and conductive surfaces in the room are tied to a common ground bus with large (#10) grounding conductors that are not looped between receptacles or surfaces.

Lighting

General illumination. Various levels of lighting intensity are required in the ICU patient room, depending on the type of activity. For example, the performance of visual tasks such as routine physical examinations or observations can be accomplished with recessed ceiling fluorescent fixtures that provide illuminance of 30 to 75 footcandles. Flexibility in lighting levels is usually achieved with multiswitched bulbs or fluorescent dimmers. The color spectrum of room lighting should also be considered; one example of this is to select wide-spectrum bulbs for patient rooms to ensure that facial color does not appear distorted.

Task illumination. The performance of visual tasks of low contrast or those that entail a small field of vision, such as I.V. manipulations, over a prolonged period of time may require increased illuminance of 100, 200, or more footcandles. This requirement may best be met through specialized or supplemental lighting, such as procedure lights or directed task lighting used occasionally and on demand. If used, task lighting should be served by emergency power circuits.

Night lighting. At the other end of the spectrum, night lighting in the ICU is usually 10 to 20 footcandles, rather than the low-intensity (i.e., less than 1 footcandle) found in general patient areas. One approach to the design of night lighting capability, however, is to provide an area of high-contrast task lighting for nurse charting off to the side of the room.

Natural lighting. The recuperation of patients in the ICU setting has been linked to the ability to perceive the difference between day and night (Beck and Meyer, 1982). Thus, the ICU design should incorporate exterior windows in proximity to patient spaces. This does limit such spaces to building perimeters, so some innovations may be necessary in the form of glass partitions or other transparent barriers that will allow daylight to reach the patient from more remote exterior windows.

Plumbing Fixtures

Handwashing sinks. The prime vectors for the transmission of microbial contamination are the personnel who work in ICUs, and the main route of contamination is direct contact (see Chapter 2). Proper aseptic technique consists of several precautions, but by far the most basic is handwashing. Failure to practice proper technique is most often the result of inadequate numbers or inconvenient locations of handwashing sinks. Therefore, these sinks should be installed in each patient room and at every major functional space.

Toilets. Toilets are not normally found in ICU patient rooms because patients are generally not ambulatory. If encouraging early ambulation or providing the staff with convenient waste disposal is desirable, a Pullman-style toilet within a cabinet may be installed. Otherwise, provision should be made for adequate staff and visitor facilities.

Heating, ventilation, and air conditioning. The design of an HVAC system to supply air to or to remove air from an intensive-care unit must meet certain common, and some specialized, criteria. The system should, insofar as possible, provide air movement from "clean" to "less clean" areas. This movement is controlled primarily by the amount of air supplied to or exhausted from individual rooms or spaces and the volume relationships between adjacent spaces. For example, isolation rooms have more air exhausted from them than supplied, thus producing a negative pressure relative to normal atmospheric pressure. If the adjacent space (e.g., the corridor) is pressure neutral, then air flows into the room from the corridor. Such isolation is often specified for patients with communicable or infectious disease.

In other situations, such as rooms for burn patients or organ transplant recipients, a reversal of these pressure and air flow relationships is required. One design provides for user-controlled variable exhaust, which allows a given space to be used as either a standard or reverse isolation space, depending on the need. In this case, verification of positive or negative pressure can be achieved through the use of a display anemometer. In addition to air flow, guidelines exist (AHA, 1982; AIA/HHS, 1987) for a number of other HVAC operational parameters for ICU design, including air changes (Table 6.3).

Cooling load calculations are based on the heat dissipation of lights, people, equipment and building face exposures. Air to all areas for inpatient care, treatment, or diagnosis and areas providing direct service or clean supplies should travel through two filter beds with efficiencies of 25 percent and 90 percent gross particulate removal, respectively, to extend the life of the final stage filter.

Air supply diffusers should be designed and located so as not to produce significant drafts directly over patient beds or areas over staff work stations. On the other hand, concentrated, localized cooling and air flow may be desirable for fixed equipment such as central station monitoring mainframes. Note that radiators and convectors are considered room recirculation units and should not be used because of cleaning difficulty and the potential for buildup of contamination. Recirculation and refiltering of up to 80 percent of air via central air handling systems is permitted in many states, which is an important energy saving consideration because the cost of heating, cooling, and handling air is substantial.

Piped Medical Gases

The availability of a continuous supply of oxygen, medical vacuum, and other piped gases, particularly in the case of special care facilities such as the ICU, is a significant consideration to the overall design. The task of the design team is to determine the quantity and location of appropriate piped medical gas outlets in relation to the patient and the number and types of devices that will require the simultaneous supply of these gases. The team should keep capacity limitations for supply systems in mind. The amount of gas that can be delivered to (or, in the case of a vacuum, drawn from) an individual outlet is determined by pipeline diameters and lengths going all the way back to primary sources such as bulk (liquid) oxygen tanks, vacuum pumps, and air compressors.

All outlets must be configured in such a way as to physically prevent inadvertent connection to the incorrect gas. This is accomplished through the use of one of several commercially available outlet configurations, such as diamond quick-connects or the diameter-indexed safety system (DISS). Even with the use of indexed outlets, it is absolutely essential to perform tests prior to the use of any newly installed or modified piped medical gas system.

Table 6.3 HVAC Guidelines for Air Movement

Area Designation	Air Movement Relationship	Min. Fresh Air Changes	Min. Total Air Changes	Recirculation by Room	All Air Exhausted
Patient Room	Neutral	2	6	No	-
Isolation	In	-	6	No	Yes
Reverse Isolation	Out	-	6	No	-
Corridor	-	-	2	-	-
Medication	-	-	4	-	-
Clean Utility	-	-	4	-	-
Soiled Utility	In	-	10	No	Yes
Bathroom	-	-	10	-	-

Intensive-care patient rooms should have a minimum of two oxygen outlets, two vacuum outlets, and one medical air outlet. These numbers may increase if it is anticipated that more oxygen (for ventilators, blenders, nasal cannulae, etc.), vacuum (gastric suction, chest tube drainage, tracheal suction, etc.), or medical air (ventilators, blenders, etc.) will be needed simultaneously.

Communications

Provisions should be incorporated into the design for a number of definite or possible communications lines to ICU patient bedsides and throughout the ICU. These communications systems include the following:

Nurse call. A variety of options are available and need to be considered, for example, two-way voice and signal communication between each patient's bedside and the nursing station; emergency call capability from each patient's bedside; and capability for nurses to summon additional help from other areas, such as the staff lounge, medication room, or even outside of the unit.

Telephones. Clearly, telephones at the nursing station, charting area, head nurse's office, and staff lounge are required. Telephones at each patient bedside may be considered, especially for patients who are recovered to the extent that lucid verbal communication is possible.

Bedside monitors. Cabling from bedsides to central station equipment must be provided. In the process, special attention should be paid to the routing and concealment of cabling to desk-mounted central displays.

Entertainment/education. Cabling, powering and mounting of televisions for use by patients as entertainment (cable TV) or education (closed circuit) and by staff for in-service education should be considered.

Other data transmission. The need for additional cabling related to such systems as bedside patient data terminals, centralized ECG management systems, laboratory test ordering and result retrieval are also important to consider. If none of these systems currently exists, the installation of empty small diameter conduit and junction boxes at strategic locations will greatly facilitate future installations.

Paging systems. Overhead hospital paging speakers; nurse "all-call" capability, and beepers should be considered.

At this point in the design process, a number of details still remain to be addressed. These include reflected ceiling plans, finish materials, and color selections. At this stage, the "packaging" of utility service outlets in the patient vicinity is of particular importance to clinical engineering. Several options are available to accomplish this:

Permanent installation within cubicle/room walls. This option utilizes the least amount of floor space but has the disadvantage of difficult and costly future modification.

Prefabricated headwalls. In this case, all utility outlets are located within a predesigned unit that is attached to the headwall with relatively simple connections at the top of the unit above the finish ceiling. These headwalls allow for modification (addition, deletion, or relocation of service outlets) in the future with minimal "demolition," but they restrict these service outlets to locations behind or on the side of the patients head.

Prefabricated service columns. These columns are designed and assembled in the same manner as prefab headwalls but can have service outlets on four sides and can be placed away from the walls, thereby allowing access to the patient from all four sides of the bed (Figure 6.9). The service column will impede access to the patient only at its closest point to the bed. An example of the layout of a prefabricated service column is illustrated in Figure 6.10, and its position in an ICU room is shown in Figure 6.11.

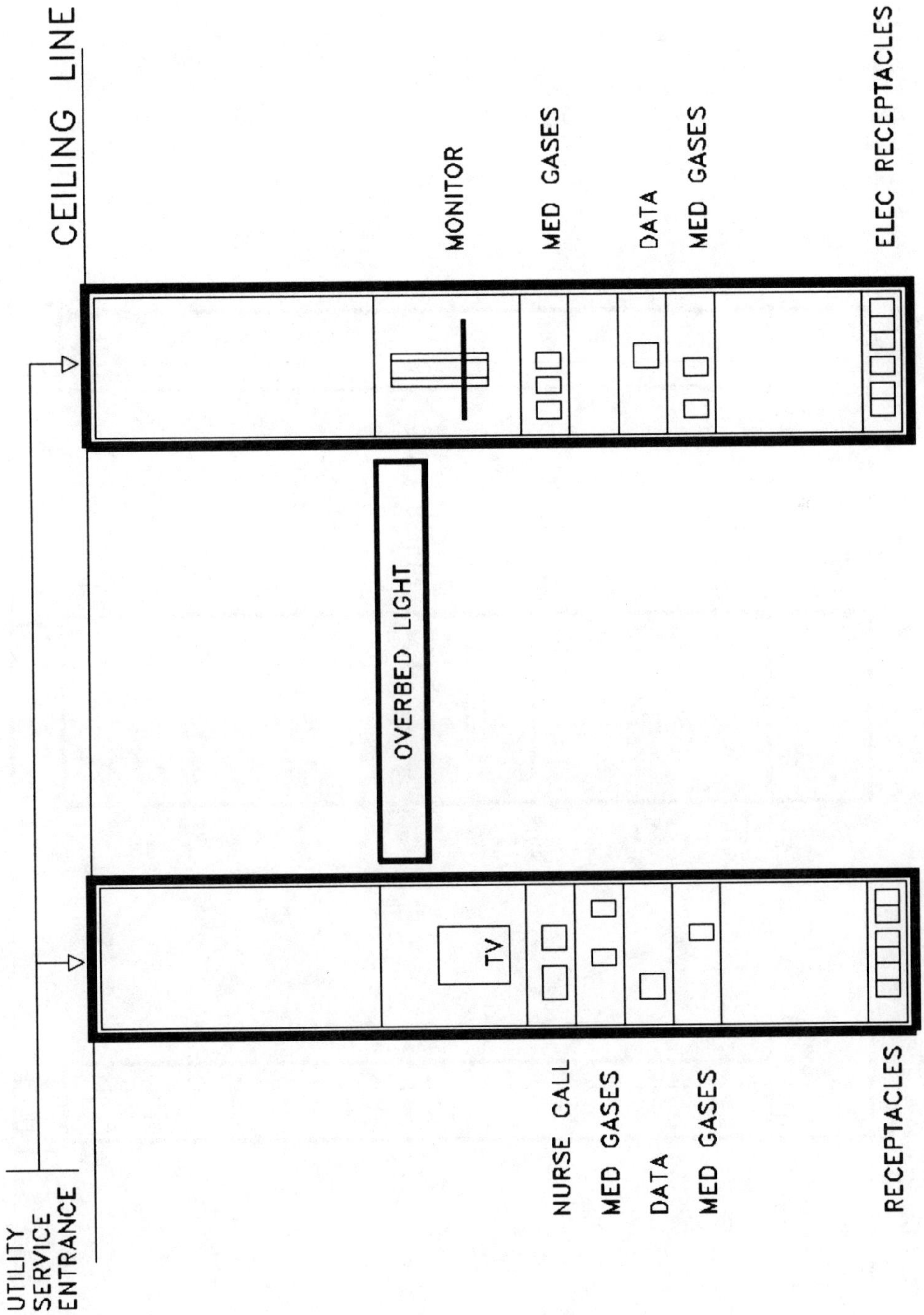

Figure 6.9: Line drawing of prefabricated service columns.

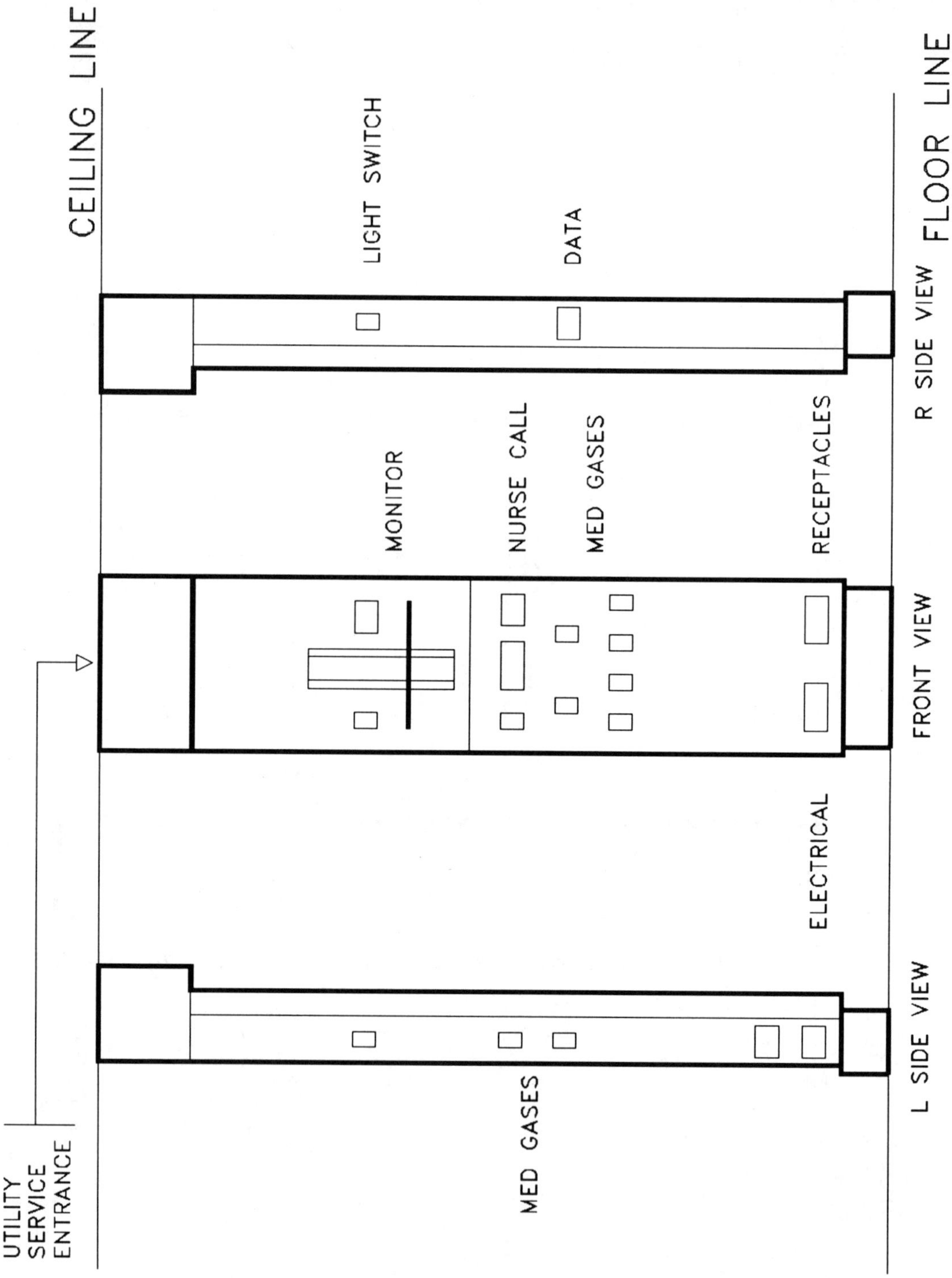

Figure 6.10: Three views of prefabricated service column indicating locations of specific services.

Rail systems. These systems provide the greatest flexibility in terms of moving service outlets around to adapt to changing needs. If adequate capacity is included in the initial installation, additional service outlets may be added with ease. Rail systems are limited to walls, as are the first and second options.

General Patient-Care Areas

The differences in design considerations between intensive-care areas and general patient-care areas are primarily a matter of degree. All of the functions described in the previous section that are necessary for the operation of an ICU are also found in the general-care unit (GCU). The required adjacencies of ICU functions also holds true for the GCU functions.

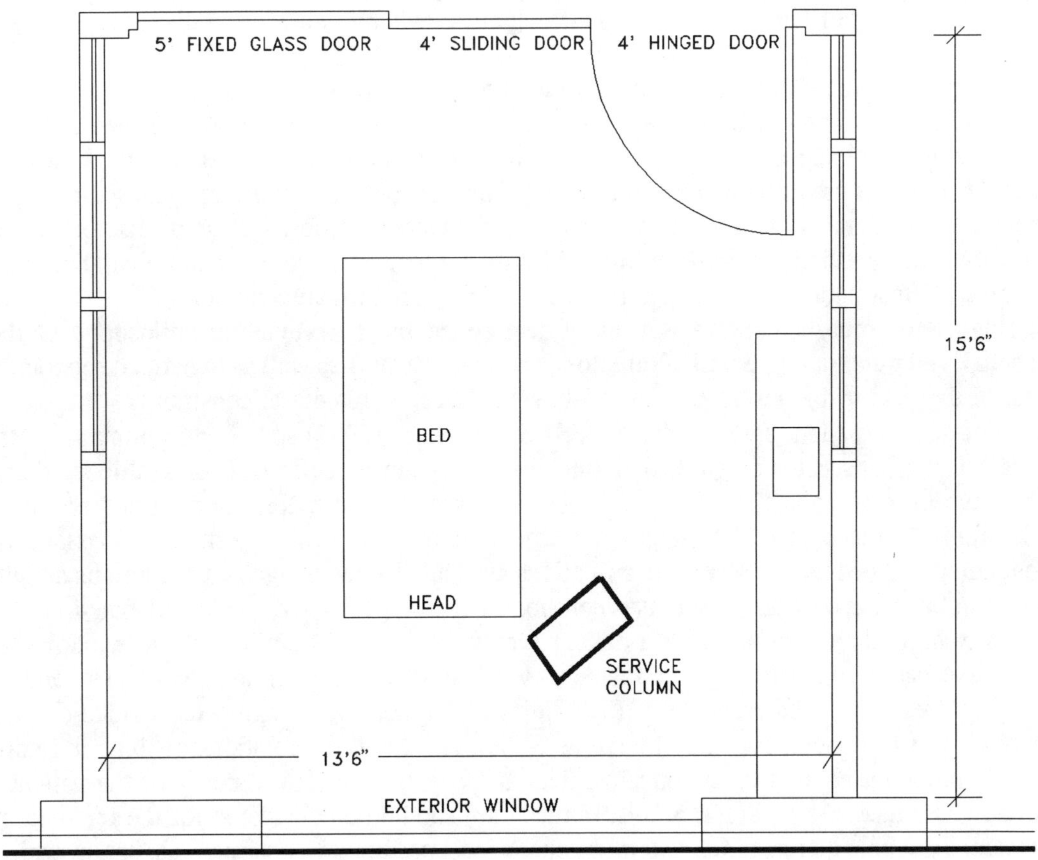

Figure 6.11: Floorplan of an ICU patient room indicating general room lay out and the position of prefabricated service column in relation to the bed.

In carrying over the design criteria from ICU to GCU, however, three factors should be kept in mind:

1. **Size.** Because the utilization of technology and labor resources is lower, the total amount of space dedicated to each patient bed in the GCU is smaller than that required in the ICU. Conversely, the total number of patients being cared for in a GCU is generally larger than in an ICU, so that certain support service spaces, such as the medication room, nourishment station, or soiled utility room, may actually be proportionately larger.

2. **Density of utility services.** Because there is less equipment and fewer and less complicated procedures are performed, the quantity of utility service outlets is significantly reduced.

3. **Increased patient awareness.** Less acutely ill or recuperating patients are much more aware of their surroundings. Therefore, considerable design attention should be paid to minimizing the effects of confinement, loss of privacy, disruption of way of life, and separation from family and friends, which are inevitable with hospitalization.

Most GCU rooms found in U.S. hospitals today are configured as either "private" or "semiprivate" (two beds). Surprisingly, studies conducted both here (Beck and Meyer, 1982) and abroad do not support the perception that most patients prefer a private room. Although single-bed rooms provide the maximum level of privacy possible in the hospital setting, they represent considerably greater expense in terms of construction cost, energy utilization, labor, and upkeep, especially housekeeping. Multibed rooms are more economical but may adversely affect patient comfort due to noise, odors, or roommate incompatibility. The mix of single- and multibed rooms is usually determined by the prevailing philosophy of the hospital's administration, board of directors, and medical staff as well as logistical, economic, and, in the case of the renovation of existing facilities, architectural constraints.

For general patient care rooms, AIA/HHS guidelines (1987) specify a minimum of 100 square feet of space for single-bed rooms and 80 square feet per bed for multibed rooms exclusive of toilet rooms, closets, wardrobes, alcoves, or vestibules. In multibed rooms, a minimum clearance of 44" is required at the foot of each bed to permit the passage of equipment and beds. These area specifications are intended as recognized minimums and do not prohibit the use of larger rooms where required for specialized needs and functions.

Any accommodation housing a patient for more than 24 hours must have windows or vents that can be opened from the inside to vent noxious fumes or smoke products and to bring in fresh air in emergencies. In buildings designed with engineered smoke-control systems, however, windows may be fixed. Whereas the diurnal rotations of light and dark are an important adjunct to the physiological and psychological well-being of the patients, window treatments (e.g., drape panels, blinds, etc.) should be considered for the removal of unwanted daytime glare and for general aesthetic reasons. In new constructions, handwashing facilities must be provided in each patient room. In renovation and modernization projects, the lavatory may be omitted from the bedroom when a water closet and lavatory are provided in a toilet room designed to serve one single-bed room or one two-bed room. This exception does not apply to postpartum rooms, which must have a lavatory within each bedroom. Each patient should have access to a toilet room without having to enter the general corridor area. One toilet room shall serve no more than four beds and no more than two patient rooms.

The toilet room should contain a toilet and a lavatory, and the door should swing outward or be double-acting. The lavatory may be omitted from a toilet room, if each patient room served by that toilet contains a lavatory for handwashing.

Each patient should have within his or her room a separate wardrobe, locker, or closet suitable for hanging full-length garments and for storing personal effects. In multibed rooms, visual privacy (e.g., cubicle curtains) must be provided for each patient. The design for privacy must not restrict patient access to the entrance, lavatory, or toilet.

The layout of patient room walls (commonly depicted as "elevations" on design and construction prints) is developed from the viewpoint of specifying and locating various utility service outlets and equipment mountings, coordinated with the placement of moveable equipment, particularly the bed, bedside cabinet and chairs. Electrical receptacles should be quantified on the basis of an analysis of anticipated moveable equipment utilization and location. Examples include a receptacle for the bed behind the head of the bed and receptacles to the side of the bed for infusion pumps, enteral feeding pumps, sequential compression devices, passive motion machines, portable three-channel ECG machines, or any number of other devices that may be used on a continuous or intermittent basis. At least one receptacle for each bed should be connected to the critical branch of the essential electrical distribution system (emergency power).

A minimum of one oxygen outlet and one medical vacuum outlet (DISS or other interconnect prohibitive configuration) should be accessible to each bed. Installation of medical air outlets is optional but should be carefully considered in relation to developments and practice patterns in respiratory therapy. Each patient room must be served by at least one nurse call station for two-way voice communication. Each bed should be provided with a call device (e.g., push-button call cord) that will activate a visible signal at the patient's door and audible or visible signals in the clean utility room, in the soiled utility room, and at the nursing station. If telephones are provided for patient use, wall jacks should be located to accommodate desk phones on bedside cabinets. Some bed manufacturers include built-in telephone capability.

Within the general care unit, it is also necessary to consider properly mounting sphygmomanometers to eliminate the need for floor space–occupying rolling units and locating overbed (reading) lights, television mounting brackets, and any other equipment as required. Reflected ceiling plans are often used to lay out patterns for general lighting, specialized lighting, air supply diffusers, cubicle curtain tracks, I.V. tracks, and sprinklers. At least one light in each room (ceiling or wall) should be connected to an emergency circuit. In the GCU, general illumination levels should range around 100 footcandles, with reading and night lighting at considerably lower levels. Patient rooms should have a ventilation rate of at least two room changes per hour, and temperature should be controlled at 70 to 75 F. Toilet rooms must have a minimum of ten air changes per hour, must be under negative pressure in relation to adjoining rooms, can have recirculation by means of a radiator, and must have all air exhausted directly outdoors. There should be at least one isolation room designed to minimize infection hazards to or from the patient for every 30 acute-care beds or fraction thereof. In view of the recent increases in infectious disease rates (AIDS, hepatitis, tuberculosis, etc.), a higher ratio may be warranted, especially if local epidemiological demographics indicate the need.

Table 6.4 Operating Rooms

Types Based on Specialties

- General surgery
- Gynecology
- Otorhinolaryngology (ENT)
- Plastic surgery
- Dental surgery
- Cystoscopy and genitourological surgery
- Orthopaedic surgery
- Cardiovascular and thoracic surgery
- Neurosurgery
- Ophthalmic surgery
- Combinations (e.g., trauma)
- Emergency ("stat")

Surgical Suites

Operating rooms have traditionally been the most complex from the viewpoint of design (U.S. Dept. HEW Publication, 1973). The exacting medical standards associated with surgical procedures are, in essence, carried over to room design specifications. The advancement of surgical and anesthetic techniques have literally transformed the OR environment from a simple large room with an amphitheater for observation to a high-technology space loaded with equipment, highly trained professionals, and a need for strict environmental control. The design of the OR must now accommodate four distinct user groups: patients, surgeons, anesthesiologists, and surgical nurses and technicians.

Let us begin the discussion of surgical suite design by outlining the wide variety of functions that must be accommodated within an OR suite. The wide variety of surgical suites becomes apparent when one reviews the various types based on medical specialty, as illustrated in Table 6.4. Some function areas are common and necessary to all or most OR room setups, regardless of specialty. In addition, other specialty areas may be necessary or desirable given the particular functions of the hospital, i.e., teaching. Examples of such areas are presented in Table 6.5.

As the number of operating rooms and the range of surgical subspecialties increases within a medical facility, there is a significant decrease in the ability to maintain adequately appropriate adjacencies of the above listed functions within a given space and geometry (suite perimeter shape). Several internal design configurations have been developed over the years in an effort to adjust to ever-larger suites.

For smaller departments (up to six ORs), the central corridor or "hotel" layout works well. Access into operating rooms is provided from a single straight, L-, or T-shaped corridor with rooms on one or both sides of the corridor. For moderately sized departments (seven to 16 O.R.s), the double central corridor ("inner racetrack") and peripheral corridor ("outer racetrack") designs accommodate both substantial traffic and a separation of "clean" and "dirty" activities. For large departments (more than 16 ORs), the cluster or grouping plan has met with moderate success. In this configuration, groups of ORs, segregated by subspecialty, are clustered together with dedicated support spaces (Figure 6.12).

Table 6.5 Function Areas Common to most Operating Rooms

- Scrub stations
- Instrument processing (central vs. decentralized "substerile")
  - Soiled receiving
  - Instrument wash
  - Terminal sterilization
- Equipment storage
  - General or generic equipment
  - Surgical subspecialty equipment
  - Anesthesia equipment
  - X-ray equipment
- Clean supply storage
- Clean linen
- Soiled utility
- Waste streams
  - Normal trash
  - Biomedical waste
- Pathology (e.g. frozen section room)
- Anesthesia workroom
- Dark rooms
- Preoperative holding
- Post anesthesia care nnit (Recovery room)
- Physician lounge and lockers (male and female)
- Nurse/technician lounge lockers (male and female)
- Dictation.
- Classroom or conference area.
- Clinical engineering maintenance/support
- Housekeeping.
- Patient support service personnel (orderlies, aides).

How to conduct an analysis for a total operating room suite design is beyond the scope of this chapter and, perhaps, beyond the needs of the practicing clinical engineer. The design of an individual operating room is, however, within the purview of the clinical engineer. Therefore, let us discuss the major factors that are considered in the design of an operating room.

Size. The current standard minimum size for operating rooms is 400 square feet. This could be 20' x 20' square, although rectangular and even circular designs have been developed. Perhaps a better way of stating the standard is that no single dimension should be less than 20 feet. Typically, the operating table, surgical team, scrub nurse, and instrument tables occupy most of that distance in one dimension, with the operating table, anesthesiologist, and anesthesiology equipment occupying most of the 20 feet in the second dimension. The addition of any specialized equipment such as cardiopulmonary bypass, laser, or video equipment, will immediately extend the required size of the room beyond the 20 foot minimum. With today's sophisticated procedures, operating room sizes up to 25 or 30 feet in one or both dimensions are often needed. Whether rooms of this size can be accommodated within a suite plan is a major difficulty. Usually, compromises between size and quantity of rooms have to be made.

The location of equipment is also very site-specific. For example, anesthesia equipment must be located at the head end of the table; fiber optic headlight light sources must be to the side of the table and behind the surgeons; video equipment must be placed so that the surgeons can see the monitors; and the scrub nurse must be able to access the instrument tables and the surgeon's outstretched hand simultaneously. Room dimensions are thus determined by equipment and personnel access factors.

Utility Services. The operating room requires high-density utility services. The design challenge here is to provide these services without producing a jungle of wires, cables, and hoses.

Electrical power. With the exception of pressurized gas-driven turbine tools, almost all of the equipment in the operating room requires electrical power. For the more technology-intensive specialties, such as open heart surgery, load capacity to the room should be sufficient to accommodate any contingency, typically in the 50 to 75 amp range. Although no longer required, many operating rooms still have isolation transformer supplies and line-isolation monitors, a remnant of the era of flammable anesthetizing agents. As stated in the section on ICU design, isolated power does provide a certain level of protection against macroshock hazard and a warning of equipment faulting. Many facilities have opted to retain this capability. The number of receptacles in the room is determined by the equipment load. The receptacles are typically of the locking type so that devices are not inadvertently unplugged. Electrical outlets are often suspended from the ceiling from droplines (with extra heavy duty strain reliefs) or service columns so that there are fewer power cables on the floor to trip over.

A liberal number of circuits should be dispersed throughout the room so that circuit failure can be rapidly alleviated by plugging into adjacent receptacles. The surgical lights and all convenience outlets must be connected to emergency power. Furthermore, as a location where invasive procedures are performed, operating rooms must be equipped with equipotential grounding.

Lighting. A high level of general illumination is required because visual tasks of low contrast and very small size need to be performed, such as the manipulation of very small sutures by the scrub nurse. Although, the choice of a surgical light is subjective, several objective criteria should be part of any evaluation. These include light intensity, light color, lamphead maneuverability, choice of mounting (multihead central hub, multiple hubs with single lampheads, lampheads on tracks), light color temperature; focusing capability and range, degree of shadow production, ease of maintenance (especially bulb changing), heat production and dissipation, and ease of cleaning.

Many surgeons supplement ceiling-mounted surgical lights with fiber-optic headlights, which are particularly useful when shadow production is high or work is performed in areas of the field where light penetration from the ceiling is virtually impossible. The use of these lights is essential when surgical light-mounted cameras are to be employed. For example, consider the use of endoscopic procedures, especially laprascopic cholecystectomy. Rather than removing the gall bladder through a large open abdominal incision, specialized laprascopes, endoscopic instruments, and video equipment are used, eliminating the need for general surgical lighting (as well as placing the entire procedure in a virtual ambulatory surgery setting).

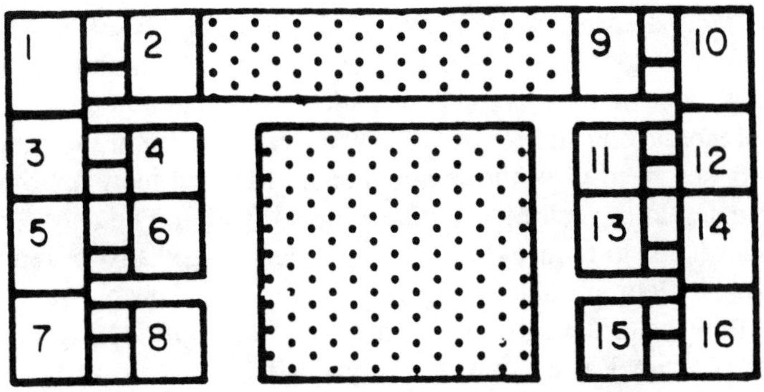

Figure 6.12: Group or Cluster plan diagram. Operating rooms are numbered, core support areas are shaded.

Plumbing. The need for fixtures within an operating room is practically nil, with the possible exception of some specialized applications, such as the hot and cold water used for cooling and reheating open heart patients through a bypass pump heat exchanger (many systems are now self-contained) or the cooling water and drain needed for high-powered medium- to low-efficiency lasers. Of course, there are significant plumbing requirements in other parts of the surgical suite, such as scrub and utility sinks and instrument processing systems.

Medical gases. The greatest concentration of medical gas outlets in the hospital occurs in the operating room. At the very least, each room requires a minimum of two oxygen, three medical vacuum and two medical air outlets. Often, additional outlets are required depending on the circumstance and procedure. Other additional piped medical gases, such as 200 pounds per square inch nitrogen for turbine tools and carbon dioxide or helium, are often needed. When used, most gas supplies are suspended from the ceiling with the exception of medical vacuum, which requires a stabilized horizontal mounting for a regulator, and suction canisters, which should be lower than the patient so that the system is not fighting gravity as well. Although nitrous oxide is still typically piped into operating rooms, it appears that this analgesic gas will eventually be replaced by other anesthesia agents.

Waste anesthesia gas scavenging. The **National Institute for Occupational Safety and Health (NIOSH)** has published guidelines for limiting the exposure of operating room personnel to anesthetic agents that have escaped from the anesthesia machine breathing circuit, piped gas supplies, or vaporizers. For example, exposure to nitrous oxide should not exceed 25 parts per million over an 8-hour period (time-weighted average (TWA) basis), and volatile halogenated agents (e.g. halothane, ethane, forane) should not exceed 0.5 ppm over an 8-hour TWA. A scavenging system which will collect and safely dispose of these waste gases is required in every inhalation anesthetizing location. If the HVAC system in the OR is 100 percent nonrecirculated, then the exhaust or return duct system can be used for this purpose. If there is some degree of recirculation, then a self-contained portable collection system, a dedicated exhaust ductwork system, or a medical vacuum must be utilized. Whichever system is chosen, all waste gas must be exhausted to a safe location, such as a building roof, where there are no personnel or nearby air intakes.

Heating, ventilation, and air conditioning. Specifications for general operating rooms include positive pressure in relation to adjacent rooms and corridors; a minimum of three room changes per hour of fresh air and a minimum of 15 room changes per hour of total air with high filtration; no recirculation by room units; relative humidity of 50 to 60 percent; and temperature control of 70 to 75 degrees (F) (a source of consternation for surgeons who say the range is too high, but perhaps correct for patients who have impaired thermoregulation capability). Central monitoring and control of HVAC and temperature systems allow each OR to be independently set up to meet the requirements of the surgeon and procedure. Supply ducts should be located in the ceiling over the surgical field and be constructed with widely dispersed small vent holes to reduce drafts and turbulence. Exhaust or return grilles should be located low to the floor on side walls as far apart from each other as possible, thus producing an air flow pattern in the room that tends to continuously draw contaminants produced by room personnel away from the surgical field.

Laminar flow systems, either vertical or horizontal, are often requested by surgeons who perform procedures, such as total joint replacements, that are subject to increased risk of serious wound infections. Because these systems are very expensive, consume a great deal of energy resources, and must be meticulously maintained, their acquisition and installation must be subjected to careful scrutiny.

Finish materials. Walls should be hard, relatively seamless, nonporous, and easy to clean. Ceramic tile has been the traditional material of choice, although the grouting has been perceived as a site for the buildup of contamination. In recent years, laminated walls and newer vinyl wall coverings have achieved wider acceptance.

In the absence of flammable anesthetic agents, conductive flooring is no longer an issue except in the sense that, if it already exists in an OR, it must still be tested according to NFPA criteria. Floors should be hard, seamless, nonporous, and easy to clean.

Finish ceilings should be washable and prevent any debris from the utilities or slab above from filtering into the operating rooms. There are several choices, each with their specific advantages and disadvantages. Fixed, permanent ceilings, such as plaster, meet the above criteria, but access to services above may be difficult and costly. Metalized ceiling tile and grid systems offer greater ease of access but may allow debris to filter down if not properly sealed and maintained.

Cabinets for storage of supplies inside the room should not intrude on available floor space. In addition, they should have glass sliding doors with wire shelves (solid shelves collect dust and could be a source of contamination) and adequate but reasonable capacity, and they should be readily accessible to the circulating nurse. Stainless steel has been the most common choice for cabinet material, but other options are available.

Communications. Communications systems incorporated into an OR design should include a voice intercom to the control desk with a stat call feature for summoning immediate emergency assistance. In addition, a communications link (intercom, telephone) to pathology should be provided to obtain results such as blood gas analyses or biopsy test results. Data terminals, if such systems are in place, and telephones for use by physicians and staff should be provided, although they should not be within the operating rooms themselves.

Obstetrical Facilities

In many respects, the functions required within the labor and delivery suite are very similar to those in the operating room suite. The primary difference in design criteria is to be found in current attitudes toward the childbirth process. Not long ago, the typical delivery room suite consisted of separate labor, delivery, recovery, and postpartum rooms occupied by mothers in sequence as they went through the stages of childbirth. The delivery rooms were essentially designed and built as general operating rooms, and the use of anesthesia during delivery was quite common. Today, the concepts and attitudes are very different. The vast majority of births are achieved without major medical intervention and occur in an environment resembling the home rather than the hospital. The design of "birthing rooms" is predicated on the notion of permitting the mother to progress through the first three major steps of childbirth in the same room and the same bed and in a room that looks like a home bedroom (but is, in fact, fully equipped to handle most deliveries.) The operative delivery room is still used when complications occur, and the potential need for an emergency (or elective) Caesarean section remains.

The physical plant resources for the birthing process, as it is now practiced, focus as much on ambience and decor as they do on utility. The space in a birthing room needs to accommodate first and foremost the mother and her spouse or partner. In addition, space is required for the obstetrical nurse to fulfill her role as care-giver, the obstetrician (who, if all goes well, spends less time in the room), and the baby. The pieces of equipment found in the room would typically be a specialized birthing bed, which can be configured for general rest, labor, delivery and recovery; a procedure lamp (a portable unit brought into the room when needed or concealed in the ceiling; an obstetrician's stool; an instrument table; a fetal monitor, and an infant warmer. Provision should be made for personal belongings: a toilet, lavatory and possibly a sitz bath, subdued as well as bright lighting, oxygen and medical vacuum for mother and child, and storage for supplies and linen. Wood finishes (such as light oak trim and oak furniture) are common. The number, location, and style of utility service outlets are again determined by personnel and equipment needs. A further extension of this concept is the labor/delivery/recovery/postpartum (LDRP) room, in which the mother spends her entire hospital stay. This concept has become logistically possible because of the ever-decreasing length of stay for a normal delivery.

Imaging Suites

Regardless of how a hospital is organized, design features for individual imaging rooms are determined primarily by the specific imaging technologies involved. These include the following:

- General radiographic systems.
- Radiographic and fluoroscopic systems.
- Ultrasound.
- Special procedures (invasive noncardiac imaging and therapeutics).
- Cardiac catheterization.
- Nuclear medicine.
- Computerized axial tomography.
- Magnetic resonance imaging.
- Positron emission tomography.

A common denominator of these imaging suites is the fact that the room is designed around equipment that is big, heavy, and expensive. These characteristics shift the designer's attention toward questions that don't usually arise in other inpatient or special-care facilities. For example, consider the following:

- Will structural characteristics of the building support the weight of the equipment?
- Will unusual utility services be required to operate the equipment? Most new systems require clean, regulated, 480-volt, three-phase power, a commodity often not readily available in existing buildings. Structural modifications may be necessary to bolster existing support mechanisms, or siting of the equipment may be limited to ground or lower floors.
- This equipment is generally fixed in place. Will service access clearances be sufficient? Space limitations or structural boundaries may compromise service access.
- Will there be special data collection, manipulation, and transmission capabilities that will need computer support or networking? As digital imaging and picture archiving and communications systems gain wider acceptance, the need for computer hardware, software, and networking capabilities will continue to demand additional resources.
- Does the equipment produce ionizing radiation or other forms of radiating energy that require shielding? Seven of the nine major technology categories listed above require shielding of radiating energy.

CASE STUDY: DESIGN OF A CARDIAC CATHETERIZATION LABORATORY

The design of a specific imaging suite provides a good example of how the participation of the clinical engineer can enhance the process of facility design. At Hartford Hospital, the administration decided to purchase and install a new adult cardiac catheterization imaging system. The prime factors supporting this decision were (1) an increase in patient volume, which placed a severe burden on the two existing adult catheterization rooms, and (2) advancements in diagnostic and therapeutic techniques, such as percutaneous transluminal coronary angioplasty and valvuloplasty, which required imaging characteristics exceeding the capacity of one of the existing catheterization systems. With this decision made, the next step was to identify the space this unit would occupy. This required ensuring not only that the space would be adequate for the procedure room (including the primary equipment configuration of the fluoroscope and patient table as well as ancillary equipment) and necessary adjacent support functions, but also that it would have the appropriate adjacency to the existing catheterization suite and procedure rooms, supply rooms, patient waiting room, film processors, film reading rooms, offices, and clerical space. During the course of the study, it was determined that the only feasible space was an area occupied at that time by the pulmonary function laboratory, located in an adjacent wing of the hospital. If the pulmonary lab could be relocated, then the project could proceed. As is often the case with renovation or expansion projects within an existing building, design possibilities were defined by the building shape rather than by the equipment and function requirements (Figure 6.13).

After going through the lengthy process of obtaining a state certificate and internal budget approval for the funding of equipment and renovations, final equipment selection was completed. Once a contract was signed with the chosen vendor, the detailed design and development team consisted of an architect, a planning associate, a representative of the cardiology physician users, the nurse supervisor, and the clinical engineer. The design of space for sophisticated imaging systems must be coordinated very closely with the manufacturer's installation representative, who is most knowledgeable of the environmental, space, and utility requirements of the system to be installed.

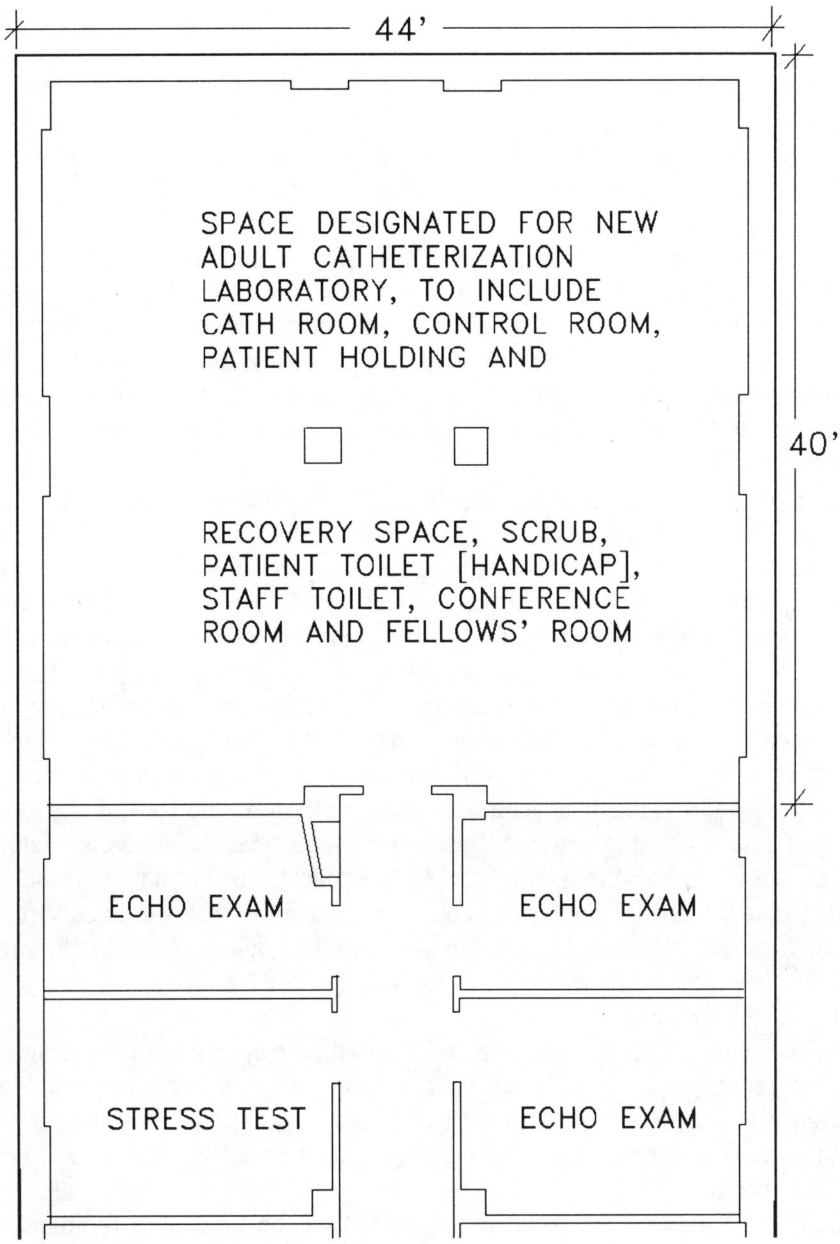

Figure 6.13: Floorplan of existing space allocated for cadiac catheterization laboratory.

The system chosen included installation of several components, each with specific location, clearance, and proximity requirements:

- A floor-mounted fluoroscopic C-arm with high heat capacity liquid-bearing X-ray tube and multispot size (9", 6", 3") image intensifier. This unit required that a 1"-thick, precisely dimensioned floor plate be recessed in the concrete slab and anchored in a manner appropriate to support the weight of the unit (1,610 pounds) and the moment arm resulting from the horizontal extension of the C-arm. Power and control cables were to run to the pedestal from the ceiling. In addition, this unit would be situated in the room in a manner that allowed appropriate rotation of the C-arm in all axes for imaging of the patient's heart in several planes.

- A floor-mounted, pedestal-base radiotranslucent table with X-Y tabletop movement capability. This unit required a heavy, recessed, and precisely dimensioned floor plate that could accommodate the weight and moment arm of the tabletop as it was extended into the axis of the C-arm alignment. This plate would also have to be precisely positioned on the center line of the C-arm pedestal floor plate, be precisely level (off by no more than 1 millimeter at a radius of 12 feet), and be placed a precise distance (12' 3-5/8" center-to-center) from the C-arm plate. All power and control cabling (including cabling to the interface box mounted to the procedure table for physiologic transducers such as ECG and invasive pressure measurement) would run into the pedestal base from below the floor slab.
- The floor plate location requirements of these components produced the first design challenge. The total width of the wing where the procedure room was to be placed was only 44 feet, and when other ancillary support spaces were established by block diagram into appropriate adjacencies, the procedure room dimensions measured 25'6" by 17'6". This was deemed an adequate space for the equipment, people, and supplies. However, ideal positioning of the C-arm/table combination was not possible because a structural beam was located directly beneath the proposed table location, preventing floor plate anchoring and cable access. The entire combination could be shifted 2 feet in either direction to miss the beam. The design team rejected a shift in the "foot" direction because this would result in inadequate clearance around the foot of the table for the passage of staff and equipment. A shift toward the "head" direction appeared, at least on paper, not to be feasible because the C-arm pedestal would not clear the far wall.
- As it turned out, a pilot hole was drilled in the floor slab at the site to confirm the exact location of the underlying beam, and it was determined that the C-arm/table combination would fit (just barely) when shifted toward the head end, thus leaving additional clearance at the foot end.
- Various rack cabinets for equipment associated with the operation of the imaging system, such as, a generator, a high tension tank, a power distribution unit (including voltage regulation and surge suppression systems), an X-ray tube control system, frontal geometry control system, digital imaging control systems, TV chain, and image intensifier controls.
- The location of these racks could either be within the procedure room itself or in a separate room (within the manufacturer-specified distance limit). Having these cabinets within the procedure room would facilitate servicing, with simultaneous visual and tactile access to both the C-arm/table combination and supporting rack cabinets. Placing the cabinets in a separate room would provide additional space in the procedure room, was more aesthetically pleasing, and transferred the heat load (and subsequent cooling capacity) to a different location. In this case, the design team decided to place the rack cabinets within the procedure room because they did not want to utilize additional remote space at the expense of adjoining support functions.
- Ceiling-suspended monitors, for viewing the live fluoroscopic image, image recall screen, a digital "road-mapping" screen, and a remote physiologic monitoring system display.

The suspension system required rails parallel, to the C-arm/table axis and attached to a unistrut-style frame affixed to the upper structural slab. The placement of the rails was critical to providing the close visibility required by the physician performing the procedure without interfering with patient access and C-arm maneuverability.

- An operator's console located in proximity to the physiologic monitoring system. The location of both the operator's console and the monitoring system must allow visual access to the procedure table without interfering with staff movement around the table.
- Control monitors duplicating the suspended monitors, control consoles, high- resolution recording equipment, and consoles to allow review and manipulation of digitized images, all located in the control room. The physician users felt strongly that the control room should be large enough to accommodate significant teaching activities so that house officers and visiting physicians could monitor all activities during a procedure without crowding into the procedure room itself.
- A large computer mainframe cabinet, housing hardware necessary for digitizing, storing, replaying, and manipulating the large number of images obtained during procedures. A large capacity was required because of the rapid frame acquisition and replay rates (up to 60 frames per second) necessary for coronary angiography. The heat load of the computer cabinet alone accounted for nearly half of the entire imaging system load, so this unit was assigned to a dedicated enclosed space with its own cooling system.

In addition to the imaging system and its components, the following functions and equipment needed to be designed in as well:

General Procedure Equipment

- Handwashing sink.
- Catheter storage cabinets.
- Medication cabinet.
- Nursing supply cabinet and work counter.
- Instrument tables.
- Dye injector.
- Crash cart.
- Defibrillator.
- Ceiling-suspended shielding for physicians and nurses at the procedure table.
- Portable shielding for the nurse or technician operating the generator control console and physiologic monitoring system.
- Ceiling-suspended procedure light.

Control Room Equipment

- Large desk for accomodating monitors, control consoles, tape recorder, and writing space, facing the procedure room and separated by a large, shielded (leaded) viewing window.
- Floor space for up to ten observers.
- A computer terminal connected to the department-wide local area network.
- Additional catheter storage cabinets.

Toilet

- Water closet.
- Lavatory with mirror.
- Handicap accessibility.

Scrub

- A two-position scrub sink.
- Storage for scrubbing accessories and waste.
- Wall protection from splashing.
- Floor treatment to prevent slipping.

Patient Waiting/Recovery

- Two individual areas.
- Cubicle curtains.
- Oxygen and vacuum service outlets.
- Space for appropriate access to the patient for such procedures as control of bleeding around catheter insertion site.
- Storage and supplies.
- Writing surface.
- Handwashing sink.

Conference Room

- Conference table large enough to accommodate six people.
- Chairs.
- Film viewing capabilities.
- Slide projector and screen.
- Storage cabinets and bookcases.
- Two small desks.

The final design floorplan is shown in Figures 6.14. A reflected ceiling plan is shown in Figure 6.15 to illustrate some of the special considerations, especially lighting. The ability of the physicians to clearly see images during a catheterization procedure can be adversely affected by a poorly designed lighting scheme. In this design, seven different lighting light sources are provided, each independently controlled:

- Primary left side procedure downlights (on dimmer).
- Secondary right side procedure downlights (on dimmer).
- Technician console downlight (on dimmer).
- Nurse workstation downlights (on dimmer).
- Control room downlights (on dimmer).
- General recessed fluorescent lighting with parabolic diffusers.
- High intensity procedure light suspended above the procedure table.

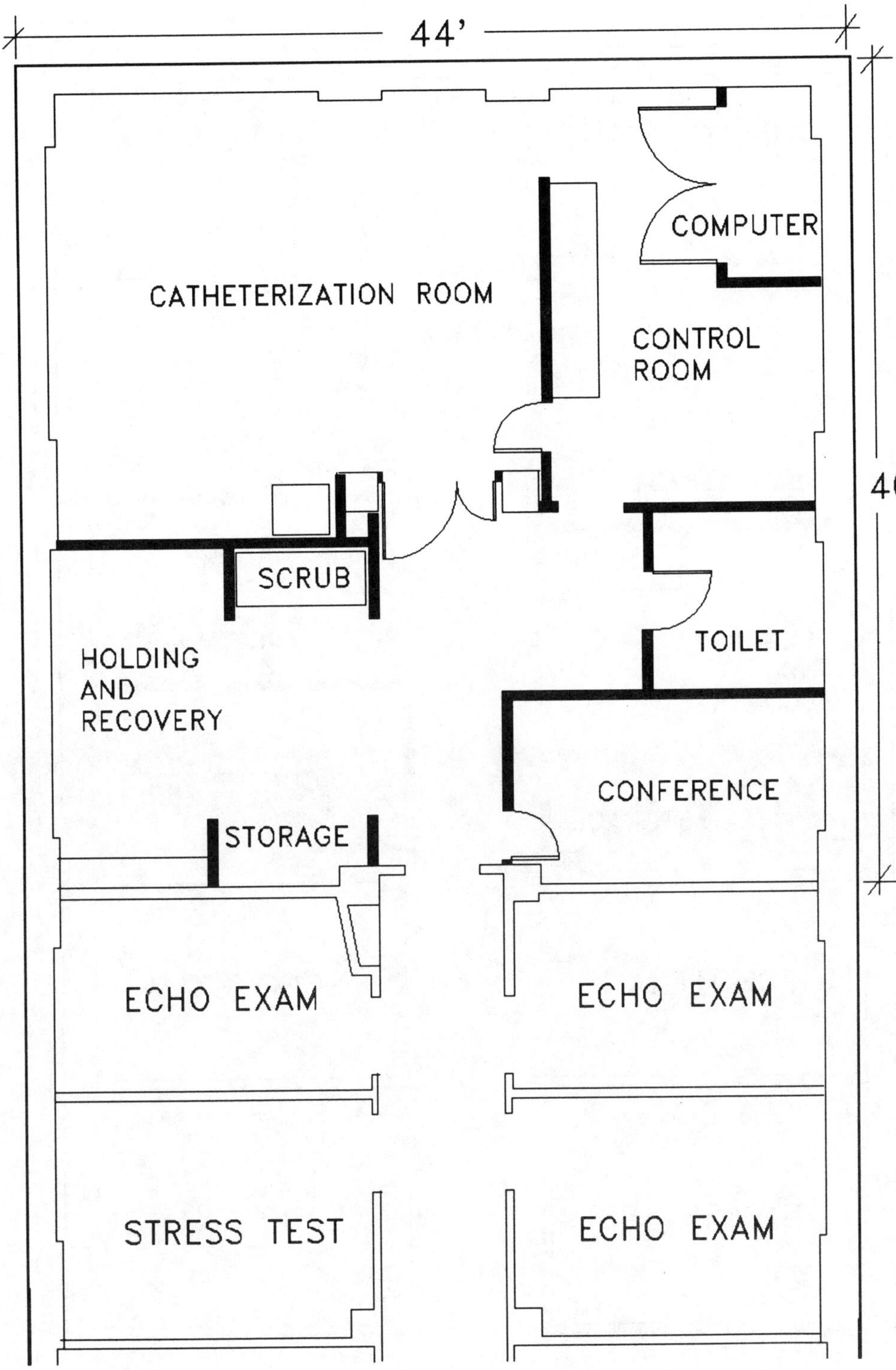

Figure 6.14: (a) Final design floorplan for cardiac catheterization laboratory.

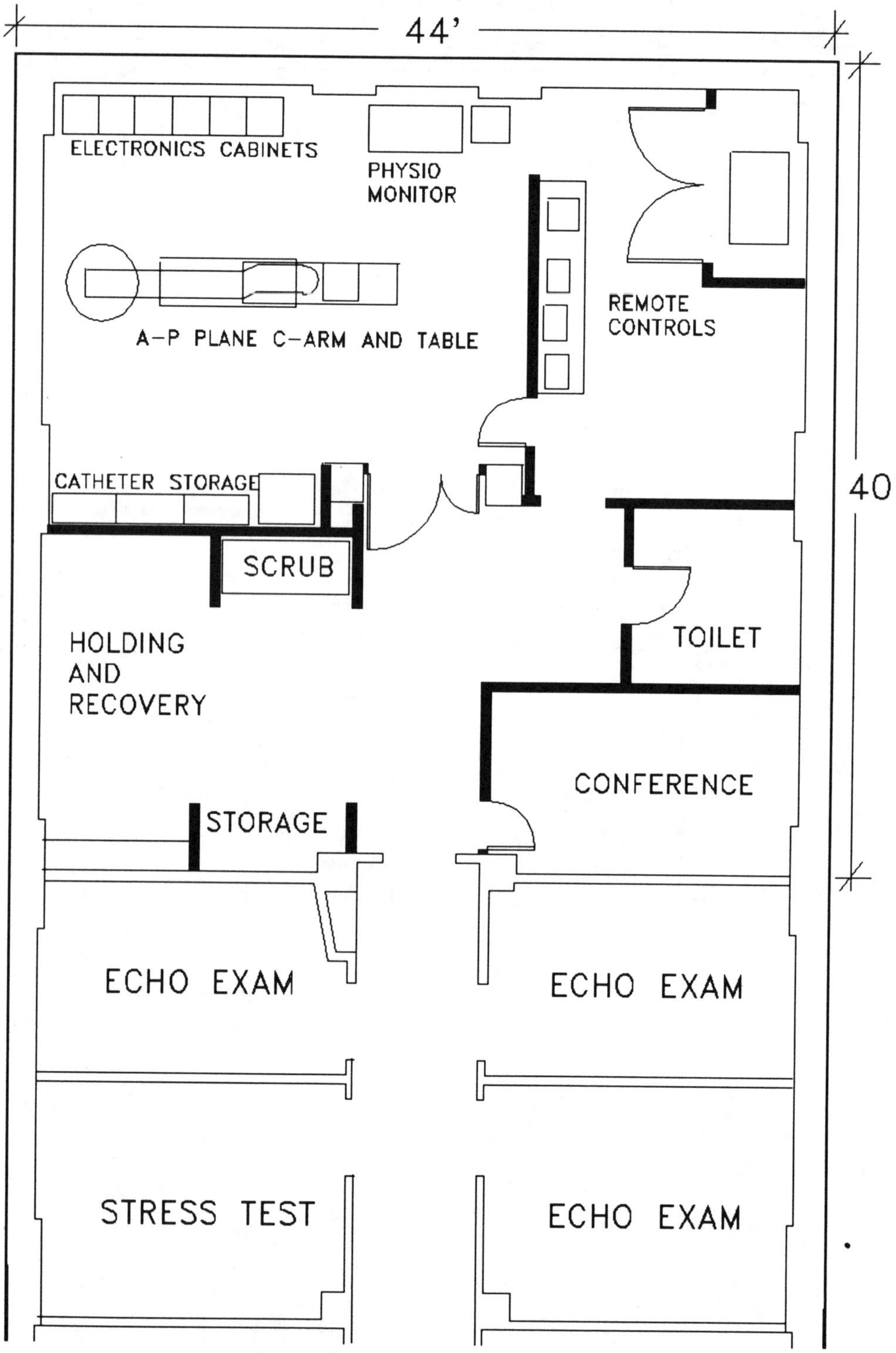

Figure 6.14: (b) Final design floorplan of the cardiac catheterization laboratiry indicating the position of specific major equipment and support furniture.

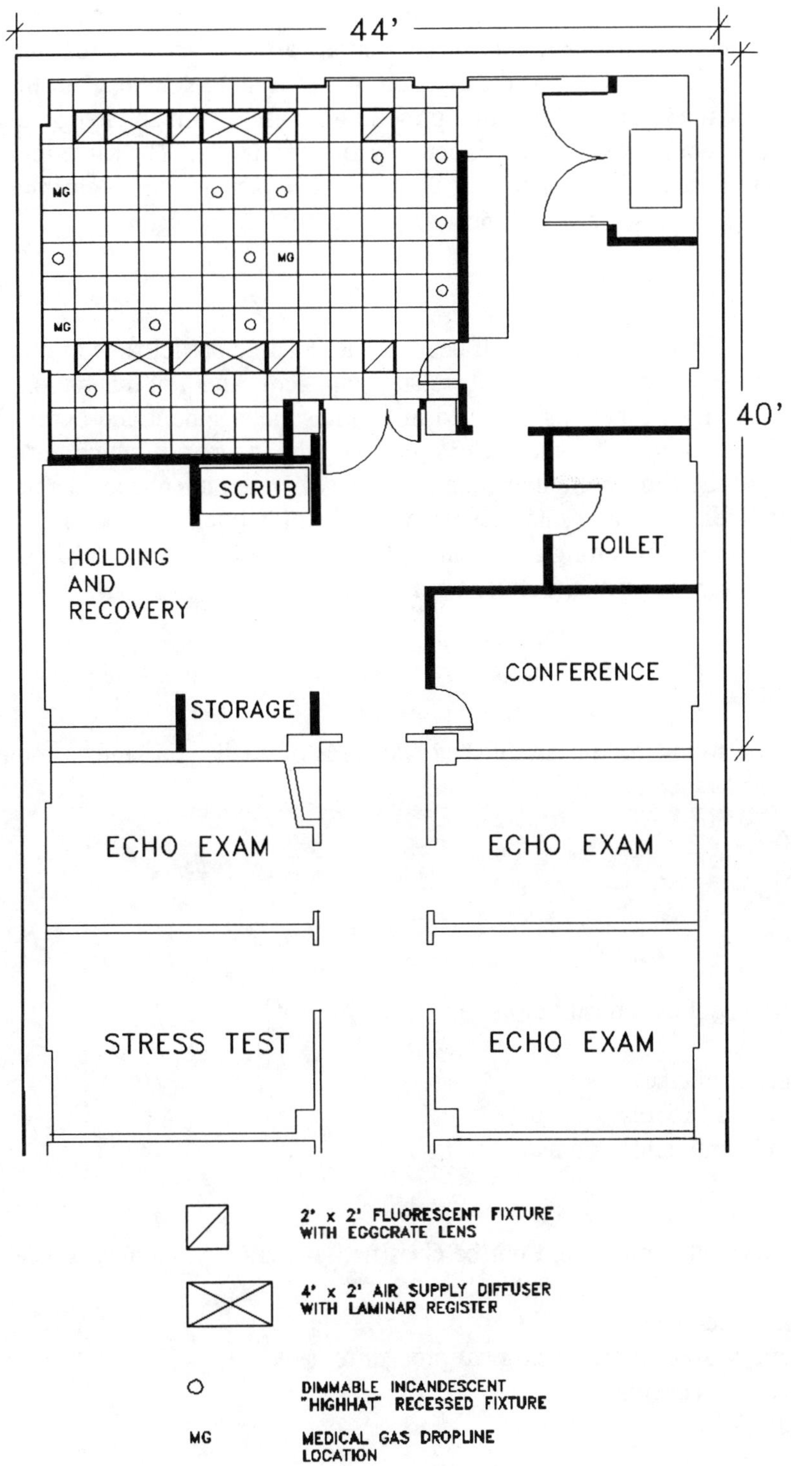

Figure 6.15: Reflected ceiling plan of cardiac catheterization laboratory.

This lighting plan was designed to minimize glare on monitor screens and to provide flexibile lighting for the various tasks. The participation of the clinical engineer in this design project provided an opportunity to incorporate a broad set of skills into the design. The result of this incorporation was the creation of a procedure suite that fulfilled the initial goals of the hospital administration while providing all users with an environment in which quality health-care could be delivered effectively and efficiently. The same logic that led to the involvement of the clinical engineer in this project, applies to the involvement of clinical engineers in design issues for any clinical area in a medical facility.

SUMMARY

In the future, clinical engineers will become more active participants in facilities design and management, especially those aspects related to patient care. For this reason, this chapter has presented the major functions involved in facilites management and outlined the issues related to facilites design. The chapter has indicated the manner in which the special skills and knowledge of the clinical engineer can effectively be used to enhance the design process of clinical facilities. As a result, the departments of clinical engineering and facilites management must develop strong cooperative and collaborative links to fulfill their missions within the health-care facility effectively and efficiently.

EXERCISES

1. Which of the following has established standards of quality that must be met for air to be classified as medical air?

   (a) NFPA
   (b) CGA
   (c) JCAHO
   (d) AMA

2. Which area requires a positive pressure environment?

   (a) Nuclear medicine
   (b) Patient ward rooms
   (c) Patient examination rooms
   (d) Surgical suites

3. Which of the following would not be classified as regulated medical waste?

   (a) Hypodermic needles
   (b) Tissue removed during a surgical procedure
   (c) Laboratory reagents
   (d) Bloody gauze

4. Regulated medical waste disposal is governed by

   (a) state law.
   (b) federal law.
   (c) local law.
   (d) Any combination of the above.

5. Describe the basic requirements of the Life Safety Code (NFPA 101). Discuss why these requirements are so important in a medical treatment facility?

6. Design and draw a sketch of the headwall in a labor/delivery/recovery/postpartum room.

7. Compare the advantages and disadvantages of adapting a clinical facilities design to an existing building.

8. What codes, standards, and regulations affect the design of an operating room?

9. List the design factors you might consider when renovating a 1950-vintage emergency department treatment room.

10. List all of the equipment that you would include in a new ICU patient room.

11. Sketch a reflected ceiling plan for a postanesthesia care unit.

12. When designing a clinical facility, what utility systems should be considered? What other factors affect the feasibility of utilizing existing systems?

13. Equipment and technology management is the more traditional purview of the practicing clinical engineer. Define the advantages for professional development that involvement with clinical facilities design would provide.

14. A long-range planning tool used to prioritize minor and major construction projects necessary for the operation, maintenance, and future development of the hospital is called

    (a) a statement of construction.
    (b) a facility master plan.
    (c) a facility utilization study.
    (d) hospital strategic plan.

15. (a) You are converting a wing of administrative offices into an intensive-care unit. What major facility medical systems must be installed or upgraded? Discuss your rationale.

    (b) This area will be completely remodeled. Discuss your selection of floor and wall coverings, and provide a rationale for your selection.

REFERENCES

AHA *Hospital Engineering Handbook*, AHA, Chicago, 1980.

AHA *Evaluation Methods for Intensive Care Unit Systems*, AHA Hospital Technology Series, Guideline Report No. 4, AHA, Chicago, 1982.

AHA *Maintenance Management for Health Care Facilities*, AHA, Chicago, 1990.

AIPE *Guide to Better Facilities Management*, American Institute of Plant Engineers, Cincinnati, 1990.

American Institute of Architects/U.S. Department of Health and Human Services. *Guidelines for Construction and Equipment of Hospital and Medical Facilities*, AIA Press, Washington, D.C., 1987.

Beck, W.C., and Meyer, R.H. *Health Care Environment: The User's Viewpoint*, CRC Press, Boca Raton, FL, 1982.

DeChant, T.A. *Managing Hospital Space as an Asset*, AHA, Chicago, 1988.

Grattendick, J. *Project Delivery Approaches: Different Options, Different Objectives*, AHA, Chicago, 1990.

IEEE. *Recommended Practice for Electric Systems in Health Care Facilities*, Institute of Electrical and Electronics Engineers, New York, 1986.

Kaiser, H.H. *The Facilities Manager's Reference*, R.S. Means Co., Kingston, MA, 1989.

Laufman, H. *Hospital Special-Care Facilities: Planning for User Needs*, Academic Press, New York, 1981.

Lee, L.D. *Waste Management Policy for Health Care Facilities*, AHA, Chicago, 1990.

Magee, G.H. *Facilities Maintenance Management*, R.S. Means Co., Kingston, MA, 1988.

Martin, P. *Electrical Distribution System: A Program for Optimal Preventive Maintenance in the Health Care Setting*, AHA, Chicago, 1987.

Martin, P. *Hospital Security Service Generates Positive Return on Investment: A Shared Service Success Story*, AHA, Chicago, 1991.

Mills, G. *Space Allocation Committee: Backbone to Facility Management*, AHA, Chicago, 1990.

Moderow, R.R. *The Quest for the Perfect Patient Unit Design*, American Society for Hospital Engineering, Technical Document Series, Chicago, 1991.

NFPA. *No. 70, National Electric Code*, National Fire Protection Assoc., Quincy, MA, 1990.

NFPA. *No. 99, Standard for Health Care Facilities*, National Fire Protection Assoc., Quincy, MA, 1990.

Peglow, T.M. *Use of Microcomputer-based CAD and Project Management Systems*, AHA, Chicago, 1987.

Ruga, W. *Selecting Interior Design Finishes and Furnishings to Create a Successful Health Care Environment*, AHA, Chicago, 1989.

Slack, G.D. *Medical Gas and Vacuum Systems*, AHA, Chicago, 1989.

Sloane, R.M. and Sloane, B.L. *A Giude to Health Care Facilites*, 3rd ed., Health Administration Press, Ann Arbor, 1992.

U.S. Department of Health, Education and Welfare. *The Surgical Suite: Functional Programming Worksheets*, U.S. Dept. of HEW Publication No. (HMS) 73-4005, Rockville, MD, 1973.

CHAPTER 7

MANAGEMENT AND SUPERVISION

For clinical engineers to manage their departments successfully they must not only be concerned about the technical aspects of this function, they should possess skills that will enable them to manage people and other resources as well. At the onset, it is important to identify two major factors that affect the development of managerial skills. The first factor is the basic personality of the manager. Although **management** is a process, **managers** are individuals. As a result, each individual manager, based upon his or her own personality and values, may apply the same set of management principles and practices differently. It has been said that "*we manage because of what we are, but how we manage is because of who we are*," (Bennett, 1987).

The second factor is the organizational structure or framework in which one must manage. Figure 7.1a illustrates a traditional organizational framework. Management (which appears at the top of the organization chart) is responsible for such activities as **planning, organizing, leading**, etc., and employees are responsible for the implementation of the manager's plans. In this organizational structure, information flows both from the top down and from the bottom up. This approach is dramatically different from a more contemporary managerial framework, which utilizes the manager as a facilitator and involves employees at all levels in many, if not all, aspects of the management process (Figure 7.1b). Although both organizational models clearly recognize that management has the responsibility for identifying the broad goals and objectives of the organization, the difference between them lies in the implementation of the goals developed by management.

In either case, the effective manager uses the implementation process provided by the organization to enable departmental personnel to contribute successfully to the overall goals of the department. Therefore, to be effective, managers must properly plan, organize, lead and control employee activities and, at the same time, establish good lines of communication with all employees. This chapter discusses in detail some of the important factors that clinical engineers must take into account in order to become effective managers.

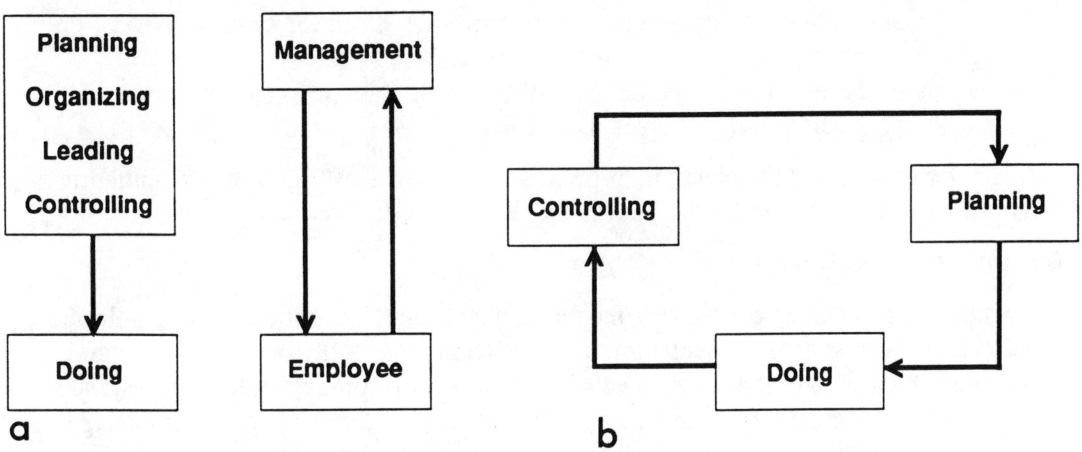

Figure 7.1: (a) Traditional top-down management structure. (b) The manager as facilitator.

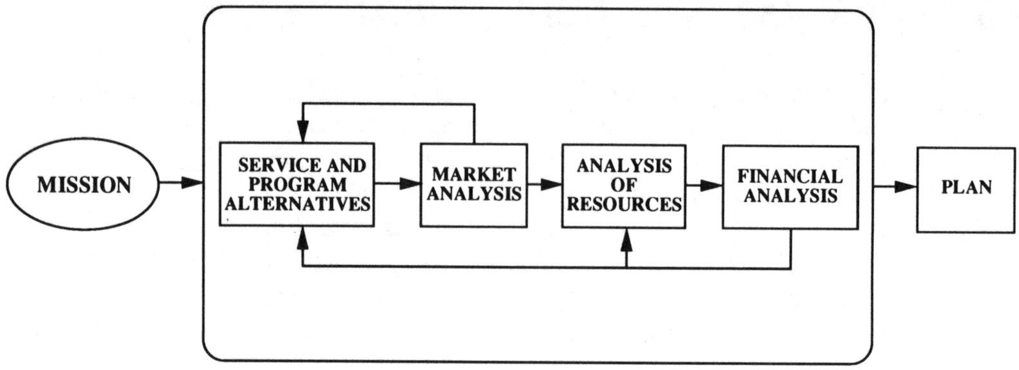

Figure 7.2: The planning process: The plan is important. The process is paramount. (reprinted with permission: *The Douglass Group*)

PLANNING

By definition, a plan is a specific design to achieve a desired future. It is a formal means of documenting where you have been, where you want to go, and the steps you intend to use to get there. Planning meals, trips, or purchases are common human activities. In a business and management context, however, planning is usually an ongoing, formal process. Good managers never stop planning, whether planning new projects or reviewing previously made plans. In any enterprise, the planning document is called the **business plan** (Anderson, 1990). In developing a business plan, managers think through all of the various aspects of the business, commit them to paper, and essentially chart the direction of that business (Marwick, 1984). In the context of this chapter, we will focus on the development and use of a business plan in clinical engineering departments. As a management function, planning should follow a defined set of steps (Figure 7.2):

- Development of a mission statement.
- Identification of services or programs to achieve the stated mission.
- Analysis of markets, competitors, and roadblocks.
- Analysis of the resources required, including people, facilities, and equipment.
- Analysis of the financial resources required.

The output from this planning process, which involves information gathering and synthesis, is a plan. Although the plan is important, the process is paramount.

Mission Statement

As discussed in Chapters 1 and 6, the mission statement is a critical starting point for the development of any plan of operation. The mission statement for a clinical engineering department focuses primarily on medically related end products or services, such as technology management which, in turn, may include such activities as contract management, repair and preventive maintenance, quality control, record maintenance, and equipment evaluation and acquisition.

In developing a business plan for a clinical engineering department, it is often desirable to use the regulatory and accreditation standards that all hospitals must meet as specific goals. For example, the Joint Commission on the Accreditation of Healthcare Organizations specifies that hospitals must have ". . . equipment management programs designed to assess and control the clinical and physical risks of fixed and portable equipment" (JCAHO, 1990). Therefore, by establishing a goal of "medical equipment management" (as required by JCAHO), the clinical engineering program supports the mainstream efforts of the hospital to achieve accreditation, identifies the necessary role clinical engineering plays in the accreditation process, and gives validity to the clinical engineering program.

Because the mission statement guides the entire planning process, there are both opportunities and pitfalls in the selection of services and programs to achieve the overall goal. For example, "medical equipment management" is an appropriate goal for a clinical engineering department. Because the accreditation standards specified by JCAHO ask for an equipment management program (without distinguishing between medical or nonmedical equipment), the goal of "medical equipment management" may present an opportunity for the entrepreneurial manager. If used in its broadest context, the term "equipment management" enables the clinical engineering department to become involved in the management of all major pieces of equipment. To achieve this goal, the department simply can state that it will monitor the equipment's maintenance history and ensure that repairs are accomplished in a timely and cost-effective manner. In this way, the clinical engineering manager does not claim that the department has the expertise to maintain all medical and nonmedical equipment, but rather the expertise necessary to manage the equipment maintenance programs necessary for major pieces of equipment. This approach subtly opens the doors of opportunity, for clinical engineering departments.

Identification of Clinical Engineering Services and Programs

Once the mission statement of the department has been developed, it is essential to identify the specific services (programs) that the department will provide. Figure 7.3 illustrates the major steps usually taken by clinical engineering departments during this part of the planning process. This activity permits the department to review all of the various services that it may offer to its users, ranging from new services to make the hospital more competitive to the traditional services of preventive maintenance and repair.

First of all, specific questions related to newly targeted programs are addressed. For example, questions like, "Are there specific high technology programs that the hospital has targeted that offer the opportunity for contributions from clinical engineering?" need to be answered in light of the hospital's mission statement.

Next, it is necessary to review the range of in-house and contract (outside) services that the department may provide. To accomplish this, certain pieces of information are helpful. These data include the following:

- Trends and utilization rates of outside services for equipment maintenance from both manufacturers and third-party service companies.
- Interviews with potential client departments that focus on (1) their perception of quality versus cost of current maintenance programs, (2) their commitment to the existing program, whatever that program might be, (3) their expectations from a maintenance service vendor, and (4) their impression of strengths and weaknesses in the current equipment maintenance program.

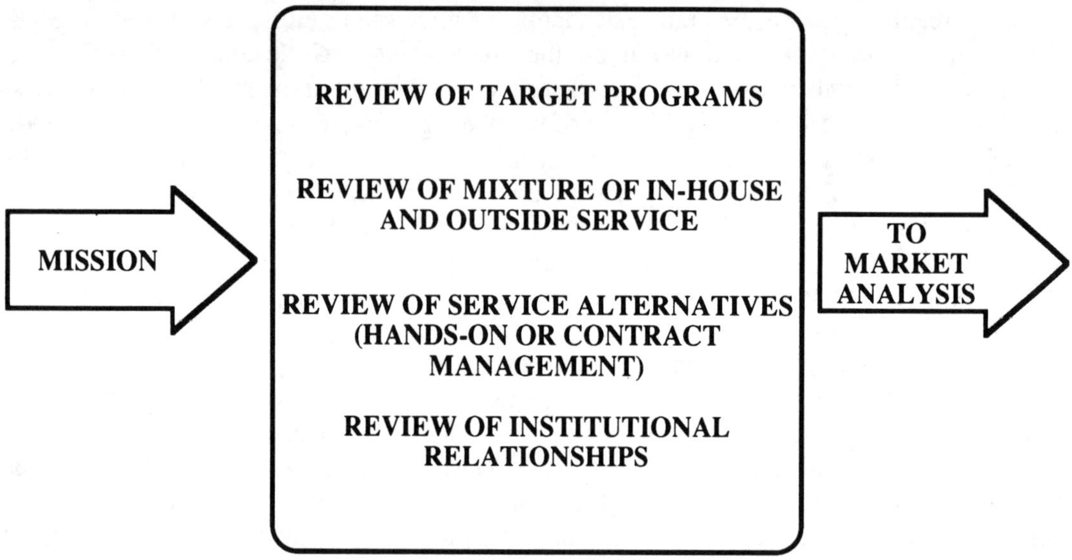
MISSION
REVIEW OF TARGET PROGRAMS
REVIEW OF MIXTURE OF IN-HOUSE AND OUTSIDE SERVICE
REVIEW OF SERVICE ALTERNATIVES (HANDS-ON OR CONTRACT MANAGEMENT)
REVIEW OF INSTITUTIONAL RELATIONSHIPS
TO MARKET ANALYSIS

Figure 7.3: The clinical engineering department's role is defined by the services it provides. These are specifically listed in the business plan. (reprinted with permission: *The Douglass Group*)

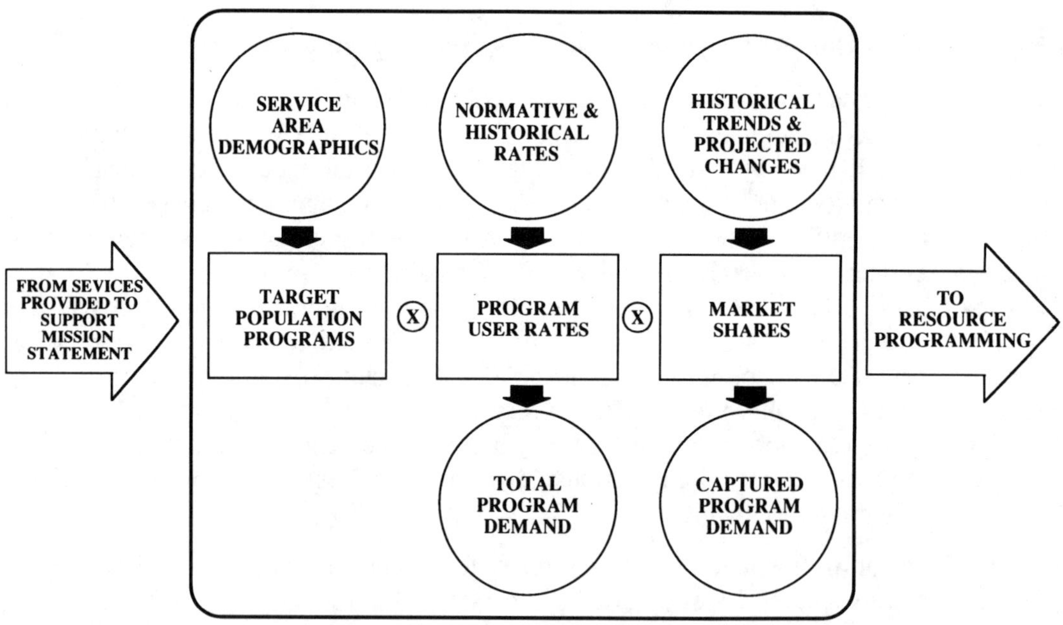

Figure 7.4: Market analysis diagram used to identify potential client hospitals or departments for programs offered by the clinical engineering department. (reprinted with permission: *The Douglass Group*)

By engaging in a careful data collection and analysis effort, the department will be able to identify the strengths and weaknesses of the current maintenance program, perceived gaps in service, unmet needs, and unserved departments. In this way, the department can become aware of both the opportunities and "threats" that it faces. With this information available, planning activities related to the development of future programs and services or even a revision of the department's mission statement can be undertaken.

Market Analysis

Although clinical engineering departments in medical institutions do not usually consider themselves to be corporations with actual products or services to sell, it is important to change this mode of thought. Once clinical engineering departments understand that they are similar to a business enterprise, they will be able to engage more successfully in marketing their services to their respective clinical users. Market analysis requires that each specific target program defined in the mission statement be examined (Figure 7.4).

This requires obtaining data regarding (1) service area demographics, i.e., demographic information on service competitors; (2) normative and historical rates of utilization, i.e., an assessment of equipment use in all clinical departments (e.g., treatments administered by a respiratory therapy department or tests performed by a laboratory and, relatedly, the equipment used in those treatments or tests); and (3) historical trends and projected changes in the use of certain medical procedures and related equipment.

To this point, we have intentionally used the word "equipment" and not "technology." That is because the word "technology," as applied to health care, covers such a broad spectrum of meaning in terms of activities and devices (Goodman, 1991). For example, the term "medical technology" usually includes surgical techniques, drugs, and intensive-care units. The hospital itself can be considered a technology, i.e., one designed to bring together under one roof a broad spectrum of specialists and their tools. Therefore, any analysis of historical trends and forecasts of future developments must include medical technology in its broadest terms.

The results obtained from this market analysis process includes a definition of the service areas in which the departmental programs can successfully operate, an inventory of existing service resources in the demographic area studied, and a description of the present and future utilization rates of major equipment users.

Resource Programming

The resources that individuals manage include people, equipment, and facilities. Resources are usually measured in terms of some standardized unit so that comparisons can be made. For example, people are measured in terms of workloads, hours, full-time equivalents (FTEs), or similar units; equipment is measured in terms of quantities and types, and facilities are measured in terms of space (i.e., square feet). In evaluating workloads for hospital departments, on the other hand, such measures as procedures performed (e.g., in respiratory therapy) or tests performed (e.g., in the clinical laboratory) are often used. Within the clinical engineering department, such activities as preventive maintenance and equipment repair are commonly measured in terms of FTE hours. In using this type of measure the estimated FTE hours used for scheduled maintenance are usually accurate, but those values used for unscheduled maintenance are often unpredictable. When faced with uncertainty, clinical engineering managers must rely heavily upon past history and personal experience.

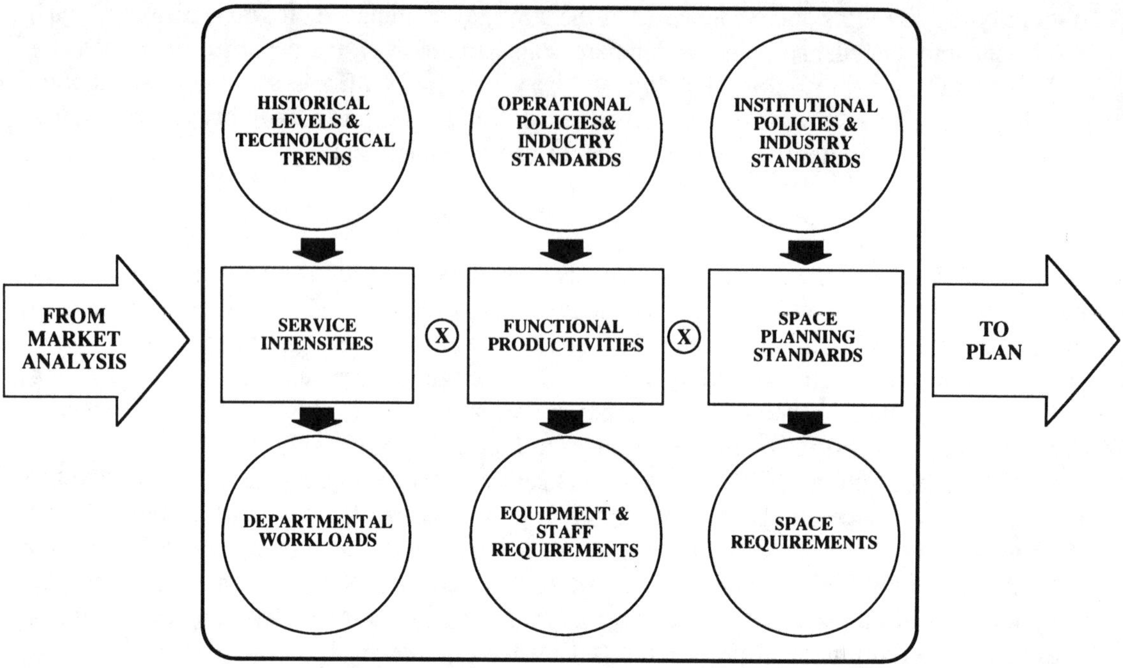

Figure 7.5: Resource programming diagram used to identify required resources to provide clinical engineering services offered. These resources are determined from the output of the market analysis. (reprinted with permission: *The Douglass Group*)

Resource programming, like market analysis, also requires data collection and analysis (Figure 7.5). In the case of resource programming, however, targeted client departments are the subjects of the analysis, and "technological trends" and "industrial" standards serve as the focus of the data collection and analysis steps.

Industry-wide standards are, many times, technology driven. For example, the monitoring of oxygen saturation via noninvasive techniques (pulse oximetry) has quickly evolved as a standard of care for any patient receiving anesthesia, especially during the postanesthesia recovery period. The rapid diffusion of this device is directly related to the efficacy of the technology itself, i.e., it is noninvasive, accurate, and simple to use, has instantaneous readout. Furthermore, pulse oximetry has virtually no impact on physical space and requires little user training. For these reasons, pulse oximetry has been extensively utilized and has become a standard of care for specific patients.

In considering resources necessary to provide specific services, it is essential to investigate the interdependency of certain technologies. For example, consider the case of creating a new service: a new coronary care unit. To provide this new service, one must consider its impact on other clinical programs (Figure 7.6). In this case, it is necessary to provide for (1) the initial receipt of coronary patients (which affects emergency room procedures), (2) the immediate diagnostic evaluation of these patients (which affects cardiac catheterization laboratory activities), and (3) surgical treatment of patients not treatable medically in the coronary care unit or invasively in the cardiac catheterization laboratory (which affects the surgical department). Therefore, in each of these other clinical areas, the resources (i.e., people, facilities, and equipment) needed to support the addition of a new coronary care unit must be carefully considered and evaluated in order to determine accurately whether or not the new service and program can indeed be implemented.

Financial Analysis

The final step in the planning cycle involves estimating the costs associated with the services and programs specified by the department (Figure 7.7). This process converts the resource requirements developed in the previous section into dollars, e.g., FTEs become technician's salaries, additional square footage becomes construction costs, etc. This financial information enables the department to develop a yearly operational budget of people and supporting supplies and a capital budget of equipment and facilities.

During the financial analysis step, it is also essential to identify income sources (i.e., funding). How clinical engineering departments obtain operating funds is critical. For example, if the clinical engineering program is to operate on a fee-for-service basis, then projected salary expenses must be offset by projected revenues. If this is the case, then the fee-for-service concept should be part of the business plan, and both anticipated expenses and anticipated revenues should be projected for a two to three-year period.

The results of the financial analysis phase of the planning process should include a one to three-year operating budget, a corresponding capital budget, and, if revenues are expected, a current and projected summary of profit and loss.

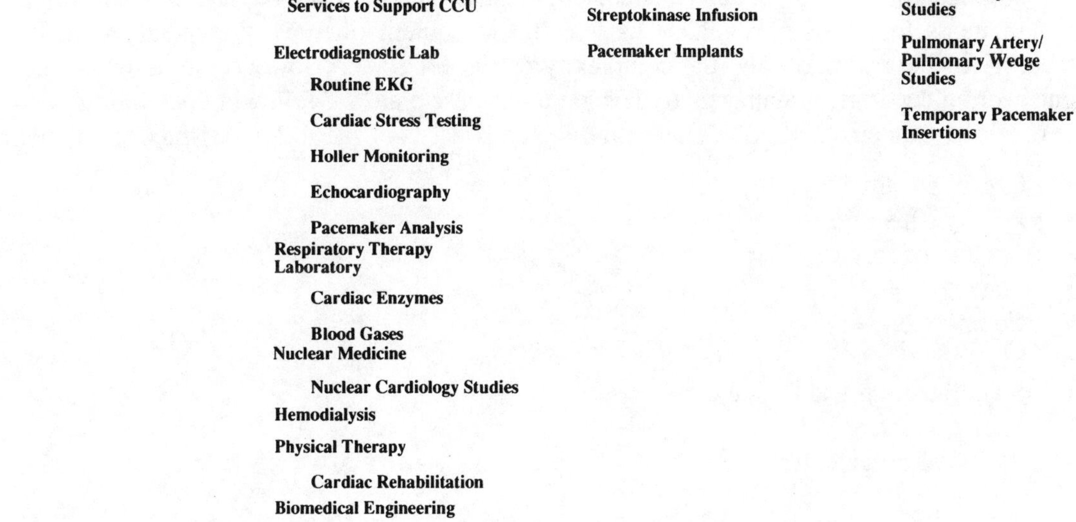

Figure 7.6: Impact on other services as a result of additional cardiovascular services.

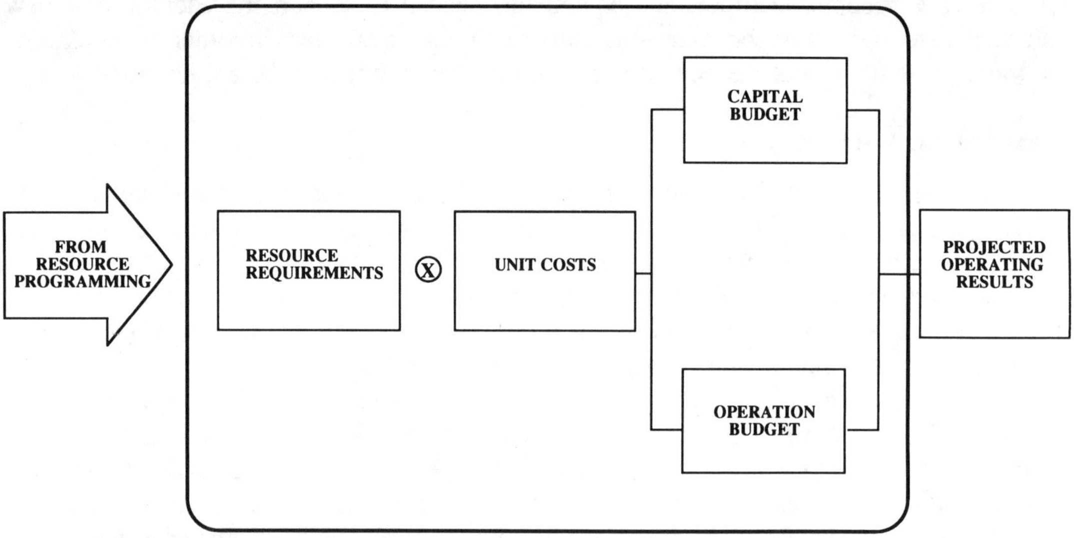

Figure 7.7: Financial analysis diagram. The ouput from resource analysis are given dollar values and sources of revenue are identified sufficient to cover the expected demands on the clinical engineering department. (reprinted with permission: *The Douglass Group*)

PREPARING A BUSINESS PLAN

A well-structured business plan consists of a series of mileposts that serve as a gauge of departmental progress and performance, and it indicates the funding required for operation of the department. In the case of the clinical engineering department, the development of the business plan provides the manager with an opportunity to capture the interest of both administrators and prospective client departments.

Although preparation of such a document is important, there are no hard and fast format requirements for a business plan. Its length and content often vary, depending on the maturity of the operation and the complexity of the program. However, to assist clinical engineering department managers to develop a business plan, the following planning format is provided (Anderson, 1990). The business plan consists of the following major sections:[1]

- Executive summary.
- Business history.
- Product or service.
- Market.
- Competition.
- Marketing.
- Manufacturing and operations.
- Management.
- Financial Projections.

---

[1]Reprinted with permission from: *An Entrepeneur's Guide to Developing a Business Plan*, Enterpise Group. © copyright 1990 by Arthur Anderson, Arthur Anderson and Company, S.C. All rights reserved.

Upon completion, the business plan must be presented administration of the institution and, perhaps prior to that, to various departments or key personnel of the health-care team for input and commentary. The way in which the plan is presented can contribute significantly to its success or failure. For this reason, some basic concepts of both written and oral presentation are also presented plan.

The executive summary is usually a two to five-page summary, i.e., an overview, of the key elements of the business plan. At a minimum, the executive summary should include the following:

- A description of the business (e.g., the clinical engineering department) and the target markets for each of its products or services. After stating whether the business (department) will compete in a large existing market or create a new one, the executive summary should compare each product or service of the department with the competition and stress its own niche in the market.
- A description of the departmental management team, emphasizing the relevant experience and special skills of each key executive. If there are management weaknesses, they should be cited along with how and when they are expected to be corrected.
- A summary of key financial projections for the next three to five years.
- A summary of funding requirements outlining when, and for what purpose the department will need varying amounts of capital.

Business History

If the business plan is being developed solely for internal use, the discussion of the history of the business may be omitted. However, it is often important to understand the department from a historical perspective. As a result, this section of the plan should include the following:

- A discussion of when the business (department) was founded, its progress to date, and a brief biographical sketch of the founders.
- The organizational structure.
- A discussion of products or services the department has developed or marketed over the years.

If it is believed that the company's past performance is not a reliable indicator of its potential, the reasons should be cited in this section.

Product or Service

The purpose of this section is to define precisely what the department intends to provide in terms of products or services. Its length varies, depending on the number and complexity of the services. This section should be written in language easily understandable by a lay person and should include, as appendices, any lengthy or detailed diagrams, technical documents, or descriptions that are important to a comprehensive understanding of the company's products.

Market

Because a comprehensive description of the department's opportunities (markets) is important to management, it is important to answer the following questions:

- Who are the users or customers (e.g., manufacturers, other client departments, etc.)?
- What is the historic (last five years) and forecasted (next five years) rate of growth for each market segment or service provided?
- What are perceived future markets?
- How will each market segment be serviced, e.g., for a specific client, who are the decision makers, what services can be offered to them, etc.?
- At what level are purchasing decisions made (e.g., senior management, operating management, technical management, administrative management, purchasing agent)?
- How does each user/client purchase the product, e.g., annual or long-term contract, unit purchases, etc.?
- What are the critical product/service characteristics, e.g., availability, price, service?
    - Does the market have any special characteristics, e.g., seasonal, cyclical, etc.?

Competition

In any business enterprise, it is important to identify competitors, indicating the special strengths, weaknesses, and market share of each. In this section, the principal competitive factors in the marketplace should also be cited. These include product performance, reliability, durability, service, and price.

Marketing

Marketing goals are usually summarized in this section. Such goals should be quantitative, realistic, and consistent with the marketing analysis performed. For example, to develop a pricing strategy the following questions should be addressed: How do you plan to price your products? How will your prices compare with the existing price structure in the marketplace? How do you expect competitors to react to your pricing strategy? What impact is their action likely to have on your financial projections?

This section of the business plan also should outline methods used to monitor the market on a continuing basis in order to assess the impact of changing competitive strategies and whether any product evaluations, pricing comparisons, or market-share analyses are needed.

Operations

This section of the business plan summarizes the nature, quality and extent of available facilities. It should indicate the strengths and limitations of these facilities. Furthermore, the timing, cost, extent and importance of any planned expansion and related financing issues should be included here.

Management

This section emphasizes the experience and competence of each key manager. If a major goal is to strengthen the management team, an outline of the planned management structure in chart form, providing detailed job descriptions and minimum qualifications for each unfilled slot should be provided here. In addition, this section should include when and how each open position will be filled and the level of compensation. It also is helpful to include job descriptions, compensation data, and detailed resumes on all managers who are already in place. Although an internal business plan often does not include such information, it may be of interest to key administrators. Personal data on key managers, therefore, should include all relevant business experience, educational background, patents or copyrights, significant awards, and any other information that would help a prospective client department conclude that the necessary management and technical resources are available.

Financial Projections

In this section, all of the assumptions and quantitative data presented elsewhere in the business plan are put to a numerical test. In other words, all of the company's sales, market, and cost projections should be provided in a summary-type financial format.

At a minimum, the following should be included:

- Past financial statements.
- Profit and loss statements.
- Current financial statements.
- Profit and loss projections on a monthly or quarterly basis, if possible, for the first two years and annually for the three subsequent years.

These financial projections serve a dual purpose: (1) to guide your management team and (2) to inform prospective clients. An illustration of the practical use of a business plan for a hospital-based clinical engineering department is provided in the case study at the end of this chapter. The clinical engineering department described is a part of the University of Texas M.D. Anderson Cancer Center, located in Houston, Texas. As a state-supported institution, certain references in the business plan are unique to the state method of funding. However, the concept of the plan and the strategy used in its preparation are applicable to any clinical engineering department.

Presentation of the Plan

Thus far, this chapter has presented the processes a clinical engineer undertakes to gather, review, and compile the data necessary to justify the establishment or expansion of a clinical engineering program. At some point the clinical engineer will need to present this information to others. Unfortunately, most clinical engineering curriculums do not include a course on presentation skills or public speaking. This may put the clinical engineer at a disadvantage when attempting to secure resources. A good presentation may not guarantee success, but a bad presentation will certainly guarantee failure. The purpose of this section is to educate the reader in the art of making a good presentation.

Loosley defined, a presentation occurs whenever a person or group communicates information to another person or group. Presentations are either written or oral, short or long. The most important rule to remember when making any presentation is to **know your audience.**

Written Presentations. Understanding the cultural perceptions of the audience is paramount in any communication effort. Generally, engineers tend to provide too much detail in written presentations to nonengineers, especially to members of the hospital administration. To illustrate this point, consider a comment made by a hospital vice-president: "*Any written communication over one page is a report, not a memo; and most administrators don't read reports.*" The implication here is not that administrators simply discard the reports that they receive; rather, they typically don't read the detail in a report.

Two lessons for effective written communication can be learned from this. First, any important information presented in written form to hospital administrators should be kept to one page. Second, supporting data should not be presented in paragraph form unless absolutely necessary. Do not infer from this that one can always present a complicated situation in only one page or that anyone will commit significant resources based on a single page of information. Rather, recognize that hospital executives usually do not have the time to closely review every piece of information that comes across their desks. They rely on the fact that the people surrounding them are competent and understand their professional responsibilities. In such an organization, executive decisions are be based upon a summary of pertinent information. In light of this, the manner in which such a summary is presented can significantly influence the reception of the proposal. To be effective, clinical engineers must be able to organize complete arguments into concise one page summaries known as **executive summaries**. As a general rule, the executive summary should be composed only after assembly of all other components of the report or proposal.

The assembly of reports (or proposals) begins with the summarization of the supporting data. Graphs are an excellent means of providing lots of information in a limited amount of space. (Remember the old axiom: A picture is worth a thousand words.) Each type of graph has particular advantages and limitations for the presentation of data. Line graphs are useful for illustrating continuous trends or for comparing two or more sets of trends. Figure 7.8 illustrates an effective way to present information on the rise in total capital assets over a period of several years. Figure 7.9 is a line graph illustrating the relationship between productivity and mean time to repair over a two-year period. Note that this graph utilizes dissimilar axes to enhance visual comparison of this data.

Bar graphs are a useful for illustrating trends over disjointed periods. These graphs can be very informative when segmented data are incorporated into the trended information. Figure 7.10 presents three graphical representations of the maintenance costs for patient care equipment from 1987 through 1991. Note that from 1987 to 1989 the hospital relied primarily on outside vendors for the majority of equipment support services and that in 1990 the clinical engineering department was extensively expanded. The first graph illustrates the total expenses for each year. The second graph shows exactly the same information, however; the Y-axis has been modified to present only data from the top quarter of the first graph. This technique accentuates the differences in expenses between each year and dramatizes the savings realized between FY89 and FY90. The reverse technique can be used to minimize the graphing of negative trends. For example, if the rise in expenses from FY87 to FY88 could not be explained by an increase of equipment within the hospital (see Figure 7.8), then it would be better to use the first graph when making a presentation of this data. The third graph presents essentially the same information as the first two, but with greater detail. The total expenses for patient-care equipment maintenance have been broken down into major categories for each year. This presentation allows visualization of key information concerning the relative costs of salaries and contracts.

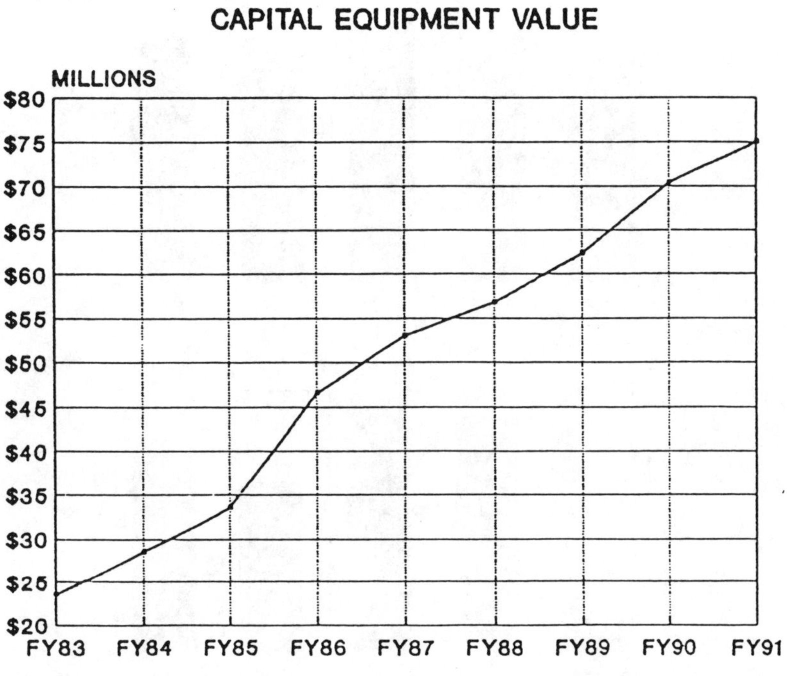

Figure 7.8: **Line graph illustrating growth of capital assets value from FY '83 to FY '91.**

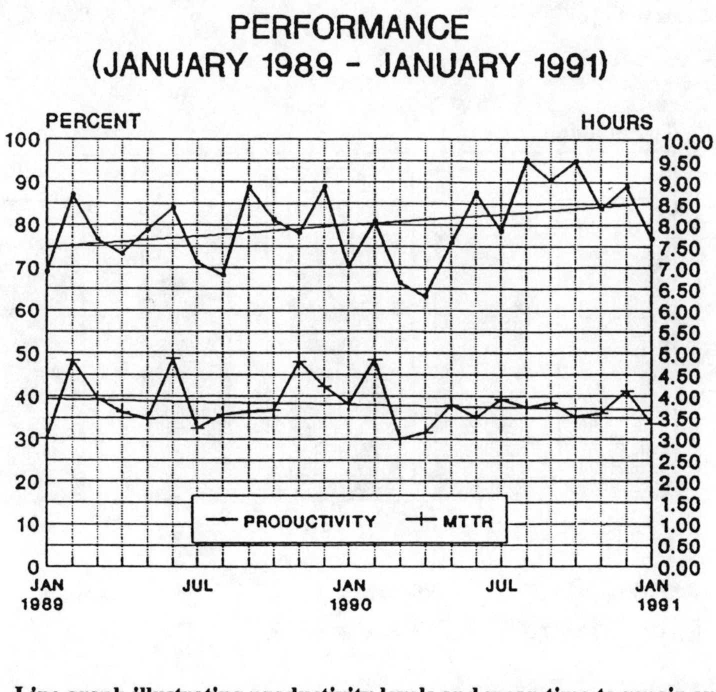

Figure 7.9: **Line graph illustrating productivity levels and mean time to repair over the period 1/89 to 1/91.**

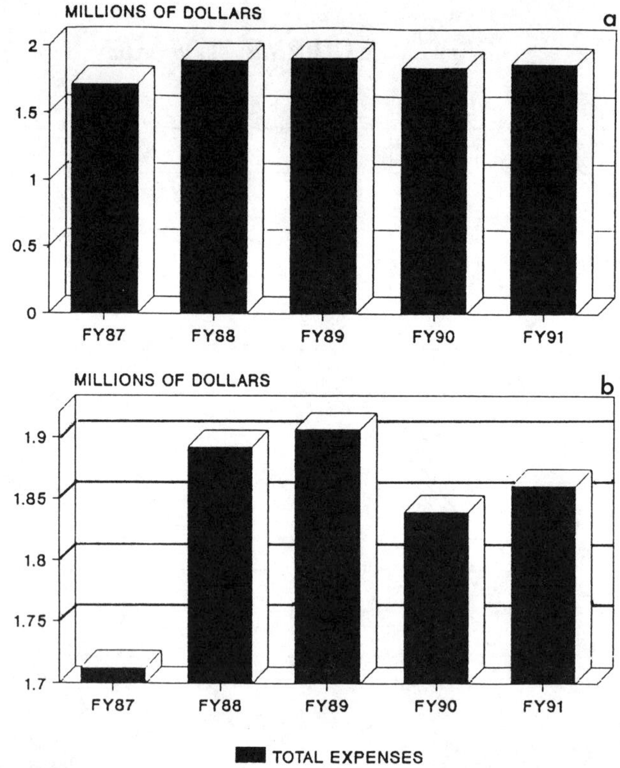

Figure 7.10: Bar graphs illustrating the aggregate maintenance costs for clinical engineering for the five-year period 1987 to 1991 (a). Noth the effect that changing the Y-axis scale has on the visual appearance of this data (b).

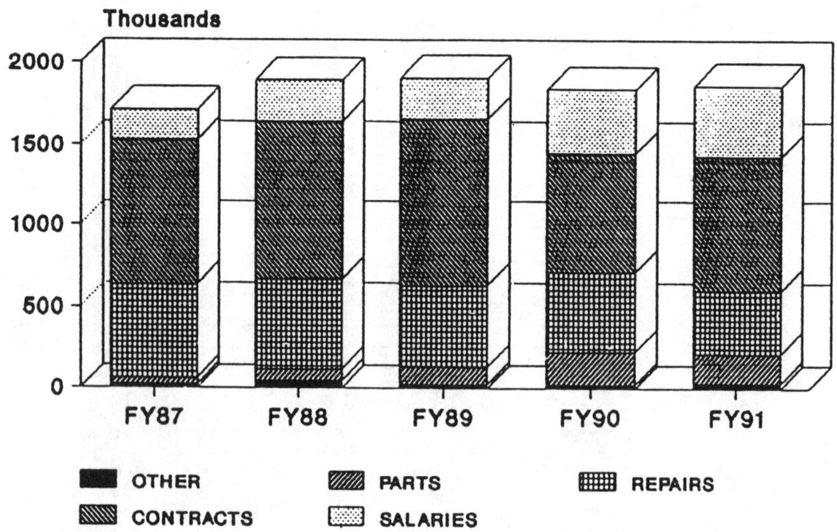

Figure 7.10: (c) Bar graph illustrating the aggregate maintenance costs for the same period as above broken down to reflect all factors involved in overall maintenance costs.

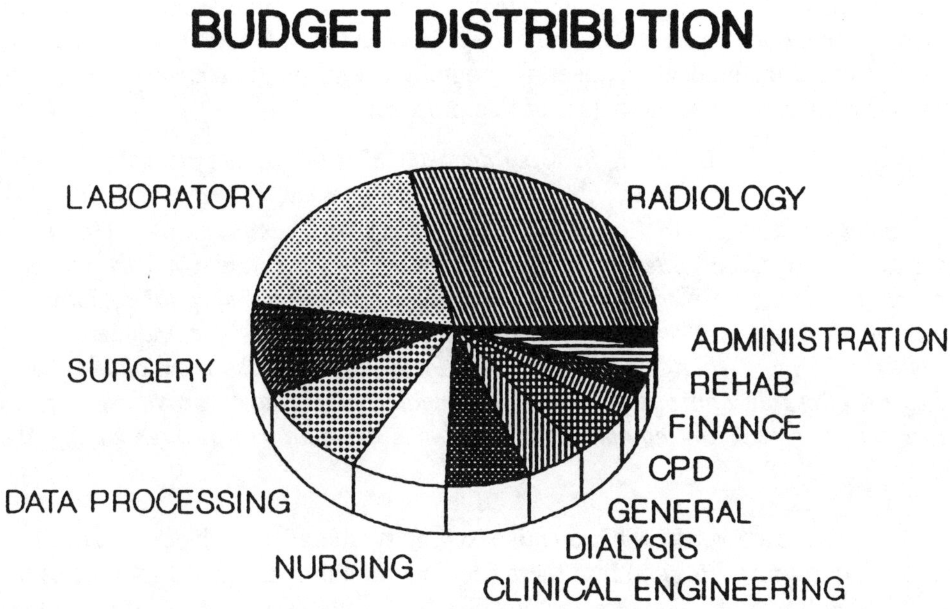

Figure 7.11: Pie graph illustrating the distibution of maintenance expenses by department.

Pie graphs can be effectively utilized to illustrate the relative value of "static" data. For example, a pie graph could be used to show the relative expenses of each hospital department (in a decentralized system) for a given year (Figure 7.11). However, it would be inappropriate to present the data in Figure 7.10c as a series of pie graphs because the data change from year to year.

Graphs are not the only method of presenting a large quantity of data on a single page, charts and tables can serve the same purpose. If one wanted to present comparative data on various maintenance support alternatives for ventilators, centrifuges, blood gas analyzers, and radiology equipment, a chart such as that shown in Table 7.1 would be quite useful. This chart shows the current cost of support and the anticipated expenditure under a proposed alternative. Numbers shown in parentheses in the far right column equate to the potential savings of the alternative and resultant changes in technician positions are also shown.

Sometimes even a chart may need to be more than one page. For example, if one wanted to illustrate the calculations for determining the appropriate number of FTEs for the clinical engineering program for every device type, this would require more than one page. Including this information as a table in a written presentation, however, is perfectly acceptable. The clinical engineer simply needs to understand that this information is presented as back-up material for reference and verification purposes only.

The final step in completing the written presentation is construction of the executive summary. After all the background work has been organized and the graphs and tables generated, the executive summary should be relatively easy to write. The executive summary should contain the following four parts: (1) the introduction; (2) the list of objectives; (3) the list of resources; and (4) the statement of benefits/closing. It should be no longer than one page.

The introduction should be a single paragraph that defines for the reader the **who, what** (goal), and **why** (background) of the document. If pertinent, references to other documents or resources should be made. The following introductory paragraph was taken from a proposal to expand the clinical engineering program at a hospital. The who, what, and why are clearly communicated at the outset of this proposal.

> *The purpose of the clinical engineering department is to provide prudent, cost effective management over the utilization of patient care equipment and related high technology equipment at this Medical Center to ensure its safe and continued use. Unfortunately, as stated in a recent internal audit, current procedures and controls inadequately address the . . . processes necessary to ensure the servicing of hospital equipment in the most efficient manner which has resulted in expenditures for maintenance being considerably more than the industry standard suggests that they should be. This proposal offers an approach to expand clinical engineering to provide greater direct involvement in reducing equipment maintenance expenditures throughout the Medical Center"*(Brody, 1989).

The next two sections of the executive summary should list objectives and required resources. The information in both of these sections should be presented as a series of brief statements in outline form. This method enables the presentation of a maximum amount of information within the space allotted (about 1/4 page for each section). Furthermore, it serves to emphasize the points presented.

An **objective** is a specific statement that describes the results that must be achieved to attain a desired goal. An objective should be defined by a specific action, which identifies a desired result, to be realized within specific time-frame. Most importantly, achieving the end result of an objective should lend itself to assessment by tangible measurement as a means of determining the level of success.

An objective is very different from a goal, which is defined as a broad statement outlining a result and which serves as an indicator of the direction to pursue. Goals tend to be open ended, challenging one to stretch. Conceptually, goals are equivalent to dreams and aspirations, and objectives require structure and planning. The following are a few examples of objectives related to the goal of developing a quality clinical engineering program for a hospital.

- To reduce the total medical center expenditures for equipment maintenance by $25,000 annually, starting within this fiscal year.
- To create an inventory of all equipment used for patient care within the medical center by December.
- To complete 95 percent of all preventive maintenance jobs assigned within three months of assignment during this year.

Note that each example objective follows this four-part formula:

To (action verb) + (desired result) **By** (measurement) + (time unit).

If the clinical engineer wished to present more detail about this objective, an extended outline format could be used:

Table 7.1 Comparison of Current and Anticipated Costs

ANTICIPATED STAFF	SALARY	EMERGENCY REPAIRS	PARTS ALLOTMENT	CURRENT EXPENDITURE FOR:	CONTRACTS	REPAIRS	DIFFERENCE
BMET II (DIALYSIS)							
	$29,277						
		$3,000	$2,000	DIALYSIS MACHINES	$18,509	$6,062	
		$1,000	$1,000	O.R. CELL SAVER	$8,250	$0	
		$2,000	$3,000	CENTRIFUGES	$5,000	$5,000	
	$29,277	$6,000	$6,000	subtotal:	$31,759	$11,062	($1,544)
BMET II (RESPIRATORY)							
	$29,277						
		$ 500	$1,200	VENTILATORS-INFANTS	$2,960	$1,000	
		$1,500	$13,300	VENTILATORS-ADULT	$47,025	$3,000	
	$29,277	$2,000	$14,500	subtotal:	$49,985	$4,000	($8,208)
BMET III (OR/ANES)							
	$32,697						
		$5,000	$8.000	LASERS	$35,025		
			$500	HEART LUNG MACHINE	$2,907		
		—	—	LASER FIBERS	—	—	
	$32,697	$5,000	$8,500	subtotal:	$37,932	$0	$3,265
BMET III (RADIOLOGY)							
	$32,697						
		$75,000	$15,000	GENERAL	$0	$130,000	
	$32,697	$75,000	$15,000	subtotal:	$0	$130,000	($7,303)
BMET III (LABORATORY)							
	$32,697						
		$5,000	$5,000	CELL COUNTER	$21,000		
		$10,000	$5,000	BLOOD GAS ANALYZER	$4,000	$35,000	
		$5,000	$2,000	GENERAL		$15,000	
	$32,697	$20,000	$12,000	subtotal:	$25,000	$50,000	($10,303)
BMET III (CRIT CARE)							
	$32,697						
		$0	$0	BMET II SALARY	$29,277	$0	
		$1,000	$1,000	IABP	$6,000	$0	
		$1,000	$500	CATH LAB MONITOR	$9,700	$0	
	$32,697	$2,000	$1,500	subtotal:	$44,977	$0	($8,780)
BMET I							
	$23,437			BMET II SALARY	$29,277		($5,840)
				TOTAL SAVINGS			($38,713)

To reduce the total medical center expenditures for equipment maintenance by $25,000 annually, starting within this fiscal year.

- By reducing expenditures for radiology equipment maintenance by $10,000.
- By reducing expenditures for laboratory equipment maintenance by $8,000.
- By reducing expenditures for general patient-care equipment maintenance by $7,000.

The outline format should also be used to present the list of resources required to successfully complete the proposed goal. Consider the following example used to explain the specific costs involved in the immediate purchase of specialized test equipment totalling $18,500.

- $11,000 for general test equipment.
- $6,000 for radiology test equipment.
- $1,500 for laboratory test equipment.

It is extremely important that both the objectives and the resources presented in any proposal are realistic. Objectives that are too easily attained may serve to weaken the justification of the resources requested. Conversely, objectives too difficult to meet lead to failure. Requesting realistic resources tied to measurable objectives also adds credibility to the document as it is reviewed.

The final section of the executive summary is the closing, which includes a summation of the benefits to be derived from the program presented. The closing should briefly explain (in a paragraph) what the successful completion of objectives would mean to the hospital and should offer any additional benefits. The following is an example of a closing paragraph used in a proposal for expansion of a clinical engineering program:

> *This proposal reflects only a portion of the savings potential ultimately available by expanding the clinical engineering department. Additional benefits include a stronger technical presence in clinical areas, better adherence to regulatory guidelines and stronger ties with the risk management department. All of these factors, coupled with the immediate financial gains, clearly demonstrate the need for this program.*

The closing may be strengthened by the inclusion of a short list of assumptions used in preparing the document. The following are examples:

- Vendor costs will increase 4 percent per year.
- Salaries will increase 3.5 percent per year.
- Employee benefits are estimated at 17 percent of salary.
- The budget proposed herein is for existing equipment only. Newly arriving equipment may require additional funding.

Once completed, the document should be carefully put together. Pages should always be numbered, and if the document contains a lot of material, it should include a table of contents. A professional-looking title page can serve to enhance a document. Most hospitals have a logo that can be copied onto the title page for a truly professional look. For a major proposal, a unique title page carrying the words "Copy for (name)" or "Prepared for (name)" should be generated for each recipient. This will indicate that the work enclosed was generated specifically for the person indicated. The use of colored paper for the title and blank end page of a stapled document will also add to the professional look of the document.

Oral Presentations. The only way to become a good public speaker is to practice. Good oral presentations are the result of five factors: (1) knowing the material, (2) knowing the audience, (3) using a good voice, (4) using positive body language, and (5) being comfortable with visual aids.

The first two factors, knowing the material and knowing the audience, have been consistent themes throughout this chapter and will not be rediscussed here. The third factor, voice, is enhanced by introducing inflection to highlight specific points. The volume of one's voice should be varied according to each situation. For example, in a small group setting use a lower volume that forces the audience to listen more intently. Conversely, in a lecture situation, one must project the voice so that the audience can hear the presentation easily. If a microphone is used, it should be placed discreetly so that the presenter can talk normally.

Body language is a strong communication tool that is frequently overlooked. Posture and placement can send strong subliminal messages that, at times, can overpower the spoken presentation. The physical location of the speaker can be used to convey authority (i.e., a judge on the bench, a manager behind a desk, a speaker at the front of the room, a committee chairperson at the head of the table), or subordination (i.e., being on the witness stand, sitting in the chair opposite the manager's desk, appearing before a committee). Placement can also be used to minimize authority (i.e., the cafeteria, a hallway).

Body positions can have the same effect as body placement. Authoritative positions include standing, sitting while leaning forward, standing or sitting squared off/eye to eye, and standing or sitting with arms crossed. More neutral positions include leaning against a wall or a piece of furniture, sitting relaxed toward the side or back of a chair, or sitting slightly sideways.

Eye contact is another form of body language. Good eye contact is extremely important for good communication. During one-on-one situations (i.e., interviews, performance evaluations, casual conversations, etc.) or small group meetings, the speaker should always have direct eye contact with the person he or she is addressing. As groups get larger, the good speakers will scan the room; stopping briefly to make eye contact with one person as they move on to the next person. Eye contact assures the listener while pacing the speaker.

Body language can be a very effective communication tool; however, it can only be mastered through experience. Students are encouraged to experiment with different body placements and positions and to observe the reactions of others.

The final key to being a good speaker is the effective use of visual aids. Because we retain only 10 percent of what we hear but over 50 percent of what we see, visual aids should be developed to enhance a presentation, not repeat it.

The three most common mistakes made when using visual aids are (1) reading material directly from the media, (2) using visuals that include images that are too small, and (3) forcing too much information into a single visual. The first issue is easily corrected if the speaker knows the material. Problems with image size, however, require that the speaker take time planning the presentation. Here are a few simple hints for developing presentation visuals:

- Graphs make better visuals than tables.
- Minimize detail.

- Accentuate shapes, line widths, and colors.
- Use a dark background.
- Limit each visual to one thought or idea.
- All text should be legible if the slide is read at arm's length without projection equipment.
- For transparencies, copy the image at 78 to 80 percent of original size, and center the image to ensure that information at the edges is not lost.

One solution to the third problem is to prepare a series of individual visuals that can be overlaid, one on top of the other, to build an image in conjunction with the evolution of the argument being presented. In addition, the speaker should always be aware of the placement of the media equipment being used. This is especially important when using a variety of equipment. Slide projectors and overhead projectors focus at different distances. Position the projection screen or chart to the side of the speaker so that the speaker can see the projected visual while continuing to face the audience. Immediately before a presentation ensure that all of the equipment works and that ancillary equipment (i.e. markers, pointers, remote controls, etc.) is available.

Today, video and computer-generated visual aids are becoming increasingly popular. The use of a computer system can enhance presentations beyond the capability of standard slides by incorporating special effects. The general tips for creating computer images are the same as those for other visual media. In most cases a good-quality 21-inch monitor will suffice for a 20' x 30' room. Additional monitors should be added for larger rooms. Projection monitors are also available and will provide the best image for a large audience.

ORGANIZING AND LEADING

Organizational Chart

Before the business plan can be implemented, an organization scheme, framework, or chart must be in place. As discussed in the introduction to this chapter, the organizational framework directs the flow of information between management and subordinate employees. However, if the organization in question is a subsection of a much larger organization, such as a department within a hospital, the basic framework may already be defined by senior-level management, and the internal structure of the department may be constrained by a budget that limits the number and level of personnel available to the department.

Job Description

Regardless of the structure used, however, the basic principles of sound management remain the same. They essentially begin and end with effective communication between those who manage and those who are managed. At a minimum, the manager must provide a written organizational chart that identifies levels of authority and paths of communication. In addition, the manager must develop job descriptions that clearly state the educational and experience level required, the basic duties, and the level of authority of the job. The job description of a clinical engineering program head, for example, is presented in Chapter 1. For other positions, *The Journal of Clinical Engineering* is an excellent source for job descriptions and salary levels of clinical engineers and biomedical equipment technicians.

Performance Appraisals

"Weakness in human resource management can be traced to an attitude that the worker is a cost factor to be minimized rather than as an evolving human resource that has to be educated" (Bennett, 1987). Managers can facilitate that education by conducting an appropriate performance appraisal during which the manager's expectations of the employee are clarified, and the focus is on performance. Although the performance appraisal may be the most difficult and discomforting role of a manager, it will be effective if the performance appraisal is the following (Bennett, 1987):

- A positive experience.
- An objective process.
- A partnership in development.
- A joint responsibility.
- A progressive review of the future.
- An experience that concentrates on performance rather than dollars.

To assist both the manager and the employee, clear guidelines are necessary. For this reason, job descriptions are important and should be used as a guideline for the development of performance appraisal criteria. Too often, the performance evaluation criteria are ill-defined and reflect some inappropriate combination of skills and attitude ratings that provide no guidelines for the employee's continued professional growth.

It has been reported that once basic needs for adequate pay and job security are fulfilled, esteem-related factors, such as advancement opportunity, become more salient. Although performance reviews typically address financial aspects and allude to the potential for growth and promotion if weaknesses are overcome, they almost never provide a clear picture of professional growth, i.e., performance expectations from entry-level through senior-level positions. An example of an appropriate performance evaluation matrix is presented in Table 7.2. To use this matrix properly it is important to understand the guidelines which were used to establish it (Goodman, 1980): *This guideline documents the criteria used in the evaluation of employees in technical positions. In all cases, it is the intent of the Department to guide all technicians toward a performance proficiency level that will qualify them to become Certified Biomedical Equipment Technicians (CBETs) by the International Certification Commission.*

Evaluation of all technical employees centers on five major areas. These are:

1. *Job Knowledge and Skills*
2. *Quality of Work*
3. *Initiative/Degree of Supervision Required*
4. *Attendance*
5. *Supervisory Skills (for Group Leaders and Supervisors Only)*

Job Knowledge and Skills is further divided into the following areas:

1. *Departmental Policies and Procedures*
2. *Medical Terminology*
3. *Codes and Standards*
4. *Equipment Servicing*

Table 7.2 Portion of the Evaluation Matrix for Medical Terminology

Medical Terminology and its demonstrated application will include the following.	Outstanding	Above Average	Average	Below Average
1. All technicians will complete the programmed text on Medical Terminology by the end of the first year of employment.	Can converse comfortably with medical personnel.	Frequently uses.	Completed. Uses in daily work occassionally.	Incomplete
2. Identify the following surgical procedures including:				
2A. A brief description of the procedure.	Uses in-depth knowledge in daily work.	In-depth knowledge. Uses occassionally.	Understands procedure and can identify major concepts.	Lacks knowledge to perform.
2B. The surgical suite most likely to be used.		Demonstrates understanding of special ancillary equipment or facilities needed.	Can identify.	Lacks knowledge to perform.
2C. The type of instrumentation most likely to be used.		In-depth knowledge of equipment and application.	Able to identify and explain general applications	Lacks knowledge to perform.
2D. Typical problems encountered with the above instrumentation in clinical usage.	In-depth knowledge.	Can identify and explain in general terms.	Can identify problems.	Lacks knowledge to perform.
2E. The recovery area the patient will mostly likely use.		Demonstrates understanding of special ancillary equipment or facilities needed.	Can identify.	Lacks knowledge to perform.
2F. The type of instrumentation most likely to be used.		In-depth knowledge of equipment and application.	Able to identify and explain general applications.	Lacks knowledge to perform.
2G. Typical problems encountered with the above instrumentation in clinical usage.	In-depth knowledge.	Can identify and explain in general terms.	Can identify problems.	Lacks knowledge to perform.

* All ratings for Equipment Technician level.
For BMET level, move all ratings one position to the left.
For Senior BMET and above, move all ratings two positions to the left.
BID 6/79

Certification is not required. It is used as a guide because of its recognized acceptance as an indicator of proficiency. Evaluation criteria are defined for all of the above areas. In particular, the four sub-areas under Job Knowledge and Skills are described in a schedule, which relates specific skills to both proficiency level and job or pay grade.

The portion of the evaluation matrix related to medical terminology is shown in Table 7.2. It will be noted that a performance level of "outstanding" for an entry-level equipment technician is only above average for an intermediate-level BMET. Senior BMETs, on the other hand, should have an excellent working knowledge of medical terminology and therefore are evaluated heaviest for equipment servicing abilities.

Leadership

In addition to evaluating employee performance, managers must be effective leaders. Therefore, they must be conscious of their leadership responsibilities. It is important to emphasize that there is no single all-purpose leadership style. Successful leaders are those who can adapt their behavior to meet the demands of their own unique situation. However, there is a recognized approach called situational leadership theory, developed by the Center for Leadership Studies (Center for Leadership Studies, 1976) that may be helpful. Situational theory is based upon an interplay among (1) the amount of direction (task behavior) a leader gives, (2) the amount of socio/emotional support (relationship behavior) a leader provides, and (3) the "maturity" level that employees exhibit on a specific task, function, or objective.

In this approach, task behavior is defined as the extent to which a leader engages in one-way communication with employees to explain what they must do as well as when, where, and how tasks are to be accomplished. Relationship behavior, on the other hand, is the extent to which a leader provides psychological support and facilitating behaviors (Figure 7.12).

Maturity is defined as the capacity to set high but attainable goals (achievement-motivation), a willingness and ability to take responsibility, and the achievement of additional education or experience. The level of maturity should be considered only in relation to a specific task to be performed. That is to say, an individual or a group is not mature or immature in any total sense. People tend to have varying degrees of maturity depending on the specific task, function, or objective that a leader is attempting to accomplish through their efforts. Thus, a biomedical equipment technician may be very mature in the way he or she approaches and completes a bench repair but may not demonstrate the same degree of maturity in preparing a report. Therefore, it may be appropriate for the clinical engineering manager to provide little direction and help on bench repairs yet provide a great deal of close supervision and direction over written report preparation.

According to situational leadership theory, as the level of maturity of the employee continues to increase in terms of accomplishing a specific task, the leader should begin to reduce task behavior and increase relationship behavior. This should continue until the individual or group reaches a moderate level of maturity. As the employee begins to move into an above-average level of maturity, it becomes appropriate for the leader to decrease not only task behavior, but relationship behavior as well. At some point, the follower will not only be mature in terms of the performance of the task but also psychologically mature.

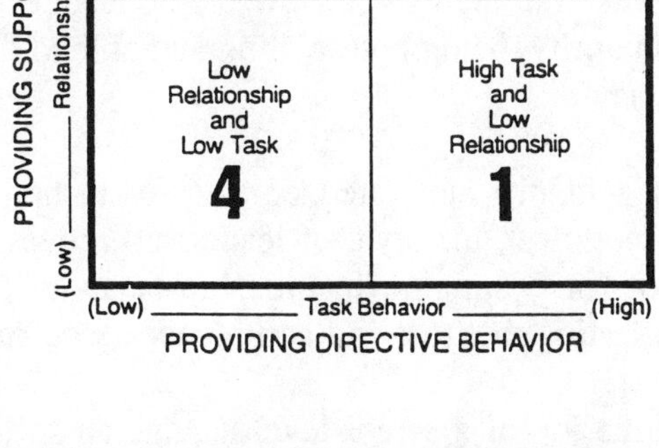

Figure 7.12: Chart of the four basic leader behavior styles. (reproduced with permission: *Leadership Studies, Inc.*)

Figure 7.13 illustrates the relation between task-relevant maturity and the appropriate leadership styles to be used as the follower moves from immaturity to maturity. This figure illustrates two different phenomena. The appropriate leadership style for given levels of follower maturity is portrayed by a curvilinear function in the four leadership quadrants. The maturity level of the individual or group being supervised (maturity of followers) is depicted below the leadership model as a continuum ranging from immature to mature. In referring to the leadership styles in the model in Figure 7.14, situational leadership theory uses the following shorthand designations: (1) high task/low relationship is referred to as leader behavior style S1; (2) high task/high relationship behavior is leader behavior style S2; (3) high relationship/low task behavior is leader behavior style S3; and (4) low relationship/low task behavior is style S4.

Low relationship behavior does not mean that the manager is not friendly or personable to the subordinate. Rather, the manager, in supervising the subordinate's handling of technical report preparation, for example, should spend more time directing the person in what to do and how, when, and where to do it than providing socio/emotional support and reinforcement. Increased relationship behavior should occur when the subordinate begins to demonstrate the ability to handle technical report writing. At that point, a movement from style 1 to style 2 would be appropriate.

While it is important to keep in mind the definitions of task and relationship behavior given earlier, the labeling of the four styles of situational leadership theory, as in Figure 7.14, is sometimes useful:

1. **High task/low relationship leader behavior** (S1) is referred to as "telling." This style is characterized by one-way communication in which the leader defines the roles of followers and tells them what, how, when, and where to do various tasks.

2. **High task/high relationship behavior** (S2) is referred to as "selling." With this style, most of the direction is still provided by the leader. He or she attempts through two-way communication and socio/emotional support to get the followers psychologically to buy into decisions that have to be made.

3. **High relationship/low task behavior** (S3) is called "participating." With this style, the leader and followers now share in decision-making through two-way communication and much facilitating behavior from the leader because the followers have the ability and knowledge to do the task.

4. **Low relationship/low task behavior** (S4) is labeled "delegating." The style involves letting followers "run their own show." The leader delegates because the followers are high in maturity, being both willing and able to take responsibility for directing their own behavior.

Consider the case of a highly motivated entry-level technician. As the technician develops technical skills (maturity), the style of leadership moves from one of "telling" or direct supervision to one of "delegating." Relationship behavior changes from a high-task to a low-task emphasis, reflecting the trust and confidence associated with the delegation of responsibilities.

If, on the other hand, the job of a senior-level technician shifts to include supervisory responsibilities, then the individual is once again at an entry level of job experience, i.e., a new supervisor.

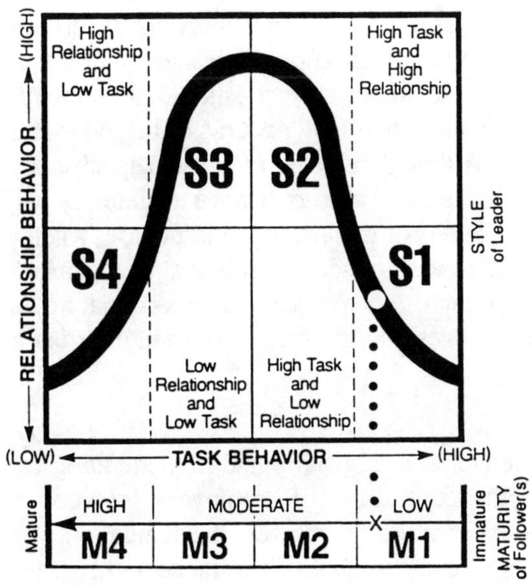

Figure 7.13: Illustration of the use of the behavior style chart to determine appropriate leadership style. ***(reproduced with permission: Leadership Studies, Inc.)***

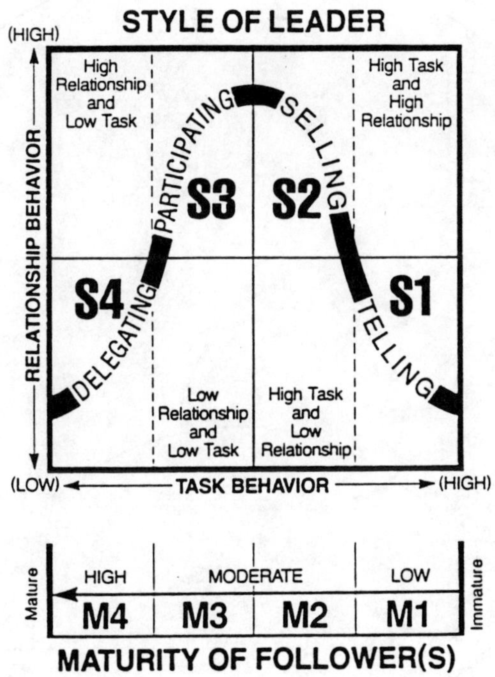

Figure 7.14: Use of the behavioral style chart for situational leadership. ***(reproduced with permission: Leadership Studies, Inc.)***

Leadership style should now adjust to one of high task/direct supervision, a "telling" management style. Without this shift, the new supervisor is left without proper guidance.

In summary, effective leaders must know their staff well enough to utilize effectively their ever-changing abilities and maturities. It should be remembered that followers, as individuals and as groups, develop their own patterns of behavior and ways of operating, i.e., norms, customs and mores. Although a leader may use a specific style for a particular work group, that leader may quite often have to behave differently with individual followers because they are at different levels of maturity. In either case, whether working with a group or an individual, situational leadership theory warns that changes in leadership style from S1 to S2, S3, and S4 must be gradual. The process, by its very nature, is evolutionary, resulting in gradual developmental changes and the creation of mutual trust and respect.

CONTROLLING

In the context of this chapter, establishing and implementing control implies regulating and policing. Although the controlling of employees is accomplished through the job description and performance appraisal processes, the regulation of the clinical engineering department functions leads directly to quality assurance and risk prevention. This section, therefore, deals with procedures that analyze and regulate the end products of the clinical engineering program.

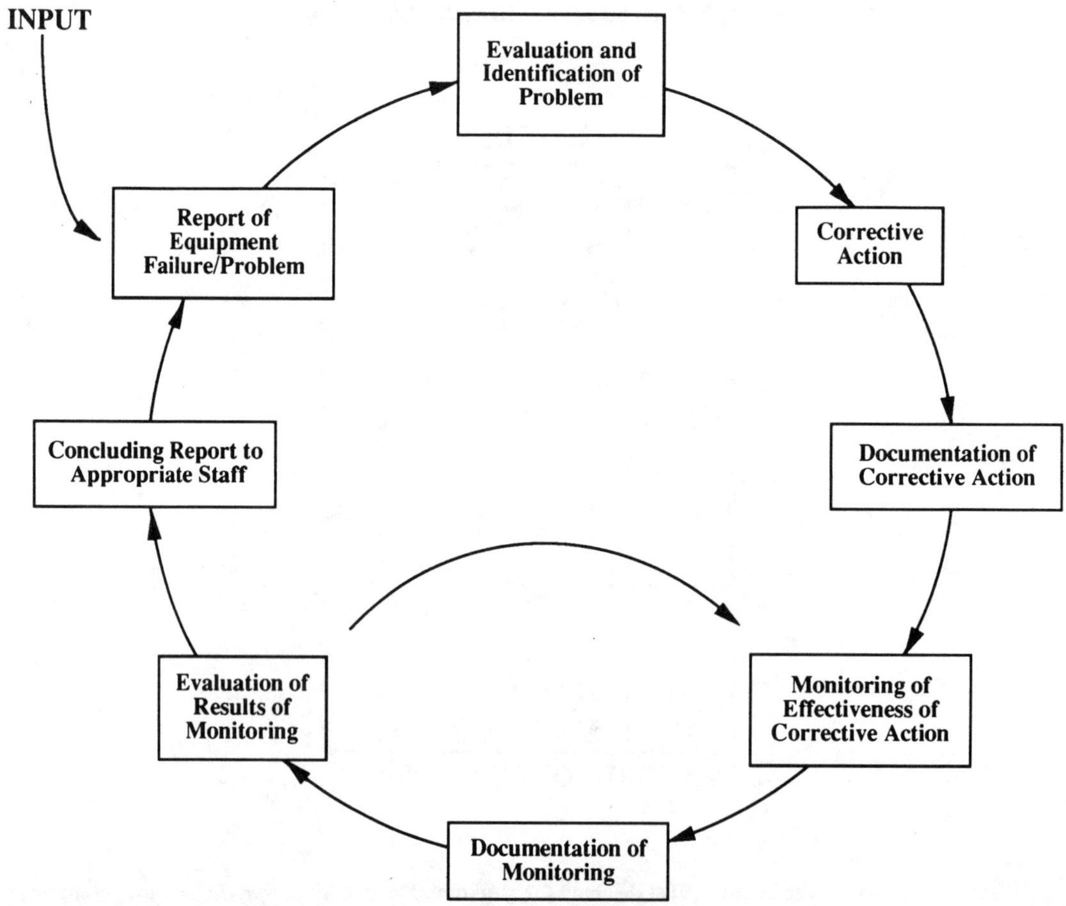

Figure 7.15: Illustration of the steps involved in a closed-loop quality control assurance review.

Quality Assurance and Risk Prevention

In Chapter 5, it was noted that the accreditation criteria of the Joint Commission on the Accreditation of Healthcare Organizations include requirements for procedures for identifying and correcting equipment malfunctions (JCAHO, 1990). Therefore, clinical engineering departments must document (1) corrective actions taken, (2) assurance that the action was effective, and (3) the need for continuation of monitoring. The resulting system is a closed-loop, quality assurance review program, which is illustrated in Figure 7.15. In this illustration, a typical equipment failure is the input to the loop. The equipment failure is analyzed, corrective action is taken, the corrective action is documented according to the repair documentation system used, and the repaired equipment is returned to service.

Does the repair episode end there? Not according to JCAHO. The corrective action itself (the repair) should be monitored to ensure that the reported problem has been successfully addressed. This can be as simple as monitoring repeat service calls (repeat failures in a piece of equipment within a specified period of time (e.g., one month following a repair). Finally, the results of the monitoring program should be documented, and if no further action is required, a concluding report is issued.

The management steps one can take in operating quality assurance (QA) and risk prevention programs are formally addressed by the JCAHO. They propose a ten-step model designed to promote a planned and systemic approach to the monitoring and evaluation of medical equipment (JCAHO, 1988). The process can be functionally differentiated into two distinct phases:

- Setting up a structure or framework.
- Actually implementing the program.

Steps 1 through 5 of the process include the initial procedures of identifying what to include in the program and identifying indicators and thresholds. The actual implementation and evaluation of the program are included in steps 6 through 10 (Resek, 1990). The ten steps are summarized below:[2]

1. **Assign responsibility.** The organization must assign overall responsibility for the program, specifying what indicators of performance will be used and who will collect data, evaluate service, take action, and report findings.
2. **Delineate scope of service.** In order to delineate the scope of service, the clinical engineering department must specify those services it will provide to the hospital community, e.g., preventive maintenance, equipment repair, etc.
3. **Identify important aspects of service.** Once the scope of service is delineated, the list must be prioritized. The most efficient use of resources will focus monitoring and evaluation activities on those aspects of service that have the greatest impact on patient care. For example, a high-volume service, such as equipment repair, will likely have a significant effect on a large number of patients. In the case of a low-volume service, such as testing of emergency electrical power, however, only if there is a high risk associated with it, should it be given a high priority for inclusion in the services to be monitored.

---

[2] © Copyright 1990 by the Joint Commision on Accreditation of Healthcare Organizations. Adapted with permission from an article in PT&SM, Number 1, 1990.

4. **Identify indicators.** To allow for evaluation of service, specific indicators of performance need to be identified. These indicators are then used to define the measurable, objective characteristics of each important aspect of service. The Joint Commission defines an indicator as a measurable variable related to the structure, process, or outcome of care. Structure includes the elements that support services, such as resources, equipment, or number of staff. Process is the actual procedure or activity, and outcome is the result of the process. In the example of a fire drill, indicators of structure might reflect the presence of alarms, fire doors, and properly functioning extinguishers. Indicators of process should measure the actual activities of the drill, such as an extinguisher being brought to the site, the code being called, and the alarm being pulled. Indicators of outcome should denote the results of the drill, such as an overall rating of the drill's effectiveness.
5. **Establish thresholds.** The last step in setting up the structure for a QA plan is to establish thresholds for evaluation. A threshold for evaluation is the level or point at which intensive evaluation of a service is triggered. A threshold can be expressed as a percentage, ratio, or number. Given that specific services cannot meet expected standards at all times, thresholds define the level of service that is considered acceptable. In general, the higher the risk involved, the closer the threshold will be to 0 percent or 100 percent.
6. **Collect and organize data.** Data sources should include existing documents whenever possible. When data are not available, the following factors should be considered in selecting an appropriate data collection method:

- The source of the information.
- Whether the data is retrospective or concurrent.
- The number in the sample.
- The frequency of data collection.
- Whether appropriate data collectors have been used.

7. **Evaluate service.** When a threshold is met, it is an indication that further evaluation is necessary. Even when a threshold is not met, it is important to analyze data for the presence of certain trends to ascertain whether or not there are any deviations in the patterns of service. Because the goal of evaluation is to improve service, instead of asking what went wrong, staff members should ask how they can do better and should have as their target a higher threshold.
8. **Take actions to solve identified problems.** If a problem or opportunity for improvement is identified, it is necessary to decide what corrective action is needed. Such an action plan should specify the following:

- What actions are expected to occur.
- Who is responsible for implementation.
- When change is expected.

9. **Assess actions and document improvement.** Corrective action alone often does not ensure problem resolution. The effectiveness of actions should be assessed and documented. If corrective action does not resolve the problem, the action may not have addressed the actual problem, and a new action plan should be established.

10. **Communication and report information.** Unless information regarding QA activities are shared, much of their potential benefit can be lost. Excellence is seldom achieved alone. For example, the results of monitoring and evaluating PT and SM activities should be reported to the safety committee, the organization-wide QA program, the governing body, and the individual departments involved. These reports should always reflect conclusions, recommendations, actions, and follow-up. It has been clearly shown that when QA information is integrated, organization-wide improvements in patient services occur.

Quality indicators appropriate for a clinical engineering program have been identified by the JCAHO and the Clinical Engineering Management Committee of the Association for the Advancement of Medical Instrumentation (AAMI, 1990). In this latter document, the processes required to implement the closed-loop quality control review depicted in Figure 7.15 were defined for the hospital-based clinical engineering program. Quality indicators for clinical engineering include the following:

1. **Compliance measurement.** Degree of compliance with established schedules for routine activities, such as preventive maintenance inspections. Compliance may be weighted by the sophistication or risk factor of the equipment. For example, life-support equipment is given the highest risk factor, and consequently, this equipment requires the highest degree of compliance with established inspection schedules.
2. **Inspections performed.** The types of failures found during the inspections are the focus of this indicator. Both numbers and types of failures serve as specific measures.
3. **Documentation.** All work performed by the clinical engineering department must be documented. Accreditation agencies such as the JCAHO require written verification with their standards. Quality indicators can also include the presence or absence of required documentation and their completeness and accuracy.
4. **Equipment repair.** Quality indicators for the equipment repair service include turnaround time of repairs, numbers of repeat failures, total downtime due to a repair, and type and frequency of certain repairs. Each of these indicators, in turn, can be further broken down into subindicators. For example, repair turnaround time subindicators include parts availability and technician productivity. Repeat failures subindicators include repeat failures of a certain type, repeat failures in a certain type of equipment, and repeat failures in the same device. Turnaround time subindicators include repair turnaround time and a measure of total out-of-service time.

It is important to have input into the quality assurance process from the technicians who are performing the preventive maintenance and repair work. This often serves as a motivational tool, allowing technicians to have direct input into the management process. One such mechanism to facilitate this process is shown in Figure 7.16. Figure 7.16a shows the reporting form to be completed by technicians assigned to preventive maintenance. The form requires the technician to condense the information from the preventive maintenance inspections into a summary of significant events. These forms then become the input for the section monthly report (Figure 7.16b).

Clinical Engineering Department
Preventive Maintenence Status Report

Month: ______________

EQUIPMENT TYPE: ____

USER DEPARTMENT(S): ________________________
____
____

TOTAL NUMBER SCHEDULED FOR INSPECTION : ______

NUMBER PASSING INSPECTION : ______
NUMBER FAILING INSPECTION : ______

TOTAL INSPECTED : ______

TOTAL REMAINING TO BE INSPECTED : ______

SUMMARY OF FAILURES (summarize number and types of failures, ie. defective power cords; use back of sheet if necessary):

INSPECTING TECHNICIAN'S RECOMMENDATIONS:

COMPLETED BY: ____

Figure 7.16 (a) Example of a preventive maintenance status report form that is filled out by the technician responsible for the specific piece of equipment.

Clinical Engineering Department
Section Monthly Report
(to be completed by Senior BMET and/or Coordinator):

1. PM completed per the established schedule. The report should briefly discuss any problems encountered and solutions either in progress or completed. PM should be reported by equipment type and department location, with actual numbers of items tested, untested, and failing PM.

2. PM past due with an estimate of resources (manpower,test equipment or parts) needed to complete the work. An appraisal of why the PM is past due is required from the standpoint of lack of resources, equipment repair load, or inaccessibility of equipment. Again, specifics are required.

3. Estimate of the probability of completing on-time the PM scheduled for the next month (both new and past due PM). Again, with a focus on resources needed.

4. An estimate of excess manpower available for the next month to assist other sections. <u>A reporting of work in progress (ie-logged into computer but not completed) is needed for this report.</u>

5. Major repairs of any type which have been completed and that you deem significant to report to the owner department (ie. high dollar cost of parts, labor, or both; incident report generated as a result of the failure).

Figure 7.16: (b) Example of a clinical engineering department monthly report form. Information for this report is derived form the preventive maintenance status report forms.

The forms, therefore, provide a mechanism for individual technicians to have input into a formal monthly review of work they had completed, and they enable inspecting technicians to identify significant repairs (high cost, unusual failure, physical damage) for review by management. In this way, the department head is presented with a "snapshot" of maintenance work performed during a monthly period, with supporting documentation stretching back to the originating individual technician.

Productivity and Cost Control

Controlling program costs is an important function for any clinical engineering manager. To be effective in this area, managers need information about two specific measures of cost-control: employee productivity and expense versus revenue ratios.

Productivity is the measure of how specified resources are managed to accomplish timely objectives (Riggs and Felix, 1983). Methods designed to monitor and improve productivity of hospital-based clinical engineering departments have been reported (Furst, 1986; David, 1986). The reports have identified the following:

- **% Productivity**: All productive hours, whether direct or indirect, calculated as

  (Repair Hrs. + Preventive Maintenance Hrs. + Other Productive Work Hrs.)/ (Available Hrs.) x 100

- **% Overtime**: Calculated as

  Overtime Hrs./Available Hrs.

- **% Labor Recovery**: Shows how well the staff is charging for its service, calculated as

  Charged Hrs./Available Hrs.

- **Backlog Days**: The average amount of time needed to service incomplete orders carried over from one week to the next, calculated as

  Carryover Hrs. Estimated/Available Hrs./ Day

- **Repair-Turnaround Days**: The average length of time a piece of equipment is out of the client's department for repairs, calculated by noting the time of receipt in the repair shop and the time of equipment return to the client department.

Analysis and interpretation of these indicators also includes assessing possible interactions. For example, if overtime is high and productivity is low, this may indicate the presence of scheduling problems, or that employees are simply delaying routine work in order to benefit from overtime wage rates. A closer supervision of employees may be warranted under these circumstances.

Expense versus revenue figures can be obtained in a more straightforward manner. A simple profit and loss summary such as that presented in the executive summary of the business plan (as illustrated in the case study at the end of the chapter) may be sufficient as a gauge of financial performance of the department. Each of the major profit and expenditure categories can be expanded to give greater detail.

For the clinical engineering departments that charge client departments a service fee, a more business-oriented financial report may be necessary (Chapter 3). To begin with, the service fee should be based on all of the department's expenses that affect the department's ability to provide its services. As presented in the Financial Data Section of the sample business plan, this includes all direct costs (personnel salaries and benefits, nonchargeable repair supplies such as solder, training) and indirect costs (office supplies, utilities, or other overhead expenses). The labor cost per hour is then calculated as follows:

Cost per Hour = Total Department Budget/Productive Hrs.

Note that productive hours = [total hours available] – [vacation hours + estimated sick hours + coffee breaks + nonbillable work hours, e.g., training, report preparation]. Typically, only 75 to 80 percent of a technician's time can be considered as productive, chargeable time. The balance is departmental overhead.

If there are no financial transaction related to the services provided by the department, then some other measure of financial benefit from the clinical engineering program will be needed. Departmental operating costs can then be compared to one of the following:

- Cost of outside service contracts for the equipment under the clinical engineering program.

- Cost of outside service based on the average hourly rate charged by manufacturer or third-party service companies times the number of repair hours generated by the clinical engineering department.
- Some combination of the above.

These financial comparisons can be comprehensive, focusing on the services of the clinical engineering program.

A CASE STUDY:

The Biomedical Instrumentation Department at the University of Texas M.D. Anderson Cancer Center [3]

An illustration of the practical use of a business plan for a hospital-based clinical engineering department is provided here. This illustration is based on an actual business plan prepared by the clinical engineering department of the University of Texas M.D. Anderson Cancer Center, located in Houston, Texas. However, portions of the original have been edited to provide the general considerations of any such plan. The Past History section is not included in this example because such a section is, by nature, specific to the individual case. Also, because UTMDA is a state-supported institution, certain references in the business plan are unique to the state method of funding. However, the concept of the plan and the strategy used in its preparation are applicable to any clinical engineering department.

Department Mission

The Biomedical Instrumentation Department at the University of Texas M.D. Anderson Cancer Center provides a centralized department responsible for the care of medical instrumentation and the aiding of hospital personnel who use this equipment. The Department's range of equipment responsibilities includes the inspection, repair, and preventive maintenance of medical instrumentation and engineering consultation for the purchase of new equipment.

Goals and Objectives

The Department will organize itself to perform four major equipment-related services: prepurchase evaluation, preventive maintenance testing, repair, and in-service training. A maintenance documentation system will be established and maintained in order to provide a database of maintenance histories and costs to client departments and hospital administration.

All services will ensure hospital compliance with standards promulgated by the Joint Commission on Accreditation of Healthcare Organizations.

The Department will operate on a predetermined fee-for-service basis for all preventive maintenance testing and repair service work.

---

[3] Adapted with permission from: the University of Texas M.D. Anderson Cancer Center, Biomedical/Clinical Engineering Department.

Executive Summary

Year-end Financial Analysis
Annual Profit and Loss Statement
Biomedical Instrumentation Revolving Fund

	FY '85	FY '86	FY '87	FY '88
Billings	$	$	$	$
Less: Expenses	$	$	$	$
Net Profit (Loss)	$ (xx,xxx)	$ (xx,xxx)	$ (xx,xxx)	$ (xx,xxx)

Background

The maintenance of patient care equipment at the University of Texas M.D. Anderson Cancer Center started as a specialty shop within the Physical Plant Department. In September of 1986, the Biomedical Electronics Shop was separated from the Physical Plant Department and established as a separate department within the Facility Services Division.

With this independent program status, it became possible for the management of Biomedical Instrumentation to establish goals and identify resources needed to discharge the unique nature of patient-care equipment maintenance. This business plan identifies those goals and resources.

The Department of Biomedical Instrumentation is seeking to establish itself as the manager of all medical and research instrumentation resources for UTMDA. In this capacity, the Department would provide the following services:

- Contract management.
- Equipment/instrumentation repair.
- Testing and preventive maintenance.
- Risk management and quality control.
- Acquisition and equipment evaluation.

The Product

Biomedical Instrumentation (BI) is in the health-are business of managing medical equipment resources. To provide this product, the Department must provide the following equipment-related services:

- Contract management.
- Repair.
- Testing and preventive maintenance.
- Risk management and quality assurance.
- Acquisition and evaluation.
- Monitoring of vendor-provided services.
- Single-point record maintenance.

At least a portion of this program is mandated through the Joint Commission on Accreditation of Healthcare Organizations (JCAHO). For patient-care equipment, the JCAHO requires a system that includes a master inventory of equipment, performance testing procedures, documentation of testing against the procedures, documentation of equipment status reporting, a procedure for identifying and correcting equipment malfunctions, and an audit trail for each function and piece of equipment.

This business plan seeks to institutionalize the responsibility for medical equipment resource management with the Biomedical Instrumentation Department. This responsibility must begin at the acquisition phase of the equipment's life cycle and continue through installation, warranty, routine maintenance and planned replacement.

The system to be put in place would be systematically evaluated by Biomedical Instrumentation. BI would then recommend the best mix of maintenance resources required to meet an individual department's needs. These maintenance resources would include outside service contracts, maintenance insurance, time and materials contracts, or in-house service.

Maintenance contracts would be negotiated, purchased, and managed by Biomedical Instrumentation. All maintenance costs would be paid directly by Biomedical Instrumentation, thus providing a quality assurance link. Departments would be billed by Biomedical Instrumentation for these costs once the work is satisfactorily completed.

The benefit to the client department is in having a single contact point for all maintenance activity. The benefit to the Institution is in having a unified database of all maintenance costs. The benefit to both individual departments and the Institution is the maximization of maintenance resource dollars by the reduction of direct maintenance costs.

The Market

The market for biomedical equipment services has grown in proportion to the increase in the use of electronic devices. Equipment services can be segregated by both type of service and potential customer as follows:

1. **Repair services only** are required for physician offices and small clinic operations where accreditation standards do not exist and where the equipment, while often sophisticated, is sold through a network of dealers who cannot provide repair services.
2. **Repair, testing, and preventive maintenance** are required for outpatient clinics, etc. that are under the accreditation requirements of Medicare/Medicaid.
3. **Equipment management services** are required for inpatient hospitals under the accreditation requirements of the JCAHO.

A number of service options are available, including direct factory service, third-party independent service companies, shared service organizations affiliated with a particular hospital or hospital group, and in-house service organizations. Service costs can be based on a fixed price contract, a time-and-materials agreement, or maintenance insurance in conjunction with a time-and-materials agreement. The cost/benefit of the above provider and payment methods depends entirely on the individual circumstances of the equipment owner.

The University of Texas System. The customer base within UTMDA for equipment management services includes . . . The expected rate of growth in services required by the customer base is difficult to predict. A significant increase in the market for biomedical services should also occur through the involvement of the Department in replacing service contracts with in-house service, the development of equipment maintenance programs where no program presently exists, and the development of support programs for administration and finance, including the preparation and review of equipment bids and contract monitoring.

The Competition

Evaluation of the competitive environment as seen by the Department must be divided between in-house competition and outside service options.

In-House Competition. By design, Biomedical Instrumentation is an independent departmental entity within UTMDA, administratively separate from any potential client department. Potential conflicts of interest are avoided in the prioritization of service work and the administration of the fee-for-service program.

There is no other department that seeks to or has the expertise to provide the umbrella service of medical equipment management. Certain high-technology departments have in place resident equipment maintenance personnel. The extent of these departmental repair programs varies considerably, from complete repair responsibility to preventive maintenance only programs.

Rather than view the other departments as competitors, these in-house service programs are perceived as resources additional to the Institutional need for repair services. Biomedical Instrumentation would seek to monitor these activities, documenting the level and type of work performed. Biomedical Instrumentation would seek to involve these groups in an ancillary operation of providing service to other components of the UT system. This would serve the important single point overview, umbrella coverage, of these functions, thus providing critical single system tracking of instrumentation maintenance.

Outside Service Competition. Outside service competition includes the traditional manufacturer service center and independent third-party service companies. In addition, two hospitals are offering repair services in the for-profit market. Corporate-owned hospitals within the greater Houston area are free to procure service from whomever they choose. Other institution-affiliated hospitals are likewise free to purchase service on the open market, although some of these have long considered providing such services.

Institution-affiliated hospitals are too committed to their parent organization to warrant a marketing effort.

Market Share

The targeting of market shares that Biomedical Instrumentation can expect to capture should follow the same planning, regardless of whether the potential customer is an in-house department or an outside customer. Specifically, the business factors (start-up costs, profitability, etc.) related to pursuing a potential customer are the key issues. Equipment types for which no outside service alternative is available are ideal for an initial thrust.

Marketing/Planning

In-House Market. The service nature of the Department's business requires an initial marketing emphasis based upon customer word-of-mouth recommendations. It is exactly this lack of support that has limited to date the effectiveness of moving the program into new areas and further developing existing areas.

This customer referral network is needed particularly among the laboratories, both clinical and research, in which the number of independent equipment users is such that they cannot be reached as a group.

Coincident with the formalization of the Department's program as outlined in this plan, a public information campaign should be initiated through existing UTMDA publications to foster an awareness of the program as it presently exists, emphasizing the program's scope and ongoing programs, including periodic updates on the Department's activities.

Outside Market. Marketing to any outside customers should be directed to that institution's chief executive officer, purchasing agent, and nursing director. The outside customers should be limited initially to UT system institutions in order to control liability problems and to limit costs. A detailed marketing plan would be developed in order to identify markets, establish marketing strategies, and obtain the necessary internal approvals. Interim pricing policies and work control policies and procedures would be the same as those for in-house clients.

Management

The Biomedical Instrumentation Department's organizational structure is a matrix, with line responsibility for specific equipment programs assigned to senior level technicians and line and staff responsibility for hospital departments assigned to technical managers. A matrix-type structure was deemed necessary because of the following:

- A wide range of equipment, equipment technology, and clinical applications, necessitating technician and manager specialization.
- Overlapping technologies (similar equipment used by different medical specialties for different purposes or with different techniques), necessitating crossover between technical and clinical knowledge.
- The need of client departments for rapid turnaround of equipment repairs.
- Limited resources of both technicians and back-up equipment, necessitating prioritization of service demands.

The management team needed to carry out the long- and short-range aspects of this plan would require the following:

Financial Data

Development of Fee-for-Service. The fee-for-service requirement of the Department should include the following in the calculation of the service fee:

1. Salary and benefits of all departmental employees charging back labor.
2. Maintenance and operating costs.
3. Capital equipment requirements.
4. Parts inventory costs (cost of goods sold).
5. Overhead, including material requisition, software/hardware for operations, and records management.
6. Retirement of negative balance (debt amortization).

The department faces a problem in that a debt from prior years of operation must be retired. Retirement of existing debt should be accomplished by the inclusion of the existing debt as an additional factor in the determination of the service fee. This should be done, however, over a reasonable period of time.

Where it is cost-effective, the program would provide in-house technical support with service work billed to client departments on a time-and-materials basis. The hourly labor rate would be determined by the operating costs of the Department. Parts would be billed at cost plus a handling fee. It is expected that the in-house cost of service would be at least 60 percent below the commercial labor rate and approximately 20 percent below the commercial parts rate. Additional in-house savings are possible from the elimination of service-related travel costs and off-shift service costs. The following service fee guidelines would be used for all clients:

Determination of First-Year Service Fee (If All Costs are to be Recovered)

1. Salary and Benefits	$ xxx
2. Maintenance & Operation	$ xxx
3. Equipment	$ xxx
4. Parts	$ xxx
5. Debt as of x/x/xx	$ xxx
Total	**$ xxx**

An hourly service fee of $xxx would be counterproductive to the further development of thc in-house program. This is in spite of the average outside service fee of $xxx per hour. As detailed in the balance of this business plan, we would seek to keep the hourly service fee between the present $xxx figure and $xxx.

Capital Equipment. At present, the Department owns approximately $xxx in test equipment, furniture, and furnishings. Additional test equipment needed to initiate this program are minimal. Equipment needs at present are limited to test meters and hand tools.

Laboratory Space. Any expansion of the activities of the Department would require additional laboratory space.

Impact of Proposed Reorganization. Financially, the implementation of this program is possible due to the magnitude of the existing program and the resources already in place. Although no dollar figure is available to compare the costs of the existing in-house program with an outside service alternative, the program at present has responsibility for the following departments: **in FY '87-'88, State funding for a portion of the Maintenance and Operations expense was budgeted at $xxx, and the State personnel was budgeted at $xxx.**

Because of the need of the Institution to meet certain JCAHO requirements in regard to patient-care equipment and because of the overhead costs of a state-operated institution, a portion of the total funding for the Department should be provided from State funds. In FY '88-'89, it is expected that nonbillable staff personnel would be assigned to the state personnel account, and billable technicians would be assigned to the revolving fund account. Our staffing plan is so aligned. The additional state funding would provide JCAHO-required records management and consulting expertise for the entire Institution's use.

Continuation of the existing program and implementation of this plan would have the following financial impact on the hourly service fee at the start of the new program. A service fee of $xxx per hour would be used for the first year of operation under this plan (effective September 1, 1988), with an increase to $xxx per hour to be made effective with the start of FY '89–'90.

Determination of Service Fee (If Partial State Funding is Provided)

Salary budget as of x/x/xx	$xxx
Add: Clinical Engineer	$xxx
Technical Supervisor	$xxx
Add: Benefits at xx percent	$xxx
Total Salary Budget	**$xxx**
Maintenance and Operations Budget	$xxx
Equipment Budget	$xxx

Parts Inventory Additions	$xxx	(Add: One-Fifth of Current Debt = xxx)
Contingency at x%	$xxx	
Total Expenses	**$xxx**	
Less: State Maintenance and Operations	$xxx	
State Personnel (All Nonbillable Staff)	$xxx	
Parts Sales (Cost Times 1.2)	$xxx	
Net Overhead	$xxx	
Hourly Service Fee	$xxx/xxx Hrs. (12 FTEs) = $xxx/hr.	

SUMMARY

The introduction to this chapter noted that "*we manage because of what we are, but how we manage is because of who we are.*" This chapter has addressed the part of management that goes with the title of manager; the "*what we are.*" "Who we are," our personality and likes and dislikes is an aspect of management that is often overlooked. Interpersonal management skills, team building, mentoring, motivating others — these are concepts that individual managers of people should use to guide their continuing management education.

As clinical engineers assume greater responsibilities for all phases of technology management within health-care institutions, they must pay particular attention to the development of managerial skills. For this reason, the primary managerial tasks of planning (development of the mission statement and the business plan) and organizing (delegaton of responsibility for implementation of the mission statement to department personnel) have been examined in detail. Although each manager has a particular style of managing which is dictated by the personality of both the manager and the personnel being managed, mastery of the specific managerial skills presented in this chapter will help ensure that management of the department will occur in an effective manner.

EXERCISES

1. In Chapter 1, you were asked to prepare a mission statement and a list of objectives for a clinical engineering department. In addition, you were asked to prepare an organizational chart of a hospital depicting the reporting lines of the clinical engineering department. Review and reframe your mission statement as necessary based on the information provided in this chapter. Revise your organizational chart to reflect these changes.

2. With the mission statement from Question 1, prepare in outline form the questions you must resolve in each section of a business plan intended to implement your stated goals.

3. You are the director of a hospital-based clinical engineering department presently providing in-house repair services on patient monitoring equipment, and ancillary equipment from the operating rooms. You have been successful in your program and are now being asked to provide the same coverage for radiographic equipment. Prepare a mission statement for this program. Following the steps in the planning process, outline the issues and questions that must be assessed. Your analysis should include an evaluation the current maintenance program and an analysis of the impact the proposed program on present operations.

4. Discuss the purpose of performance appraisals. What can be done to make this process a worthwhile experience for both the manager and the employee?

5. Based on the leadership styles presented in figure 7.14, provide examples of the situations in which you would employee each of the described styles.

6. Identify the ten steps necessary to develop and implement a quality assurance program. Provide an outline of such a program to handle equipment repair.

7. Equipment maintenance quality assurance indicators include repeat failures, repeat repairs, high cost of repairs, and operator errors. Discuss the significance of each of these indicators to an equipment maintenance program. How would each of the factors affect client department confidence in your maintenance program?

REFERENCES

AAMI. "Design of Clinical Engineering Quality Assurance and Risk Management Programs," Association for the Advancement of Medical Instrumentation, 1990.

Arthur Anderson and Company. "An Entrepreneur's Guide to Developing a Business Plan," 1990.

Bennett, A. "10 Rules Key to Developing New Managers," *Hospitals*, 88, September 20, 1987.

David, Y., and Rohe, D. "Clinical Engineering Program Productivity and Measurement," *Journal of Clinical Engineering*, 11(6):435–443, 1986.

Furst, E. "Productivity and Cost Effectiveness of Clinical Engineering," *Journal of Clinical Engineering*, 11(2):105–113, 1986.

Goodman, G. "Professional Development of the BMET," *Journal of Clinical Engineering*, 5(3):215–219, 1980.

Goodman, G. "Technology Assessment, Transfer, and Management: The Implications to the Professional Development of Clinical Engineering," *Journal of Clinical Engineering*, 16(2):117–122, 1991.

JCAHO. "Guide to Quality Assurance", Joint Commission on Accreditation of Healthcare Organizations, Chicago, 1988.

JCAHO. "Plant, Technology and Safety Management", *Accreditation Manual for Hospitals*, Joint Commission on Accreditation of Healthcare Organizations, Chicago, 1990.

"Business Planning," A Publication of: The Private Business Advisory Group - Peat, Marwick, Mitchell & Co., 1984.

Resek, J. "Applying the Ten-Step Process to Plant, Technology, and Safety Management," *Plant Technology and Safety Management Series: Measuring Quality in PTSM*, Joint Commission on Accreditation of Healthcare Organizations, Chicago, 1990.

Riggs, L., and Felix, G.H. "Productivity by Objectives," Prentice-Hall, Englewood Cliffs, NJ, 1983.

Situational Leadership, University Associates, Escondido, CA, 1991.

CHAPTER 8

DEVELOPMENT AND OPERATION OF A CLINICAL ENGINEERING DEPARTMENT: A PRACTITIONER'S PERSPECTIVE

Having presented the fundamental concepts of clinical engineering in preceding chapters, it is now appropriate to examine the question, "*How can these concepts be applied in the modern health care-setting.*" The purpose of this chapter, therefore, is to weave these basic concepts together with some practical examples to illustrate how a clinical engineering department is actually developed and managed. With this in mind, this chapter presents the basic steps necessary to (1) identify the clinical engineering services required by the institution, (2) determine the costs (resources) associated with these activities, (3) communicate these requirements effectively to the administration, and (4) create a productive work environment.

DEVELOPMENT OF A CLINICAL ENGINEERING PROGRAM: INITIAL STEPS

The first step in developing a hospital-based clinical engineering program is to ask two basic sets of questions. The first set will assist in assessing the scope of the clinical engineering program in relation to the needs of the hospital and the resources that will be provided. The second set will assist in the continuing effort to evaluate the clinical engineering program. For the first set of questions, there are four primary considerations:

1. How many pieces of equipment are to be serviced by the clinical engineering program?
2. What is the total acquisition price of this equipment (i.e. what is the total capital asset value of this equipment)?
3. What services does the hospital administration expect the clinical engineering program to provide?
4. What is the current expenditure for the clinical engineering services now being provided?

There is a continuing debate among clinical engineers about the scope of "equipment" that should be managed by a clinical engineering program. There are those, for example, who contend that clinical engineering programs should only support patient care equipment or, as defined by the JCAHO, the equipment that is "*used to treat, monitor, or diagnose patients*" (1989b). Others believe that clinical engineering programs should support both patient care equipment and other high tech electronic equipment (such as PCs). Still others extend the coverage to include office equipment, telecommunications equipment, and a host of facilities-related systems. Because every hospital is different, it is extremely important for the clinical engineering director and the hospital administrator to agree upon exactly what is to be supported by the clinical engineering program.

Having established the scope of coverage desired, the clinical engineer must develop an inventory of all equipment to be serviced. This inventory process can be as simple as verifying existing equipment lists or as complicated as physically identifying every item.

Conducting an Inventory Review

In small hospitals, a physical inventory is desirable even if a current inventory list exists. By performing a physical inventory, the clinical engineer can quickly gain firsthand knowledge of the condition of the equipment as well as its specific location. This process also helps to introduce the clinical engineer to the various equipment users. This initial visibility serves to develop the foundation for good interpersonal relations, which can be of significant value later when revising or implementing equipment-related policies.

In a medium or large hospital, the performance of an initial physical inventory is often impractical. In such situations, one must find other ways of procuring the necessary information. Although the hospital may not have a specific list of the equipment in question, all hospitals keep a listing of their total physical assets. This list is typically called a **depreciation register** or a **capital assets register** and is usually found in the financial services department. The depreciation register is a line item listing of every capital item the hospital has ever purchased. It includes the land, buildings, renovations, patient-care equipment, office equipment, general equipment, utility systems, furniture, and furnishings (drapes, carpet, etc.). The purpose of this register is to keep track of the value of these assets for reimbursement purposes. Therefore, most hospitals attempt to keep this list current. As a result, this document represents a primary information source for establishing the purchase prices of various inventory items.

Because this register incorporates a variety of entry types (i.e., land, buildings, equipment, etc.), exact items are not always specified. For example, a new Hewlett Packard® defibrillator purchased for the emergency room a few years ago may be listed on the depreciation register only as:

Log Entry	Description	Date	Cost
#4621	Defibrillator	01/01/90	$6,500

Without a model or serial number it may be impossible to link this entry to a specific piece of equipment. However, it is important to remember that the goal here is not to identify specific items, but simply to quantify the number of items to be supported. From the register entry listed above it is clear that there is one defibrillator to be supported. Unfortunately register entries are not always clear. Consider the following:

Log Entry	Description	Date	Cost
#4622	Total ER Addition	01/01/90	$153,200

In this case there is no way of extrapolating the cost of the defibrillator from the cost of construction and other equipment.

When a physical inventory is not practical and the depreciation register is too general to be useful, one must make a best-guess approximation of the inventory. For a new clinical engineer this may be a little difficult, but not impossible. One starts by making a list of common device types similar to those listed in Table 8.1. This list should then be distributed to existing clinical engineering personnel and a wide variety of equipment users throughout the medical center with a request to indicate how many pieces of equipment are in their areas. By collecting the lists and summing the responses for each device type, a reasonable approximation of the equipment inventory can be derived.

Table 8.1: SAMPLE DEVICE TYPES

- Absorbance Detector
- Alarm Module
- Amplifier, Audio
- Analyzer, Laboratory
- Analyzer, Test Equipment
- Anesthesia Machine
- Bacti-Cinerator
- Calculator
- Camera, Baby
- Camera, TV
- Capnometer
- Cardiac Output Computer
- Cart, Resuscitation
- Cell Washer
- Central Monitoring Station
- Centifuge
- Cervical Traction Device
- Compressor, Medical Air
- Cryo-Opthalmic Unit
- CT
- CVT
- Defibrillator
- Dermatome
- Diathermy
- ECT
- EEG
- Electrocardiograph
- EMG
- External Pacemekers
- Eye Tester
- Fetal Monitor
- Flame Photometer
- Flow Meter, Blood
- Furnace
- Heart/Lung Machine
- Heat Probe Unit
- Heater, Isothermal
- Hemodialysis Machine
- Homogenizer
- Hood, Anaerobic
- Hood, General
- Hot Plate
- Hydromassage
- Hydrotherapy Tank
- Hypo/hyperthemia Machine
- IABP
- Illuminator, Film Panel
- Impedance Phlebograph
- Incubator, Infant
- Injector, Angiographic
- Insufflator
- Intercom System
- Laser
- Laser Fibers
- Late Potential Detector
- Mamograph
- Magameter
- Microscope, Laboratory
- Microscope, Surgical
- Monitor, Holter
- Monitor, Oxygen
- Monitor, Physiologic critical
- Monitor, Physiologic general
- Monitor, Physiologic infant
- Monitor, Physiologic apnea
- Monitor, Telemetry
- MRI
- NIBP
- Nurse Call
- Opthalmoscope
- Otoscope
- Pacemaker Accs.
- Paging System
- pH Meter
- Phonic Meter
- Photic Stimulator
- Power Supply
- Pulmonary Function Analyzer
- Pulse Oximeter
- Pulse Volume Recorder
- Pump, Blood
- Pump, Drainage
- Pump, Holter
- Pump, IV
- Pump, Suction
- Pump, Syringe
- Radiation Therapy Unit Blood
- Radiation Therapy Unit Human
- Recorder, Physiologic
- Reverse Osmosis, Fixed
- Reverse Osmosis, Portable
- Sequential Compression Device
- Spectrometer
- Spectrphotometer
- Spinner, Test Tube
- Spirometer
- Sterilizer
- Stethoscope, Ultrasonic
- Stimulator, Muscle/Nerve
- Stress Test Unit
- Telecaption Unit
- Thermometry Unit
- Timer
- Tissue Processor
- Titrator
- Tympanometer
- Ultrasonic Cleaner
- Ultrasound Unit
- Ventilator, Adult
- Ventilator, Humidifier
- Ventilator, Infant
- Ventilator, O_2 Monitor
- X-Ray Camera
- X-Ray Generator
- X-Ray Portable
- X-ray Portable, C-Arm
- X-Ray System, Fixed

The only caution here is that the user list should be distributed to only one key contact per area to prevent the double counting of devices.

If it is found that the depreciation register is too general or inaccurate to be used for the clinical engineering equipment inventory, then it may also be of little use to the finance people. Therefore, as a current inventory list is generated, this information should be made available to the finance department. The inclusion of specific device identifiers, such as serial numbers or hospital tag numbers, in the register will enhance the future usefulness of this document.

Estimating Equipment Costs

Determining the cost of equipment listed on the inventory is also important. There are basically two methods of reporting equipment costs. The clinical engineer should carefully select one method and use it consistently. The first method involves documenting the acquisition cost (i.e., the amount paid at the time of purchase). This is in contrast to the second method, which is to record the replacement cost of the equipment (i.e., the cost to replace the unit today). Although utilization of either method is acceptable, the use of acquisition cost is preferable because the replacement cost method may artificially inflate (or deflate) the value of the equipment, thereby introducing error when computing direct service costs and depreciation values.

The depreciation register may also be a good source of information regarding the cost of equipment because it lists the actual equipment acquisition cost (from which depreciation is calculated) as well as the estimated replacement cost. Other sources include (1) a review of actual purchase orders for the equipment in question and (2) contact with the companies that originally sold the equipment to the hospital, using comparison guides such as the ECRI *Product Comparison System.*

The ECRI *Product Comparison System* consists of loose-leaf pamphlets that are categorized by device type and provide basic information on the function of the device, stage of development, and known problems. They also list the known manufacturers of the device and provide comparative data including, the list price. Because these comparisons are up-to-date, the costs presented should be categorized as replacement costs and used accordingly.

If the current inventory includes the cost information for only some equipment then an attempt should be made to use available known information to fill in the remaining blanks. This can be done by extrapolating the equipment costs of a similar manufacturer. None of the methods described above should be considered to be mutually exclusive. Each one may be useful in gathering data for the equipment inventory.

Determining Services to Be Provided by the Clinical Engineering Department

Having determined the extent of the equipment to be supported as well as its capital value, the third question presented earlier, i.e., *What services does the hospital administration expect the clinical engineering program to provide?* can be examined. To answer this question properly, the clinical engineer needs to assess fully all potential functions of the clinical engineering program, as identified in Chapter 1 (Figure 8.1). Not every clinical engineering program can provide all of these functions. The mix of services actually provided will vary from hospital to hospital based upon available resources. The mix of functions provided by each job classification within the program may also be different for each hospital. For example, according to information published in the *Journal of Clinical Engineering*, general biomedical equipment technicians, or BMET IIs, spend about 75 percent of their time doing a combination of corrective maintenance and assurance inspection activities (Pacela, 1990). Junior BMETs, or BMET Is, spend more than 80 percent of their time on these activities, and senior BMETs, or BMET IIIs, spend less than 70 percent of their time involved in repairs and inspections. The job responsibilities and corresponding percentages for the major clinical engineering job classifications are listed in Figure 8.2.

- **Technical Prepurchase Evaluation**
- **Incoming Inspection/Acceptance Testing**
- **Equipment Inventory Control**
- **Training Assistance**
  - Equipment Operation
  - Electrical Safety
- **Performance Assurance Inspections**
  - Performance Testing
  - Preventive Maintenance
  - Routine Calibration
  - Electrical Safety Testing
- **Corrective Maintenance**
  - Administer Service Contracts
  - Technically Oversee Vendor Maintenance
  - Perform In-House Repairs
- **Condition Review for Excess**

Figure 8.1: Functions of a clinical engineering program relating to the equipment life cycle.

Determining the Cost of Clinical Engineering Services

It is important to know what the hospital is currently paying for the services that the clinical engineering department is to provide. These costs include service contracts, emergency repairs, and possibly engineering consulting fees, etc. Because a single list of current expenses may not exist, approaches similar to those used for obtaining an inventory list should be followed. This process is often difficult because there are many ways in which hospitals can allocate funds for equipment maintenance. Some hospitals have centralized equipment maintenance budgets within the clinical engineering program, although most distribute the budget for equipment support to the departments who own or use the equipment. In a medium or large hospital this means that maintenance expenditures may originate from as many as 50 to one hundred different places. Investigating each of these sources individually can be as time consuming as conducting a physical inventory determination. Fortunately, there are other ways of gathering this information.

For tracking purposes, most hospitals categorize expenditures into utilization groupings. These groupings, typically referred to as **expense codes**, form the basis for line-item budgeting. In line-item budgeting, each entity must justify the expenditure request needed to support a particular activity, such as salaries, supplies, travel, photocopying, and equipment maintenance. If the hospital uses a slightly more sophisticated system, then separate expense codes may exist for such items as service contracts, general vendor support, and in-house support. With the assistance of the financial services and computer departments it should be a relatively easy task to compile a listing of the budget for all maintenance-related expense codes from every cost center for a given period.

Although this budget information is helpful (and can be used for developing approximations), what is really needed is the actual cost of maintenance, i.e., a listing of what was actually spent to support equipment for the given period. The process for obtaining this information should not be much more difficult then the process of obtaining budget information. Again, one must know the right questions to ask. To obtain a listing of current maintenance-related expenditures, the clinical engineer should ask for a report of payments made from the expense codes relating to maintenance. This report should provide expense code information by department, vendor, and purchase order number and should be sorted in that order. The report may also include data elements for vendor invoice number, vendor invoice date, hospital check (or voucher) number, date of payment, and amount of payment. A sample list of these elements is shown in Figure 8.3.

(A) BMET I Job Responsibilities (%)	
Repairs	36.4
Scheduled PM or Safety Testing	42.0
Clinical Support	2.5
Design; Modifications; R & D	0.4
Supervision of others	0.3
Incoming Testing	6.4
Coordinate Outside Services	0.7
Give Training and Inservice	0.7
Receive Training and Inservice	4.4
Purchasing and Requisitions	3.0
Prepurchase Evaluation	0.5
Department Development	0.9
Other	2.1

(D) BMET Supervisor Job Responsibilities (%)	
Repairs	18.5
Scheduled PM or Safety Testing	9.8
Clinical Support	5.7
Design; Modifications; R & D	2.0
Supervision of others	26.8
Incoming Testing	2.7
Coordinate Outside Services	5.3
Give Training and Inservice	4.5
Receive Training and Inservice	2.2
Purchasing and Requisitions	6.0
Prepurchase Evaluation	4.4
Department Development	9.3
Other	2.8

(B) BMET II Job Responsibilities (%)	
Repairs	42.2
Scheduled PM or Safety Testing	33.2
Clinical Support	3.2
Design; Modifications; R & D	1.1
Supervision of others	0.6
Incoming Testing	5.2
Coordinate Outside Services	1.9
Give Training and Inservice	1.8
Receive Training and Inservice	3.2
Purchasing and Requisitions	4.1
Prepurchase Evaluation	1.1
Department Development	1.3
Other	1.1

(E) Clinical Engineer Job Responsibilities (%)	
Repairs	18.8
Scheduled PM or Safety Testing	12.0
Clinical Support	12.5
Design; Modifications; R & D	13.3
Supervision of others	2.5
Incoming Testing	3.0
Coordinate Outside Services	4.4
Give Training and Inservice	4.2
Receive Training and Inservice	2.9
Purchasing and Requisitions	4.8
Prepurchase Evaluation	7.5
Department Development	10.0
Other	4.1

(C) BMET III Job Responsibilities (%)	
Repairs	45.1
Scheduled PM or Safety Testing	25.5
Clinical Support	4.6
Design; Modifications; R & D	2.3
Supervision of others	1.3
Incoming Testing	4.0
Coordinate Outside Services	2.5
Give Training and Inservice	2.6
Receive Training and Inservice	2.2
Purchasing and Requisitions	3.9
Prepurchase Evaluation	1.8
Department Development	2.2
Other	2.0

(F) CE Supervisor Job Responsibilities (%)	
Repairs	4.4
Scheduled PM or Safety Testing	1.8
Clinical Support	9.5
Design; Modifications; R & D	4.4
Supervision of others	27.6
Incoming Testing	1.7
Coordinate Outside Services	6.7
Give Training and Inservice	5.2
Receive Training and Inservice	1.8
Purchasing and Requisitions	5.6
Prepurchase Evaluation	7.5
Department Development	18.6
Other	5.2

Figure 8.2: Job responsibilities as a percent of total time for various staff positions. (reprinted with permission from: *The Journal of Clinical Engineering, C, 1990, Quest Publishing, Brea, CA)*

EXPENSE CODE	VENDOR NUMBER	VENDOR NAME	P.O. NUMBER	VOUCHER NUMBER	INVOICE DATE	INVOICE NUMBER	AMOUNT
18311020	2259	FEDERAL EXPRESS CORP		032384	43091	4–293–31785	96.50
	2259	FEDERAL EXPRESS CORP		034072	51491	4–306–39772	57.50
18311020							154.00
18313580	0149	ALEXANDER BATTERY CO	400228	035486	50391	8223	187.80
	0149	ALEXANDER BATTERY CO	208805	033743	51591	8578	58.52
	0670	BAXTER HEALTHCARE CO	208319	032771	50391	4047283	8.29
	0670	BAXTER HEALTHCARE CO	208319	035199	50791	4202418	8.29
	0679	BAYMEDICAL INC	208868	034308	50991	108356–00	95.32
	2123	ELECTRONIC ASSEMBLY	250002	033627	50991	126584	57.50
	2770	HEWLETT PACKARD	208772	032508	50291	6BH1922	790.00
	2770	HEWLETT PACKARD	208892	035740	51791	6BR2038	2,815.00
	4232	MAREC INC	208437	03232	41591	4474	71.51
	5321	P.C.		044179	50191	PETTY CASH	6.52
	5321	P.C.		044198	51391	P.C.REIMB.	1.46
	5321	P.C.		044219	52891	P.C.REIMB.	4.70
	8172	VALLEYLAB INC	208907	034992	52091	I402644 91	609.85
	8678	CARL ZEISS INC	208742	031816	42991	91032109	29.00
18313580							3,953 76
18315020	0380	AMERICAN STERILIZER	412007	032528	42291	1087752	80.00
	0380	AMERICAN STERILIZER	412007	033364	42491	1090300	68.78
	0380	AMERICAN STERILIZER	412007	035502	50991	1103090	95.65
	0682	BAY STATE ANESTHESIA	412379	035511	43091	56926	447.00
	0682	BAY STATE ANESTHESIA	412379	035512	43091	56936	1,779.50
	1226	CASTLE-M D T BIOLO	426325	035541	50991	282347	394.68
	1226	CASTLE-M D T BIOLO	426325	032554	41591	280937	460.80
	1226	CASTLE-M D T BIOLO	426325	032555	41691	015654	394.34
	1226	CASTLE-M D T BIOLO	426325	032556	41891	016132	103.16
	1226	CASTLE-M D T BIOLO	426325	032557	41291	280833	720.00
18315020							4,440.75
18315920	1769	CYBEX	330760	035579	52191	309920	357.61
	1823	DATA CARD CORPORATIO	400066	034166	50891	517646	200.00
	2029	DYNATECH NEVADA	331442	035708	51591	51899	250.00
	2770	HEWLETT PACKARD	438948	034201	50291	45V7G85	990.00
	2770	HEWLETT PACKARD	330746	034202	50991	030Q8R93	602.50
	5136	OLYMPUS CORP OF AMER	331447	035622	52891	0831669	230.00
	5136	OLYMPUS CORP OF AMER	331447	035623	52891	0831668	230.00
	7848	TEK NET INC	330778	031990	42391	TN 92968	255.08
	8275	UNITED BUSINESS MACH	400182	032994	42391	14240	65.19
	8275	UNITED BUSINESS MACH	400182	034257	42391	14241	65.19
18315920							3,245.57
							11,794.08

Figure 8.3: Sample expense report

There are four things to remember when reviewing this report:

1. Understand how credits are annotated on the list to ensure that they are correctly counted.
2. Expect that the list will contain expenditures for equipment not considered part of clinical engineering's responsibility. If some of these expenses originate from specific departments, such as facilities maintenance or environmental services, simply extract the value of these departments from the total.
3. Anticipate that departments may use budgeted funds other than those identified in the maintenance-related expense codes for maintenance activities. If there is an expense code for miscellaneous, supplementary services, or other, then it would be wise to include these in at least the first report run. If there is no evidence of hidden expenses from these categories, then they can be deleted from future reports.
4. Understand that some services may have been paid outside of the period being examined. It is quite common to find two- and three-year service agreements that are paid in full upon the signing of the agreement. By working closely with people from the purchasing department and department heads from the areas who own or use the equipment, it should be possible to account for these expenses.

DETERMINATION of REQUIRED RESOURCES

There is a saying among the personnel who work at any one of the 142 Veterans' Administration Medical Centers: *"Once you've seen one VA Medical Center, you've seen only one VA Medical Center."* This saying can be applied to most hospitals. Each has its own personality and culture. As a result, what works at one institution may not work at another. Because of this, it is important that the clinical engineer determine the resources required to provide the range and level of services needed by the specific hospital.

The first step in determining the available resources for clinical engineering services is to categorize the equipment listed in the inventory into groups based on device type (Table 8.1). These device types should be specific enough to include only equipment that is similar in function, physical risk, and maintenance requirements. Note, however, that only major variations should exclude an item from any device type to ensure that the total number of different device types remains manageable (approximately 150 to 350). Consider the following questions:

- Should a defibrillator with a built-in ECG monitor be categorized separately from a defibrillator with no integral ECG monitor?
- Can adult physiological monitors, pediatric physiological monitors, and infant physiological monitors be categorized together?
- Is it necessary to identify every type of system module (plug-in)?
- Does every item in a radiology suite need to be conspicuously identifiable?

The answers to these questions may be different at each hospital. However, answering such questions will guide the clinical engineer in developing the appropriate list of required resources for the particular hospital. Furthermore, the device type list should not be a static document; rather, it should be revised continuously as new equipment is put into use.

Once the list of equipment to be supported has been completed, the next step is to determine the resources required to provide this support.

Required resources can be broken into four major categories: personnel, maintenance, general recurring, and start-up resources.

Personnel Resources

Personnel costs typically represent from 20 to 60 percent of the clinical engineering program's budget; thus, it is appropriate that personnel needs be calculated first. The personnel needed to support a known quantity of inventory can be determined as follows:

Number of People = (Number of Pieces of Eqipment) x (Time Value of Maintenance)/ (Hrs. Worked per Person)

It is difficult, however, for those who have not monitored workers for an extended period of time to come up with statistically valid time values on their own. Fortunately, time values for a wide variety of device types and different activities are available from several sources (ECRI, 1984; AHA, 1982, 1988). The most common activities listed in these references are repair and inspections (Table 8.2).

Using the annual time value per unit of device from this reference one can quickly calculate the annual hours needed to support a specific device or piece of equipment. For example, if a hospital owns eight electrocardiographs, how many hours are needed annually to support this equipment? From Table 8.2, we can see that inspection tests for each electrocardiograph require 1.4 hours per year. Because repairs to this equipment are estimated to take 2.9 hours, an annual support time of 4.3 hours is required. Although the table also shows that each electrocardiograph will be repaired 2.1 times during the year, this number does not enter into the calculation because it is included in the annual repair hours given. Therefore, calculating the annual hours necessary to support the eight electrocardiographs can be calculated as follows:

8 Electrocardiographs 4.3 Hrs./Yr. = 34.4 Hrs./Yr.

If this computation is made for each device type, the total personnel hours required to provide repair and inspection services for all equipment on the inventory list can be obtained. The values listed in Figure 8.2 can then be used to obtain the total number of people needed based upon the various job levels.

Assuming all staff to be at the BMET II level (repairs = 42 percent of job responsibility, inspections = 33 percent of job responsibility), the total number of hours, **M**, needed to provide 100% of clinical engineering's services is obtained by the following:

M = (Total Hrs. — Maintenance and Inspection)/(0.42) x (0.33)

Many managers and supervisors would like to be able to use **M** to calculate personnel needs because it assumes that everyone works at full capacity all of the time with 100 percent productivity and that no one takes vacation time. Reality, however, requires that both productivity and vacation time be included in the calculation.

There are many sources from which productivity factors for clinical engineering positions can be derived (AHA1, 1982; AHA2, 1988; Lodge, 1991; Mahachek, 1989; Betts, 1989; Bauld, 1987). Although the highest productivity factor considered to be practically attainable by most of these references is 85 percent, the value used for determining resources may need to be somewhat higher in order to justify resource requests to the hospital administration.

Table 8.2 Labor Time Estimates for Specific Device Types

Class Code	Description	Labor per each Scheduled Maint. (hours)	Annual Labor Requirements (hours) Sched. Maint.	Correct. Maint.	Total Maint.	Annual Parts Cost	Annual # CM's
320M	Blood Gas Analyzer	2 - 4	5 - 7	9 - 16	14 - 23		
420M	Cardiac Output Computer	0.6	1.2	1.1	2.3	.40	0.7
430M	Central Monitoring System	1.3	2.6	7.2	9.0	2.10	0.6
435M	Centrifuge	0.5 - 2	1 - 4	1 - 6	2 - 10		
505M	Defibrillator	0.7	1.4	1.7	3.1	6.90	1.4
510M	Defib/Monitor	0.8	1.6	1.5	3.1	25.30	0.4
605M	Electrocardiograph	0.7	1.4	2.9	4.3	20.00	2.1
610M	Electrocardiograph Scanner	0.9	1.8	8.7	10.5	49.00	5.9
645M	External Pacemaker	0.6	1.2	0.6	1.8	.20	0.7
905M	Heart/Lung Bypass Machine	1.1	2.2	0.9	3.1		
910M	Hemodialysis System	2.0	4.0	10.7	14.7	82.00	4.5
1025M	Intra-Aortic Balloon Pump	0.8	1.6	1.8	3.4		
1735M	Physiologic	0.7	1.4	1.8	3.2	7.40	0.4
2215M	Volume Ventilator Monitor System	1.2	2.4	1.8	4.2	22.40	1.1

The total number of hours, **P**, needed to provide 100 percent of clinical engineering's services with personnel performing work at the 85 percent productivity level is calculated by

P = M/(0.85)

The last thing to be considered is paid time away, which includes both vacation and sick time. Most companies provide employees with two to six weeks of vacation per year plus paid holidays (i.e., Christmas Day, New Year's Day, etc.) and allow this vacation time to be accumulated from year to year. In addition, employees receive sick time allowances that vary greatly between institutions. The human resources department of the hospital, however, should be able to provide an average paid time away percentage for the institution. Consider the following example in which the average paid time away is 5 percent. The total number of hours, **V**, needed to provide clinical engineering services with personnel who perform at the 85 percent productivity level and are at the hospital 95 percent of the time can be calculated as

V = P/(0.95)

Up to this point, all calculations have yielded a number in hours/year. Before proceeding with further calculations it is necessary to define the term full time equivalent (FTE). FTE is utilized to allow managers and supervisors flexibility in filling positions. For example, an employer with one FTE can hire one person full time, two people half time each, etc. One FTE is usually defined as 2,080 worked hours per year. This value is roughly equivalent to 173.3 worked hours per month or 40 worked hours per week. The number is derived by taking an eight-hour workday and multiplying it by the number of workdays in the period.

The number of FTEs needed to provide the clinical engineering program with personnel who perform at an 85 percent productivity level and are at the hospital 95 percent of the time can be determined by dividing the total hours calculated for **V** by 2,080:

FTE = V/2,080

Extrapolating all of these calculations backwards gives

FTE = (1.65) (Hrs. for Maintenance and Inspection)/2,080

The number of FTEs derived in this manner represents only the technical staff needed based upon the device types used. If the calculations are performed for all of the device types to be supported by the clinical engineering program, then the final FTE value should approximate the total number of FTEs needed to provide direct equipment support. However, this calculation does not take into account the abilities of individuals to be cross-trained on multiple device types. To get a more accurate picture of the FTEs needed to provide the appropriate personnel skills mix, these calculations should be performed individually for small groups of similar equipment and should be evaluated before being summed together. In this way, the department will know that 0.83 FTE is needed to service respiratory equipment, 0.50 FTE to service dialysis equipment, 1.25 FTE to service radiology equipment, etc.

In addition to the technical staff just calculated, some estimation of the amount of administrative staff needed to run the program on a daily basis will also be required. In this computation, the first thing to consider is whether the clinical engineer will provide direct equipment support. If so (as will likely be the case for a small program), then some of the clinical engineer's time has already been accounted for in the preceding calculations, and only the remainder may be added. If the clinical engineer's function is purely administrative then all of that time must be added.

A resource factor for supervisors and clerical support must also be added. In a very small clinical engineering program, there may be no formal supervisor beyond the clinical engineer, although in most larger clinical engineering programs (more than five people) there is at least one supervisor in addition to the director.

To determine the actual number of supervisors needed, one must decide if some of the supervisor's time has already been included in the preceding calculations because some percentage of that time will be spent in the direct support of equipment. It is quite common for a supervisor's position to be created consisting of 0.5 FTE supervisor + 0.5 FTE specialty equipment technician when neither position would be justifiable on its own. Supervisors with some direct equipment support activities should be able to supervise five FTEs effectively, and those individuals with only supervisory responsibilities may be able to supervise as many as 15 FTEs effectively. The average number of FTEs per supervisor is about ten people.

Required clerical resources (i.e., secretaries, receptionists, data entry clerks, etc.) vary significantly from hospital to hospital. In a small hospital it is unusual for every department to have its own secretary. Clinical engineering is no exception. Yet, as the size or complexity of a clinical engineering program grows, adequate clerical support is critical to the continued success of the program. Once the size of a clinical engineering department reaches five technicians or engineers, the documentation requirements generally warrant one clerical FTE. Another clerical FTE should be added for every five to seven additional technicians. More clerical support may be needed for additional clinical engineers, who will likely generate more technical documents than the routine documentation generated by technicians. In a large program, the director of the clinical engineering program may even need a personal secretary. This is especially true if the director actively participates on several hospital committees.

The calculations for transference of total required FTEs into dollar resources goes beyond the scope of this chapter. Salary evaluation is a function that should be performed by a compensation analyst, who is usually found in the hospital's human resource department. The clinical engineer should not be left out of this process, however, because medical compensation analysts may be unfamiliar with clinical engineering job requirements and may grade them against criteria for facilities engineering or trades positions. However, to work effectively with the compensation analyst, the clinical engineer must have a basic idea of how salaries are determined for different positions.

According to a survey performed by the American Compensation Association, more than 79 percent of technical jobs are rated using a quantitative system (Greene and Nash, 1989). About 14 percent of technical jobs are rated based upon a market survey of the salaries for similar positions within the facility or at nearby facilities. One example of the type of quantitative system that may be used to grade clinical engineers and biomedical equipment technicians is the **National Position Evaluation Plan** (NMTA Associates, 1980). This plan utilizes 11 factors to establish a score for any job category. This score is then compared to the score of other jobs to establish pay grades. In this manner, dissimilar jobs with equal levels of difficulty should fall into the same pay grade, thereby ensuring pay equity throughout the organization. A higher score corresponds to a higher grade and more pay. The 11 factors (including some examples of relative point values) are as follows:

- **Knowledge**: Measurement of basic knowledge or "scholastic content" essential as background training prior to learning the position. This knowledge is often expressed in terms of educational equivalents

  45 Points for 2 years of college
  60 Points for 4 years of college
  75 Points for 6 years of college

- **Experience**: Measurement of the length of time usually or typically required to perform effectively in the position under the normal supervision levels.

  60 points for 1 to 3 years
  100 points for 5 to 7 years
  140 points for more than 10 years

- **Complexity of duties**: Measurement of the extent to which responsibilities of the position are circumscribed by standard practice. Consideration is given to the degree of independent action permissible, the impact of decisions, the amount of resourcefulness needed, and the amount of personal planning required.

  45 points for general judgment based upon standard practices
  75 points for conceptual judgment based upon issues with little precedent

- **Supervision received:** Measurement of the degree to which a supervisor outlines the methods or procedures to be followed in completing the job or the results to be obtained. Consideration is given to the proximity of the supervisor and the extent and number of supervisory contacts.

  20 points for planing and doing own work under general supervision
  60 points for establishing own performance standards

- **Errors**: Measurement of the position's responsibility for preventing errors based on the degree to which work is checked or verified and on the potential impact of errors.

  20 points for errors that may have a serious effect within the organization
  40 points for errors that will have a serious external effect on the organization

- **Contacts with others**: Measurement of the responsibility for meeting, dealing with, or influencing others and the impact of such contacts on the organization.

  5 points for no contacts other than supervisor
  40 points for inside/outside contacts with great influence on organization

- **Confidential data**: Measurement of the integrity and discretion required by the position in safeguarding confidential data and the impact of disclosure of such data on internal, external, community, or competitive relations.

  5 points for little or no exposure
  20 points for exposure to highly sensitive material

- **Mental or visual demand**: Measurement of the degree of mental and visual attention involved in the performance of normal duties, including manual dexterity and the fatigue resulting from such duties.

  5 points for needing attention at intervals
  10 points for continuous general attention
  25 points for unusually high coordination skills required

- **Working conditions**: Measurement of the extent to which the surroundings or physical conditions might make the position undesirable. This factor typically affects only positions outside of an office environment.

  5 points for normal office environment
  15 points for somewhat undesirable conditions
  25 points for extremely undesirable conditions

- **Sphere of influence**: Measurement of the degree or kind of supervisory responsibilities required by the position and the placement of the position in the formal hierarchy of the organization. For the purposes of this factor, "supervisory responsibilities" include control over costs, policies, and personnel.

  5 points for general supervision with no cost or policy responsibilities
  20 points for independent work with total responsibility for a department

- **Scope of supervision**: Measurement of the number of personnel directly supervised by the position. This factor is not considered when grading staff positions.

  5 points for supervising 1 to 2 people
  10 points for supervising 3 to 10 people
  15 points for supervising 11 to 25 people
  20 points for supervising 26 to 50 people

If the hospital does not have the capability to perform quantitative job analysis and a market survey approach is to be used, there are salary surveys done specifically for clinical engineering positions (Pacela, 1989, 1990, 1991) that can provide general information about the salary corresponding to specific job titles. These surveys even provide data on salaries for various regions of the U.S., for teaching versus non-teaching hospitals, and for union versus nonunion hospitals. However, these data are very static and cannot adequately reflect the "*many intangibles that influence both salaries and responsibilities in a particular hospital*" (Pacela, 1991) so they should be used carefully as a guide, not an absolute. The data from these surveys can also be used for comparison against salaries determined by the quantitative approach.

Although most biomedical equipment technicians are hired from the local geographic market, an increasing number of quality hospitals are recruiting on a national level. With an understanding of the job grading process, the clinical engineer can ensure that any positions being established are paid at a rate that will enable the recruitment and retention of the best qualified people.

Maintenance Resources

Equipment support is the major objective of any clinical engineering program, thus, the direct expenses for maintenance should be the second resource to consider. Direct maintenance expenses include the following:

- The cost of service contracts.
- The cost of vendor-provided as-needed services.
- The cost of parts used by clinical engineering personnel.

Service Contracts. As discussed in Chapter 3, "service contract" is the term used for any agreement between the hospital and a vendor that provides specific services at a specific cost over a specific period. Because of the high cost of supporting equipment with service contracts, these should be reserved for highly complex technologies, vital one-of-a-kind equipment, and aging problematic equipment. There exist a wide range of service contract types, and the services and costs of these contracts vary accordingly. Care should be taken to explore all of the various options available prior to entering into any service contract agreements with outside vendors. In general, service contracts fall into one of the following four categories:

- **Full-service contracts,** in which the vendor has been hired to perform all necessary services to the equipment for the life of the contract. These contracts typically cost about nine - 11 percent of the purchase price of the equipment.
- **Preventive maintenance (PM) only contracts,** in which the vendor is hired to perform only preventive maintenance to the equipment on a preset schedule for the term of the contract. The number of visits and the work to be performed during these visits is carefully spelled out in the agreement. PM contracts with some limited emergency service coverage also exist. The cost of PM only contracts typically runs 4 to 9 percent of the purchase price of the equipment.
- **Maintenance insurance contracts,** which are written with a third-party insurer who provides brokerage services. This insurer is paid a fixed price, or premium, against a list of services for identified equipment just as with other types of insurance. When equipment service is needed, the hospital secures that service and passes the bill along to the insurance company. The cost of maintenance insurance ranges from 6 to 8 percent of the purchase price of the equipment.
- **Retainer Contracts,** in which the vendor is given a purchase order to be used for any services that the hospital requires at a fixed cost for those services. Typically, the vendor agrees to a fixed price for hourly service during regular business hours and another fixed price for overtime service and often offers a discount on parts. Unlike the other types of contracts described, the hospital pays against a retainer contract only when it actually receives work. Because this type of agreement offers more security to the equipment user than having no contract at all, it is becoming popular among clinical engineers as an intermediate step to wean equipment users away from longstanding vendor dependencies. Estimates for the cost of retainer contracts range from 5 to 10 percent of the purchase price.

Although this section is concerned with calculating resources, a few general notes about contract management are in order. First, when generating either a full-service or a PM only contract, one should be careful to identify when preventive maintenance visits are to occur so that they can be tracked during the term of the contract. Failure to identify inspection dates can result in "creeping" in which the inspections get close together toward the end of the term of the contract. In some cases, the "creeping" can become so extensive that the last scheduled visit cannot be performed during the term of the contract. In this case, the hospital should ask for a refund or credit toward the cost of the next contract period.

Second, the cost of parts included in a contract and the payment terms can have a major impact on the total cost of the contract. For the novice it may be best to include all parts in a contract to fix the cost even though it may be possible to reduce contracts by 2 to 5 percent if parts are excluded and paid for as needed. Also, most companies now charge a premium of as much as 6 percent of the contract cost for semiannual, quarterly, or monthly billing. This cost must be weighed against the knowledge that withholding payment may be the only means of negotiating with a company that is providing poor service after the contact is signed.

Third, the per-item cost of a contract can often be reduced by adding more items or agreeing to a longer contract term because these situations make it easier for the vendor to plan resource utilization. Again, this savings must be weighed against the knowledge that withholding payment or short-term cancellation of the contract may be the only means of negotiating with a company providing poor service after the contact is signed.

Finally, as mentioned in Chapter 3, contract management is an important part of the clinical engineer's function. The signing of a service contract to support a piece of equipment does not absolve the clinical engineer of any responsibility for that equipment. In fact, more than one foolish clinical engineer has been left wondering how they could have grossly underestimated their contract expense needs simply through a failure to monitor hidden contract costs.

Vendor Services. It is virtually impossible for any clinical engineering program to support all of the hospital's equipment internally 100 percent of the time. Service contracts offer one method of subsidy for extended periods. However, as the hospital needs specialized service for specific equipment on a limited basis, formal service contracts become impractical. When these situations occur, a service vendor is hired by the hospital to perform the task. The tasks performed by this vendor can include any of the services that the internal clinical engineering program may provide but are usually limited to infrequent preventive maintenance, nonroutine calibrations, and emergency repairs.

Because vendor services are provided randomly to many different types of equipment, it is difficult to quantify the exact cost of these services. A good approximation would be 6 to 8 percent of the purchase price of the equipment likely to be supported in this manner, i.e., all equipment to be supported by the clinical engineering program less those items known to be supported by service contracts and those items for which clinical engineering personnel can unquestionably provide support. Basic statistics demonstrate that the larger the equipment base of the hospital, the more accurate this approximation will be.

Parts. The last major resource to be estimated is the cost of the parts to be used by clinical engineering personnel in the course of their work. The most accurate way to estimate parts cost would be to contact the manufacturer of every piece of equipment on the inventory list and ask them for a list of necessary replacement parts and their cost. For a small hospital this may be possible, in the case of most hospitals, it is not.

To estimate the cost of parts one can again refer to tables designed for this purpose (Table 8.2). Using such a table, the estimated cost of parts can be calculated in the same fashion as personnel resources were calculated, i.e., by summing the calculated parts cost for every device type included in the inventory.

Example. If a hospital owns 20 defibrillator/monitors, what is the estimated annual parts cost for this equipment? Table 8.2 shows that each defibrillator/monitor requires an average of $25.30 worth of parts per year. The total parts cost then equals $506.00 per year. This method provides a good first approximation and can be utilized when multiplied by some regional and inflationary factors.

Overall, the cost of routine parts ranges from 20 to 60 percent of salary expenses, which already include regional variances. Clinical engineering programs that support highly mechanical devices (ventilators, beds, dialysis machines, sterilizers, etc.) or devices that contain glassware (X-ray units, billiblankets, etc.) should estimate at the high end. Conversely, programs that support predominantly electronic devices (physiologic monitors, defibrillators, etc.) can estimate lower.

To supplement any of these methods it may be possible to contact manufacturers for the exact pricing of parts used for scheduled preventive maintenance of particular devices. By knowing the frequency of preventive maintenance and the cost of the manufacturer's PM kit one can validate the approximated values or those presented in published tables.

General Recurring Resources

In addition to the resources necessary to provide direct equipment support, the clinical engineering department needs funding for general expenses, which are known in the business world as **overhead**. Overhead expenses generally fall into two categories: **physical** and **nonphysical.**

Physical overhead refers to rent (space), heat, electricity, and telephone costs. Most hospital-based clinical engineering programs are not concerned with these expenses because they are included in the total hospital budget. Guidelines for space estimates for a clinical engineering program can be found in the **Veterans' Administration DM & S Construction Guidelines for Hospitals, Manual H-08-9**, Chapter 230. An abridged copy of these recommended minimum space requirements is presented in Table 8.3

Table 8.3 Guidelines for Space Requirements

Repair and Development	**400 sq. ft./employee**
Receiving and Holding	**100 sq. ft./employee**
Storage	**100 sq. ft./employee**
Conference and Library	**150 sq. ft./employee**
Director's Office	**150 sq. ft.**
Secretary and Waining Area	**120 sq. ft. (+) 80 sq. ft./additional employee**
All Others	**85 sq. ft./employee**
Toilets	**40 sq. ft./employee (+) 5 sq. ft./employee**

(from: The Veterans Administration DM&S Construction Guidelines for Hospitals.) (H-08-9, Chapter 230).

Indirect overhead includes such items as books and manuals, cleaning supplies magazines and periodicals, general medical supplies for testing (i.e., fluids, IV tubing, electrodes, etc.), membership dues, minor tool replacement, office supplies, photocopying, postage and shipping, professional development and travel. These costs vary directly with the size of the clinical engineering program. A good approximation can be obtained by calculating 8 percent of salary expenses.

Start-Up Resources

If a clinical engineering program is being established where one did not previously exist, then additional resources will be needed for start-up services and supplies. These start-up services may be as trivial as painting the walls of work areas and installing phones or they may be more integral to the function of clinical engineering. A list of some start-up equipment and supplies and their estimated cost appears in Chapter 7 (Table 7.1).

Justifying Resource Requests

According to *Hospitals Magazine*, "*most healthcare executives don't know how much their hospital spends in support of equipment each year*" (Hard, 1991). The efforts necessary to uncover maintenance cost information, which were described earlier in this chapter, support this statement. Because the cost of equipment support can represent as much as 1 to 2 percent of the yearly operating expenses for a hospital, such ignorance can be very costly.

To say that health-care executives do not want to know or don't care about the cost of equipment support is to oversimplify the problem. The problem relates more to (1) administrators who are naive about the cost-control possibilites embodied by equipment support alternatives, (2) department managers who are unable to devote large amounts of time to equipment support activities, and (3) clinical engineers who are unable to communicate effectively. Problems 1 and 2 should have a positive impact on the clinical engineer's ability to justify resources for a clinical engineering program. "*Success, however, will only come to those who properly communicate the right information to the right people in a manner that they can understand*" (Brody, 1988).

"*Unfortunately, many clinical engineers believe that hospital administrators have an inherent responsibility to understand the role and benefits of clinical engineering*" (Greenstein and Phillips, 1989). They may become frustrated at the need to describe continually to administrators the benefits of a clinical engineering program. For the new clinical engineer, this attitude is a dangerous trap that should be avoided. "*The clinical engineering manager must accept the major share of the responsibility for developing a credible clinical engineering program*" and then demonstrate the benefits of the program to hospital department managers, clinicians, and senior administrators (Greenstein and Phillips, 1989).

Understanding differences in perspective and perception among individuals and groups is instrumental to any clinical engineering program's success. Consider the education of a clinical engineer. Clinical engineers are trained to think in analytical terms. In the hospital environment, decisions made by a clinical engineer will be centered around medical equipment and based upon safety, regulatory compliance, available support alternatives, and costs. Physicians and nurses are taught to assess patient status by integrating the information from medical equipment with that derived from chemical, physiologic, and physical indicators. It is important to these clinicians that the equipment work correctly and consistently. The staff may also find themselves quite overwhelmed by the myriad of bedside technology now in use at most hospitals and may be concerned about their ability to operate this equipment properly. It is unlikely that these individuals will be especially interested in hearing explanations of extended downtime versus cost and thus may be unwilling to hand over functioning equipment for routine testing.

In contrast, administrators are concerned with the cost of treatment, reimbursement (DRGs), liability, compliance with regulatory standards, and community perceptions. Department managers, who answer to both clinicians and administrators, may have hybrid views and conflicting priorities. By designing a program around clinical, nursing, and administrative goals and objectives, clinical engineers further their own professional credibility as well as that of the program (Greenstein and Phillips, 1989).

Having assembled all of the necessary facts and figures, the clinical engineer must now translate thes data into a persuasive argument designed to overcome these problems. Perhaps the strongest and most persuasive argument available to the clinical engineer is that of cost containment, supported by a thorough analysis of expenses and alternatives. With a complete analysis of the costs and alternatives in hand, the clinical engineering director can promote the department functions as the best-case alternative on the grounds of cost containment. One simply has to look to the literature or attend a conference on clinical engineering to see numerous examples of the cost savings possible through an effective clinical engineering program (Brody, 1988, 1991a; Hasper, 1991; Baumeister, 1987; Furst, 1986; Cohen, 1982).

At this point, one must remember that good intentions do not cover miscalculated expenses. If clinical engineering is given central control of equipment support and all of the services that are currently available to equipment users cannot be provided with in-house personnel then some money must be allotted to cover these external expenses. To illustrate this point consider the following example:

> Assume a hospital owns five Intra-aortic balloon pumps (IABPs) and currently services them under contract for $7,200. According to Table 8.2, these devices require an average of 1.6 hours of preventive maintenance and 1.8 hours of corrective maintenance time per IABP per year. Assuming that only preventive maintenance can be performed by the clinical engineering program, 8 hours of a technician's time will be required per year to support the equipment. If the technician earns $15 per hour, the annual cost of preventive maintenance services to this equipment will be $120. Given that the vendor charges $100 per hour for service calls, the anticipated corrective maintenance charges will be $900. If each preventive maintenance action requires $200 in parts, then another $2,000 will be needed for semiannual preventive maintenance of the five units.

Estimating the cost of vendor-installed parts is the hardest part of this process. Circuit cards can range from a few dollars to a few thousand dollars. To be effective, the clinical engineer must be willing to take some risks and depend upon the law of averages to ensure that major components do not fail in all systems every year. For this example, assume that the most expensive replacement component in the IABP is a $1,500 circuit card. The next most expensive item is an $800 circuit card, followed by several $100 mechanical parts. Assuming that a total of one of each circuit card and five mechanical parts will need to be replaced each year gives an estimated cost of vendor parts of $2,800.

DIGITAL VOLT METER (DVM)	PER TECHNICIAN	$150
ELECTRONIC WORK BENCH	PER TECHNICIAN	$1,400
MINOR TOOLS WITH CASE	PER TECHNICIAN	$1,000
PHYSIOLOGICAL SIMULATOR	PER TECHNICIAN	$1,200
SOLDERING STATION	PER TECHNICIAN	$130
VENTILATOR TESTER	ONE + ONE PER EVERY 15 TECHNICIANS	$7,000
ESU OUTPUT METER	ONE + ONE PER EVERY 10 TECHNICIANS	$2,000
INFUSION PUMP ANALYZER	ONE + ONE PER EVERY 10 TECHNICIANS	$3,200
MECHANICS TOOL SET	ONE + ONE PER EVERY 10 TECHNICIANS	$1,200
DEFIBRILLATOR OUTPUT METER	ONE + ONE PER EVERY 8 TECHNICIANS	$2,500
ELECTRICAL SAFETY ANALYZER	ONE + ONE PER EVERY 5 TECHNICIANS	$6,500
FREQUENCY GENERATOR	ONE + ONE PER EVERY 5 TECHNICIANS	$600
MICROCOMPUTER	ONE + ONE PER EVERY 5 TECHNICIANS	$3,200
POWER SUPPLY	ONE + ONE PER EVERY 5 TECHNICIANS	$300
DESOLDERING STATION	ONE + ONE PER EVERY 3 TECHNICIANS	$250
OSCILLOSCOPE, GENERAL	ONE + ONE PER EVERY 3 TECHNICIANS	$8,000
DRILL PRESS	ONE	$500
GRINDER	ONE	$300
LASER OUTPUT METER	ONE	$3,000
MAINTENANCE MANAGEMENT SOFTWARE	ONE	$5,000
OSCILLOSCOPE, MULTIFUNCTION	ONE	$20,000
OSCILLOSCOPE CAMERA	ONE	$500
TACHOMETER	ONE	$400
ULTRASOUND POWER METER	ONE	$2,500
X-RAY OUTPUT METER	ONE	$10,000
X-RAY TEST PATTERN	ONE	$2,000
CMOS LOGIC CHIP SET	INITIAL ORDER	$1,300
GENERAL ELECTRONIC COMPONENTS	INITIAL ORDER	$3,500
GENERAL ELECTRONIC HARDWARE	INITIAL ORDER	$1,200
PARTS BINS	INITIAL ORDER	$8,000
TTL LOGIC CHIP SET	INITIAL ORDER	$1,800

Figure 8.4: Suggested list of start-up equipment and supplies.

Calculating all of the expenses yields:

Clinical Engineering Labor	$ 120
Clinical Engineering Parts	$2,000
Vendor Labor	$ 900
Vendor Parts	$2,800
TOTAL	**$5,820**

This analysis indicates that in-house servicing of this equipment would result in a savings of $1,380 over the current cost of supporting this equipment. However, only $120 of this cost is labor, the remaining $5,700 must still be in the budget to cover the vendor's cost even though these are not contract costs.

Table 8.4 presents a program-wide example of how current costs can be reallocated to cover anticipated costs and indicates that the transfer of a service contract to some degree of in-house support is not the only option available. Significant savings are possible by eliminating contracts and opting for services on a time-and-materials basis for those pieces of equipment requiring infrequent contact. This option should not be overlooked.

Although contracts are costly, many department managers feel that the expense is worthwhile because it relieves them of the burden of managing service activities on a day-to-day basis (Bouley, 1991). It is important for the clinical engineer to understand the impact of equipment downtime on a busy laboratory or radiology department. Because of the high dependence of such areas on the technology a series of events occurs whenever equipment breaks down. First, medical tests that utilize the equipment are delayed and staff must be reassigned to other tasks to remain productive. Next, clinicians begin to complain that their patients cannot be adequately diagnosed. Therefore, tests may need to be done elsewhere at a cost to the hospital. Other procedures may also be delayed if the primary tests are unavailable. Finally, if the equipment remains down, the public's opinion of the quality of care provided by the hospital diminishes.

Each of these events causes a reduction in the quality of patient care provided or has an associated loss of revenue or cost (i.e., staff who are idle but are still being paid; external testing) that the department manager must be concerned with. Therefore, if managers feel that a service contract will guarantee minimal downtime at a fixed cost and will require only a simple phone call to repair problems that arise with the equipment, they are likely to enter into such a contract. This is especially true if a contract is the only alternative that ensures the prompt, quality equipment support necessary. However, if clinical engineering can demonstrate the ability to provide an equal or a greater level of support at a reduced cost, then a good department manager should be willing to listen.

There are two ways to gain the support of department managers; one is by evolution and the other is by revolution. In the evolutionary process, the clinical engineering program moves forward like an inch worm. The program extends itself to take on one type of activity at a time (i.e., maintenance to a particular type of equipment or maintenance to all equipment within a given department). Once the new activity has been thoroughly integrated into the clinical engineering program, the program extends itself to another activity. Each time that clinical engineering succeeds with such an integration, the credibility of the program is enhanced. If the program consistently succeeds or the effects of failures are minimized then integration into new areas becomes increasingly easier. In fact, there may be a point at which department managers seek out clinical engineering services rather than vice versa.

This evolutionary process is recommended for all new clinical engineers and is very easily accomplished in hospitals that allow clinical engineering to charge back for their services.

For experienced clinical engineers in hospitals where there are decentralized equipment support budgets, there may come a time when maintenance spending appears to have gone beyond reasonable levels. In this case, the hospital administration may decide to centralize patient-care equipment support under one entity. If this decision is made unilaterally and is binding to all hospital departments, this is an example of a revolutionary change. If the clinical engineering program has been effective and has good credibility within the hospital, then this type of change can bring about dramatic quality improvements and cost savings in a very short period of time. If not, then the results can be disastrous. It is for this reason that the evolutionary approach should be the method of choice for the integration of clinical engineering services into any hospital.

Additionally, there may be times when the clinical engineering department finds that the revolutionary approach has been thrust upon them. Consider the increasingly common scenario in which a large, well-established hospital forms an affiliation with another, usually smaller, hospital to keep both institutions financially viable. What is the response of the clinical engineering department when it is instructed by senior management to support the equipment of the affiliated hospital when

(a) There is no clinical engineering program at the second hospital?
(b) The department managers at this hospital are moderately satisfied with the service that they are receiving by a third party vendor or the original equipment manufacturer?
(c) The cost of equipment support at this hospital is quite high?

This scenario is no different from the case where the clinical engineering department is instructed to make revolutionary changes within its own institution. The clinical engineering department must establish credibility at the second hospital. This should be a very straightforward process, arising from recognition of the effectiveness of the existing program at the primary hospital.

PROGRAM MANAGEMENT

Having documented the need for clinical engineering services and successfully presented this information, the clinical engineer must now manage the program. To accomplish this, policies, procedures, and standards of practice must be established as a framework for the program. Consideration must be given to three basic areas: fundamental work, materials handling, and expected performance levels. It is critical that the clinical engineer understand the appropriate flow of activity in these areas so that effective direction toward positive outcomes occurs.

Monitoring the Work Flow

The consistent theme of this book is that the fundamental work of a clinical engineering program is the management of technology within a hospital or health-care setting. "*To assist clinical engineering in evaluating effectiveness, the JCAHO has developed a general model of technology management and data analysis that stresses the use of empirical data from all those who deal with the equipment*" (Keil and Camplin, 1987). The process of technology management begins with the basic decision to acquire a new device and ends when that device is permanently removed from service (Keil and Camplin, 1987). During the life span of the device, records must be kept that document that the device has been routinely tested according to "written procedures" and that note any failures or malfunctions. A block diagram of the JCAHO process is shown in Fig. 8.5.

A simple scoring system to determine if scheduled maintenance should occur and at what frequency is presented in detail in Chapter 3. For the system to work effectively, the equipment management (EM) number described should be calculated independently at every hospital for each device type used by that hospital in creating its equipment inventory (see Table 8.1). Likewise, the cutoff for inclusion of a device into the equipment control program should be developed independently by every hospital using the value of 12 as a guide, but not an absolute cutoff. After developing the inclusion list, the clinical engineer should present the data and the rationale for the list to the hospital's safety committee or QA board for approval. Once identified, most computer systems will allow the scheduled maintenance inclusion list to be maintained as a subset of the master inventory list by adding a Boolean identifier field to each inventory record. The EM number can also be maintained as a field on the device type list. In this way, future equipment can quickly be identified for inclusion or exclusion from scheduled maintenance by comparing it with the standard for established device types. Furthermore, if new equipment cannot be categorized into an established category, a new category can easily be created.

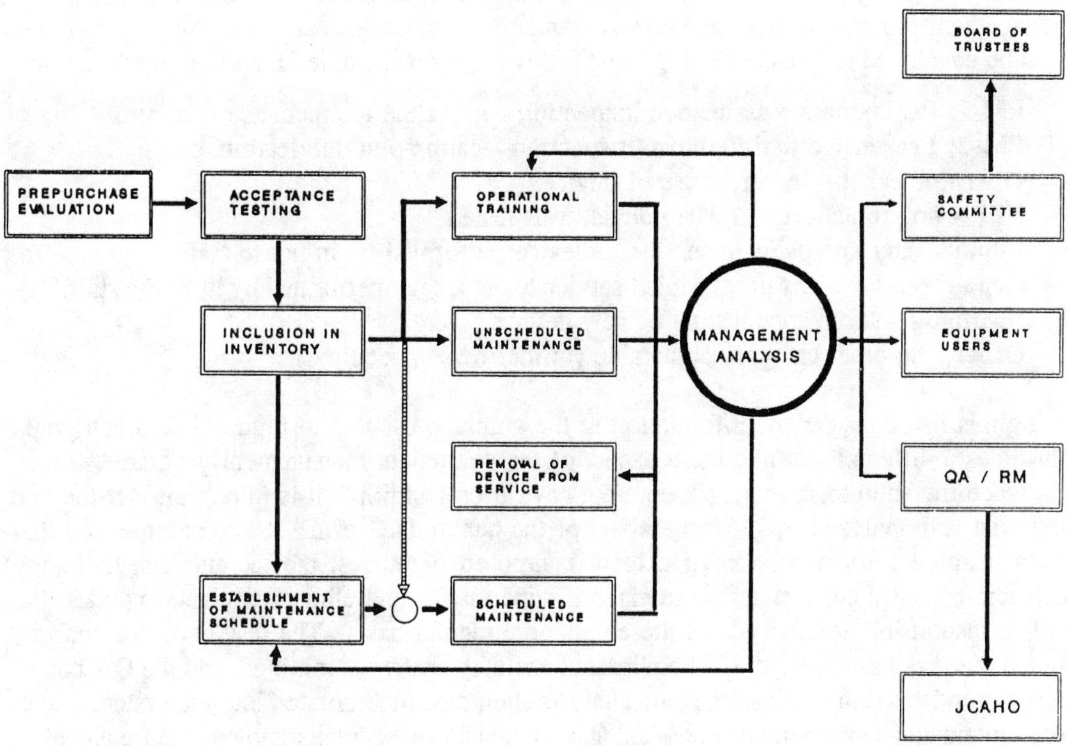

Figure 8.5: Flowchart illustrating the equipment management program.

The JCAHO standards also mandate that "*equipment management programs should be able to assess and control the clinical and physical risks of equipment*" (1989a). Most hospitals utilize some form of work order or job ticket that is completed by the person performing the work to monitor activities associated with the equipment management program. There are probably as many variations of work orders as there are hospitals, but basically, a work order is a uniquely identifiable record of work performed on a uniquely identifiable piece of equipment and includes some detail about the work performed. Work orders can be as simple as an entry in a log book or as complex as a series of codes stored on a computer system. For work orders to be effectively used to analyze the equipment control program they should include at least the following information:

- A unique identifier for the equipment.
- A field or link establishing the device type.
- A field or link establishing the owner department of the device.
- The name of the technician performing the service.
- A classification for the type of work performed.
- The cost of parts or outside services used.
- The total hours used.
- The beginning and end date for the service.
- A description of the problem.
- A description of the solution.

By evaluating groups of these items, important information about the equipment management program can be learned. A standard set of classifications for work performed must be developed before continuing. The following is an example of a set of classifications:

- **PM-1: Performance assurance inspection**—no actual maintenance required.
- **PM-2: Preventive maintenance inspection**—calibration, lubrication, etc.
- **Operator error**—incorrect use of device.
- **NPF**—no problem found when device was tested.
- **Repair**—any unscheduled service to device performed by in-house staff.
- **Repair/vendor**—any unscheduled service to device not performed by in-house staff.
- **Incoming**—acceptance testing of new device.
- **Other**—no other category applicable (further review required).

Using this list, consider the information in the graphs presented in Figure 8.6. Each graph illustrates a different and important aspect of the equipment management program.

Once the equipment management data have been compiled, it is important that they be reviewed and analyzed by other members of the health-care team. It is recommended that every hospital form a collaborative team composed of nurses, lab technicians, radiology technicians, instructors, materials managers, supervisors, and clinical engineering staff that will be responsible for analysis of these data on a regular basis. The results of this analysis should then be disseminated to all equipment users, the safety committee, and the QA board. Recommendations made from the data analysis should be incorporated into the system. Such recommendations might include increasing or decreasing scheduled maintenance frequencies, providing additional training on a specific device, or removing a specific device or device type from service.

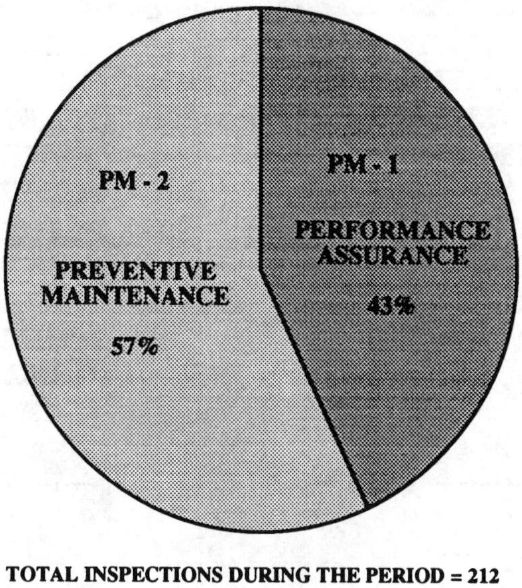

Figure 8.6a: Pie chart illustrating PM-1 and PM-2 as a percent of total inspections made.

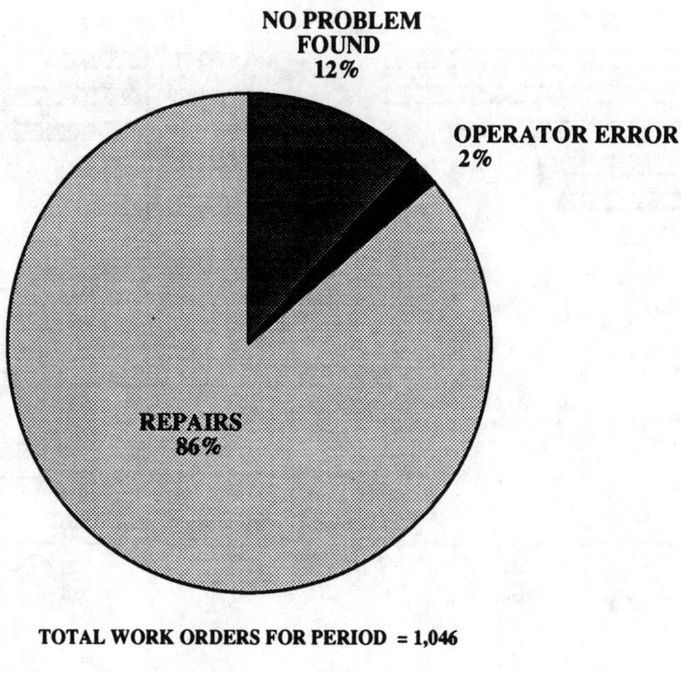

Figure 8.6b: Pie chart illustrating relative percentage of operator error, repair, and no problem found work order.

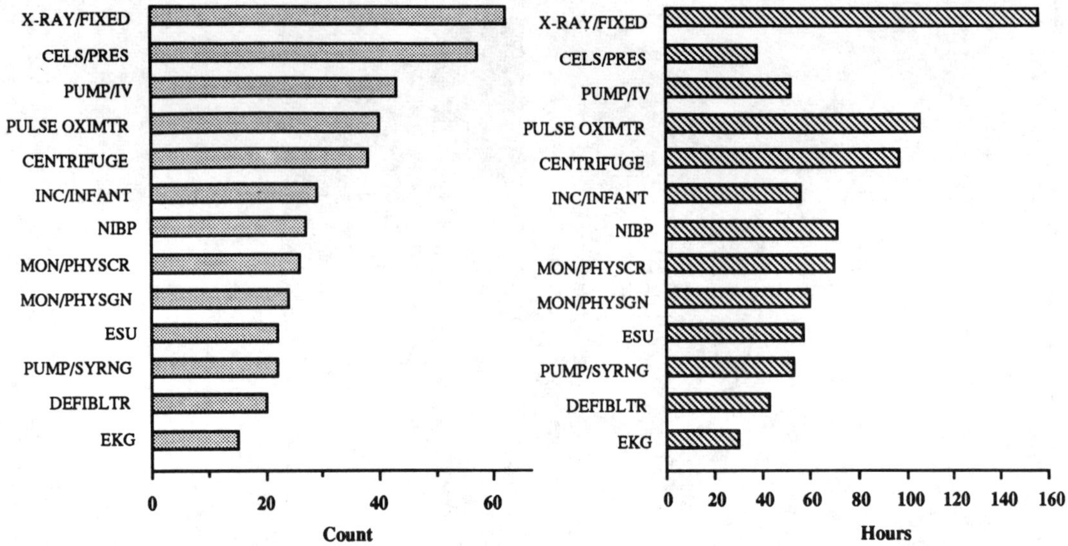

Figure 8.6c: Bar graphs illustrating the number of total repairs, operator errors, and no problem found work orders by device type.

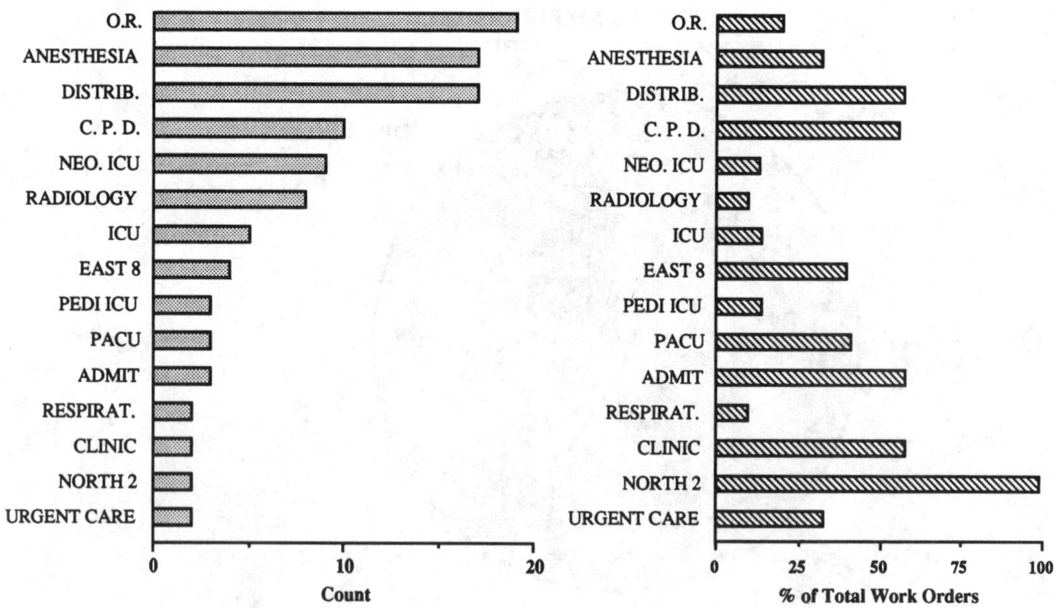

Figure 8.6d: Bar graph illustrating the number of operator errors and no problem found work orders by department.

It is important that clinical engineers develop an effective process to identify significant events in the data collected during the course of equipment management activities. High technology carries with it a fixed requirement for support. To provide less than the technology in place requires will, over time, erode the quality of the environment that has been developed. Conversely, the U.S. health-care system costs as much as it does because it was built in such a manner that it requires extensive clinical engineering support. (Keil and Camplin, 1987). The challenge for future clinical engineers will be to continually evaluate the support being provided to ensure that quality is maintained while providing that support with decreasing resources.

Monitoring Materials Flow

In order for a clinical engineering program to function in a hospital, it must have access to goods and services from outside the hospital. The system for acquiring these goods and services can be very complex, as outlined in Figure 8.7. To start with, most hospital departments cannot formally acquire anything from outside of the hospital. They must request that the goods or services be acquired by the hospital's purchasing department. This is done to prevent just anyone from acting as a representative of the hospital to a vendor. Most large corporations and universities also employ this system.

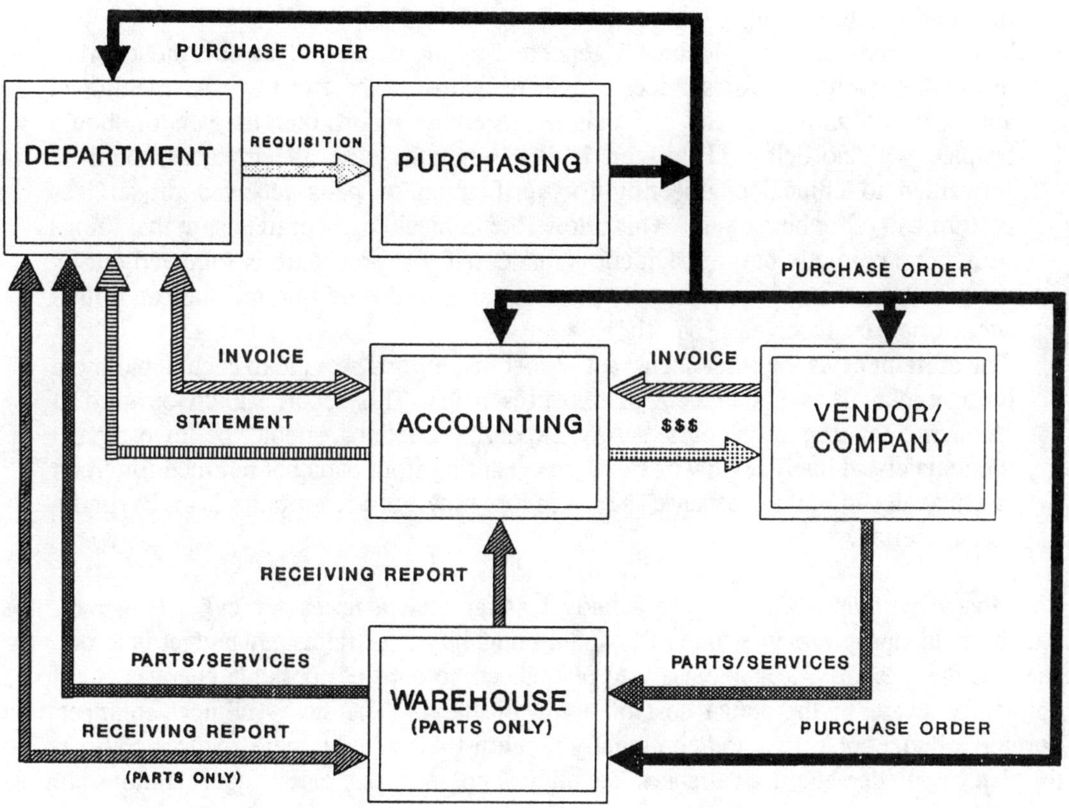

Figure 8.7: Flowchart illustrating materials handling and paperwork routing.

For clinical engineers to make effective use of this system, they must be able to monitor each step of the process. The following list of generic documents is presented to give the student an idea of how to monitor this system:

- **The requisition,** is an internal document requesting that purchasing place an order on behalf of someone. Most institutions use an official form. Some may accept telephone calls, and others use computer systems.
- **The Purchase order (PO),** is the basic document controlling what is ordered. This document is sent to all parties involved in the transaction. The PO is also the primary document of the transaction for legal purposes. Therefore, the accuracy of this document is extremely important. A purchase order number is assigned to the PO and used by all parties (including the vendor) for tracking and billing purposes.
- **The receiving report,** documents that the goods or services have been received in good order and have been accepted as such. In the case where a vendor provides service at the institution, the vendor's service ticket may represent the only receiving report. However, when a part is received through the institution's warehouse, there is usually a formal receiving report that is checked by the warehouse staff against the PO. It should be rechecked by the clinical engineering staff to ensure accuracy. **Note:** Clinical engineers should not allow their staff to be held responsible for any transactions that they are not allowed to recheck and initial on a receiving report. However, once initialed, a receiving report should be used to generate payment to the vendor automatically.
- **The invoice,** is the only document generated by the vendor. This document serves to bill the institution for services rendered against a specific PO. As mentioned above, if accounting already has a signed receiving report, then the vendor should be paid with no delay. However, if this is not the case, the invoice should be forwarded to clinical engineering for verification of parts received or services performed before being paid. This allows the clinical engineer to ensure that things were done correctly before payment is made. (If this procedure is followed during the purchase of new equipment it will also serve to ensure that manuals and other accessories are received promptly.)
- **The statement,** is the final document. Most institutions provide to each department on a regular basis a statement of expenses paid. This report should be used to reconcile department records. Any expense variations should be investigated immediately. Timely review of variations resulting from parts not returned for credit is especially important because most vendors may not accept parts back beyond a certain period.

Most department heads regard a budget as, at best, a necessary evil. However, this attitude is inappropriate in a time of hospital budgetary constraints. A budget is a tool. To use a budget properly, it is necessary to plan ahead, to consider possible changes, and to be constantly aware of the actual cost of doing business. The savvy clinical engineer will develop a budget plan first and continually monitor the actual budget expenses compared to the plan. By understanding variances, the clinical engineer exercises a conscientious attitude toward budget control. This allows a common level of communication with administrators (who are more aware of a clinical engineering program's financial performance than of its technical performance) and further attempts to justify future activities (Steifel, 1987).

Monitoring Performance

The performance of a clinical engineering program depends upon two things: (1) the collective performance of staff members and (2) the individual performance of staff members. As one might expect these two factors are interdependent.

The JCAHO has developed a ten-step model for monitoring and evaluating hospital programs. This model defines a number of performance indicators, which include percentage of inspections performed, accuracy of documentation, turnaround time, and frequency of repeat repairs. Typically, these indicators are looked at only macroscopically, i.e., for the program as a whole. To generate positive change, one must look at these same indicators on a microscopic level (i.e., one staff member at a time). The employee performance systems now in use at most hospitals are criteria-based. This means that the performance of each staff member is tied to specific job functions. For clinical engineering staff, general performance criteria include inspections, repairs, documentation, vendor interaction, training, and department development. In addition to criteria-based standards, the clinical engineering staff may also have goal-related criteria as part of their performance standards. Goals can be related to such issues as financial performance or professional development (successful completion of the Certified Clinical Eengineer or Certified Biomedical Equipment Technician exam, for example). Under a performance management system, individual performance follows the same pathway as program performance. First, objective criteria should be established with threshold indicators. This activity is best done by a team composed of staff and management to promote consensus on the final product. Next, monitoring occurs. To achieve the best results, monitoring should be continual. Finally, evaluations are completed. However, contrary to traditional performance evaluation techniques, evaluation of the clinical engineering staff should be conducted regularly and at short intervals. This is not to say that every employee should be given a formal performance review each month. Rather, every employee should receive regular feedback on aspects of their performance. Thus, if productivity is calculated for the clinical engineering department on a monthly basis, then each technician should be given their productivity data at the same time. The same is true for mean time to repair, turnaround time, frequency of repeat repairs, timeliness or accuracy of submitted documentation, etc.

W. Edwards Demming's concept of **total quality management (TQM)** is probably the most exciting and important topic in American health-care today. The 14 Points towards quality management, which form the basis of this concept, provide a foundation on which to build. Demming's **continuous quality improvement (CQI)** regimen of **Plan → Do → Check → Act** is paramount for success. However, **TQM** is achievable macroscopically only if **CQI** is operating at a microscopic level. "*By reviewing individual performance with each staff member on an on-going basis, unfavorable trends can be quickly quantified, explored and resolved before the quality level of the entire program suffers. Equally, positive performance can be acknowledged and promoted so that it continues and extends to others*" (Brody, 1991).

SUMMARY

This chapter has presented a practitioner's perspective of the basic considerations that clinical engineers must be cognizant of to manage effectively the creation, development, daily operation, and growth of a clinical engineering program. From this perspective, the goal has been to provide practical insight into the ways in which the clinical engineer can make significant contributions to the overall mission of the hospital, which is the efficient and cost-effective delivery of health-care services.

EXERCISES

1. List the four basic questions to be asked at a hospital when preparing to set up a clinical engineering program.

2. When reviewing prior maintenance expenses, the clinical engineer should ask for a list of

   (a) line item budgets.
   (b) actual invoices.
   (c) report of payments.
   (d) expense code identifiers.

3. Given that BMET IIs get two weeks of vacation per year plus eight paid holidays and that they take two 15 minute breaks per day, how many hours per year is each technician available for work?

4. Which of the following is **Not** a direct maintenance expense?

   (a) The cost of service contracts.
   (b) The cost of technical personnel.
   (c) The cost of vendor provided services.
   (d) The cost of parts used during service.

5. "Success will only come to those who ________________ the right information to the right people."

6. "The ________________ approach should be the method of choice to integrate clinical engineering into a hospital."

7. You have just received a phone call from a service vendor who claims not to have been paid for services rendered. Explain what steps you would take to resolve this problem. List any assumptions made.

8. Develop two performance indicators for a clinical engineering program and explain how they would be monitored.

9. Develop two performance indicators for a clinical engineering technician and explain how they would be monitored.

10. List W. Edwards Demming's 14 Points towards Quality Management, and describe each one.

REFERENCES

AHA. "Maintenance Management for Medical Equipment," American Hospital Association, Chicago, IL, 1982.

AHA. "Maintenance Management for Medical Equipment," American Hospital Association, Chicago, IL, 1988.Bauld, T.J., III. "Productivity: Standard Terminology and Definitions," *J. Clin. Engin.*, 139–145, March/April 1987.

Baumeister, J., "Hospital Financial Audit of Medical Equipment Maintenance: A Case Study," *J. Clin. Engin.*, 197–201, May/June 1987.

Betts, W.F. "Using Productivity Measures in Clinical Engineering Departments," *Biomed. Instr. Technol.*, 120–127, March/April 1989.

Bouley, A.J. "Letter to the Editor," *Hospitals*, June 20, 1991.

Brody, M.S. "Reducing Maintenance Costs Through Increased Communications," *Proc. 23rd Ann. AAMI Meeting*, AAMI, Arlington, VA, 1988.

Brody, M.S. "A Simple Computerized Approach to Incorporate Individual Technician Productivity into a Quality Assurance Program," *Proc. 26th Ann. AAMI Meeting*, AAMI, Arlington, VA, 1991a.

Brody, M.S. "Letter to the Editor," *Hospitals*, June 20, 1991b.

Cohen, T. "The Cost of Biomedical Equipment Repair and Maintenance: Results of a Survey," *Medical Instrumentation*, 16:269–271, 1982.

Demming, W.E. "Out of the Crisis," MIT Press, Cambridge, MA, 1986.

Emergency Care Research Inst. "Health Devices Inspection and Preventive Maintenance System," ECRI, Plymouth Meeting, PA, 1984.

Furst, M. "Productivity and Cost Effectiveness of Clinical Engineering," *J. Clin. Engin.*, 105–113, March/April 1986.

Greene, R.J., and Nash, N.M. "Survey of Job Evaluation Practices," American Compensation Association, Scottsdale, AZ, 1989.

Greenstein, A.S., and Phillips, K.A. "Enhancing Clinical Engineering Credibility and Visability in a Medical Center," *Biomed. Instr. Technol.*, 283–285, July/August 1989.

Hard, R. "A Little Know-How Can Help Reduce Service Costs," *Hospitals*, 68, April 5, 1991.

Hasper, K., Jr. "Centralized Maintenance Responsibilities: A Case Study," *J. Clin. Engin.*, 191–206, May/June 1991.

JCAHO. "Implementing the 1989 JCAHO PTSM Standards: Case Studies," Joint Commission on the Accreditation of Healthcare Organizations, Chicago, IL, 1989.

JCAHO. "JCAHO 1990 Accreditation Manual for Hospitals," Joint Commission on the Accreditation of Healthcare Organizations, 1989.

Keil, O.R., and Camplin, C.R. "Quality Assurance," *J. Clin. Engin.*, 153–158, March/April 1987.

Lodge, D.A. "Productivity Efficiency and Effectiveness in the Management of Healthcare Technology: An Incentive Pay Proposal," *J. Clin. Engin.*, 29–34, January/February 1991.

Mahacheck, A.R. "Productivity Measurement: Taking the First Steps," *Biomed. Instr. Technol.*, 16–20, January/February 1989a.

Mahacheck, A.R. "The Clinical Engineering Budget," *Biomed. Instr. Technol.*, 276–282 July/August 1989b.

NMTA Associates. "National Position Evaluation Plan," NMTA Associates/Management Association of Illinois, Westchester, IL, 1980.

Pacela, A.F. "1989 Survey of Hospital Salaries and Job Responsibilities for Clinical Engineers and Biomedical Technicians," *J. Clin. Engin.*, 313–329, July/August 1989.

Pacela, A.F. "1990 Survey of Hospital Salaries and Job Responsibilities for Clinical Engineers and Biomedical Technicians," *J. Clin. Engin.*, 269–286, July/August 1990.

Pacela, A.F. "1991 Survey of Hospital Salaries and Job Responsibilities for Clinical Engineers and Biomedical Technicians," *J. Clin. Engin.*, 241–258, May/June 1991.

Steifel, R.H. "Use of A Spreadsheet to Develop and Track Budget Performance," *J. Clin. Engin.*, 133–137, March/April 1987.

Walton, M. "The Demming Management Method," Putnam Publishing Group, New York, 1986.

CHAPTER 9

COMPUTER SYSTEMS OF INTEREST TO CLINICAL ENGINEERS

Today, computer technology is involved in almost every facet of human activity, yet this technology is still considered to be in its infancy. This observation is especially true for the use of computer technologies in the clinical environment. Computers have essentially revolutionized the practice of medicine by:

- Providing completely new insights into the anatomy and physiology of the human organism through computerized imaging techniques.
- Facilitating patient surveillance and the delivery of controlled medication in intensive-care units.
- Assisting health professionals in various aspects of clinical decision making using advances in artificial intelligence technology.
- Optimizing the collection, retrieval and display of a wide range of patient-related information through automation of the clinical laboratories and development of hospital information systems (Jenkins, 1978; Bronzino, 1982; Anbar, 1987; Shortliffe et al., 1990).

As a result of these efforts, many of these medical computing systems:

- Provide clinicians with access to sophisticated and often widely dispersed resources.
- Simplify the assembly of patient-related data for review by all types of health-care professionals.
- Assist health-care professionals in making fundamental decisions about patient health-care strategies.

Patients are no longer dependent on the knowledge of a single physician, since up-to-date medical knowledge is now available via the nearest computer terminal. For example, the latest medical knowledge and literature have been automated into the *Index Medicus* by the **National Library of Medicine**. In the process, an entirely new discipline—"medical informatics"— has emerged to enhance the organized dissemination of, and access to this wealth of medical information (Kriewall and Long, 1991).

As already discussed in Chapter 1, a major emphasis of biomedical/clinical engineering activities has always been the development of medical instrumentation (such as advanced monitoring systems, transducers for clinical or laboratory use, and image enhancement devices for use in radiology). In recent years however, many of the new advanced medical devices and systems are essentially computer-based. This fact, coupled with the increasing responsibilities for the acquisition and modification of computer hardware and software in the hospital, has made it critical for clinical engineers to become familiar not only with advances in computer technology, but those computer applications which directly affect patient care and the management of medical technology.

In recent years, the medical computing systems of interest to clinical engineers have included the following:

- Clinical laboratory analysis.
- Acquisition of patient data.
- Establishment and maintenance of computer-based medical record and information retrieval systems.
- Automated patient monitoring.
- Diagnostic support systems, including artificial intelligence technology.
- Medical imaging.

This chapter, therefore, focuses on those medical computing applications which are of special interest to clinical engineers. Although it is not possible within the scope of this chapter to discuss each of the above-mentioned medical computing systems in great detail, they are so important to modern clinical engineering that each will be briefly examined. Furthermore, since the processing of information regarding equipment acquisition and maintenance information is of particular interest and importance to clinical engineering departments, the use of clinical emergency information-management systems to assist in such functions as the processing of work orders and service requests, the tracking medical of equipment inventory, and preventive maintenance scheduling will also be presented. However, before launching into specific computer applications, it is important to highlight some of the basic computer concepts that illustrate how computers manage to perform such a large variety of applications with essentially a few basic operative functions. With this in mind, let us review the main components of computer hardware, the different kinds of software, and some essential computer jargon.

BASIC COMPUTER CONCEPTS

Initially, the computer was designed as a tool to manipulate numbers and thus solve arithmetic problems. However, during its development, researchers recognized that any machine that can manipulate numbers can also manipulate any symbol that can be represented in numeric form. This feature is extremely important, for humans create, use, and manipulate many symbols that represent events and facts in the world about them. These symbols and the concepts they represent are essentially termed "information" (Bronzino, 1982).

A computer, then, is essentially an information-processing machine. It is a device capable of performing computations and making logical decisions at speeds much faster than are possible for their human counterparts. Modern computers range in size from the miniaturized microprocessors in hand-held calculators; to personal computers (PCs), which are small, relatively inexpensive, single-user machines; to the large main frames that are operated and maintained by professional computing personnel in national computer centers. However, regardless of their physical characteristics or applications, most computers have a common organizational structure. That is, a computer must accept information (in the form of instructions and data), store this information so that it can be retrieved as desired, perform calculations (and other manipulations) on the data, and provide the results of the computation process, all in a controllable fashion.Thus, to process information a machine must contain the following:

- The **input** of a computer accepts information entered by humans from various input devices for processing by other units in the machine.
- The **memory**, or storage unit, retains the information entered by the input device so that it is available to the processing units as needed. In addition, information that

has already been processed is stored here until it is placed into the appropriate output devices.

- The **central processing unit** (CPU), performs computations. It consists of two major components: the arithmetic and logic unit (ALU), and the control unit. The arithmetic and logic unit performs all the arithmetic calculations, such as addition, subtraction, multiplication, and division. These four operations are all used in a variety of ways to perform other calculations. In addition, the ALU can perform logical operations, such as comparing information entered from the input unit to information already stored in memory. The control unit, on the other hand, directs the overall functioning of all of the other units and controls the flow of information among them during the processing procedures. In turn, the instructions written into the machine in the form of a computer program control this unit.
- The **output unit** takes the information processed by the machine and displays it in various formats (tables, graphs, etc.) for review by humans.

Modern computing systems employ the latest advances in solid-state electronics to provide an extremely accurate, reliable, versatile, and high-speed tool. But how does this information-handling process actually take place? The answer to this question is necessary to provide some explanation of the internal operation of digital machines; from the machine language that enables the computer to enter and handle information, to the interaction of the various components that process this information in a manner prescribed by the operator.

The BINARY NUMBER SYSTEM

Digital computers are electronic devices capable of manipulating bits of information under the control of sequenced instructions stored within their memory. Electronic devices, of course, respond to electrical signals. Therefore, to enable these signals to represent information, recognizable codes that are easily and reliably deciphered within the device are necessary. In a digital computer these codes are based on the binary system, which uses two binary digits (1 and 0) so that one number (1) represents the presence of an electrical signal at a given time, and the other (0) denotes the absence of a signal. Binary signals then can represent both instructions and data; consequently, the binary number system provides the basic language of the digital computer.

We live in a decimal system. The selection of the base (in this case, ten) establishes the number of symbols (digits) available and the positional value each of the digits in any decimal number. The number 4,102, for example, is simply a convenient way of expressing the following sum:

$$
\begin{array}{rrcrcr}
 & 4 & \text{x} & 1000 & = & 4{,}000 \\
+ & 1 & \text{x} & 100 & = & 400 \\
+ & 0 & \text{x} & 10 & = & 0 \\
+ & 2 & \text{x} & 1 & = & \underline{2} \\
 & & & & & 4{,}102
\end{array}
$$

As can be seen, in the decimal system the positional values are increasing powers of the base ten, beginning with ten raised to the zero power ($10^0 = 1$).

Using the binary system, the process is same except that the base power is two, not ten. Counting in the binary system, then, is identical to counting in any other system except for the obvious inconvenience of running out of symbols more quickly. For example, consider the binary number 10110 represented in the following way:

$$
\begin{array}{lrcr}
 & 1 \times 2^4 & = & 16 \\
+ & 0 \times 2^3 & = & 0 \\
+ & 1 \times 2^2 & = & 4 \\
+ & 1 \times 2^1 & = & 2 \\
+ & 0 \times 2^0 & = & \underline{0} \\
 & & & 22
\end{array}
$$

Thus, the binary number 10110 represents the decimal number 22. In a similar manner, any binary number can be converted into its more familiar decimal equivalent.

The most elementary piece of information in the binary system is one binary digit, or *bit*. Note that the word *bit* is derived from *binary digit*. A group of eight bits is known as a *byte*. These two terms are used quite commonly and form an important part of computer jargon. The number of bits used to define a particular number or symbol is important for another reason: it defines or limits the number of possible arrangements of 1's and 0's, e.g., sixteen different meanings can be communicated using four bits. In general, if n bits are used, then 2^n meanings can be established. One of the most common computer codes involves the use of eight bits, thereby providing 256 possible meanings.

The octal system has eight as its base and operates in a similar manner. In this case, however, we can use eight symbols, zero to seven, and determine the potential value by using powers of eight. For example, The octal number $(201)_8$ can be converted to its decimal equivalent as follows:

$$
\begin{array}{lrcr}
 & 2 \times 8^2 & = & 128 \\
+ & 0 \times 8^1 & = & 0 \\
+ & 1 \times 8^0 & = & \underline{1} \\
 & & & 129
\end{array}
$$

Therefore, $(201)_8 = (129)_{10}$.

Any *number* can be represented in binary, octal, or decimal notation. In binary notation, however, large numbers require such a long string of symbols that they are often difficult to read. As a result, the bits used to represent the numbers are often assembled in succeeding groups of threes. For example, let the string 010110110100011 be grouped into the following subsets: 010 = 2, 110 = 6, 100 = 4, and 011 = 3. By placing these subsets in consecutive order we have $(26643)_8$; that is, we have generated a number in the octal system. In this way, the length of the string has been shortened three-fold, and the monotonous succession of 0's and 1's is relieved. Thus, an octal number is a short equivalent of a rather lengthy binary number. This feature is important because the conversion from binary to octal is far easier than the conversion from octal to decimal.

Since any decimal number can be converted to binary notation, this information can be entered into the computer and appropriate arithmetic operations can be performed within the machine, again by using binary notation. However, we do not deal solely with numbers; we also handle alphabetic information. In order for letters or certain characters to be properly interpreted and communicated to a machine that deals solely with long strings of 0's and 1's, it is necessary to develop the notion of *coding*: the code relates data to a fixed array of binary digits or bits so that the specific arrangement has only one meaning. The system of expressing decimal digits in an equivalent representation is known as *binary coded decimal* (BCD). An early BCD system developed by IBM, for example, represented the letters of the alphabet as shown in Table 9.1.

Table 9.1: BCD code letters of the alphabet.

A	110001	*J*	100001	*S*	010010
B	110010	*K*	100010	*T*	010011
C	110011	*L*	100000	*U*	010100
D	110100	*M*	100101	*V*	010101
E	110101	*N*	100101	*W*	010110
F	110110	*O*	100110	*X*	011000
G	110111	*P*	100111	*Z*	011001
H	1101000	*Q*	10000		
I	1101001	*R*	101001		

BINARY LOGIC: HARDWARE

Working with long string of 0's and 1's would be cumbersome for humans, but it is simple for the digital computer. Composed mostly of parts that are essentially on/off switches, machines are perfectly suited to binary computation. When a switch is open, it corresponds to the binary digit 0; closed, it stands for the digit 1. But how does the computer make sense of the binary numbers represented by its open and closed switches?

At the heart of this answer is the work of the gifted 19th century mathematician George Boole, who devised a system of algebra, or mathematical logic, that can reliably determine whether a statement is true or false. Since a Boolean proposition is either true or false, by using Boolean algebra there are only three logical functions needed to process true and false statements (or, in computer terms, 1's and 0's). These functions are **NOT, AND, OR**, and their operation can be readily duplicated today by inexpensive integrated circuits containing multiple electronic switches or transistors. These devices and the functions they represent are called **logic gates.** Incredible as it may seem, such gates can, in the proper combinations, perform all of the computer's high-speed prestidigitations.

The NOT function is the algebraic means of representing the logical complement of any other state. The NOT circuit is a very simple one because its response is the inverse of any input, such as *A*. The result of such an operation is the symbol $\bar{A}$, which means, "*not A*". The electronic device or "gate" that performs the NOT operation is called an **inverter** (Figure 9.1).

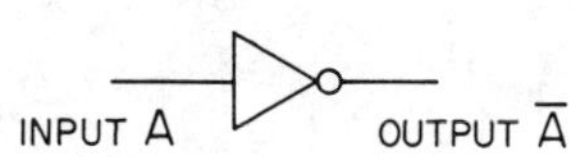

INPUT A	OUTPUT $\bar{A}$
0	1
1	0

Figure 9.1: Symbol and associated truth table for the NOT (inverter) operation.

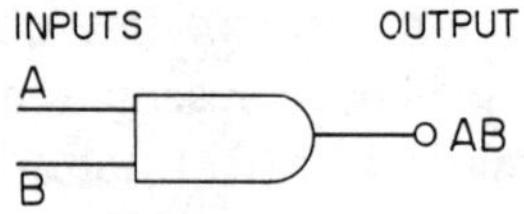

AND Truth Table

A	B	AB
0	0	0
0	1	0
1	0	0
1	1	1

Figure 9.2: Symbol and associated truth table for the AND operation.

AND and OR gates can be obtained in the following way. If two switches, A and B, are connected into a circuit, they can be arranged in two different ways, either in parallel or in series (Figure 9.2). In the series arrangement, both A and B must be closed (TRUE) for a circuit to be conductive. In Boolean terms, this would be expressed as $A \wedge B \equiv C$ where the symbol $\wedge$ is the logic symbol for AND and the symbol $\equiv$ means "identical to." Therefore, the AND operation of the two variables A and B is 0 if either A or $B = 0$, and 1 if both A and $B = 1$. Figure 9.2 shows the functional relationship between the input and output variables. This logical "truth table" as it is called, represents the switch closed, conductive, or the arithmetic expression $1 \times 1 = 1$. Therefore, the AND statement is the logical equivalent of multiplication and can be written as $A \bullet B \equiv C$.

In the parallel arrangement, on the other hand, A or B must be closed (true) to enable the circuit to conduct. In Boolean terms, this is written as $A \vee B \equiv C$. The OR operation of the variables A and B is 1 if both A and $B = 0$; and 1 if either A or $B = 1$. Figure 9.3 shows the symbol for the OR gate and illustrates the truth table describing the relationships between its input and output variables. As can be seen, when either A or $B = 1$, or both A and $B = 1$, the normal, or INCLUSIVE-OR gate gives 1. However, it will be recalled that in binary arithmetic $0 + 0 = 0$; $0 + 1 = 1$; and $1 + 1 = 0$, with carry = 1. To implement the carry operation, the normal OR gate is not used. Rather, the EXCLUSIVE-OR gate, illustrated in Figure 9.4, is employed and is the equivalent of binary addition. This function may be represented by $A \oplus B \equiv C$ with the $\oplus$ symbol representing the EXCLUSIVE-OR gate.

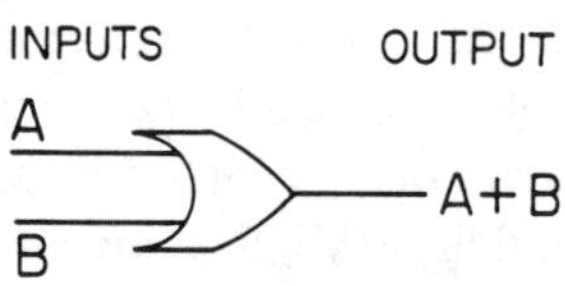

OR Truth Table

A	B	A+B
0	0	0
0	1	1
1	0	1
1	1	1

Figure 9.3: Symbol and associated truth table for the OR operation.

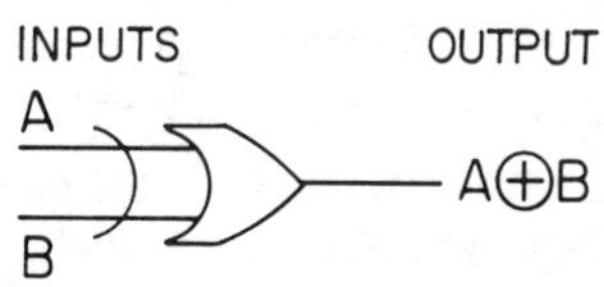

EXCLUSIVE-OR Truth Table

A	B	$A \oplus B$
0	0	0
0	1	1
1	0	1
1	1	0

Figure 9.4: Symbol and associated truth table for the EXCLUSIVE-OR operation.

The design of electronic hardware to treat electrical signals as if they represent numbers constitutes the **hardware** aspect of the computer. The design begins with a statement of the functions (such as arithmetic operations: addition, multiplication, and so on) to be performed and the constraints placed on these functions by the digital logic circuits. A computer, therefore, comprises a very large number of electronic components arranged to handle information (such as numbers) in binary format and to follow a sequence of instructions dealing with the processes to which this information will be subjected.

Computer Software

Digital computers have been defined as machines capable of manipulating bits of information under control of sequenced instructions called **computer programs** stored within the memory of the machine. These programs—the software—guide the computer through an orderly series of steps to assure that the information is processed according to a desired procedure specified by computer programmers. Since the computer requires instructions in order to solve specific problems, computer programming is the process of telling the computer when and how to utilize its various components to solve these problems.

The process of generating programs, or software packages, consists of a number of distinct steps: (1) defining the problem, (2) determining the operations that the computer must perform in a sequential manner to solve a particular problem, (3) selecting a "language" (or code) that is both appropriate and available for preparation of the program, (4) coding the operations to be performed in accordance with the rules of that language, and (5) entering the program into the computer's memory. Once it is in the memory of the machine, this stored program is processed to achieve the desired results whenever it is called into action.

Since computers can perform these programmed instructions at speeds thousands and even millions of times faster than humans, the resultant computations, although followed one after the other, are completed in a relatively short period of time. In recent years, considerable research has yielded interesting results in parallel programming, i.e., the use of multiple processors running in parallel which have greatly enhanced the ability of computers to solve complex problems.

Digital computers not only perform computations, but also have the ability to make logical decisions. This decision making-ability means that when the computer has two possible actions it can be programmed to select one or the other, depending on the outcome of a previous event. For example, consider the use of the computer to monitor the heart rate of a patient in an intensive care unit. In this case, one supplies the monitored heartbeat, and the computer calculates the heart rate. If the calculated value of the heart rate is above or below a preselected value, the computer activates an alarm to alert the attending staff that a problem exists. If the value is within preselected values (often called a **window**), the computer continues to calculate the heart rate over the next time period. The computer, however, must be programmed to decide whether to activate the alarm circuitry or simply to proceed with the monitoring process; it does not make this decision itself.

As previously discussed, computer programs are a sequence of instructions written for the computer in a language that the machine understands. Some programming languages are directly understandable by the computer, but others require additional translational steps. Although hundreds of computer languages are in use today, they all basically fall into one of three categories:

1. Machine languages.
2. Assembly languages.
3. High-level languages.

Machine language is the natural language of a particular computer. It is closely related to the actual construction of the digital logic circuits (discussed previously) within the machine. Consequently, a machine language instruction generally consists of a code in binary notation (long strings of 1's and 0's) that directs the computer via the logic gates to perform some specific operation, such as add, subtract, store, read, or write. As a result, any computer can directly understand the machine language developed for it. However, machine languages are extremely machine dependent: each computer has its own machine language. Consequently, programmers must be familiar with the basic set of instructions inherent to each machine before they can begin to communicate with it. Coding a program in machine language is difficult. Therefore, although machine languages provide a means to communicate directly with the machine, they are usually inconvenient for the majority of human operators who do not have a thorough knowledge of the computer.

Initially, machine languages were the only ones available. Therefore, anyone who wanted to work with a particular computer had to learn the special language of that machine. As a result, even a simple problem in arithmetic represented a major problem in programming. Consequently, other approaches became necessary. The first simplification was the development of symbolic languages, or mnemonics. Nearly everyone uses mnemonic symbols as a quick, easy-to-remember shorthand for longer expressions. For baseball fans, K for "strikeout" and BB for "base on balls" are familiar examples. Equally common are such symbols as RN for registered nurse, NIH for National Institute of Health, and DOD for Department of Defense. Using this concept, computer programmers developed their own shorthand codes that enabled them to write instructions in alphabetic symbols. These symbols were easier to remember than their binary equivalents in machine language, and thus significantly reduced the time necessary to program a problem.

Languages consisting of these English-like abbreviations are called **assembly languages.** In this type of language, all operation codes have a mnemonic designation, and all machine addresses and other operands in the instruction are written with symbolic notation. As an example, the letters LA, instead of a long string of ones and zeros, can represent the program instruction to load the address (i.e., location of data or instruction) into the computer's memory, and ADD can tell the computer to add two operands specified in the other portion of the instruction [using symbolic labels and instruction mnemonics, one can create the simple program in Table 9.2 to calculate the sum of two numbers, $D = A + B$].

Table 9.2: Assembler language coding form.

Location	Operation	Operand 1	Operand 2	Comments
BEGIN	MOVE	*D*	*A*	Move *A* to *D*
	ADD	*D*	*B*	Add *B* to *D*
	STOP			End of Program
A:	(value of *A*)			
B:	(value of *B*)			
D:	(value of *D*)			

However, before the computer can use this program, it must translate these symbolic instructions into machine language form. As a result, computer programs called assemblers were developed to read and translate assembler language programs to object programs in machine code. Note that in the program in Table 9.2 symbolic names designate the address or location used to store data (such as the values of *A* and *B*) or the results. Address values must somehow be assigned for them. The advantage of the assembler is that it can do this automatically for the programmer. As the assembler encounters each of these symbolic locations, it assigns it to a particular location. Therefore, this type of language helps the programmer to specify exact memory locations for the data and for the operations to be conducted. However, although this type of program does relieve the programmer of many intricate coding details, it still requires an intimated knowledge of the computer.

Macroinstructions were another big step forward. With a macroinstruction, the programmer can, with one statement, cause the computer to go through a long sequence of previously written steps. These are used for functions that keep recurring in any computer program. For example, with one macroinstruction to read a record stored in memory, the computer automatically goes through the many individual steps required, and the programmer does not have to write out each step.

Technology improved and computer speed increased so that internal processing of an instruction took only millionths of a second. Higher-level languages, along with appropriate language translation programs called compilers or interpreters, were developed to do just that, speeding up the process of programming computers significantly. **Higher-level languages** permit instructions to be written in a manner closely resembling English and contain commonly used mathematical notations such as multiply, square root, etc. As a result, these languages are much more desirable from a programming standpoint than other types of computer languages; they are easy to learn and easy to use. Although they sacrifice speed, computer time, and computer memory, they do allow ease of operation and provide extremely valuable diagnostic services (such as being able to debug the program as it is being written), which more than offset the disadvantages. A number of languages, such as **FORTRAN, PASCAL, C, COBOL, MUMPS,** and **LISP,** have been developed to permit the operator to generate rather useful and complex programs without understanding the internal operations of the computer. As a result of the advances in these higher-level languages, computer users now have a wide variety of programming aids that they can tailor to their individual needs.

THE MICROCOMPUTER

In recent years, the size and shape of the digital computer have changed as a result of the advances in solid-state electronics that preceded the development of **microprocessors,** which are essentially integrated circuits (ICs) impressed on small silicon chips possessing enormous computing capacity. These microprocessors, hooked to input/output devices and additional memory, constitute the **microcomputer**. Figure 9.5 illustrates the typical functional organization or architecture of a microcomputer. Referring to the initial definition, a microcomputer system is a digital computer containing the basic components of a computer: (1) the input unit, (2) the control and arithmetic units contained within the microprocessor, (3) the memory unit, and (4) the output unit. It is classed as a microcomputer only because of its small size and low cost. The microprocessor generally forms the central processing unit (CPU) section of a microcomputer system and regulates all the units of the system by control lines.

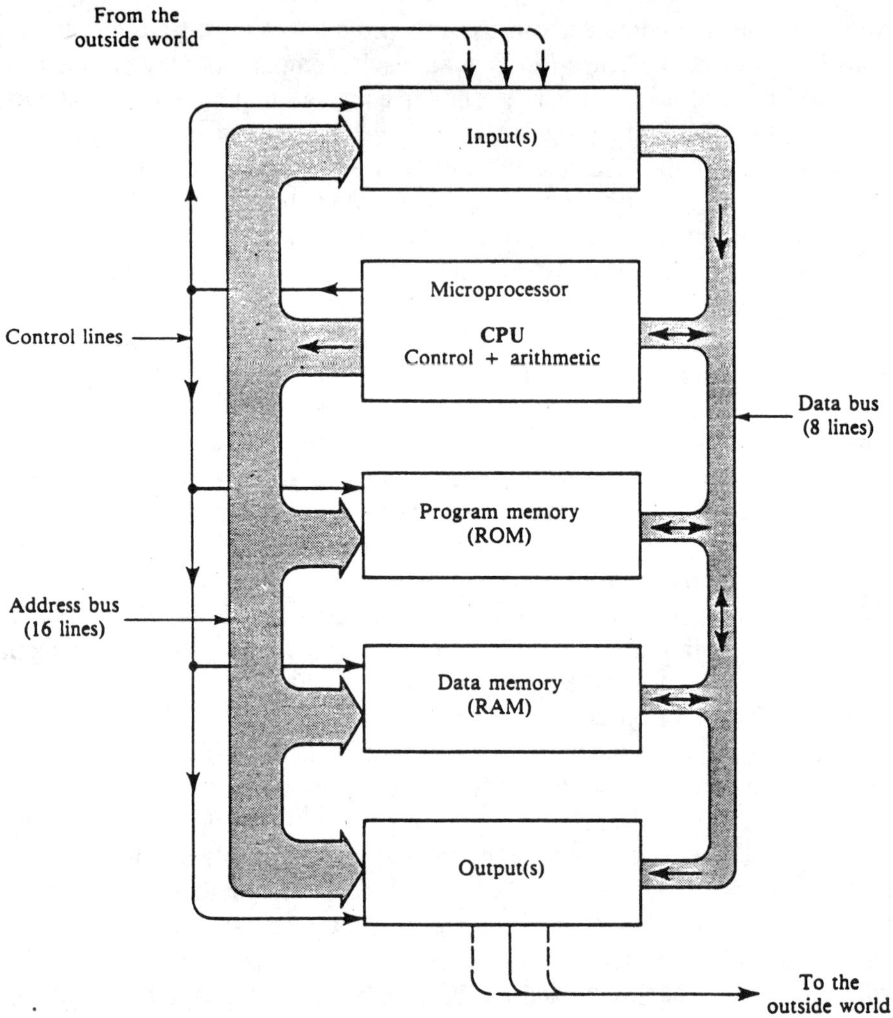

Figure 9.5: Schematic diagram of the organization of a microcomputer.

Besides the control lines, the **address bus** (the sixteen conductors in Figure 9.5) selects a certain memory location, input port, or output port. The **data bus** (the eight parallel conductors in figure 9.5) on the right is a two-way path for transferring data in and out of the microprocessor unit. It is important to note that the microprocessor unit (MPU) can send data to or receive data from memory using the data bus.

Programs can be stored permanently by placing them in a device known as **read-only memory** (ROM). Data of a temporary nature are usually stored in an IC device called a **read/write memory** (RWM). In common practice, the read/write memory is referred to as **random-access memory** (RAM). The RAM and ROM sections of memory are usually shown as separate units. Advances in semi-conductor technology have made it possible for memory units to be quite large and relatively inexpensive; for example, a 640K (1K = 2^{10} or 1024 bytes) personal computer can store 655,360 bytes of information.

MEMORY STORAGE AND INPUT/OUTPUT (I/O) DEVICES

In the context of electronics, **memory** refers to a device for storing digital information. The most widely used digital memories are read/write memories that perform read and write operations at an identical or similar rate. Important characteristics include storage capacity, cost per bit, reliability, speed of operation (defined in terms of access time), cycle time, and data-transfer rate. Access time is simply the time required to read or write at any storage location. Some memories, such as RAMs, have the same access time to any storage location, whereas serial-access and block-access memories have access times that depend on the storage location selected. Cycle time, on the other hand, is the specified minimum period of time random-access memories can complete a read/write operation, and data-transfer rate is the speed at which information is transferred to or from sequential storage locations.

Typically, programs and data must persist over long periods so that they can be reused. They are stored in the less expensive auxiliary memory provided by peripheral storage devices and are loaded into working memory when needed. Conceptually, auxiliary memory can be divided into two types: active and archival storage. Active storage is used to store data with long-term validity (for example, the medical record of a patient who currently is being treated within the hospital that may need to be retrieved with little delay (in a few seconds or less). Archival storage, on the other hand, is used to store data for documentation or legal purposes (Perreault and Wiederhold, 1990).

Currently, magnetic disks (i.e., hard or floppy) are the most common media for active storage. Each magnetic disk is a round, flat plate of material that can accept and store magnetic charge. The disk spins beneath a read/write head, much like a phonograph record spinning beneath a needle. As the disk spins, data are stored by the read/write head, which places a sequence of magnetic charges on the disk's surface along circular tracks. Similarly, the read/write head reads data by detecting the presence or absence of charge along the tracks. A disk unit consists of one or more disks—either fixed or removable, a drive system to rotate the disk, a movable read/write head to access the data, and a mechanism to position the read/write head over the surface of the disk.

Magnetic disks (designated as either hard or floppy) are less expensive than main memory, but data retrieval from them is much slower. Whereas the CPU can quickly access any data element in RAM by addressing the memory location directly, it must access externally stores data in two time-consuming steps: first, it must mechanically position the read/write head over the track where the data are stored, then it must search through the tracks sequentially, following the track as the disk rotates. Once the read/write head has been positioned correctly, blocks of data can be transferred rapidly. While data in working memory can be accessed in microseconds, access times for data stored on disk can reach several tenths of a second.

The most common medium for archival storage is magnetic tape, a ribbon of plastic covered with material that can accept and store magnetic charge. Like the disk drive, a tape drive has a read/write head that places or detects magnetic charges along the tracks of the tape. Magnetic tape is currently the least expensive means of storing archival data, but retrieval of archived data is slow. A computer operator must locate the tape and physically mount it on the tape drive, a procedure that can produce delays of minutes or hours. The tape must then be scanned linearly from the beginning until the information is located.

Optical storage is a relatively new technology that is growing rapidly in popularity. The main advantage to the use of optical disks is that huge amounts of data can be stored in a compact manner—the high wavelength of light permits a much higher density of data-carrying spots on the surface of the disk than can be achieved on magnetic media. Compact disk read/only/memory (CD/ROM) stores prerecorded information, which is read by a finely focused semiconductor laser that detects reflections from the disk. Such compact disks have become a common medium for recording and playing music. The first medical applications of optical-disk technology have been the storage of large bodies of reference material.

The choice of storage medium has a major impact on the performance and cost of a computer system. Data that are needed rapidly must be kept in more expensive, active storage (for example, hard disks). Less time-critical data can be archived on less expensive media (for example magnetic tapes or floppy disks). Because data often have to be shared, the designer must consider who will be expected to read the data, and how the data will be read. Devices that can handle standard tapes or floppy disks allow sharing of data among sites; the data are copied and are physically transported to a destination with a compatible drive. The compatibility of storage devices is less important when computers are linked into communication networks that can transport data from site to site by wire rather than by the physical movement of a storage medium.

Various input/output devices permit users to communicate directly with the computer and to view the results of the calculations it performs. The input devices transfer the information from its original form, usually a handwritten, typed, or printed document, into machine-readable form. For this purpose, video display terminals (VDTs) with associated keyboards act as primary input for data or the program. For example, during medical-history taking at a screening clinic, the patient responds directly to questions displayed at a console terminal. After the patient responds, the computer files the response and goes on to the next question. In analyzing information obtained from monitoring or laboratory equipment, analog electrical signals are converted into the appropriate digital format by analog-to-digital converters (ADCs). Optical scanners are also available to digitize a typed document, drawing, or image. Printers and teletypewriters are the most commonly used output devices, but once again it is possible to convert a sequence of digital numbers into an analog signal by means of a digital-to-analog converter (DAC) and to have the electrical signal control external devices (such as humidifiers or air conditioners that control the room environment). Thus, computers can communicate directly with other machines to achieve a specific objective (such as regulating the air temperature and humidity of incubators to ensure that premature infants have an appropriate environment).

DATA ACQUISITION AND SIGNAL PROCESSING

A prominent theme of biomedical engineering applications involves the real-time acquisition of data directly from instruments by the computer. Direct acquisition of data avoids the need for people to measure, encode, and enter the data manually. In these applications, the analog electrical signals are sampled periodically and converted to digital representation for storage and processing.

Two parameters determine how closely the digital data represent the original analog signal: the precision with which the signal is recorded and the frequency with which the signal is sampled. "Precision" describes the degree of accuracy with which a sample observation of the signal is made. It is determined by the number of bits used to represent the signal and their correctness; the more bits, the greater the number of levels that can be distinguished. Precision also is limited by the accuracy of the equipment that converts and transmits the signal. Ranging and calibration of the instruments, either manually or automatically, is necessary for signals to be represented with as much precision as possible, since improper ranging will result in the loss of information. For example, a change in a signal that varies between 0.1 and 0.2 volts will be undetectable if the instrument has been set to record changes between 0.0 and 1.0 in 0.25-volt increments.

The sampling rate is the second parameter that affects the correspondence between an analog signal and its digital representation. A sampling rate that is too low will produce poor representation. On the other hand, oversampling increases the expense of processing and storing data. According to the sampling theorem, to accurately represent any signal, you need to sample at least twice as frequently as the highest frequency component needed from the signal. This rate is called the "Nyquist frequency."

Another aspect of signal quality is the amount of "noise" in the signal (i.e., the component of the acquired data that is not due to the specific phenomenon being measured). A primary source of noise is the electrical or magnetic signals produced by nearby devices and power lines. Three techniques, often used in combination, minimize the amount of noise in a signal (Perreault and Wiederhold, 1990):

- Shielding, isolation, and grounding of cables and instruments carrying analog signals reduce electrical interference. The use of glass fiber optic cables eliminates interference from electrical machinery, because optical signals are not affected by magnetic fields.
- Since digital transmission of signals is inherently noise-free, (i.e., interference rarely is great enough to change a 1 value to a 0 value, or vice versa), conversion of analog signals to digital form provides the most robust transmission. The nearer the source the conversion occurs, the more effective this technique is. Placement of digital signal processing (DSP) chip near the signal source is now the most common way to achieve such a conversion.
- Filtering algorithms can also be used to reduce the effect of noise. Usually, these algorithms are applied to the data stored in memory. Since noise has a relatively random pattern, repetitive signals, such as an ECG, can be integrated over several cycles reducing the effects of random noise. Noise components of the signal can thus, be filtered out.

COMPUTER NETWORKS

During the past decade, increased emphasis has been placed on the development of distributed computer networks. Distribution offers flexibility in choice of software and hardware in the laboratory, pharmacy, the intensive-care unit, the business office, and so on. Technology is now available to allow linking of independent computers in networks. The most common method for communicating computer information is to use the telephone lines. A modem (modulator-demodulator) converts the digital data generated by a keyboard or a computer to analog signals within voice range. It then transmits the tones over the telephone lines—a conversion between computers occurs. At the receiving end, the tones are reconverted to the original digital signals by another modem.

Different modems support different "baud rates," or rates of information transfer. The standard transmission rate for data entry supports three-hundred baud, which is an information transfer rate equivalent to 300 bits per second (bps), or 30 characters per second. This speed is adequate for transmitting data as they are typed, but too slow for input of scanned documents or for transmitting results as they are reproduced by a computer. For these purposes, modems of at least twelve-hundred baud are needed for typed data, and to communicate information to VDTs, a baud rate of twenty-four hundred to ninety-six hundred is desirable. Since data signals become unacceptably noisy at high baud rates, dedicated telephone lines suitable for transmitting data are available. Another approach that can be more advantageous for an institution is to invest in its own local-area network (LAN), which simplifies the sharing of resources—data, software, and equipment—among multiple users.

One type of LAN is the "private branch exchange" (PBX), an extension of an organization's internal telephone system in which the telephone wires are used to transfer both voice signals and data. The exchange of data within a LAN is controlled by a set of rules; a network protocol which specifies how messages are prepared and transmitted electronically. If two people are to communicate effectively, they must agree on the meaning of the words they are using, the style of the interaction (lecture versus conversation), a procedure for handling interruptions, and so on. The protocol of the LAN settles these issues at the level of computer communications. For example, the Ethernet protocol developed jointly by Xerox, Intel, and Digital Equipment Corporation (DEC) is now an Institute of Electrical and Electronics Engineers (IEEE) standard that has been widely adopted in the private sector.

Several LANs can be interconnected to allow communication among machines that are more widely dispersed geographically or that are owned by separate institutions. In this way, two independent computer systems or connected networks can send messages through special computers that reside on both networks. The linking of LANs to wide-area networks such as BITNET make it possible to share data and resources among independent users and institutions around the world. Network users can access shared patient data (such as a hospital's medical records) or nationwide data bases (such as the bibliographic data bases of scientific literature citations). They can read electronic bulletin boards to obtain information and programs, and they can exchange mail electronically.

DATA BASE SYSTEMS

As previously mentioned, effective computer use requires timely access to large volumes of data from diverse sources. With the use of data base management software techniques, computers can provide the means for organizing and accessing vast amounts of data, such as providing summaries of laboratory results or scheduling preventive maintenance. Data base technology, therefore, enhances the integration and organization of data and assists users with data entry, storage, and retrieval of not only individual data elements but also their meanings and their relationships with other data.

Data bases are collections of data typically organized into fields, records, and files. The field is the most primitive element; each field represents one data element. For example, the data base of a hospital information system typically has fields for the patient's identification number, name, date of birth, gender, admission rate admitting diagnosis, and so on. Fields are grouped together to form records. Each record is uniquely identified by one or more key fields—for example, patient-identification number and observation time. Records that contain similar information are grouped in files. In addition to files related to patients (diagnoses, treatment, and drug therapies), the data base of a hospital information system (HIS) will have separate files containing information about charges and payments, personnel and payroll, inventory, and so on.

Once programmers know the structure and the format of a data file, programs can be written to access the data directly. A data base-management system (DBMS) is an integrated set of programs created to help users. Typically, users retrieve data from a data base in one of two ways. They query the data base directly using query language such as Structured Query Language (SQL) to extract information in an *ad hoc* fashion—for example, to retrieve the records of all male hypertensive patients aged 45 to 64 years for inclusion in a retrospective study. Thus, DBMS's often provide an alternative, simpler means for formulating such queries, called report generation. Users specify their data requests on the input screen of the report generator program. The report generator then produces the actual query program using information stored in the schema (Perreault and Wiederhold, 1990).

The computer, with all its hardware, software, and information-processing capabilities, must still be applied to specific tasks to achieve any useful purpose. Many of these applications have changed the organizations that use them, sometimes dramatically, more often subtly. In the health-care field, these applications are increasing at an incredible rate and will change the very nature of health-care delivery in the future. It is impossible here to review all the possible computer applications in medicine; consequently, we will focus our attention on those applications that are of particular interest to clinical engineers.

COMPUTERS IN THE CLINICAL LABORATORY

The primary information required for any clinical decision consists of the medical data collected during the care of patients. These data are often processed in clinical laboratories that have historically provided the chemical, hematological, microbiological, and blood banking services for hospitalized patients and outpatients (Williams, 1975). The traditional organization of clinical laboratories includes the disciplines of hematology, chemistry, and microbiology; the breakdown of activities within these disciplines is as follows (Martinek, 1972):

- **Hematology**: which is concerned primarily with monitoring the activity of a single physiological process, i.e., the formation and development of erythrocytes (red blood cells).
- **Clinical Chemistry**: which is based on the technical science of chemistry and is oriented primarily to the application of clinical methods without regard for any specific physiological system or anatomic group of organs or diseases. According to the **International Federation of Clinical Chemistry**, clinical chemistry encompasses the study of the chemical aspects of human life in health and illness and the application of chemical laboratory methods of diagnosis, control of treatment, and prevention of disease.
- **Clinical Microbiology**: which includes bacteriology, serology, immunology, virology, and other related disciplines, is concerned primarily with the detection of a large number of extraneous biological agents (the microbes). In addition, it involves blood bank operations limited to the collection and preservation of blood and its characterization for compatibility and therapeutic use.

The activities within clinical laboratories are primarily concerned with providing information regarding the presence of any "pathological" condition. If physiology is defined as the study of the normal function of cells, tissues, and organs, then pathology is the study of alterations in the human body that are induced by disease. The various laboratory procedures (which include chemical tests, microscopic examinations, tissue cultures, and the like conducted within the clinical laboratory) are vital if the appropriate health professionals are to properly diagnose and monitor the course of a particular disease. To be of clinical value, this information must be accurate, easily accessible, and processed as rapidly as possible.

Today's clinical laboratory has the primary function of obtaining medical data about a given patient for review by the attending physician. To accomplish this task, the laboratory must collect samples, process tests, report the results, and store all the relevant data collected on each patient. The performance of these steps by manual methods has become increasingly difficult as the type of determinations have grown in complexity as well as volume. In 1960, for example, clinical laboratories had an armamentarium limited to twelve or so different biochemical tests (Dickson, 1969), whereas today more than four hundred different tests are available. These tests range from a rather simple physical measurement of specific gravity to such sophisticated techniques as atomic absorption spectrophotometry. The number of such tests conducted each year has also grown at an ever-increasing rate, reaching the ten-billion mark by the mid-1980s (approximately fifty tests per year for each person in the United States). These staggering numbers illustrate the importance of medical test data in the treatment of patients (Bronzino et al., 1990).

Over the years a number of extremely successful systems have evolved to handle this type of information. In the most recent systems, microcomputers have been directly interfaced with a wide variety of laboratory instruments for on-line analysis of data. As computer technology continues to become less expensive and more flexible, computerization of the clinical laboratory will require that clinical engineers as well as laboratory personnel become involved in the conceptual planning of the computerized systems being designed for a particular laboratory. One way to view the clinical laboratory is to consider the following two levels of potential computerization:

1. The instrumental/process control level (IPC).
2. The management level: use of the central laboratory computer (CLC).

This division reflects a distinction between decentralized autonomy (which increases processing efficiency within a unit) and central regulation (which promotes patient-oriented integration of data from a variety of sources). To achieve a successful clinical laboratory system, a balance between these two levels should be obtained.

The Instrument Level

The first level, the IPC concept, consists of a set of computers or simple processors, each characterized by (1) inputs that are specimens and associated identification data, and (2) digital outputs that represent results, analytic conditions, and associated identification data. Typically, equipment such as sequential multiple analyzers and Coulter counters fall into this category, and their high-volume activity makes computerization quite attractive.

The reliability of the analytic results and the capture of all data that emerge from these devices are still important concerns in selecting computer techniques to automate these devices. More important, however, the IPC concept emphasizes:

- The modularity and pseudoindependence of individual IPC units.
- Uniformity in data protocols.
- Local control of analytic conditions where the computation process is sufficiently understood and methods are accurate, thereby ensuring confidence in results.
- The addition or modification of laboratory instrumentation without major interruption of overall system operation.

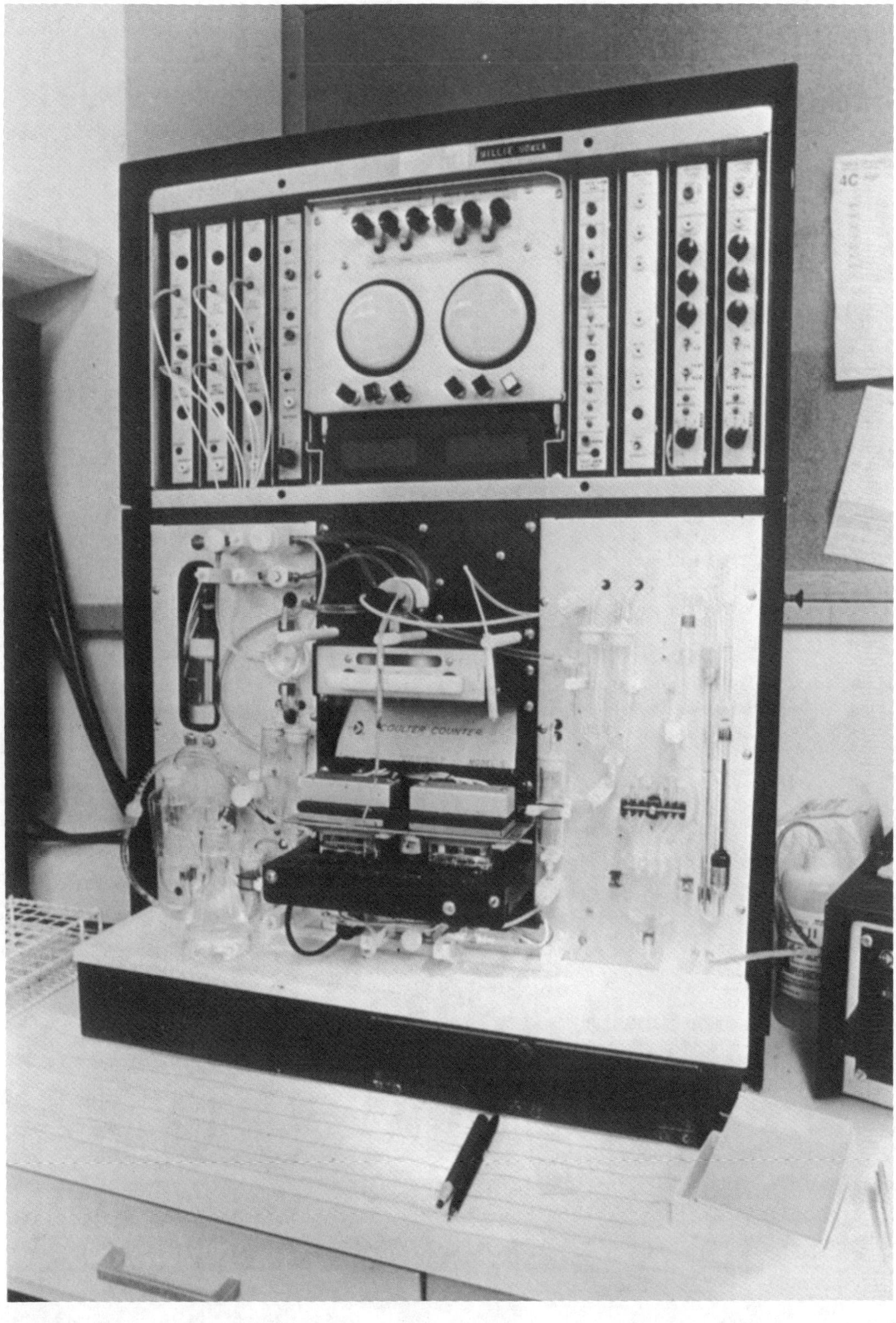

Figure 9.6: The Coulter counter.

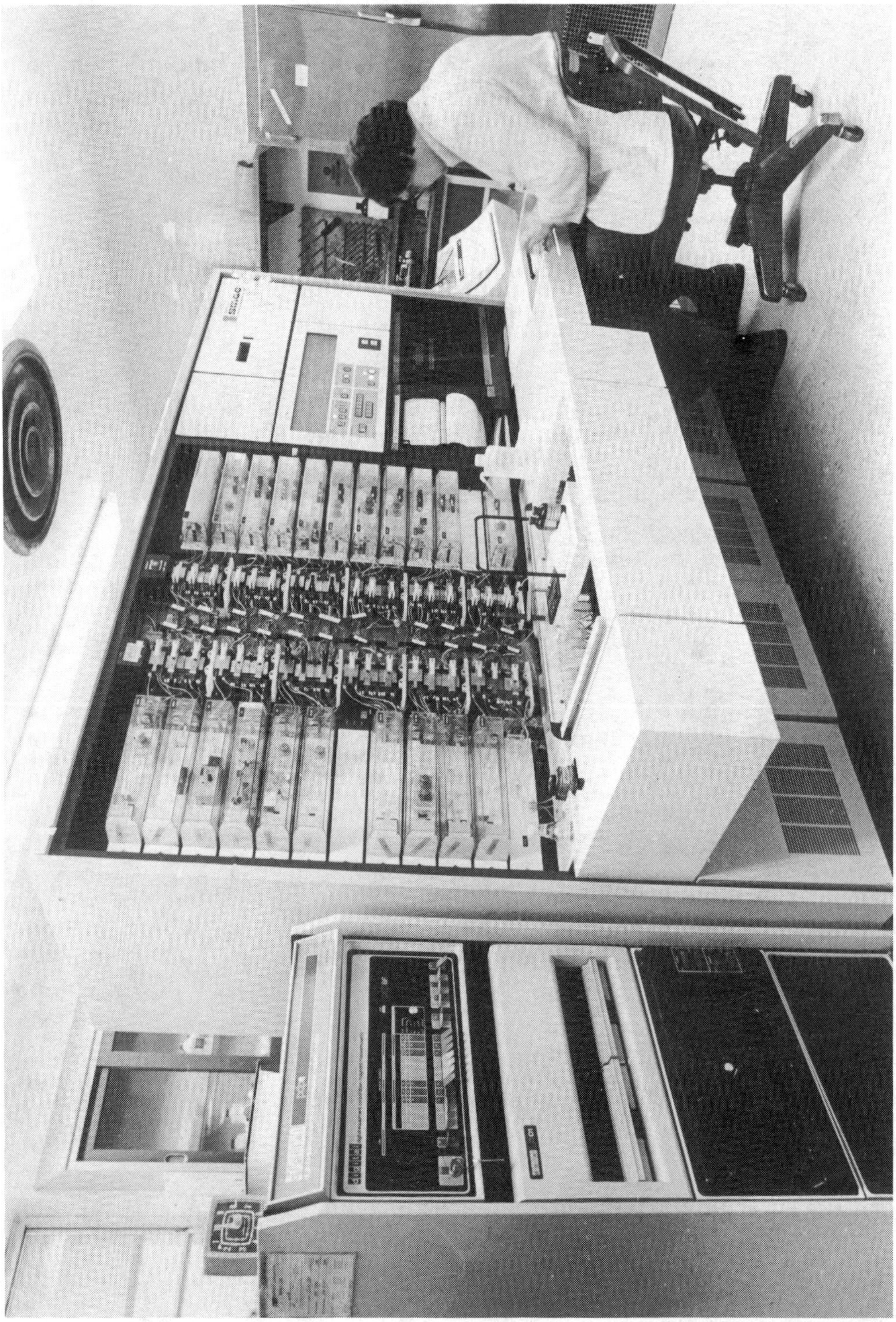

Figure 9.7: Photograph of the sequential multiple analysis plus computer (SMAC).

At the individual instrument level computerization can be made cost-effective. The program to run a Coulter counter (Figure 9.6), for example, can be essentially the same anywhere. The differences between such instrumental programs are at the input (that is, specimen identification data) and output (for example, communications protocol peculiar to the local installation) levels. Thus, each device may be designed, constructed, and programmed independently to perform its particular function.

Additionally, if the data obtained from the clinical laboratory can be combined with information pertaining to each patient, it becomes possible to generate "patient records." With this in mind, several of the presently available automatic analyzers now include small built-in computers that allow computations to be carried out and improve data presentation. One such device is the sequential multiple analysis plus computer (**SMAC**) system. The **SMAC** system (Figure 9.7) was a direct result of further development of the continuous-flow systems in which samples, separated by air bubbles, are distributed to different channels, dialyzed and heated, measured and recorded. In the **SMAC** system, however, the computer is involved in virtually every phase of system operation. For example, the computer calibrates each channel at preselected intervals, monitors all channels and modules, aids in troubleshooting, identifies samples, calculates data, and reports results. The **SMAC** system is an excellent example of a computerized laboratory instrument.

As more and more microprocessor-based instruments are introduced into the clinical laboratories it becomes possible to interface each of these with a central computer for data processing and to integrate specific test results with other pertinent patient information. Such an approach would certainly help laboratories perform their managerial functions.

The Management Level

Use of a Central Laboratory Computer (CLC). In general, the incorporation of a computerized management system permits two different functions to be accomplished. The first concerns primarily the control and integration of various laboratory instruments to transfer data processed directly from the various analytic devices into a computerized patient record. The second deals with the clerical functions of the laboratory, for example, recording, verifying, and reporting medical data, and with linking the data collected within the laboratory to other data banks. [NOTE: This concept also applies to clinical engineering management systems which will be discussed later in this chapter.]

In the first case, a CLC can be used to "call" an instrument by presenting it with an appropriate identified specimen or reference standard. The analytic device performs its tests, computes the results, and outputs a string of data in appropriate digital format. In this type of modular system, each determination is performed by a specific instrument that is specifically adapted to its own particular task and contains a digital interface, buffer, and controller. These are, *vis-à-vis* the analysis, specifically adapted to the procedure, its calibration, and the anticipated vagaries of analytic conditions. The output, on the other hand, consists of a small series of standard-length digital words that represent the result, identification, and any other parameterization data for each determination. Such output is delivered to the CLC for final processing and storage.

The integration of medical data from different laboratory instruments involves not only hardware aspects but software complexities required to properly integrate each instrument. Each device must give its data to the main computer before the data are replaced by new data. Some instruments may have more data-items per second than other instruments.

The computer is in the middle of the information exchange process, continually integrating these instruments;

> "*. . . all right number 4, tell me what you have; is that all? O.K. now number 5; is that all? O.K. now number 6—everyone wait a minute—I've finally got to talk to number 1 . . .*" and so forth.

Standardized digital circuits and connector "buses" make the task of getting the correct signals to flow more easily. Interfacing the instrumentation in the clinical laboratory in this way results in the creation of a single, overall computerized system.

In the second case, the data collected from the various analytical instruments within the clinical laboratory can be linked to other medical data bases. Figure 9.8 illustrates such a connection with the "HELP" computer system which combines clinical data from many different laboratories into one integrated data base related to the patient's health status. These data can also be used to generate reports regarding such information as volume, status, and the number of abnormal results for each of the tests conducted in the laboratory.

Available systems, however, represent only the beginning. The benefits of today's Laboratory Information Systems (LIS) derive from these systems' ability to facilitate information flow both within the laboratory and between the laboratory and the health-care personnel using the laboratory's services. Currently, LIS's are used primarily for data collection, record keeping, and process control, although more sophisticated patient-care applications are possible and some interpretive systems are being developed (Smith and Svirbely, 1990). In general, major developments will come only through the introduction of new instruments capable of detecting minute amounts of biological compounds and the incorporation of data-processing equipment and techniques designed to provide automated analysis. There is no need, however, for a large computer in most laboratories. Personal computer-based systems (PCs) have been developed that can easily assemble and accumulate one day's laboratory data at a cost considerably less than that of large machines.

This process is underway. As we move toward the end of the twentieth century, advances in medical computer technology will continue to change many instruments and the methodologies used in the clinical laboratory; with further emphasis on the following:

- Upgrading the data-handling processes within these laboratories.
- More automatic collation of test results on the same patient from all over the laboratory.
- More instrument self-monitored fault-finding and operator alerts.
- Greater availability of ongoing automatic quality-control data.
- Widespread use of effective patient and sample identification systems.

In fact, entire clinical laboratories will shortly be designed around a CLC. In the process, all analytical instruments will become computer accessories, interconnected with a central computer that will collate results for a patient from several instruments and call for the tests to be performed in logical order. The current processes used by laboratories, and others not yet even conceived of will be carried out by cheaper, faster, smaller, and more powerful computers.

Unfortunately, the development of computer systems to support other laboratories, such as microbiology and pathology, has proceeded more slowly than for the chemistry and hematology laboratories.

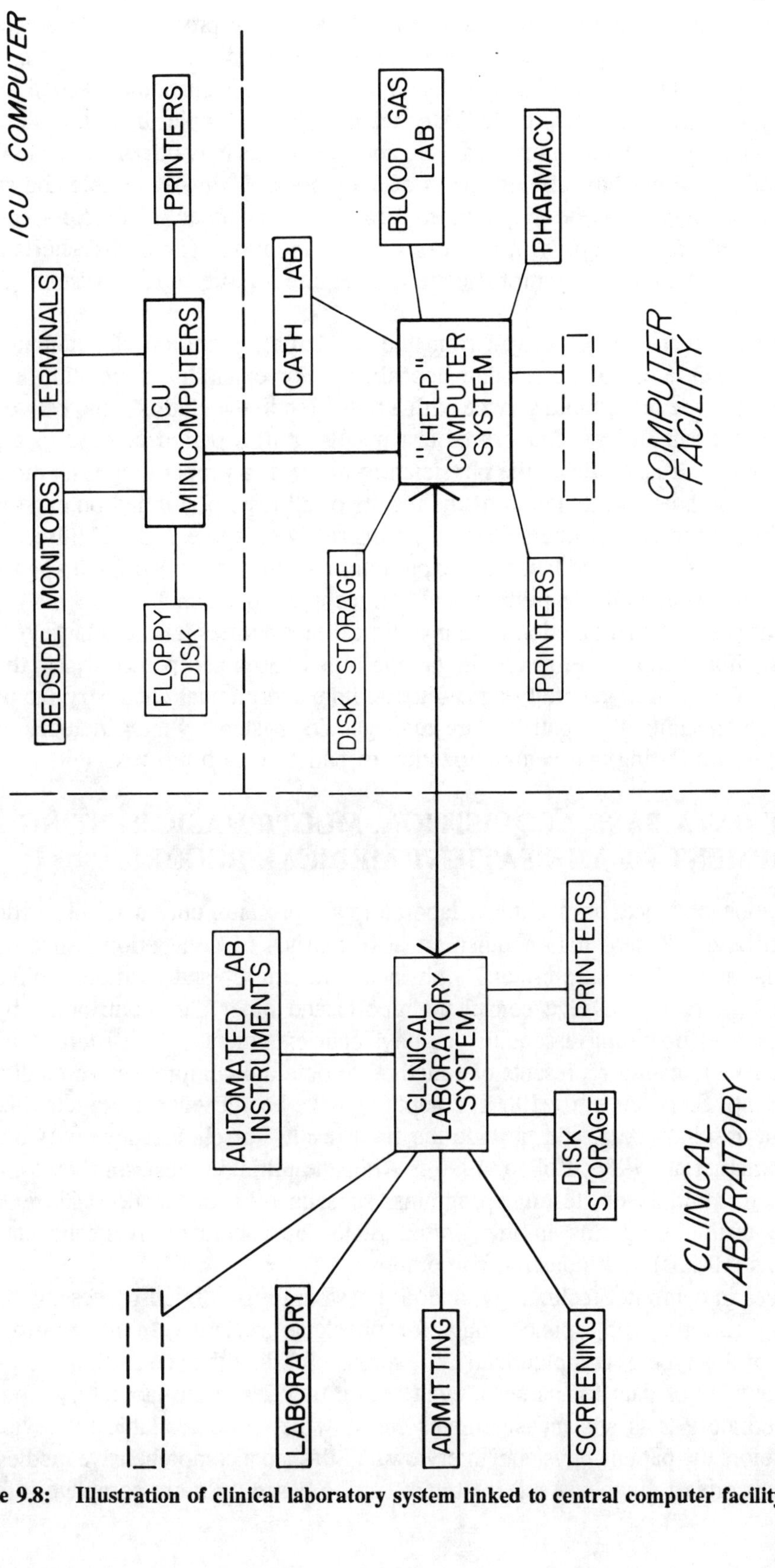

Figure 9.8: Illustration of clinical laboratory system linked to central computer facility.

Some of the difficulties derive from the nature of the testing process in these departments. First, many of the steps in processing specimens are not automated; technologists must view specimens directly, interpret findings, and summarize their conclusions. Second, the testing process may vary depending on preliminary results. For example, if initial microbiology-culture results identify an infectious organism, additional tests may be performed to determine the organism's sensitivity to different types of antibiotics. Third, a variable and sometimes long period of time may be required to process a specimen completely, e.g., some microbiology cultures are grown for weeks or even months. These characteristics of the testing process make data entry problematic and require a more flexible system (Smith and Svirbely, 1990).

The benefits that can be derived from the continuing evolution of automated clinical laboratory systems are, however, quite appealing. For example, automation enables the laboratory to provide more rapid service with a reduction in the elapsed time between receipt of the biological sample and delivery of test results from a period of days to a period of hours or minutes. It also allows the physician to arrive at a proper diagnosis more quickly as a result of computer presentation of the results of all tests performed on each patient on a single printout sheet or on the screen of an interactive display terminal. Because of the scarcity and expense of skilled labor, the exploitation of automation within this setting allows optimal utilization of available professional and technical personnel.

In recent years, the automation of many clinical laboratories has, to a large extent, been successful both in technical terms and in gaining broad-based acceptance within the medical community. Today, it is generally agreed that automated clinical chemistry facilities are a significant component of a "patient care management system" which includes automated multiphasic health testing and computerization of patient health records.

PATIENT DATA BASE ACQUISITION, MULTIPHASIC TESTING AND DEVELOPMENT OF THE PATIENT MEDICAL RECORD

Information obtained from clinical laboratories represents only a small portion of the patient data base. Patient data acquisition also consists of conventional medical history information, subjective impressions, physical findings, and various physiological measurements. It may involve consultant reports and other data contributed by various support personnel operating essentially as physician extenders. With such varied inputs, multiphasic health testing represents one method to obtain a comprehensive medical profile of each patient. Since the early 1960s, computers have been used to automate this process, assemble the resultant data, and provide the final results for clinical review (Collen et al., 1974; Freidman et al., 1986; Collen, 1990). After the initial enthusiasm, however, interest in automated multiphasic testing programs subsequently declined. Currently, most multiphasic testing programs in the United States are operated by health-maintenance organizations (HMOs) and industrial corporations.

Advances in computer technology made it possible to use digital-processing techniques in gathering and preparing patient data for physician review. In many instances the availability of this type of computerized system made feasible the acquisition and processing of large quantities of data for patients, even before they leave the laboratory. As a result, standard laboratory tests and measurements can now be made available for review by the physician before the patient-physician interview. With such a comprehensive medical profile, decisions concerning diagnosis and treatment can be based on more complete information, thereby ensuring better treatment for the patient. Early advocates, (Garfield, 1970, 1974; Collen et al., 1974), viewed **Automated Multiphasic Health Testing** (AMHT) as a "point of entry" into the health-care system, from which the consumer is directed and referred to appropriate health-care services. The availability of computerized health-testing makes it possible to introduce modern technology into primary care areas and, via telecommunications, to move this technology out of specialized central facilities into small satellite health centers.

To enter such an automated health testing laboratory simply requires insertion of a patient's identification card. Once this identification is validated, all data can be referred under the patient's unique record number (Figure 9.9). A typical multiphasic testing facility includes stations for (1) registration of patients, (2) collection of medical-history information, (3) measurement of physiological parameters (such as height, weight, pulse rate, blood pressure, ocular tension, auditory and visual acuity, pulmonary function, and muscular fitness), (4) specimen analyses (hematology and clinical chemistry tests, urinalysis, stool analysis for occult blood), (5) electrocardiography (and sometimes physician-supervised cardiovascular testing by ergometry or treadmill), (6) chest X-ray examination and mammography in women, (7) physical examination by a physician, physician's assistant, or nurse practitioner (including rectal and pelvic examinations, and cervical Pap tests for women), and (8) review and explanation of results.

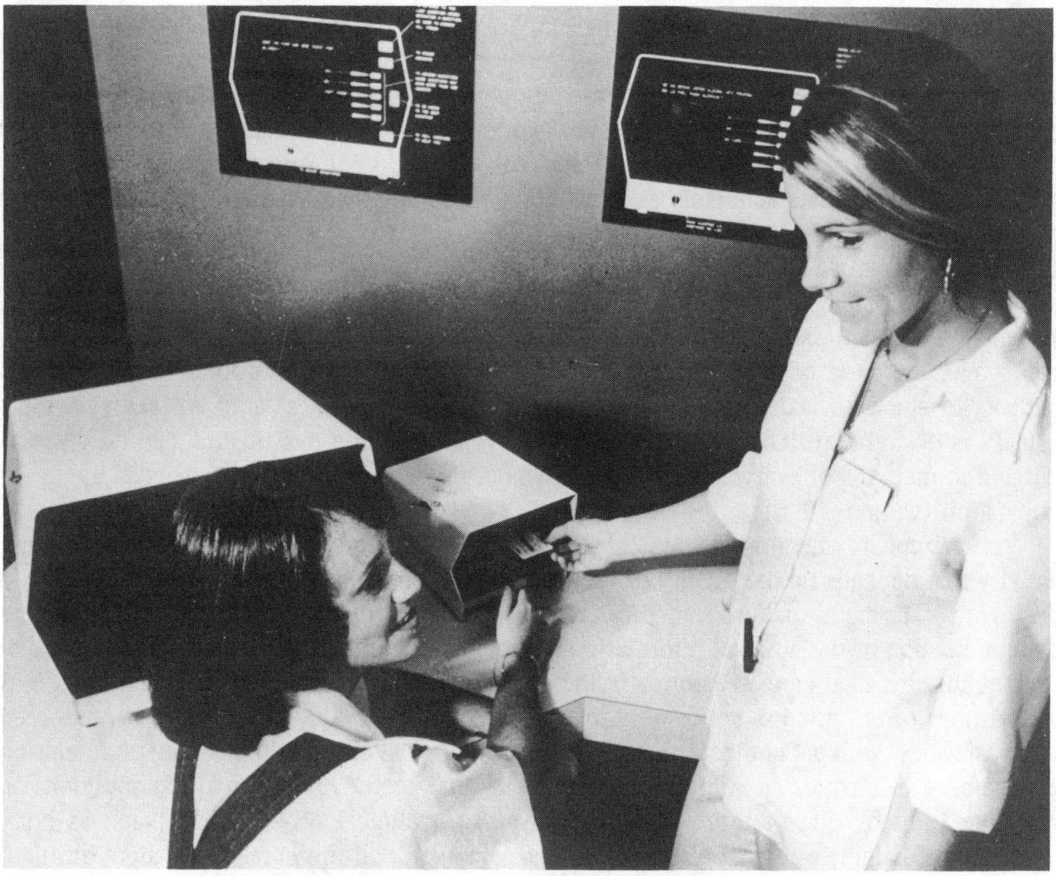

Figure 9.9: Example of the use of a patient identification card to gain access to an AMHT.

Although in the past the primary use of AMHT has been screening for disease, programs have been expanded so that this approach is increasingly being used for the following:

- Admission and preoperative examinations for hospital patients.
- Periodic health examinations for ambulatory patients.
- Evaluation of the general health of a particular population for special purposes (for example, military, industrial, insurance).
- The conduction of diagnostic surveys to evaluate the quality of care one receives from the health professionals within an institution.

The operational costs of an AMHT system depends on the number of tests performed, the number of personnel employed, the facility design, the amortization rate of capitalized equipment, the cost of supplies, the cost of facility maintenance, and so on. The most critical of factors for determining the cost unit, i.e., cost per examination (which determines the charge to users), is the AMHT system's work load (the number of examinees per day), the degree of equipment (which influences the number of personnel required to operate and manage the system), and the facility's design (which affects the efficiency of the program).

Because health-care delivery is a labor-intensive process, AMHT systems can reduce total costs by substituting automated procedures for manual procedures and by using paramedical personnel rather than physicians whenever possible. Cost per examination is further reduced because the systematic approach and the use of automated equipment improves the efficiency of operation of AMHT. An institution can perform more examinations per day with AMHT than with the traditional system of health-care delivery. Thus, the fixed costs of AMHT can be spread over a larger number of patients. In addition, automated data processing increases the efficiency of health-care personnel and the reliability of information processing by reducing the rate of data acquisition errors and by hastening the turnaround time of summary reports to physicians.

In general, small AMHT programs are unable to afford the large capital investment in automated equipment and therefore remain almost entirely manual operations. Larger AMHT systems—those that examine more than fifty persons per day (or one thousand per month)—can spread the costs of acquiring computers and computer-based instruments over enough patients to attain an acceptable cost per examination. For such a large AMHT system, it usually is desirable to have a dedicated space and information system that can be custom-tailored to meet the objectives of the AMHTS and, more specifically, the needs of the target population (Collen, 1990).

As previously mentioned, clinical medicine is inherently an information-processing activity that depends on the quality of clinical data and the speed of placing this data in and retrieving it from the patient's medical record. As a result, the **medical record** and the communication of the medical information it contains are critical elements in the practice of high-quality medical care. Historically the principal use of the medical record has been as a repository of information concerning the patient. In its most general form, it is composed of a basic sheet with patient identification and chronological data, including date of admission and date of discharge; an initial medical history and record of physical examinations in narrative form by one or more attending physicians; clinical observations (such as body temperature, height, weight, pulse, arterial and venous blood pressure, and patient attitude) recorded throughout the hospital stay by physicians, nurses, therapists, and social workers; precise therapeutic instructions in chronological order and consultation reports, including judgments and therapeutic recommendations; operation reports in narrative form; clinical pathology laboratory determination; results of functional tests, including pulmonary function studies, electrocardiograms, electroencephalograms, and electromyograms; special reports by departments that provide selective services, such as radiation therapy, physical therapy, radiology, nuclear medicine, and the cardiac catheterization laboratory; and a discharge summary that contains a synopsis of the patient's history, examination, course of treatment, final diagnosis, and outcome.

The structure of the medical record has essentially remained unchanged since the early part of the twentieth century. Recording practices still rely almost completely on the traditional manual record folder where physicians' notes are handwritten and merged with laboratory data and other patient material. It is interesting to note that only forty to fifty years ago the family physician, able to recall the family background, past medical history, and significant medical encounters (such as previous surgeries, pregnancies, and so on) was the guardian of the patient's past medical record. Today, in a mobile society with specialization in medicine, fragments of the patient's record are scattered, kept in hospitals, clinics, X-ray departments, and even by insurance companies. Consequently, by default, each patient has become the carrier of his or her own medical history, and expensive and time-consuming reconstruction of the patient's past medical history must take place every time the patient changes hospitals or visits a different doctor. More important perhaps is the fact that, over time, the quality of the medical history given by typical patients often becomes quite unsatisfactory because they cannot remember the names of drugs used, the exact diagnosis, and so forth, from previous treatments.

Trying to extract information from even modern medical records is a difficult process, even for those directly involved in the patient's care. There is little standardization and storage, and retrieval techniques are not at the frontiers of technology. Yet, the medical chart is extremely important not only for the care of patients, but for both medical/legal and quality assurance reasons. Today, a major goal of most clinical institutions is the establishment of a computerized medical information system that will:

- Enable the health professional providing medical care (doctors, nurses) to communicate individual patient data into the patient's own computer medical record. Once this record is established, it could then be communicated to other professionals (e.g., dietitian or therapist) and hospital services (for example, radiology or clinical laboratory) to inform them of the needs of the patient.
- Permit patient data obtained from subsystem components (e.g., automated multiphasic screening laboratory or intensive care unit) to be inserted into the patient's computer medical record.
- Provide a means by which clinical services (i.e., nursing stations) can communicate with auxiliary services (e.g., cardiac or radiology laboratory) regarding a particular patient.
- Establish procedures and communicate information to schedule patient, for the delivery of specific health-care services.
- Establish a data base for administrative and business functions.
- Establish a medical data base that can fulfill research and teaching objectives.

Although there has been significant progress in the development of hospital information systems (HIS) and the incorporation of relational data base technology, comprehensive computerized hospital information systems that provide all of the functions listed above do not yet operate anywhere in the world. Several large medical centers do have some subsystem components, such as AMHT, admission and bed census, outpatient scheduling, and hospital data base systems. The key is the integration of various data into a single data base system that is capable of responding in an accurate and timely fashion to a clinician's inquiry. Clinical engineering departments can play an important role in the development of these systems.

PATIENT MONITORING SYSTEMS

Patient monitoring systems have been defined as

". . . *repeated or continuous observations or measurements of patients, their physiological function and the function of life support equipment for the purpose of guiding management decisions, including when to make therapeutic interventions, and assessment of those interventions*" (Hudson. 1985).

Patient monitoring systems, therefore, should not only alert health-care personnel to potentially life-threatening events, but may also control devices to maintain life (Gardner, 1990). Any patient monitoring system consists of five basic components which include the following, (Figure 9.10):

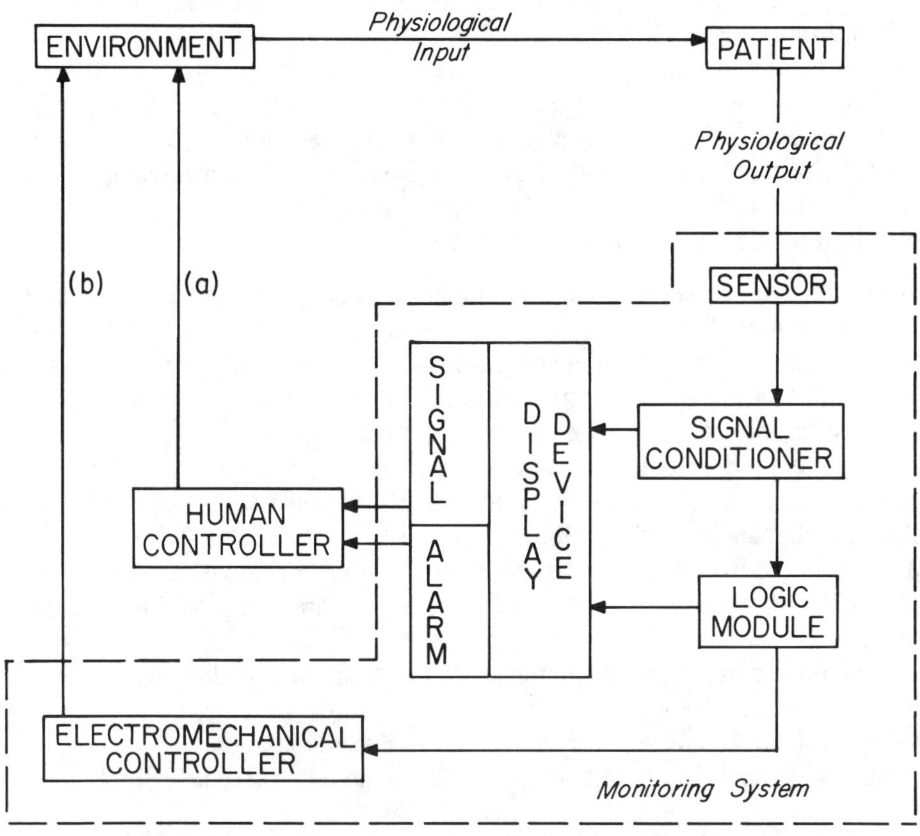

Figure 9.10: Schematic diagram of the basic components of a patient monitoring system.

The Sensor

The properties of various electrodes and transducers used to detect physiological signals are well-known. Those most commonly used in physiological monitoring systems include contact electrodes for electrocardiography and electroencephalography, light pulse oximetry, intravascular and respiratory pressure transducers, ultrasonic and electromagnetic flow-rate detectors, and chemical and pH electrodes. The output of each of these sensors is an electrical signal that is directly related to the measured physiological parameter.

One of the persistent questions facing people who monitor patients is "Should I measure a parameter continuously, or is intermittent sampling enough?" A related question is, "How often do I make the measurement?" These questions have no simple answer. If we want to display an ECG signal continuously, we must sample the signal at a rate of at least twice the rate of the maximum frequency of interest in the signal. For an ECG, the sampling rate should be at least 200 measurements per second.

When intermittent monitoring (periodic measurement of blood pH value, for example) must be performed, the overriding concerns in determining sampling rate are how rapidly the parameter can change, and how long before a dangerous change will result in irreversible damage. Sudden heart stoppage or severe dysrhythmias are the most frequent causes of sudden death. Therefore, heart-rate and heart-rhythm monitors must function continuously and should sound alarms within 15 to 20 seconds after detecting the problem. Other physiological parameters are not as labile and can be monitored less frequently. For the most part, medical measurements are made intermittently, and even continuously measured parameters are displayed at intervals. For example, heart rate can change with each beat (by 0.35 to 1 second). To provide data that a human can interpret, however, a bedside monitor usually updates its display of the rate every 3 seconds (Gardner, 1990).

The Signal Conditioner

The electrical signals available from each sensor usually require amplification and filtering before they can be transmitted for review by the clinician. The signal conditioner extracts the necessary information from the input signal and conditions it for display, recording or analysis. The signal conditioner usually consists of a number of electrical devices, such as detectors, amplifiers, filter, and other signal-transformation devices.

The Display Device

The display unit receives an electrical signal from the signal-conditioning module and converts it into an appropriate display. Various types of displays include dial indicators, digital displays, cathode ray tubes, signal lights, audible alarms, and hard-copy output. The latter may include strip-chart recorders, as well as laser printers or photographic reproductions.

The Logic Module

The logic module simply compares a signal with a reference level or performs more complex analyses. A common example of the former is the cardiac monitor, which compares heart rate with preset upper and lower rate limits. However, if computation of specific parameters, such as cardiac output, or analysis of specific components of each electrocardiogram (ECG) are desired, requirements will be greater. Then a digital computer is used. In general, the extent of the hardware and software needed to perform a particular analysis generally depends on the nature and complexity of the analysis to be performed.

The Controller

The type of control used, if any, also depends on the application. A passive control system, for example, provides for human interaction in the maintenance of a clinical state. It usually features visual or auditory alarms (or both) that are triggered whenever a physiological signal falls outside the preset range. When an alarm occurs, the intended response is that a human observer will bring the physiological signal back within its normal range by exerting some direct or indirect controlling action on the physiological system (for example, by administering drugs or instituting other therapeutic measures).

With active control systems, there is usually some form of direct feedback pathway between the logic module and a controller of the physiological input. For example, a sensor system interfaced with a digital computer can convert measured urinary output and central venous pressure to a signal that activates an infusion pump to maintain a specified fluid balance. A nonmedical example of a closed-loop control system is the thermostat on a heater. A sensor continuously measures the temperature of the air. When the temperature drops below the setpoint, the heater turns on. When the temperature rises sufficiently, the heater shuts off. This type of device has also been reported to be effective in controlling physiological parameters (Sheppard, 1980). A computer-controlled infusion pump, for example, was used to control the administration of sodium nitroprusside, a drug used to regulate blood pressure. It was shown that the controller performed more effectively than did a nurse in regulating constant blood pressure. Closed-loop drug-delivery systems are now commercially available for controlling the infusion of oxytocin (a labor-inducing drug) and insulin and dextrose (used to control the level of glucose in the blood). In the future, closed-loop systems will control the delivery of other drugs and fluids, the administration of anesthesia, and the management of patients on ventilator therapy.

In general, patient monitoring is recommended for the following categories of patients (Gardner, 1990):

- Patients with unstable physiologic regulatory systems; for example, a patient whose respiratory-control system is suppressed as a result of a drug overdose or anesthesia.
- Patients with a suspected life-threatening condition; for example, a patient who has findings indicating an acute myocardial infarction (heart attack).
- Patients with a high-risk status; for example, a patient who has just had open-heart surgery, or a premature infant whose heart and lungs are not fully developed.
- Patients in a critical physiological state; for example, a patient with multiple types of trauma.

As a result, patient-monitoring equipment is found in the following areas:

- **Diagnostic**: Clinical areas where unstable patient status requires continuous monitoring. Such areas include the emergency room, cardiac catheterization laboratories and during special radiological procedures.

- **Treatment**: Clinical areas such as operating or delivery rooms where procedures are conducted with the aim of improving patient status, but which involve some risk of patient status deterioration (Figure 9.11).

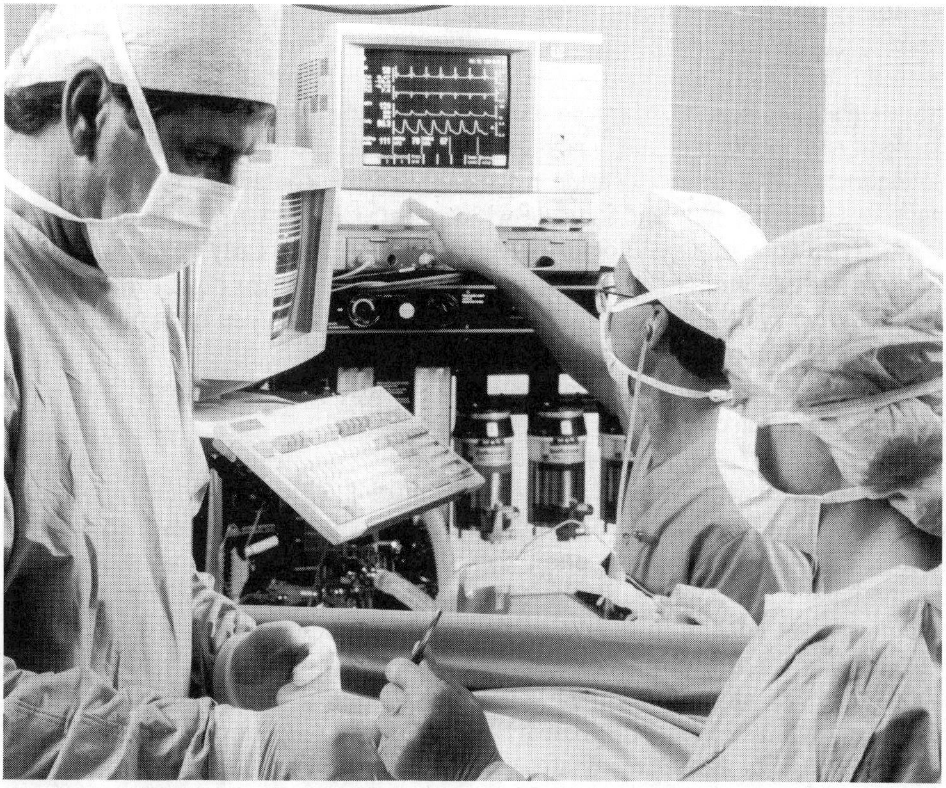

Figure 9.11: Physiological monitoring devices in use in the operating room.

- **Surveillance**: Clinical areas where patients are monitored during stabilization and recuperative periods. Surgical, medical, coronary, and neonatal intensive care units are the best known examples of such areas.

The patient-monitoring equipment used in these critical-care areas involves primarily bedside monitoring stations and some sort of central information-processing facility, usually the central nursing station. The standard bedside monitoring system is a compact and simply structured unit which provides a quick and comprehensive picture of the monitored patient's status, such as heart rate and ECG (Sondak et al., 1979; Bronzino, 1982; Gardner, 1990). The bedside monitor usually contains a small screen (CRT), which displays regularly updated critical values or waveforms. Each bedside system also sends information to a repeater screen at the central nursing station, which enables the nursing staff to simultaneously monitor all patients on the floor.

In recent years the concept of "modular" patient-monitoring equipment has gained wide acceptance and implementation, permitting clinicians to select a variety of physiologic monitoring units for individual patients based on the specific functions under surveillance. The newest bedside monitors contain multiple built-in microcomputers and, as a result, have much greater computing power and larger memories than earlier systems. These advanced monitoring systems have several advantages (Gardner, 1990):

- The ability to store waveform information permits the computer to perform sophisticated pattern recognition and feature extraction procedures that utilize waveform templates to identify the presence of abnormal waveform patterns (arrhythmias) and send an alarm to the central nursing station.
- The ability to monitor signal quality. For example, the system can monitor the degradation of ECG/skin electrode resistance. If the contact becomes poor, the system can alert the staff and indicate which electrode in an array needs attention.
- The ability to convert physiological signals to digital form early in the processing cycle. As a result, more effective waveform processing, such as digital filtering, can be done by the system; and longer periods of digitized data can be stored, thereby aiding in detection of life-threatening trends.
- The ability to transmit digitized physiological signals that are inherently noise-free, thus minimizing false alarms.

All of these factors enable modern patient-monitoring systems to detect life-threatening situations promptly, so that they can be treated before they result in irreversible damage or death. In addition, because they permit the collection of an enormous amount of data through continuous observation, health-care professionals can obtain trend or specific occurrence data in a concise and time-efficient fashion, thereby enabling them to provide quality health-care for critically ill patients.

Although general-purpose, computer-based physiological monitoring systems have not yet been widely adopted, computer-based ECG arrhythmia-monitoring systems have been accepted quickly. ECG arrhythmia analysis is one of the most sophisticated and difficult of the bedside monitoring tasks (Figure 9.12). Conventional arrhythmia monitoring, which depends on visual monitoring of displayed signals, is expensive, unreliable, tedious, and stressful to observers. The newest bedside monitors have built-in arrhythmia-monitoring systems, generally use a 16-bit architecture, waveform templates, and real-time cross-correlation techniques to classify rhythm abnormalities.

Modern computer algorithms for processing ECG rhythms take the sampled data; extract features, such as the amplitude and duration of the QRS complex; and perform feature extraction by searching the sampled data from beginning to end to locate the P wave, QRS complex, and T wave. When ECG monitoring begins, the computer-based bedside monitor initiates a learning process to determine which QRS waveform shape is seen most frequently. The learning process requires a certain number of beats from which to determine R-R intervals (the times between successive R waves) and to calculate the average interval. Waveforms are classified by shape. Of those waveforms with the most frequently occurring shape, the one having the longest R-R interval is designated the dominant shape. If at any time the dominant beat fails to occur within an interval of four beats, then the system seeks a new dominant beat by restarting the learning process. As the system detects each new QRS complex, it performs classification by comparing the waveform with stored beats called templates; the cross-correlation process seeks beats of similar shape. The first template stored is the dominant beat found in the learning process. Up to fifteen template beats are stored and are used for cross-correlation. Series of beats are analyzed to classify rhythms. Once an abnormal rhythm has been identified, the system generates an alarm, depending on the severity of the detected arrhythmia.

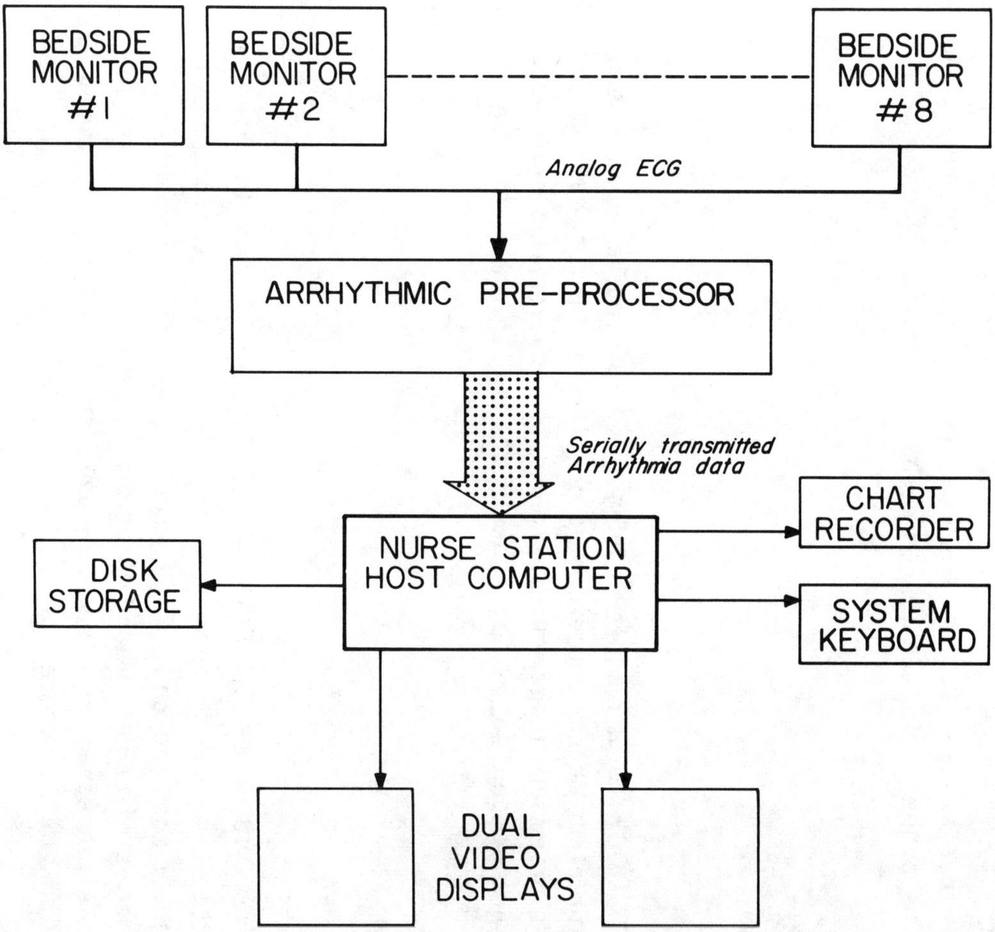

Figure 9.12: Schematic diagram of ECG arrhythmia monitoring and analysis system.

MEDICAL IMAGING TECHNOLOGY

Medical imaging encompasses those procedures that allow indirect visualization of internal body structures. Although modern medical imaging takes many forms, systems of most practical interest today include the following: film-based X-ray imaging, computerized tomography (digital radiography), nuclear medicine, diagnostic ultrasound, and magnetic resonance imaging. These imaging devices enable doctors to avoid exploratory surgery and still watch vital organs at work, identify blockages and growths, and detect the warning signs of possible future disorders.

Radiography

Film-based radiography is the primary modality used in radiology departments today. In fact, film-based radiography still account for over 80 percent of all medical imaging procedures performed—some 200 to 300 million films per year. This technique uses high-energy electromagnetic waves or photons (X-rays) to obtain information on anatomical structures (Figure 9.13).

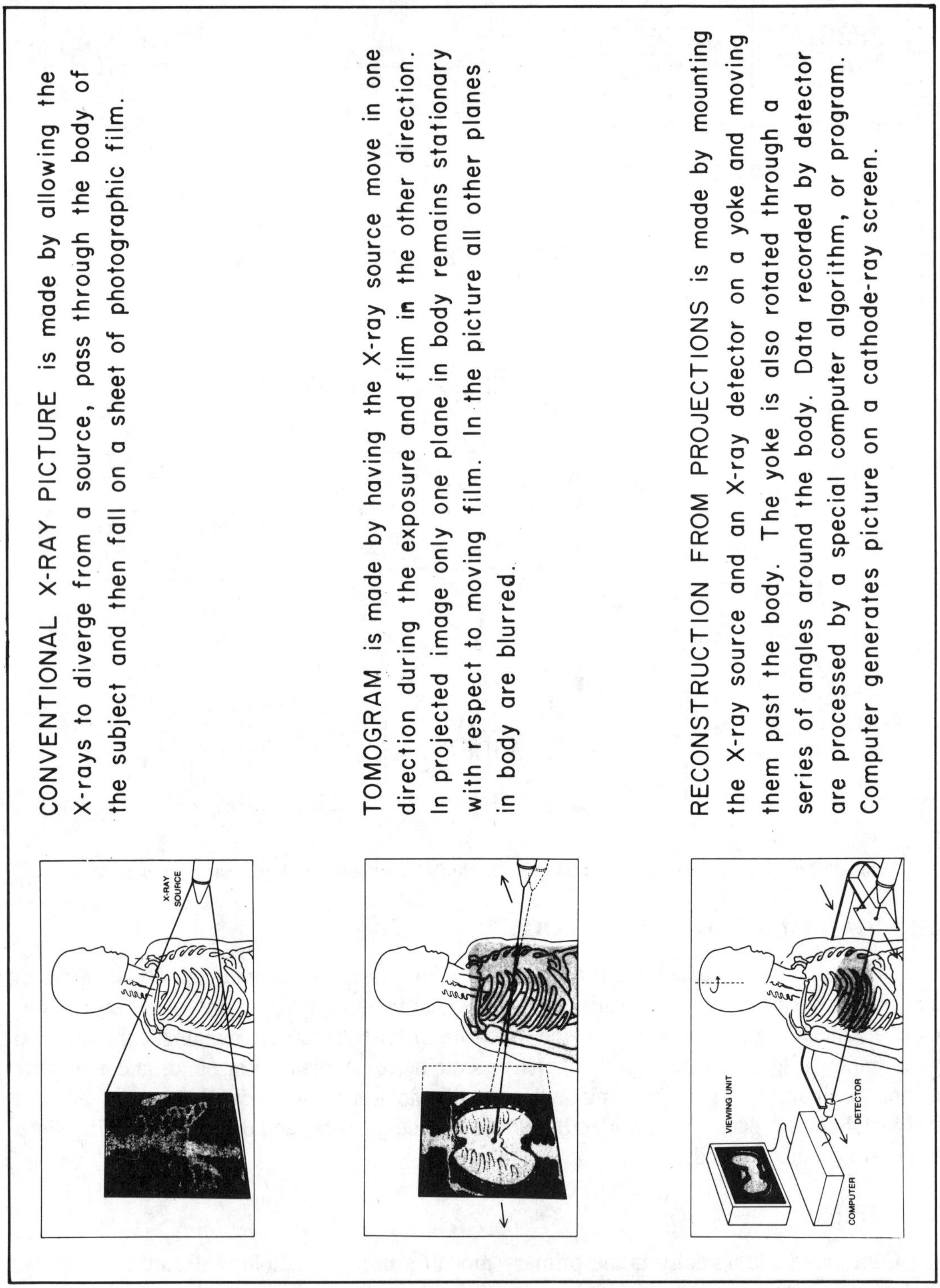

Figure 9.13: Examples of the application of film-based radiography to obtain information on anatomical structures.

The propagation of X-rays, characterized by wavelengths that are shorter than the atomic diameters of the penetrated matter, is dominated by corpuscular ray properties rather than by the wave character of light. The velocity of propagation is essentially constant for all kinds of biological tissue; thus the refractive index of all such structures is unity. As a consequence, the only mechanisms of interaction are absorption and scattering; no reflection or diffraction takes place. Thus, unlike ultrasonic waves (discussed below), X-rays travel in straight lines through the body, unaffected by tissue interfaces, and provide undistorted images of high resolution.

Digital radiography, or CT (Ledley, 1976), applies the same techniques as film-based radiography; however, the images are digitized and recorded in computer memory rather than on film. Since its introduction, computed tomography has undergone continuous refinement and development. Significant improvements have been made in several aspects:

- X-ray tube performance.
- Reduction of scan times.
- Reduction of image reconstruction time.
- Reduction and, in some cases, elimination of image artifacts.
- Reduction of patient dose.

Present CT scanners are usually integrated units consisting of three major elements (Figure 9.14):

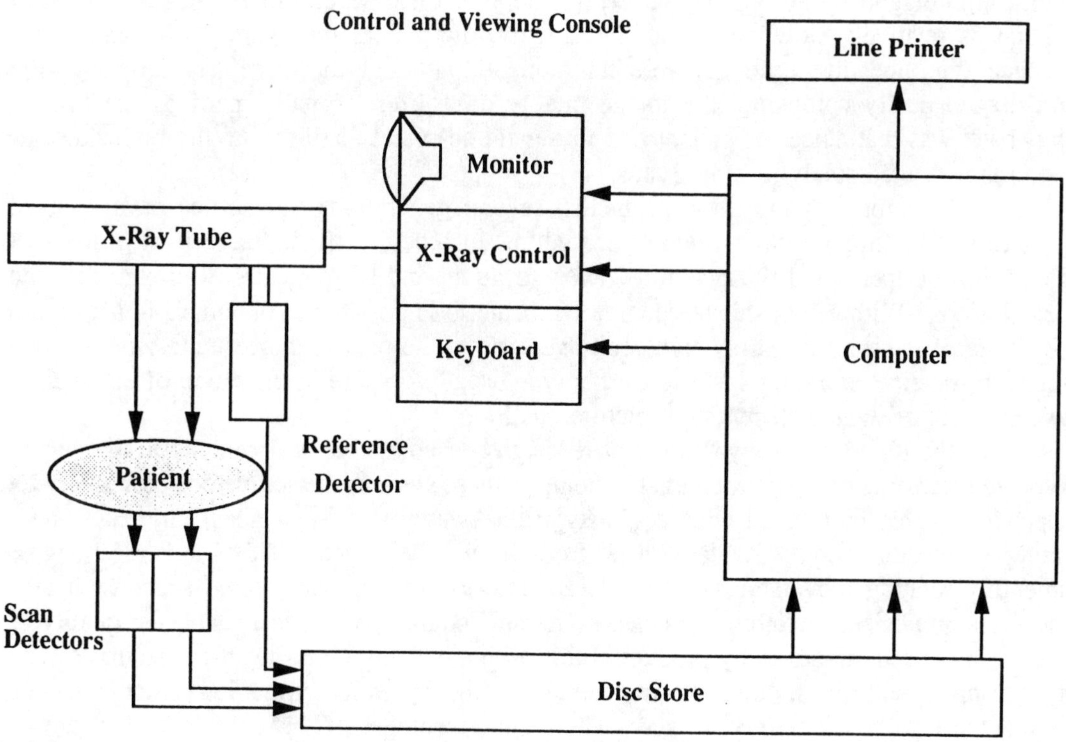

Figure 9.14: Block diagram representing the major components of a CT scanner system.

1. **The scanning gantry**, which takes the readings in a suitable form and quantity for a picture to be reconstructed.
2. **The data handling unit**, which converts these readings into intelligible picture information, presents this picture information in a visual format, and provides various manipulative aids to enhance the image and thereby assist the doctor in forming a diagnosis.
3. **A storage facility**, which enables the information to be examined or reexamined at any time subsequent to the actual scan (Walmsley, 1979).

The objective of the scanning system is to obtain enough information to reconstruct an image of the cross section of interest. All the information obtained must be relevant and accurate, and there must be enough independent readings to reconstruct a picture with sufficient spatial resolution and density discrimination to permit an accurate diagnosis. The operation of the scanning system is, therefore, extremely important.

Since the early 1970s, the CT scanner has undergone several design changes. The earliest generation of gantries used a system known as "traverse and index." In these systems, the tube and detector were mounted on a frame and a single beam of X-rays traversed the slice linearly, thereby providing absorption measurements along one profile. At the end of the traverse, the frame indexed through one degree and the traverse was repeated. This procedure continued until 180 single traverses were made and 180 profiles were measured. Using the "traverse and index" approach, the entire scanning procedure took approximately four to five minutes. The images it provided had excellent picture quality and hence high diagnostic utility. However, this approach had several disadvantages. First of all it was relatively slow, resulting in relatively low patient throughput. Second, streak artifacts (i.e., lines in the image) were common, and although these artifacts normally were not diagnostically confusing, the image quality did suffer. Finally, perhaps the biggest drawback was that since the patient had to remain absolutely still during the procedure, its use was restricted solely to brain scans.

In an attempt to solve these problems, several generations of gantries have evolved (Figure 9.15). Initially new scanning procedures included a translation step as in the first generation but permitted the scanning gantry to go around the patient (180 degrees) in ten degree steps. With use of this ten degree fan beam, it is possible to obtain a full set of 180 degree profiles by making only eighteen traverses. At the rate of approximately one second for each traverse, scanning systems of this type usually operate in the range of eighteen to twenty seconds while still retaining picture quality.

Very shortly after, however, a major redesign ensued, and a third generation of gantries evolved consisting of a pure rotational system. In these systems the source/detector unit, with a pulsing, highly collimated wide angle (typically twenty to fifty degrees) fan beam and a multiple detector array, is rotated 360 degrees around the patient. This single, 360 degree smoothly rotating movement decreases scan time to approximately three seconds; it also increases appreciably reliability because data are acquired twice, increasing the quality of the reconstructed image. A by-product of this design is that the pulsing X-ray source can be synchronized with physiological parameters enabling rhythmically moving structures, such as the heart, to be accurately imaged. The main advantages of this type of system are its simplicity and its speed; however, its fixed geometry system with a fan beam, usually established for the largest patient, makes it inefficient for profiling smaller objects, in particular head scanning.

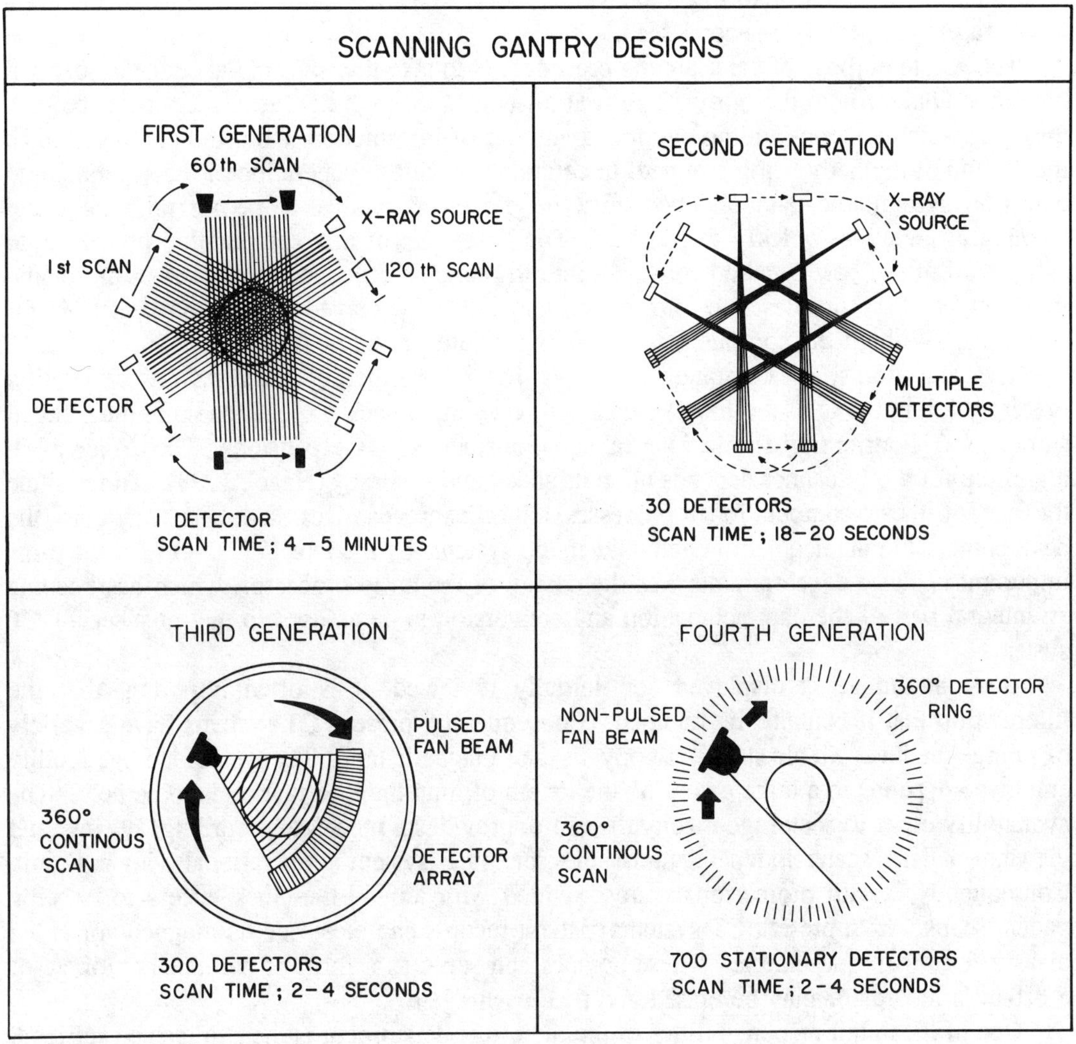

Figure 9.15: Evolution of the scanning gantry.

Consequently, a fourth generation gantry system consisting of a continuous ring of fixed detectors (usually numbering between five hundred and seven hundred) was developed. In this system, the X-ray source rotates as before but the detectors remain stationary, arranged in a full circle around the gantry. The fan beam is increased slightly so that the detectors on the leading and trailing edge of the fan can be continuously monitored and the data adjusted in case of shifts in detector performance (Maravilla and Pastel, 1978).

Recently, the bulky, noisy electromechanical rotation mechanism has been replaced by a magnetic induction system that rotates the source. This has enabled designers to attain a long-sought goal: the one-second scan.

The whole purpose of the scanning procedure is to take thousands of accurate absorption measurements through the body. Taken at all angles through the cross section of interest, these measurements provide an enormous amount of information about the composition of the section of the body being scanned. In conjunction with the operation of the scanning and detection system, the data obtained must be processed rapidly to permit producing and viewing an image as quickly as possible. The first stage of this computation process is to analyze all of this raw data and convert it into the set of profiles, normally 180 or more, and then convert these profiles into information that can be displayed as a picture and used for diagnosis. Without the computer, CT scanning would not be possible.

The algorithms, or computer programs for reconstructing tissue X-ray absorption presently fall into one of the following categories: simple back projection (sometimes called summation); Fourier transforms; integral equations; and series expansions. The choice of an algorithm for a CT scanner depends upon its speed and accuracy (Nagel, 1988). To facilitate the use of these computational processes, significant advances had been made in the development of data acquisition and conversion systems by the late 1970s. One of the most important of these developments was the design of the array processor, which has become an integral part of the data acquisition and conversion systems used in the most recent CT systems.

Once an image is displayed and initially reviewed, it is often important that the information that it contains be retained. Consequently, present CT systems have a variety of storage media available such as floppy disks or magnetic tape. The type of storage facility employed depends to a large extent on the length of time the information is to be held. The availability of various storage media, therefore, provides a means of recording, storing, and viewing patient scans independent of the scanning system's operational viewing unit. Consequently, health professionals are provided with around-the-clock access to existing patient scans. With present CT systems, patient records can be stored on magnetic or video disks in less than one minute. These devices can serve as a form of permanent storage of a patient's records or may be erased and then used again.

One of the major responsibilities of the radiology department is the storage and retrieval of medical images. At present, the majority of medical images are recorded and stored on film. Even CT scans are generally transferred to film once they have been optimized for viewing. Ultrasound records are transferred to videotape for review, interpretation, and storage. Film records of each examination are labelled with appropriate patient-identification information and placed in the patient's master film file in the film library. Each time an image is needed, the staff must locate and retrieve it from the library. As a result, film archiving requires a significant amount of space and personnel time. Digital acquisition and storage of images offers the prospect of significantly reducing the space, materials costs, and labor associated with traditional film-archiving tasks. The development of computerized-picture archiving and communication systems (PACS), represents a rapidly expanding area of medical informatics which will provide the means for rapid retrieval and high-speed transmission, via communications networks, of desired archived images from centralized image data bases. Several complex problems must be overcome, however, before PACS become practical. These include (Greenes and Brinkley, 1990):

- Standardization of image transmission and storage formats.
- Development of storage/retrieval/management schema for the enormous amount of data making up the image data base.
- Design of workstations for interpretation of digitized images that are acceptable replacements for the light boxes presently used by radiologists working with film-based images.

Management of the work flow in a radiology department involves not only the maintenance of the film library, but also includes the scheduling of examinations, registration of patients, distribution of radiology reports to referring physicians, and billing for services rendered. In addition, the manager of the radiology department must collect and analyze process-control and financial information used to prepare budgets and determine staffing requirements; anticipate equipment and purchase order needs; and maintain inventory control, quality assurance, radiation-exposure monitoring, and preventive maintenance schedules. To meet these needs, computer-based Radiology Information Systems (RIS) have been developed that are capable of automating nearly all information-management tasks within a radiology department. RIS's have been implemented as both stand-alone systems and as part of larger, centralized hospital-information systems. In both cases, for the RIS to be most effective it must be integrated with other information systems within the institution, which permits such applications as reconciliation of patient data, preventive maintenance scheduling, etc. (Greenes and Brinkley, 1990).

Nuclear Medicine

Nuclear medicine has been defined as the application of radioactive materials (tracers) to medical diagnosis and treatment. It is a classic example of a medical discipline that has embraced and utilized concepts developed in the physical sciences. In the process, the domain of nuclear medicine has grown to include studies pertaining to:

- The creation and proper utilization of radioactive tracers (or radiopharmaceuticals).
- The design and application of appropriate nuclear instrumentation to detect and display the activity of these radioactive materials.
- The determination of the relationship between the activity of the radioactive tracer and specific physiological processes (Wagner, 1975).

With the discovery of artificial radionuclides, pioneers were encouraged to employ radioactive tracer techniques to gain information regarding biological and physiological systems. One of the first physiological systems to be studied in both animal's and human's was the metabolism of phosphorus. Using the cyclotron-produced tracer ^{32}P, several investigators observed the great efficiency with which the body absorbed inorganic phosphorus and preferentially utilized it in rapidly multiplying tissues, such as those associated with malignancies. In 1936, John Lawrence, recognizing the therapeutic implications of these findings, acted. He used ^{32}P in the treatment of leukemia, and in the process inaugurated the therapeutic employment of artificial radionuclides (Wagner, 1975).

Although the early uses of radioactive materials in medicine were chiefly in radiation therapy, today most radioactive materials are used to provide useful diagnostic information. These radionuclides can be monitored within the patient *(in vivo)* or in various bodily fluids removed from the patient *(in vitro)*. For example, it is possible to inject a patient with a radioactive substance that is "taken up" by a particular organ, such as the kidney. By placing a detector over the kidneys, the amount of radioactive material accumulated by the kidney can actually be measured. This uptake test allows the clinician to monitor the activity of specific organs and to determine whether they are functioning properly. Another example of an *in vivo* study involves imaging the distribution of a radionuclide within an organ. This can be very important, especially since it has been demonstrated that abnormal tissue tends to accumulate either more or less of the radionuclide administered than the normal tissue surrounding it. In this way, radionuclide measurement can help the clinician delineate the presence of tissue abnormalities. The key to success in this application is the specificity of the radioactive material used (Bronzino, 1977). That is, the more closely the radionuclide can be tied to a specific function, the easier it is to examine the dynamic physiological system under study.

The *in vitro* category includes tests made outside the body. These tests are used to study various chemical as well as physiological processes. Today, *in vitro* tests are capable of detecting extremely small amounts of various hormones and chemicals in the blood and have been used to determine:

- Insulin dosage in diabetics.
- Whether individuals are immune to specific diseases, such as hepatitis.
- The proper dosage of digitalis required by cardiac patients.

The gamma camera system, one of the most basic instruments of diagnostic nuclear medicine (Spencer and Hosain, 1986), converts the radioactive emissions into an image (Figure 9.16). Interfacing this device with a digital computer enables clinicians to perform data collection, storage, and analyses.

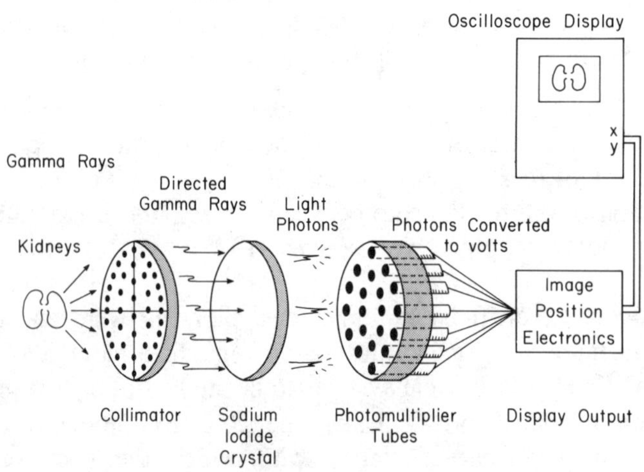

Figure 9.16: Basic components of the gamma camera system.

Gamma camera systems are large and heavy and cannot be moved easily. They are regarded as stationary cameras. Fortunately, relatively mobile versions are available with computer interfaces designed especially for cardiac studies. It is often times possible for Gamma cameras to obtain whole-body images by moving the camera head linearly along the patient bed. These so-called "scanning cameras," have replaced rectilinear scanner systems. A major innovation in gamma camera design has been the addition of an extra camera head with rotational capabilities, which is used with a computer system known as single-photon-emission computed tomography (SPECT) for carrying out optional tomographic work (Spencer and Hosain, 1986). The major thrust of the current application in nuclear medicine lies primarily in the use of radioactive tracers for both *in vivo* and *in vitro* studies to evaluate various physiological systems within a patient. Clearly, it is beyond the scope of this text to provide a complete outline of all the applications presently being utilized; however, some of the most common clinical applications of nuclear technology in studying major organs are summarized in Table 9.3.

Positron Emission Tomography

Positron emission tomographic (PET) imaging relies on the application of radionuclide-tagged biopharmaceuticals and the measurement of their decay components, detected as in gamma camera scintigraphy, but with a notable difference. The radionuclide decay consists of emission of positrons that, after losing most of their kinetic energy in tissue, are annihilated by combining with nearby electrons (see also Chapter 2: Radiation Safety). Certain isotopes produce positrons, which react with electrons to emit two photons at 511 keV in opposite directions. One photon path is shorter, and the opposite path is longer; the average signal level is the same without regard to patient attenuation or point of origin. These isotopes have two means of decay that result in the annihilation of an electron. In one case, the nucleus can capture an orbital electron that combines with one positive charge; alternatively, the nucleus can emit the positive charge as a positron that travels a short distance to combine with an external electron. The combination of the negative and positive particles annihilates the charges and masses of each, energy and momentum are conserved, and two 511 keV gamma rays are emitted in opposite directions (Siedband, 1992).

This property gives PET the ability to locate the region of origin. Instead of the multihole collimator found in most gamma cameras, two imaging detectors capable of determining X–Y position are used. Each X–Y pair is accepted if the two scintillation effects are coincident and have energy levels (pulse heights) close to the expected value of 511 keV.

Very elegant cameras have been constructed using a circular ring of many detectors that surround the patient and do not have to be rotated. As in all radionuclide imagers, the level of the radioactivity places a noise boundary on the images, which means that compromises must be made in the amount of radionuclide administered; it must be large enough to obtain a good image in the time required and small enough to minimize patient exposure to radiation (Siedband, 1992).

The advantages of PET over conventional nuclear imaging include the clarity of the cross-sectional views and the availability of positron emitters that can be compounded as metabolites that make it possible to map metabolic activity in the brain by using tagged compounds to observe uptake and clearance. The results are remarkably detailed pictures of the brain and other soft tissues, as well as high-contrast images of tumors and aneurysms produced by linking the radionuclide to biopharmaceuticals with a high differential affinity.

Table 9.3: Clinical applications of nuclear medicine imaging technology.

1. *Brain scanning*
   - (a) Detection of intracerebral-space-occupying disease: primary or secondary neoplasms, abscesses, arteriovenous malformations.
   - (b) Evaluation of cerebrovascular disease.
   - (c) Detection and localization of intracranial injury after trauma.
2. *Lung scanning*
   - (a) Diagnosis and management of pulmonary embolism.
   - (b) Evaluation of regional function in emphysema and other forms of chronic obstructive lung disease.
   - (c) Evaluation of pulmonary venous hypertension.
3. *Thyroid scanning*
   - (a) Evaluation of thyroid size, position, and function.
   - (b) Functional assessment of thyroid nodules.
   - (c) Diagnosis of functioning metastatic lesions in with known carcinomas.
4. *Liver scanning*
   - (a) Evaluation of liver size, configuration, and position.
   - (b) Preoperative search for metastatic disease when a primary neoplasm exists elsewhere.
   - (c) Functional evaluation of cirrhosis and other diffuse parenchymal processes.
5. *Spleen screening*
   - (a) Evaluation of spleen size, shape, and position.
   - (b) Detection of intrasplenic-space-occupying diseases.
6. *Pancreas scanning*
   - (a) Carcinoma of the pancreas.
   - (b) Pancreatitis.
   - (c) Miscellaneous pancreatic problems such as psuedocysts.

Ultrasonic Imaging

The application of ultrasound as a noninvasive diagnostic tool is now widely accepted within the medical community. As a matter of fact, diagnostic ultrasound studies are often the method of choice because they provide information otherwise unobtainable. The term ultrasound is used to describe sound waves (mechanical vibrations) that are beyond the range of human hearing, that is, above 20,000 Hz. Since sound waves of any frequency are essentially vibratory phenomena, their transmission from one point to another requires the presence of matter. In a vacuum the conduction of sound waves becomes impossible.

Since the composition of each substance varies, these ultrasonic or high-frequency sound waves travel through them at different velocities. Thus, it is possible to investigate the internal composition of many materials simply by studying the transmission of ultrasound through them. In addition, just as audible sound under correct conditions produces echoes, ultrasonic waves produce echoes that can be detected with appropriate instruments, and then processed and displayed. The application of these basic concepts of ultrasound transmission and echo-ranging led to the development of non-destructive testing techniques in industry, and eventually to the utilization of ultrasonic techniques in the conduction of noninvasive testing in medicine. However, although the discovery of ultrasound preceded the discovery of X-rays by twelve years, X-rays found almost immediate clinical application, while the use of ultrasound did not become widespread until much later. The primary reason for this delay is that the application of ultrasound had to await the development of appropriate technologies to detect the presence of echoes and display the information in a meaningful manner.

Real-time ultrasonic examinations are being used diagnostically to characterize normal and abnormal anatomical structures accurately in many areas of the body (Peura, 1986). Ultrasonic images of the fetus, for example, are especially useful in fetal examinations since there is no electromagnetic radiation danger, and they can be used to guide a needle to harvest ovarian material for pathological tests. Today, it is estimated that from one-half to two-thirds of the pregnant women in the United States have at least one fetal ultrasound scan, while in Great Britain and Germany fetal examination by ultrasound is required by law.

Fetal ultrasound scans are used to view the fetus and to determine whether it is developing normally. Fetal ultrasound examination allows measurement of the width of the fetal head, the size of brain ventricles (used to check for hydrocephalus), crown-to-rump length (used to determine the fetal age), examination of the spine (to check for abnormalities), the femur length (to correlate with biparietal diameter as a means of assessing proper physical development), and the detection of other fetal anomalies.

Real-time ultrasound has been used to perform interventional therapeutic techniques on the fetus *in utero*. Fetal transfusions have been performed using real-time ultrasonic visualization. Also, ultrasonic guidance has been used to drain hydrocephalus, posterior urethral valves, and chylothorax *in utero*.

The introduction of ultrasonic examinations of the heart (Figure 9.17) has had great impact on the field of cardiology, since the present real-time, two-dimensional ultrasound images or echocardiograms provide an almost unlimited number of cross-sectional image planes. Through the use of real-time scanners, additional spatial resolutions of the valve morphology as well as the cardiac chambers are now possible. The addition of Doppler flow measurements to echocardiographic imaging has enabled visualization of the movement of cardiac structures and the measurement of blood-flow velocity in the heart chambers and great vessels. Superficial structures, located less than 5 cm from the skin surface, can also be imaged in real time using ultrasound techniques. Because depth penetration is not a requirement, high-frequency transducers with resultant sub-millimeter anatomic resolution are used, thereby permitting very small lesions (two to three mm) to be observed. Superficial anatomical structures that can be imaged include the thyroid, carotid arteries, eye, scrotum, breast, and subcutaneous tissue.

Ultrasonic examinations of the eye are especially important when an ophthalmologist cannot visually examine the eye (e.g., in situations where opaque material such as blood is present or when the patient has cataracts). It would be unfortunate to have a situation in which a cataract was removed only to find that the patient had a retinal detachment or a large melanoma. The major application of ultrasonic examinations of the eye is in the evaluation of nonmetallic foreign bodies, retinal detachment, and intraocular tumors. The availability of high-frequency transducers also makes evaluating the eye for periorbital and intraorbital disorders possible.

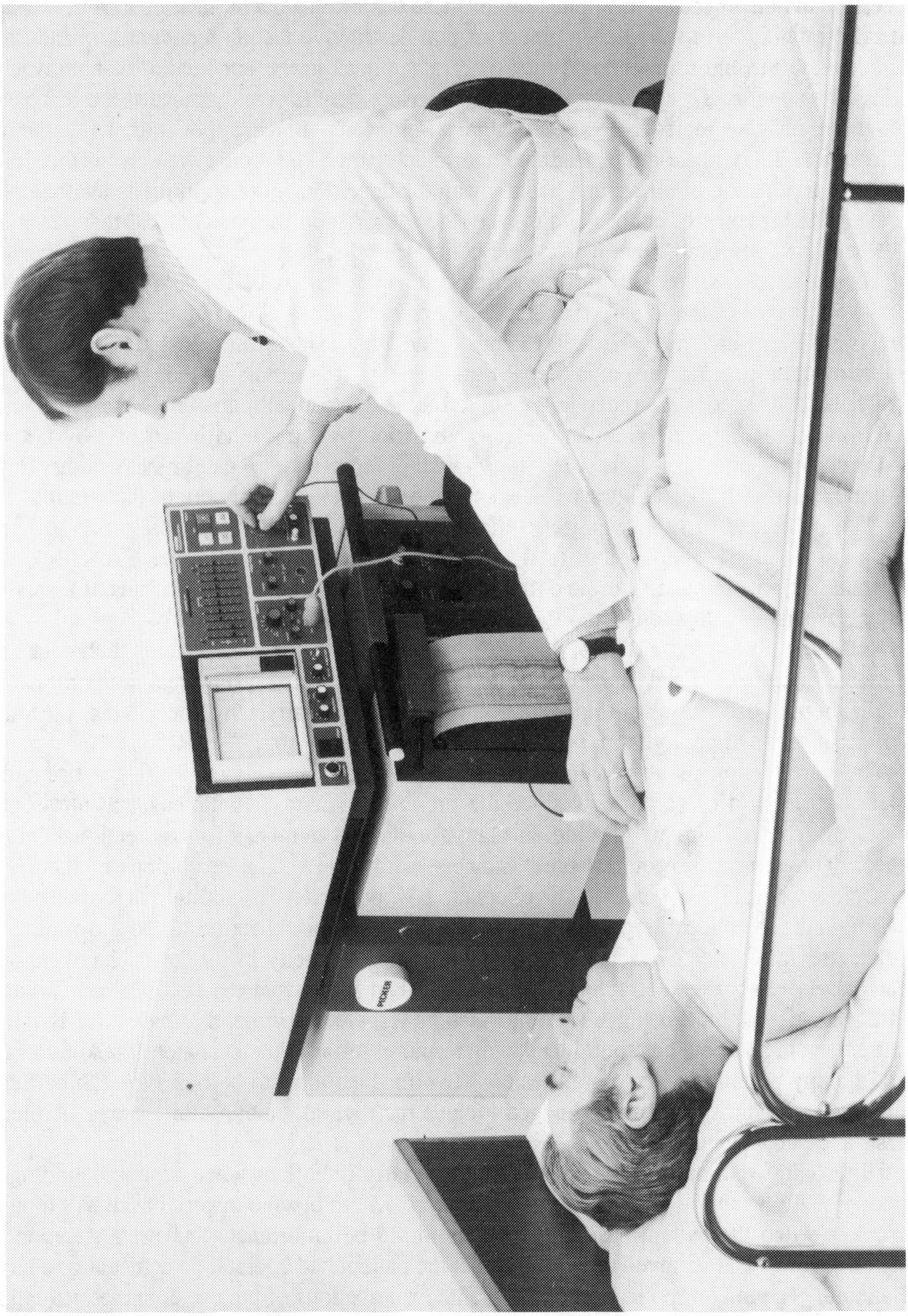

Figure 9.17: Patient undergoing ultrasound examination of the heart.

Future medical applications of diagnostic ultrasound are tied to the progress of electronic and computer technology. As electronic and computer circuits become more powerful for the same hardware volume and cost, more sophisticated ultrasonic imagers will be developed, and new medical applications will be found. The future of diagnostic ultrasonic applications in medicine is further contingent on the development of improved digital processing of the ultrasonic data. New image-processing algorithms will handle and quantify the large amounts of ultrasonic data. In present-day systems, once the data are stored in relatively inexpensive digital memory devices, they can be manipulated to improve the image quality and to make simple calculations of tissue dimensions. Further work remains in terms of improving the image quality, extracting information about the nature of the tissue, and making accurate calculations of tissue dimension, including volume, from three-dimensional measurements.

Magnetic Resonance Imaging (MRI)

In recent years, attention has focused on body-scanning devices capable of providing information on specific chemicals as well as structural information about soft tissues. These imaging technologies include Nuclear Magnetic Resonance Imaging (MRI) and Positron Emission Tomography (see above discussion). MRI, takes advantage of the magnetic properties of nuclei containing an odd number of protons or neutrons, most notably hydrogen, and perturbs these properties by introducing two magnetic fields: one to excite a resonant "precession" frequency, and the other to modulate its characteristics.

Since spinning charged particles have a magnetic moment, when placed in a magnetic field they tend to align with that field. Usually, the charged particles align themselves N to S, where N refers to the north pole of the particle's field and S refers to the south pole of the external field. However, the particles may also be oriented N to N and have the property such that a slight perturbation causes the particle to flip back to the lower-energy state. As a result, the N–to–N state is termed a "high energy state."

At any instant, there are particles in the normal state (spin up) and particles in the excited state (spin down). The quantum energy difference can be expressed as $\Delta E = hv$, where h is Planck's constant and v is the frequency. The ratio of the populations of normal to excited particles is expressed as $N_n/ N_e = e^{hv/kT}$, where k is Boltzmann's constant and T is the temperature. Actually, the axes of the spinning particles do not remain fixed in the magnetic field but rather precess, or wobble, just as a spinning top does in a gravitational field. The precessional frequency can be found from the relationship $\omega = \gamma B$, where ω is 2π times the precessional frequency, B is the magnetic field, and γ is a property of the particle called the gyromagnetic ratio. Resonance occurs when radio-frequency energy is applied at the Lamor frequency and causes particles to change state and become excited (Siedband, 1992).

In order to perform either type of imaging, the nuclei must emit a signal at the precession frequency. This is done by exciting the precessing nuclei into resonance with a radio-frequency magnetic field. When the external magnetic field is turned off, the rotating magnetic moment undergoes what is known as free induction decay (FID) as the nuclei return to the ground state. In this process, a signal emitted at the resonant frequency is usually detected by the same coils used to produce the external magnetic field. Nuclei lose their energy through two distinct relaxation processes: (1) spin-lattice, or longitudinal relaxation, characterized by the spin–spin relaxation time T_1, and (2) spin–spin, or transverse relaxation, which is characterized by spin-spin relaxation time T_2. Spin lattice relaxation involves the transfer of the excess energy from the excited nuclei to the molecular lattice by thermal interaction, whereas spin-spin relaxation involves the transfer of energy between excited nuclei and adjacent nuclei in the ground state. Typically, T_1 is on the order of one second, T_2 is greater than T_1, and therefore the FID signals induced in the coils primarily decay at the T_1 time constant. The result is a voltage associated with FID that is induced in the coils by the transfer of energy. In most imaging systems, repeated excitations are necessary to realize an adequate image signal–to–noise ratio (SNR). In most instruments, the FID signals are analyzed via Fourier spectral analysis to generate an image.

MRI produces images of lesions that can hardly be detected by other imaging techniques. Further, bone does not obstruct the MRI image of underlying tissues, unlike other imaging modalities. MRI imaging is currently more expensive than CT imaging, but because the information it provides may be unique, such as in the case of certain lesions in the brain or spinal cord, its use is growing quickly.

The ability to visualize soft internal structures *in vivo* without use of ionizing radiation has assured MRI of a quick clinical acceptance, similar to the rate at which CT scanners found favor. Since MRI can also combine biochemical with morphologic data in completely new ways, future research and experience may reveal clinical uses for this imaging technology not yet envisioned today.

DIAGNOSTIC SUPPORT SYSTEMS: EXPERT SYSTEMS IN CLINICAL CARE

The computer may also be used as an amplifier that increases the range and scope of human intelligence. In this setting, computer systems can serve as a tools to enhance human productivity by giving its user access to information to support the clinician in the decision-making process.

The science of computer systems designed to model or mimic human intelligence is refereed to as artificial intelligence"(AI) (Blum, 1984a,b). The application of AI technology to such tasks as planning, deduction, problem-solving, and understanding language (properties of human thought or intelligence) has received a great deal of attention and created considerable excitement. The term "expert system" (Waterman, 1986; Myers, 1986; Firebaugh, 1988) has been used to define a class of AI applications, which have achieved a level of performance approaching that of human experts. Of particular interest here are those expert systems that have been developed for medical use (Sandell and Bourne, 1985). These medical-expert or knowledge-based systems:

- Represent knowledge in a non-procedural form, that is, not encoded as an algorithm.
- Provide an inference mechanism that allows the application of facts (data and information) to given knowledge to produce new facts.
- Use symbolic rather than numerically coded data.
- Maintain an audit trail so that the system can justify or explain its recommendations.

Expert systems are capable of manipulating symbolic as well as numerical data and have the ability to interact with the user in something approximating natural language. They consist of two major components: the knowledge base and the inference engine (Figure 9.18). The knowledge base consists of all identifiable information relevant to the file in question. This information may include assertions, facts, relationships, and assumptions, and may be expressed in a variety of formats. The inference engine, however, is the unique design feature of expert systems; it enables them to infer the solution to a problem from a given set of assumptions or rules. The knowledge incorporated into expert systems is typically of four types:

1. Knowledge derived from data analysis; e.g, the association between gender and thyroid disease can be established as a medical fact through review (analysis) of cumulative data.
2. Subjective knowledge (judgment) derived from experience rather than theory or formal statistical analyses, but a key element in medical decision making.
3. Theoretical knowledge, such as information about causal relationships or basic mechanisms of action; for example, the effects of psychotropic drugs.
4. Strategic knowledge used in problem solving that uses strategies rather than bits of information; the rule of parsimony in developing a differential diagnosis is a strategy.

"Intelligent" computer systems do not simulate the detailed structure of the brain but rather mimic strategies followed by humans to reach a decision. For example, the "rule-based" approach assumes that human experts follow a series of logical rules that can be stated as a series of *"if . . . then"* statements.

Computer programs to support clinical decision making were first introduced nearly thirty years ago. The initial phase of research in this area, however, was based on general problem-solving algorithms that had previously been applied to mathematics and chess strategies. Therefore, the computer technology of the 1960s emphasized the use of numeric techniques to recognize patterns for modelling physical processes, the development of algorithms to deal with routine clinical chores, and the application of Bayesian statistics to determine probabilities and occurrence. The goal during this period was to develop good decision-making techniques. In the 1970s, the emphasis shifted to developing strategies of knowledge acquisition and representation, so that these systems could explain their decisions (Shortliffe, 1976). Research has led to the development of non-numerical methods of encoding information which more closely parallels the human reasoning process used in complex fields, such as medicine (Shortliffe, 1986; Rennels and Shortliffe, 1987).

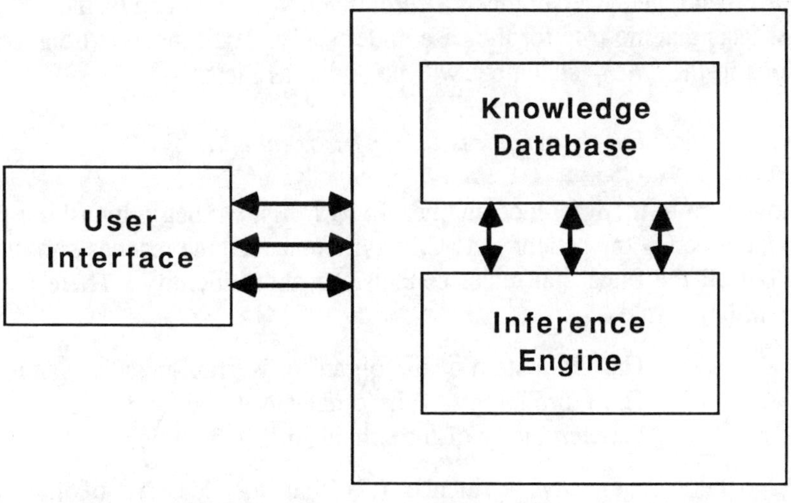

Figure 9.18: Basic components of the expert system.

Most prominent among the early applications of expert systems in medicine were **MYCIN** (Shortliffe et al., 1973; Shortliffe, 1976), **INTERNIST** (Miller et al.,, 1982), and **GLAUCOMA** (Weiss et al., 1978). Subsequently, more than 50 medical programs were developed, including **EXPERT** (Kulikowski and Weiss, 1982), **NEOMYCIN** (Clancey, 1983), **ONCOCIN** (Shortliffe et al., 1981), **QMR** (Miller et al., 1986), **BLUEBOX** (Mulsant and Servan-Schreiber, 1984; Servan-Schreiber, 1986), **DXPLain** (Barnett et al., 1987), **METHUSELAH** (Werner, 1987), and **PSYXPERT** (Shortliffe, 1986; Rennels and Shortliffe, 1987).

A somewhat different approach is taken by **OVERSEER** (Bronzino et al., 1989), a prototype expert system designed to perform quality assurance monitoring in the psychiatric hospital. OVERSEER interfaces directly with the hospital's data base and uses treatment protocols to monitor drug treatment therapy. Since it issues alert messages when clinical protocols are not followed or when other apparent problems are detected, it provides an opportunity to directly affect patient care and monitor the quality of care that patients receive from their physicians.

To illustrate how medical knowledge can be used by these systems, consider the following rule from MYCIN, a system developed at Stanford University to help physicians determine which antibiotics to use on bacterial infections of the bloodstream. To assist in this process, MYCIN's knowledge base contains four hundred to five hundred rules, each of which looks like the following:

IF: 1. The site of the culture is blood, and
2. There is significant disease associated with this occurrence of the organism,

AND: 3. The organism's portal of entry is gastrointestinal, and
4. The patient is a compromised host,

THEN: It is definite (1.0) that *Bacteroides* is an organism for which therapy should cover.

Such rules are simple "*if . . . then*" inferential statements, i.e., if we know that certain conditions have been met, we can make a certain conclusion. Each of the "*if*" assertions is tested against facts that are true for the case under study. If all the assertions are valid, then the conclusions in the "*then*" statement will be added as facts.

For example, "*the infection that requires therapy is meningitis.*"

Let us now, turn to the inference engine. In MYCIN, we begin by asking for the name of the organism infecting the patient. MYCIN's inference engine reaches into the knowledge base to pull out all the rules that make conclusions about identity. There are many such rules, one of which is rule 27:

IF: 1. The gram stain of the organism is gram-negative, and
2. The morphology of the organism is rod, and
3. The aerobicity of the organism is anaerobic,

THEN: There is suggestive evidence (.7) that the identity of the organism is *Bacteroides*.

Rule 27 is relevant in this case only if each of its preconditions has been met: the gram stain of the organism is gram-negative, the shape is rod, and it is anaerobic. How is it possible to find out if the gram stain is negative? It is possible by starting all over again, retrieving all of the rules that have anything to say about negative gram stain, and trying each in turn. This process is known as backward chaining, i.e., the inference engine starts with the suggested diagnosis and moves backward through the set of knowledge base rules to reach a conclusion. If it runs out of rules prior to arriving at a conclusion, it asks the physician to provide an additional piece of information, and continues. Thus, the inference engine searches through the knowledge base using heuristic (that is, rule-of-thumb) techniques to guide and constrain the search. Because the knowledge base is separate from the inference engine, new knowledge can be added without a major programming effort; thus the knowledge base is extensible and cumulative (Blum, 1984a). MYCIN has a number of common characteristics found in many expert systems, including:

- A performance level equivalent to human experts in the field.
- Reasoning in the face of uncertainty, a crucial part of the MYCIN system. The scale ranges from -1 (certainly wrong) to +1 (certainly right).
- Expertise derived from hand-crafted knowledge in a restricted domain, in this case, infectious blood disease.
- A special user-interface program, **TEIRESIAS**, developed for providing flexible knowledge acquisition and editing.

MYCIN also:

- Uses standard production rules rather than inference networks.
- Uses backward chaining from the diagnostic hypothesis to the data, rather than forward chaining.
- Has been a very influential research program, but to date has not been commercialized.

Another feature of MYCIN-type expert systems is that the user can interact with them to determine the rationale behind a given response of the system. For example, a physician can ask the relevance of the question that the system has asked.

MYCIN system query: *"Is the patient's illness with ORGANISM-1 a hospital-acquired infection?"*

Physician response: *"Why?"*

[i.e., Why is it important to determine whether the infection with ORGANISM-1 was acquired while the patient was hospitalized?]

The response from the system will be something like:

[2.0] This will aid in determining the identity of ORGANISM-1.
It has already been established that

[2.1] the morphology of ORGANISM-1 IS ROD
[2.2] the gram stain of ORGANISM-1 is gramneg
[2.3] the aerobicity of ORGANISM-1 is facul

Therefore, if

[2.4] the infection with ORGANISM-1 was acquired while the patient was hospitalized then there is weakly suggestive evidence
[2.5] that the identity of ORGANISM-1 is Pseudomonas
[RULE 50]

This type of explanation technology produces an audit trail by providing the clinician with a review of the system's logic steps. By keeping track of the rules that were used, MYCIN can describe how it reached its conclusion.

The power of any expert system, including MYCIN, lies in its knowledge base. In simple tests, MYCIN compared favorably with some of the experts in the field, yet the inference engine is trivial. MYCIN achieves its credible record because of the five-hundred rules stored in the knowledge base. These rules were not found in a manual of infectious disease diagnosis. They were extracted slowly from the experts, which is why it took almost six years to develop the MYCIN system.

CLINICAL ENGINEERING AND MANAGEMENT-INFORMATION SYSTEMS

Requirements of regulatory agencies, monetary pressures, and the need for quality health-care delivery demand that hospitals optimize the productivity and cost-effectiveness of each department. As previously discussed in Chapter 3, a primary concern of any clinical engineering department is the management of medical instrumentation, devices, and systems. Since most hospitals have thousands of medical instruments, devices and systems, managing the required documentation associated with each device can be quite formidable.

During the past two decades, a number of data base computer systems designed to assist clinical-engineering departments in meeting their requirements have been reported (Sherwood, 1985; Brody, 1986; Fennigkoh, 1987; Clark, 1990, Dickey, 1990). In recent years, many of these systems have been designed for personal computers (PCs). One of the most significant of these recent software packages is the current ECRI computerized **Hospital Equipment Control System (HECS)** package, developed in 1986 for IBM compatible PCs. HECS is part of a much larger comprehensive integrated medical technology management information system that permits user access to a large data base from which reliability and quality assurance data can be readily obtained. Although a complete review of these systems is not possible here, several other systems include: (1) **The Asset Information Management System (AIMS)**, introduced by Master Soft Corporation in 1983, which integrates information from multiple data bases to monitor preventive and corrective maintenance procedures of a clinical engineering department; and (2) the computer maintenance software packages marketed by **Dynatech Nevada®** and **BioTek®**, which are similar to the HECS package with the exception that these software packages accept calibration and electrical safety data automatically from their own test equipment; (3) the computerized maintenance management system **MAXIMO** developed by Product Software and Development Inc., which uses **MICROSOFT WINDOWS**.

Bio-Tek's OTIS test integration software automates test procedures for specific pieces of medical equipment and then links this information with **PROFILE,** a sophisticated equipment management software package that uses test results generated by OTIS to provide decision-making suggestions and the tools needed to take positive action. At the test site, it is only necessary for the user to enter the device control number, via bar-code wand or keyboard, and OTIS retrieves the appropriate device record and test form (procedures) to the screen of a lap-top computer. OTIS will then automatically sequence through each check item, controlling the test devices via a lap-top computer and logging all test results directly onto a hard disk. At the end of the inspection tour, the test data can be printed and/or transferred to PROFILE, which can then automatically generate work orders to assign functions for the day's activity. After providing PROFILE with equipment inventory information, preventive maintenance test procedures, and inspection cycle, it will display the list of equipment due for inspection organized by location, device type, department or cost center; provide the priority rating based on risk factor; and then generate reports ranging from failure to work analysis. This information, can then be used to initiate safety and cost decisions.

A recent survey and comparison of available maintenance-management systems illustrates a growing list of software options and significant enhancements in the use of these systems (AIPE Facilities, 1991). For any computerized system to be effective, however, clinical-engineering departments must initially determine the specific functional requirements demanded of the desired system by their department, and then evaluate the capability of available software packages to meet these requirements. The general rule is: "*If the software package meets 70–75% of their needs, buy it. If there are no available software packages that meet this criteria, then the system should be developed in-house.*"

Many of the available software systems include **Work Order, PM,** and **Inventory** applications, but how does one distinguish which package is best suited for a particular facility? To answer this question, the following factors must be evaluated: the organization, the real application needs (including short- and long-term mission), cost constraints, and future expandability. These factors combine to create the features/benefits evaluation of the computing software packages under consideration. For example:

- **Organization questions:**

  1. What is the department's overall mission?
  2. How is the department organized?
  3. What cost centers and/or users are to be included?
  4. How long, How diverse is the work? How much supervision can be given?
  5. If there is no one available now, can personnel be secured for the job? Remember, that with an automated system you will be collecting more information than before.

- **Real needs:**

  1. What is the present work flow? How are work orders initiated, completed, etc.
  2. What data files presently exist, and what format are they in? Can the current data be loaded directly into the new software?
  3. Identify the shortcomings of presently used software packages.
  4. Identify cost-tracking objectives and reporting requirements.
  5. Is expandability important? Virtually every maintenance system is likely to evolve into a bigger system with more user terminals.
  6. What systems should the new system be able to interface with—Computer Aided Design (CAD), Materials Management, Assets, Space Allocation/ Planning, Security?
  7. Identify maintenance and parts-inventory mission.

- **Cost constraints and expandability:**

  1. What are the hardware costs—CPU, monitor, keyboard, modem, printer, terminals, wiring and pulling cables, power conditioning and, back-up capacity?
  2. What are the software costs—operating system (e.g., DOS, UNIX, etc.), a run time version of a data base system (e.g., D-Base, ORACLE, etc.), applications software, communications, flexible report-writing capabilities?
  3. What will support costs be, including assembly of all components; loading of the operating system, software applications, and other utilities; systems training; data transfer from old to new system; custom modifications; software/hardware maintenance; service contracts after warranty period?

It is appropriate to start with greater capacity than is initially required. Today, hardware such as memory is relatively inexpensive, so greater capacity should be specified at the outset. Hardware should be selected in concert with the software suppliers specifications. For any system larger than a PC, the hardware supplier should assemble the system, including loading the operating system, installing all ports and digi-boards, and configuring disc partitions in accordance with the software requirements.

The above are general guidelines; now let's get a little more specific. In evaluating or designing a **Clinical Engineering Management Information System (CEMIS)** system it is important to consider a number of features, including the master file, user interface (e.g., via screen menus, input screens, specific windows) its operation, and the reports required. The "master file," which is the heart of any CEMIS, contains a record of each medical device supported by the clinical engineering department. Each record, in turn, consists of a series of files containing specific information, including the type of device, its location date of purchase, manufacturer, model and serial number, etc. The master file is essentially an unordered list (i.e., as each new item is added, an entry is created at the end of the master file). Within this file, however, a unique equipment control number is assigned to each piece of equipment, and a label bearing this information is attached to the device. This unique control number then serves as the link to all other data related to the medical device in the master file.

Two important types of ancillary files are usually associated with the master file. The first is the dictionary, which includes the equipment dictionary, the department dictionary, and the dictionary of manufacturers. The second type is the cross-reference file, which contains the control number and the index number (i.e., location within the master file) for each piece of equipment.

Most modern software packages contain a menu system that outlines the functions available to the user (Figure 9.19). A typical main menu for CEMIS allows access to specific system functions, such as the equipment menu, the reports menu, the work order menu, the operating system, or the personnel input screen (Figure 9.20) (Holden and Mueller, 1992). The equipment menu, for example, allows access to all input screens related to specific pieces of medical equipment included within the description category. The reports menu, on the other hand, permits the user to call up specific equipment reports, management reports, work order reports, and performance assurance scheduling reports. Finally, the work-order menu allows the user access to work order generation and data input screens.

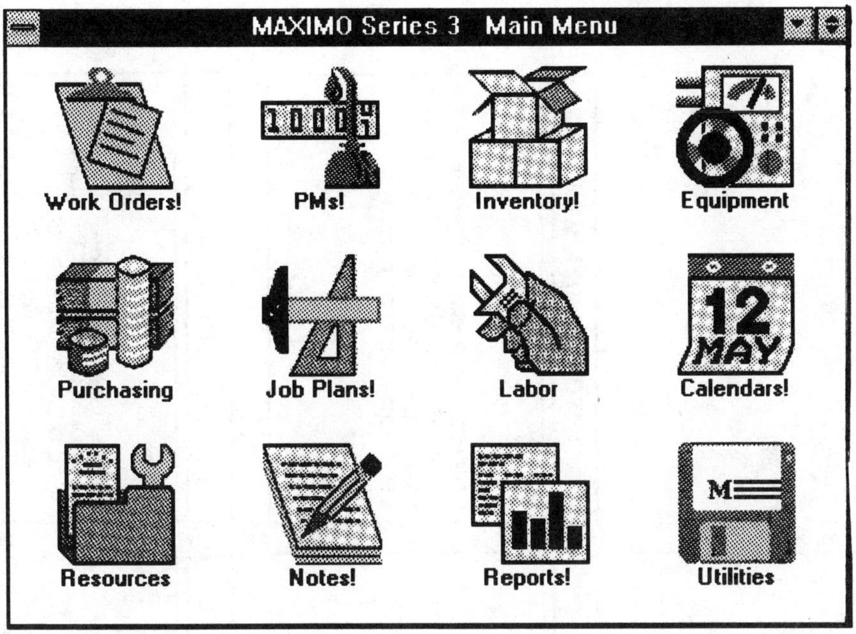

Figure 9.19: Screen presentation of the main menu provided by MAXIMO.

Input screens are used to enter, delete, or view information in the data base tables. Entering data through the supplied input screens is effective and efficient, and usually results in maintained integrity of the data base. Through the use of programmed triggers, the input screens are designed to verify correct information, format entered data, and implement help screens. As a result, most input screens employ block and cursor navigation techniques to allow a smooth, orderly, and user-friendly method for entering data into the data base (Figure 9.21). Entering data via the input screens can be further facilitated by default values that are automatically entered into the screen fields.

A recent CEMIS developed at the University of Alabama Medical Center (Holden and Mueller, 1992), has proven effective in both work order and management functions. In this system, **work order functions** consist of incoming inspections, performance assurance inspections, and service requests. An incoming inspection is performed on all clinical instruments prior to their use in the hospital. The test is to verify the instrument's conformance to manufacturer's specifications and compliance with applicable codes and standards. Repair work orders are prepared whenever a corrective or valuative action is needed on a specific device. Periodic inspections are performed to ensure proper performance of the clinical instruments. The frequency of these inspections varies depending upon the type of inspection, considerations of patient safety, recommendations of the manufacturer, and repair history.

At the end of each month, an inspection-due list is printed. Technically, this can be printed for a future month, up to one year in advance. This can be helpful in determining the workload for a given department or technician. If an unusually heavy workload is detected in advance, some of the anticipated work can be performed in earlier, less heavy months. This system then creates an inspection-due list by examining the inspection frequency and inspection start date. Consequently, any instrument that meets the criteria programmed in the report generator will be included on this list.

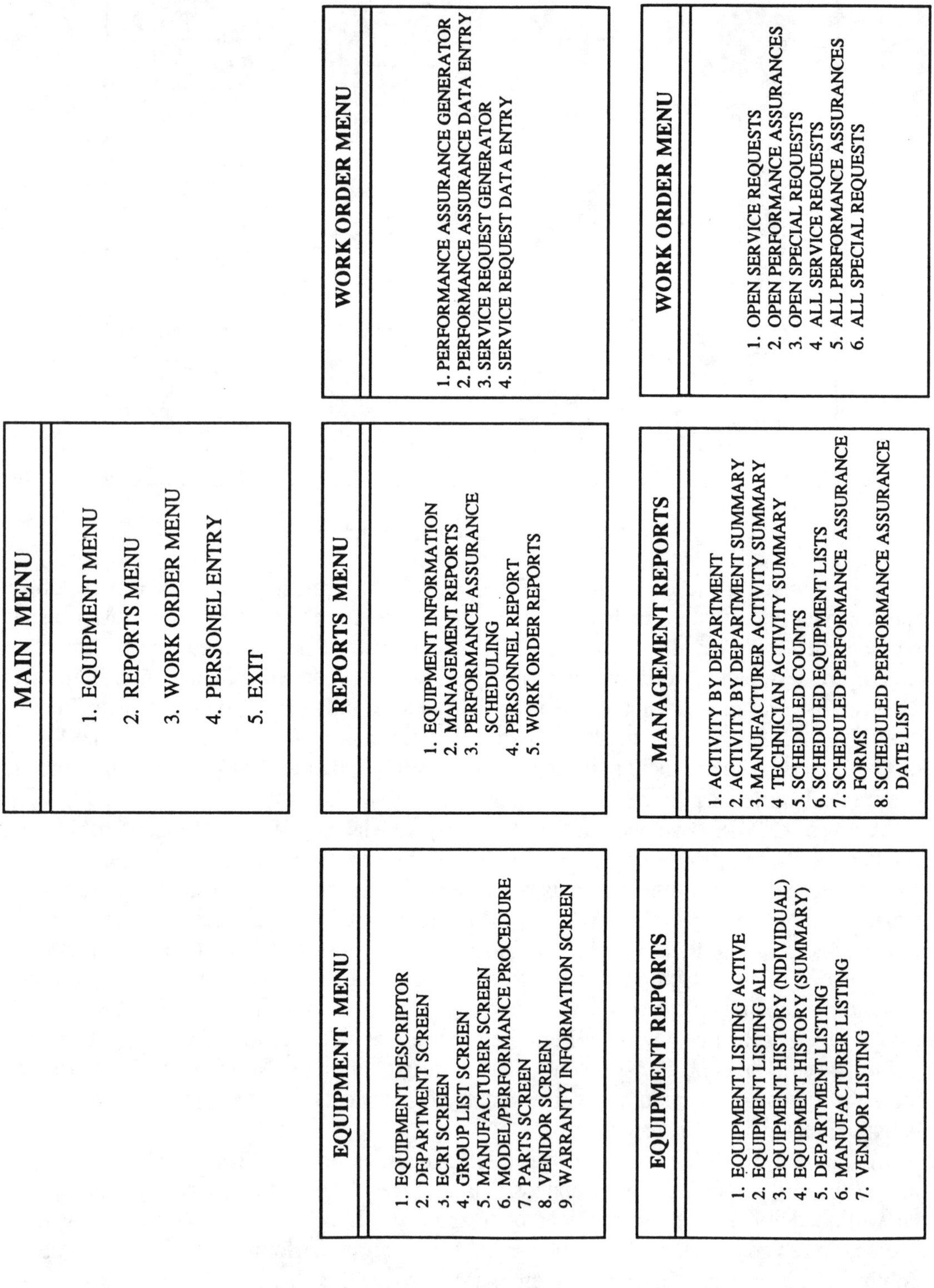

Figure 9.20: Typical screen menus of a CEMIS system.

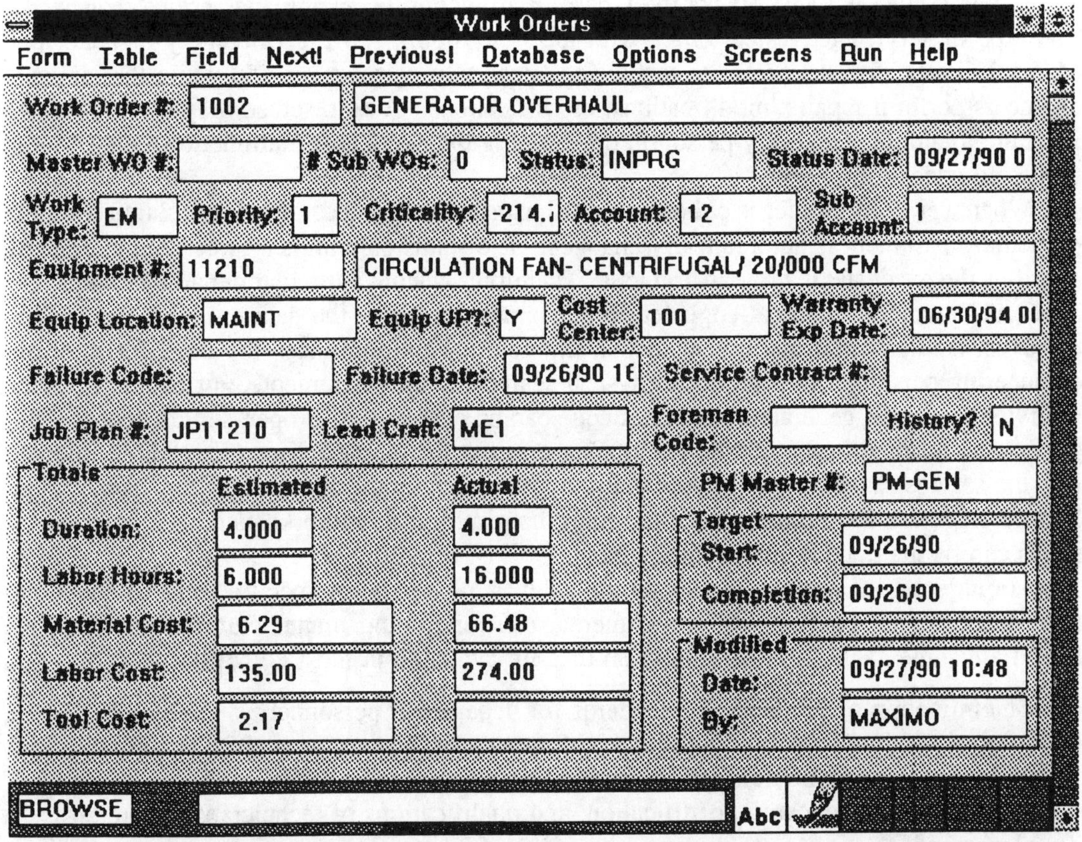

Figure 9.21: Work order screen provided by MAXIMO. The wording of each field can be modified by the user to provide the specific information needed ensure that each work order is attended to in an orderly and complete manner.

Two lists are printed; one ordered by technician number, the other by department number. Individual performance assurance forms for each instrument due for inspection are also printed. Each technician receives the performance assurance forms and inspection-due list for the equipment they are responsible for. Prior to the inspection cycle, each department receives its portion of the inspection-due list. This facilitates locating and subsequent inspection of instruments in the department's area.

The performance assurance form is used to document any incoming and periodic inspections. It can be generated upon demand or automatically for any scheduled periodic inspection. The top section of the form describes the instrument and its location. Once the form is completed, it can be entered into the system via the input screens by the technicians or data entry clerk, and serves as an outline of the proper inspection procedure.

Whenever an instrument is in need of service, the technician generates a service-request form. The top section of the form describes the instrument, its location, the reported malfunction, and the person who requested the service. In addition, the date of the last service request is noted, thereby increasing the technician's productivity and efficiency. If the date is recent, the technician can generate a copy of this service request before going out to the field to better equip himself for the task at hand.

In this system, CEMIS tracks the type of malfunction occurring and service requested. The type of service requested varies with job description. At the University of Alabama Medical Center, for example, the technicians generally perform repairs, while the clinical engineers perform repairs, modifications, or fabrications. A help screen may be invoked at any time to aid the data entry person in determining the applicable malfunction and service-requested codes.

Whenever a work order is either generated, closed, or updated, the status column for that particular instrument is automatically changed. The status column is a three-digit code that specifies the exact status of an instrument. Therefore, when a particular department inquires about an instrument, clinical-engineering personnel can query the data base and determine the exact status of the instrument at that moment. This eliminates the need for clinical engineering personnel to perform a physical search for the instrument. For example, once a service request is generated, the status code can be changed to an open-service request. If the service resulted in the instrument's being sent out for third-party service, this is entered into the service-request input screen, and the system automatically changes the status field. Since technicians have the capability to enter the results at their workbench, an instrument's status can be maintained in near real-time.

Management functions pertain to the analysis of trends for specific areas of concern, such as personnel productivity, departmental efficiency, and manufacturer dependability. Listed are some examples of information that are available in most CEMIS:

- Determination of productivity standards for department personnel.
- Analysis of time spent on repairs and performance assurances for a given department to determine appropriate staffing needs.
- Analysis of the education, certification, and qualifications of technicians for proper placement.
- Analysis of malfunction codes for a department to determine whether repairs are due to operator errors (misuse, abuse) or device errors (electrical or mechanical failure).
- Determination of the most reliable equipment manufacturers through analysis of repair costs and downtime percentages.
- Comparison of equipment service companies with each other or with in-house service (i.e., analysis costs for parts, labor, and downtime).

One of the key elements in any CEMIS is its report-generating capability. The presence of a flexible report generator is essential in order to develop the reports desired by managers at specific institutions. For example, listed below is a sample of the reports available (Holden and Mueller, 1992).

Equipment Reports

- Lists of all instruments, active and retired, ordered by the default parameters.
- An instrument history consisting of individual work orders, labor, and parts, ordered by work order number, date closed, and/or any default parameter.
- An instrument history summary consisting of total work orders, labor, and parts, ordered by work order number, date closed, and/or any default parameter.
- Department, manufacturer, and vendor listings ordered by their respective names, cities, states, assigned numbers, etc.

Management Reports

- A listing of work orders performed in a department for a specified period of time ordered by work order number, date closed, and/or any default parameter.
- A summary, for each work order type, performed in a department for a specified period of time, ordered by work order number, date closed, and/or any default parameter.
- A summary, for each work order type, performed on a manufacturer for a specified period of time, ordered by work order number, date closed, and/or any default parameter.
- A summary, for each work order type, performed by a technician for a specified period of time ordered by work order number, date closed, and any default parameter.
- The number of instruments due for inspection during a specified month, for each technician, department, and equipment classification, ordered by the default parameters.
- A list of equipment due for inspections during any specified month, ordered by the default parameters.
- The performance-assurance form for each instrument scheduled for an inspection during any specified month, ordered by technician and department and subordered by the default parameters.
- Listing of performance assurance dates for each instrument ordered by the default parameters.

Work Order Reports

- Open service requests ordered by service request number and/or default parameters.
- Open performance assurances ordered by performance assurance numbers and/or default parameters.
- Open special requests ordered by service request numbers and/or default parameter.
- A listing of all service requests, performance assurances, and/or special requests ordered by their respective identification number and/or default parameters.

SUMMARY

In this chapter, the primary objective has been to present those medical-computing applications of particular interest to clinical engineers. With this in mind, some of the basic definitions and concepts related to modern computer technology have been reviewed. In the process, terms such as "bit," "byte," "mainframe," "microcomputer," "RAM," "ROM," "baud rate," and "LAN," have all been presented in a way that makes them more familiar to the practicing clinical engineer.

After establishing a common background, specific clinical applications have been presented. The clinical chemistry and hematology laboratories, where numerous instruments are now microcomputer-based, were discussed first. The utilization of computers at both the instrument and management levels (i.e., in the form of a centralized laboratory computer) were described in an effort to stress the importance of data assemblies and integration required to provide comprehensive health status reports for clinical decision making. This concept was carried over into the discussion of automated multiphasic health-testing systems

(AMHTS), and computerized storage and recall of the patient's medical record.

The discussion of computerized patient-monitoring systems should be of particular importance to clinical engineers because of their responsibilities within intensive-care units and increased interest in self-controlling systems. The incorporation of basic instrumentation and automation techniques at the bedside makes this a hot topic for the future.

Computers are the essential component of all imaging systems. As a result, the medical imaging applications of computerized tomography (CT), nuclear medicine, ultrasound, nuclear magnetic resonance, and positron emission tomography (PET) are all briefly discussed. In the future, knowledge-based systems will hold center stage. As a result, the characteristics of an important subspecialty of artificial intelligence, namely expert systems, has also been presented.

Finally, since clinical engineers must effectively engage in all aspects of technology management, the development and use of clinical engineering information systems are discussed. These systems assist in managing work orders, service requests, equipment inventory, and scheduling preventive maintenance. As a result, they have become a critical factor in enabling clinical engineering departments achieve an effective and efficient level of operation within the hospital environment.

EXERCISES

1. For the following binary numbers, determine the equivalent representation in the decimal and octal number systems.

   (a) 11001
   (b) 101011
   (c) 1101101

2. The most elementary piece of information in the binary system is

   (a) the byte.
   (b) the number 1.
   (c) zero.
   (d) the bit.

3. If input A or B are activated in the circuit below and the circuit turns off, the circuit is call a NOR; provide a truth table for the NOR gate.

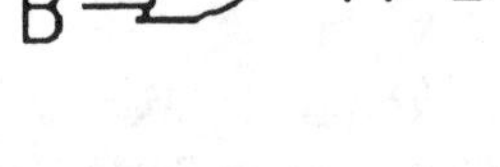

4. Which (0 or 1) enables an

   (a) AND gate.
   (b) OR gate.
   (c) NAND gate.
   (d) NOR gate.

5. For the following circuit determine the output

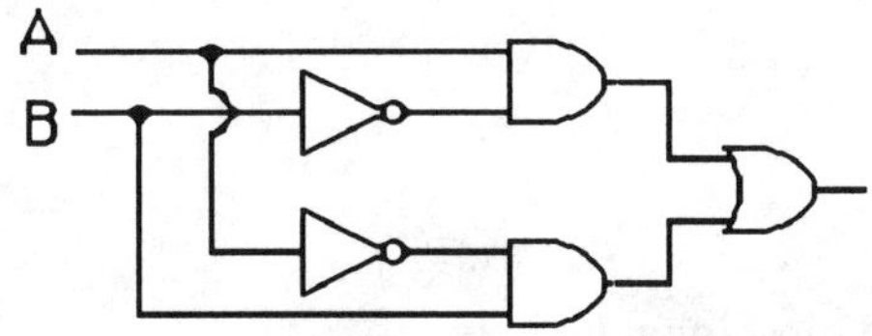

6. Identify the basic components of a microcomputer. Provide two examples of its use in a dedicated medical device.

7. Explain the reasons that data and programs are stored on auxiliary storage media rather than in the main memory unit.

8. Explain how computer software insulates the user from hardware changes. To what do you attribute the proliferation of different computer languages?

9. Describe how several laboratories within the hospital may be interconnected in a LAN. Discuss the advantages and disadvantages of such a network.

10. Design a LAN system that integrates the data from the clinical chemistry and hematology laboratories. Discuss the development of an appropriate data-base system for the information collected regarding each patient. [That is, what data elements would you select, what reports would you generate, etc.?].

11. Discuss three factors important in choosing which diagnostic tests to include in an AMHTS. What considerations are particularly relevant in deciding whether to include tests for high cholesterol level, hypertension, breast cancer, and presence of the AIDS antibody? For each condition, define the appropriate population for testing.

12. Despite the fact that AMHTS have been shown to be more economical than traditional methods for providing comprehensive screening examination, AMHTS have not achieved widespread acceptance in the United States. Discuss the sociological and economic factors that have limited acceptance of these systems in this country.

13. Discuss the physiological parameters that may be monitored during an exercise stress test. Explain the importance and/or use of each measurement. Provide a diagram of set-up.

14. Radiology departments are involved in the following activities

    (a) Film X-rays.
    (b) CT scanning.
    (c) PACS.
    (d) RIS.

15. Present CT scanners can obtain one cross-sectional image every

    (a) thirty seconds.
    (b) twenty minutes.
    (c) one second.
    (d) five minutes.

16. The field of nuclear medicine includes

    (a) Radiopharmaceuticals.
    (b) Neurotransmitters.
    (c) Stable isotopes.
    (d) X-rays.

17. The major reason that ultrasound has become such a common diagnostic tool is

    (a) It is fast.
    (b) It is accurate.
    (c) It is non-invasive.
    (d) It is inexpensive.

18. Expert systems are used in medical applications because

    (a) They are smart.
    (b) They can teach the user.
    (c) They possess a large bank of knowledge.
    (d) They are fast.

19. Provide examples of medical situations which can best be studied using

    (a) Film-based radiology.
    (b) CT scanning.
    (c) Nuclear medicine.
    (d) Ultrasonic imaging.
    (e) MRI.

20. Complete the following, emphasizing the differences between conventional and expert (symbolic) programming.

Conventional Programming	*Expert Systems (Symbolic) Programming*
Algorithms	____________________
Numerically addressed data base	____________________
____________________	Oriented toward symbolic processing
____________________	Highly interactive processing
Mid-run explanation impassible	____________________

21. Data-base systems are extremely important in the development of a CEMIS. Describe how they can be used to

    (a) Develop an inventory control system.
    (b) Provide preventive maintenance schedules.
    (c) Keep track of work orders or service requests.

REFERENCES

Anbar, M., ed. "Computers in Medicine," Computer Science Press, Rockville, MD, 1987.

Barnett, G.O., Cimino, J.J., and Hupp, J.A. "DXplain: An Evolving Diagnostic Decision Support System," *JAMA*, 258:67–74, 1987.

Blum, B.I. "Why AI?," in *Proc. of the 8th Ann. Symp. on Computer Applications in Medical Care* (G.S. Cohen, ed.), IEEE Press, Nrew York, pp.3–9, 1984a.

Blum, B.I. ed. "Information Systems for Patiet Care," Springer-Verlag, New York, 1984b.

Brody, M.S. "Fundamentals of a Computerized Clinical Engineering Management System," *Biomed. Tech. Today*, 1:42–47, 1986.

Bronzino, J.D. "Technology for Patient Care: Applications for Today, Implications for Tomorrow," C.V. Mosby Co., St. Louis, MO, 1977.

Bronzino, J.D., ed. "Computer Applications for Patient Care," Addison Wesley, Menlo Park, CA, 1982.

Bronzino, J.D., and Morelli, R.A. "Expert Systems: Basic Concepts," New Liberal Arts Program, Monograph Series, Research Foundation SUNY, Stony Brook, NY, 1989.

Bronzino, J.D., Smith, V.H., and Wade, M.L. "Medical Technology and Society: An Interdisciplinary Perspective," The New Liberal Arts Series, MIT Press, Cambridge, MA, 1990.

Clancey, W.J. "The Epistemology of a Rule-Based Expert System: A Framework for Explanation," *Artificial Intelligence*, 20:215–251, 1983.

Clark, T. "Computerized Engineering Maintenance Systems," *Health Facilities Management*, pp. 15–20, May, 1990.

Collen, M.F. et al. "Functional Goals and Problems in Large-scale Management and Automated Screening," *Federation Proc.*, 33:2376–2379, 1974.

Collen, M.F. "Health Assessment Systems," in Medical Informatics: Computer Applications In Health Care, (E.H.Shortliffe, et al, eds.), Addison-Wesley Publishing Co., Reading, MA, pp. 562–582, 1990.

Dickey, D. "Surviving and Growing in the 1990's: Managerial Methods for the Hospital-Based BME/CE Department," *Biomed. Instr. Technol.*, 23:345–354, 1990.

Dickson, J.R. "Automation of Clinical Laboratories," *Proc. IEEE*, 57:1974–1985, 1969.

Fennigkoh, L. "Management of the Clinical Engineering Department: How to Convert a Cost Center into a Profit Center," Quest Publishing Co., Brea, CA, 1987.

Firebaugh, M.W. "Artificial Intelligence: A Knowledge-Based Approach," Boyd and Fraser Publishing Co., Boston, 1988.

Friedman, G.D., Collen, M.D.F., and Fireman, B.H. "Multiphasic Health Checkup evaluation: A 16-year Follow-up," *J. Chronic Diseases*, 39:453, 1986.

Fullerton, G.D., and Cameron, I.L. "Magnetic Image Resonance Imaging," in Encyclopedia of Medical Devices and Instrumentation (J.G. Webster, ed.), John Wiley and Sons, New York, pp 1833–1840, 1988.

Gardner, R. "Patient Monitoring Systems," in Medical Informatics: Computer Applications In Health Care, (E.H.Shortliffe, et al., eds.), Addison-Wesley Publishing Co., Reading, MA, pp. 366–399, 1990.

Garfield, S.R. "The Delivery of Medical Care," *Sci. Am.*, 222:15–23, 1970.

Garfield, S. R., "The Computer and the New Health Care System," in Hospital Computer Systems (M.F. Collen, ed.), John Wiley and Sons, New York, pp. 24–31, 1974.

Greenes, R.A., and Brinkley, J.F. "Radiology Systems," in Medical Informatics (E. Shortliffe and L. Perrault, eds.), Addison Wesley, Reading, MA. pp. 324–365, 1990.

Holden, J.J., and Mueller, J.T. "Design of a Clinical Engineering Management Information System," *Biomed. Instr. Technol.*, 37:16–25, 1992.

Hudson, L. "Monitoring of Critically Ill Patients: Conference Summary," *Respiratory Care*, 30:628–630, 1985.

Jenkins, M.A. "Functions of Patient Care Computing," *Med. Instrum.*, 12:213–214, 1978.

Kriewall, T.J., and Long, J.M. "Computer-based Medical Systems," *Computer*, 24:9–12, 1991.

Kulikowski, C.A., and Weiss, S.M. "Representation of Expert Knowledge for Consultation: The CASNET and EXPORT Projects," in Artificial Intelligence in Medicine (P. Szolovitz, ed.), West View Press, Boulder, CO, pp. 21–55, 1982.

Ledley, R.S. "Introduction to Computerized Tomography," *Comput. Biol. Med.*, 6:239–246, 1976.

Maravilla, K., and Pastel, M. "Technical Aspects of CT Scanning," *Comput. Tomograph.*, 2:137–144, 1978.

Martinek, R. "Automated Analytical Systems," *Medical Electronics and Data*, 3:33–39, 1972.

Miller, R.A., Paple, H.E., and Myers, J.D. "Internist-1: An Evolving Computer-based Diagnostic Consultant for General Internal Medicine," *New. Engl. J. Med.*, 307:468–476, 1982.

Miller, R.A., McNeil, M.A., and Challino, S.M. "The Internist-1/QUICK Medical Conference Project: Status Report," *Western J. Med.*, 145:816–822, 1986.

Mulsant, B., and Servan-Schreiber, D. "Knowledge Engineering: A Daily Activity on a Hospital Ward," *Comput. Biomed. Res.*, 17:71–91, 1984.

CHAPTER 10

MORAL AND ETHICAL ISSUES IN CLINICAL ENGINEERING PRACTICE

Why should engineers, particularly biomedical and clinical engineers, be concerned with ethics? The answer to this question lies in part with the fact that innovations in medical technology have endowed modern medicine with capabilities unimagined even a few decades ago. Today's health-care providers can prolong life, prevent and cure many diseases and disabilities, and otherwise ameliorate a wide range of undesirable physical and mental conditions for which little could previously be done. However, by increasing these creative powers and possibilities, technology also increases the range of choices (e.g., reproductive technologies) available to humankind and, in the process, raises moral dilemmas for the medical staff, clinical engineers, and society as a whole. In the realm of health care technology, these moral dilemmas may involve decisions. *Which new options ought to be pursued? Which ought to be avoided? Which new ways of doing things should actually be implemented? Which should not?* Such decisions are not easy and often involve consideration of conflicting viewpoints. To address these types of decisions properly, we must turn to ethics. We must know both what our moral standards are and how they apply to the changes and possibilities created by technology. Accordingly, this chapter provides an introduction to ethics and discusses some of the moral issues of special importance to biomedical and clinical engineers.

THE ETHICAL SIGNIFICANCE OF PROFESSIONALISM

One of the major reasons for clinical engineers to be concerned with ethics derives from their status as professionals. As discussed in Chapter 1, if clinical engineers desire professional status, they must address matters of ethical significance. Benjamin Barber (1963) has noted four defining characteristics of professional occupations, three of which are particularly germane to this discussion:

1. *a high degree of generalized and systematic knowledge.*
2. *primary orientation to the community interest rather than to individual self-interest.*
3. *a high degree of self-control of behavior through codes of ethics internalized in the process of work socialization and through voluntary associations organized and operated by the work specialists themselves.*
4. *and a system of rewards (monetary and honorary) that is primarily a set of symbols of work achievements and thus ends in themselves, not means to some end of individual self-interest.*

The first of these characteristics recognizes that because of their training and education, such professionals possess knowledge and skills not possessed by laypeople and have valuable capabilities that laypeople do not possess. To practice a professional occupation, then, is to have significant power to affect the lives of others. The greater that power is, the more important it is to ensure that it is not abused and misused. Clearly then, all professionals, including engineers, need to be aware of the ethical dimensions of their activities. This awareness, however, requires more than a passing acquaintance with ethics.

This is especially true for biomedical and clinical engineers because their activities have dramatic effects on the quality and efficacy of health care which in turn has enormous impact on the quality of human life.

According to the second characteristic listed above, to be a professional is to be dedicated to using one's particular occupational skills and knowledge for the public good rather than purely for self-interest. This is not, of course, to say that professionalism requires renunciation of personal gain. It does mean, however, that professionals seek personal gain by using their occupational skills and knowledge in ways that serve society, and it requires that they reject those personally remunerative uses of their occupational skills and knowledge that are contrary to the public good. What is the public good? Which personally beneficial uses of expertise must professionals avoid? What ought a professional do when the requirements of service to the public good are inconsistent with personal gain or when meeting such requirements will result in significant personal losses? What ought professionals do when their expertise shows them that what the public wants does not promote the public good? If engineers are to regard themselves as professionals, they must face questions of this nature and to do so successfully they must draw upon the resources of ethics.

Finally, the third characteristic of professionalism requires that if the professions are to minimize the misuse and abuse of the power entailed by their expertise and if they are to carry out fully their pledge to use that power to serve the public good, then the occupational activities of their members must be regulated. This regulation will, of necessity, largely have to be self-regulation. Because their occupational activities involve knowledge that is not possessed by laypeople, it is the responsibility of the members of a profession to understand the nature and probable consequences of those occupational activities and to develop effective regulation procedures. However, if professionals are to be truly successful at self-regulation and if the public is to continue to accept oversight of professions by their members, it is essential that professionals have some grounding in ethics. Otherwise, although their efforts at self-control may be well intended and grounded in appropriate technical knowledge, those efforts are likely to fail to meet the needs of society.

CODES OF ETHICS

As a consequence of increased awareness of the ethical significance of their occupational activities, biomedical and clinical engineers and their counterparts in the other professions have promulgated codes of professional ethics. Typically taking the form of a short list of general rules, such codes express both the minimal standards to which all members of a profession are expected to conform and the ideals for which all members are expected to strive. Such codes provide a practical guide for the ethical conduct of the profession's practitioners. Consider, for example, the **code of ethics** endorsed by the **American College of Clinical Engineers** (below).

Although codes of professional ethics can be useful in promoting ethical conduct, particularly if their provisions are ethically sound and genuinely enforced, they do have limits. To be manageable, codes cannot contain all of the directives and information relevant to ethically sound conduct. Their contents, for the most part, must be brief general rules abstracted from the diversity of concrete situations that professionals face in the course of their occupational activities. Such rules obviously cannot provide ethical guidance in every situation. A profession that aims to maximize the ethical conduct of its members must not limit the ethical consciousness of its members to knowledge of their professional code alone. It must also provide them with resources that will enable them to determine what the code requires in a particular concrete situation and thereby enable them to arrive at ethically sound judgments in situations in which the directives of the code are ambiguous or simply do not apply. A better understanding of ethics is therefore essential for clinical engineers to function as professionals in the clinical environment. With this in mind, let us examine some of the basic tenets of ethics and morality.

American College of Clinical Engineering

Code of Ethics

As a member of the American College of Clinical Engineering, I subscribe to the established Code of Ethics in that I will:

- Accurately represent my level of responsibility, authority, experience, knowledge, and education.
- Strive to prevent a person from being placed at risk due to the use of technology.
- Reveal conflicts of interest that may affect information provided or received.
- Respect the confidentiality of information.
- Work toward improving the delivery of health care.
- Work toward the containment of costs by the better management and utilization of technology.
- Promote the profession of clinical engineering.

THE NATURE of MORAL JUDGEMENTS

Although the terms "ethics" and "morality" are commonly used as synonyms, philosophers interpret "ethics" as a particular kind of study and use "morality" to refer to its subject matter. The ultimate aim of ethics is to provide valid answers to questions regarding which actions ought or ought not be taken. Answers to such questions are referred to as moral judgments. Because moral judgments and the principles used to derive them represent the basic components of any morality, an understanding of the nature of ethics best begins with the nature of such judgments.

What distinguishes moral judgments from other kinds of judgments? All moral judgments are "normative judgments" and as such can often be recognized simply by their characteristic evaluative terms such as **good, bad, right, wrong, ought, ought not,** and the like. Examples of typical normative judgments include these:

- Stealing is wrong.
- Gold is an excellent investment.
- Toyota is the right choice for smart car buyers.
- Voluntary euthanasia should not be legalized.
- Everyone ought to have access to an education.

Each of these judgments expresses an evaluation, i.e., conveys a negative or positive attitude toward some state of affairs. Each, therefore, is intended to play an action-guiding function. To utter the sentence, "Everyone ought to have access to an education," is to imply that arrangements should be made to ensure that the opportunity to obtain an education is available to all who desire it. This prescriptive or action-guiding function distinguishes normative from non-normative judgments.

Although all normative judgments express evaluations and are intended to guide human conduct, not all normative judgments are moral judgments. Some normative judgments express legal evaluations, others are judgments of etiquette, and still others are aesthetic judgments. Knowing that a judgment is normative is not sufficient for defining it as a moral judgment. Clearly, actions that are illegal, impolite, or unaesthetic are not necessarily immoral and actions that are moral are not necessarily legal, polite, or aesthetic.

Moral judgments then are those normative judgments arrived at by applying moral standards rather than standards of law, etiquette, or aesthetics. Consequently the problem of distinguishing moral judgments from other sorts of normative judgments resolves into distinguishing moral standards from nonmoral standards. Ethicist Manuel Valasquez (1988) has summarized the four characteristics most often cited in the literature of ethics as the distinguishing features of moral standards. Collectively, these four characteristics should suffice in most cases to distinguish moral from nonmoral standards.

1. *[M]oral standards deal with matters that are (or are thought to be of serious consequence to our human well-being. That is, they are concerned with behavior that can seriously injure or seriously benefit human beings (or that is believed to be capable of having these consequences).*
2. *Moral standards are not made up by particular bodies, nor does their validity rest on the particular decisions of particular persons. The validity of moral standards rests instead on the adequacy of the reasons that are taken to support and justify them, and so long as these reasons are adequate, the standards remain valid.*
3. *Moral standards are supposed to override self-interest. That is, if a person has a moral obligation to do something, then the person is supposed to do it even if it is not in the person's own interests to do so.*
4. *[M]oral standards are based on the moral point of view, that is, a point of view that does not evaluate standards according to whether or not they advance the interests of a particular individual or group, but that goes beyond personal interests to a universal standpoint in which everyone's interests are impartially counted as equal.*

Concern with moral judgments is not limited to ethics. Sociology, anthropology, history, and psychology, among other disciplines, also focus upon moral judgments. Perhaps the most important difference between ethics and these other studies of moral judgments is that the latter are factual studies. That is, they seek primarily to discover, report, categorize, and explain the moral judgments that people actually have made, do make, or will make. Ethics is chiefly concerned with determining which moral judgments should be made and used as bases for human conduct. Hence, ethics is itself normative, as it seeks to evaluate moral judgments and thereby guide the activity of those making such judgments.

Traditionally, ethics has been divided into two related domains, **ethical theory** and **applied ethics**. Ethical theory, in turn, is usually divided into two related branches, **metaethics** and **normative ethics**.

Ethical Theory and Applied Ethics

Applied ethics is to ethical theory what engineering is to pure science. Like theoretical science, ethical theory is primarily concerned with extending our general knowledge. Pure science's main concern is, of course, factual knowledge, and ethical theory's main concern is generalizable knowledge of right and wrong, good and evil, virtue and vice, and the like, typically expressed in the form of general principles. Just as applied science seeks to increase our ability to act and to enhance what we can achieve, so does applied ethics seek primarily to provide implementable answers to concrete questions about how we should act, what we should choose to do, etc. Although answers to such questions have been provided, and will continue to be provided, without explicitly drawing upon ethical theory, contemporary concern with such problems tends to recognize the importance of utilizing the resources of ethical theory. The old saw that theory without practice is often empty and practice without theory is often blind applies to ethics and science alike.

For the most part, the types of ethical issues posed by engineering, including biomedical/clinical engineering, do not concern general ethical knowledge. They concern concrete choices of what to do, or not do, in the concrete situations encountered by biomedical engineers. Engineering ethics, thus, belongs squarely within the domain of applied ethics. Yet, like all areas of applied ethics, arriving at practicable solutions to concrete dilemmas requires a firm grounding in the general knowledge provided by ethical theory.

Metaethics

Metaethics is that branch of ethical theory concerned with the analysis of moral concepts and other concepts central to moral reasoning and argument. Because concepts are usually expressed by means of words, metaethics largely focuses upon clarifying moral terminology. This activity is critical to any attempt to arrive at sound moral judgments. If the terminology used to express moral judgments is not clearly understood, determining when those judgments are valid or invalid is likely to be very difficult. For example, determining whether use of a particular medical device is morally appropriate might depend upon whether such use is to be considered experimental or therapeutic. Unless the concepts of experimentation and therapy and the differences between them are clearly defined and understood, morally inappropriate uses of the device may occur. Physicians may fail to recognize that the risks that are ethically permissible in the therapeutic use of a device may differ from those that are ethically permissible in experimental use. Hence, the safeguards that are required by ethical experimentation or ethically sound therapy may not be adequately implemented. Given that human well-being and even human life can be at stake in this sort of instance, clarification of morally relevant terminology is clearly more than a mere exercise in semantics.

An understanding of metaethics begins with conceptual analysis, i.e., the determination of the necessary and sufficient conditions that must be met for the proper use of particular concepts (more strictly, for the terms used to express them). To completely analyze a concept and thereby completely illuminate its meaning, the complete set of necessary and sufficient conditions for its appropriate use must be given. Unfortunately, in many instances a complete set of necessary and sufficient conditions for valid use cannot be determined. Many concepts simply are not as precise as the concept of a rectangle, nor is their meaning as uncontested. A lesson that can be safely drawn from metaethical investigations is that many of the concepts of greatest relevance to moral deliberation are of this kind. For example, most medical ethicists agree that, except perhaps in cases of dire emergency, the ethically sound use of medical devices on competent adult patients or experimental subjects requires the acquisition of informed and voluntary consent. Nonetheless there exists much disagreement as to what constitutes informed consent. Is consent genuinely voluntary when given under the duress of the fear and suffering often accompanying illness? How much information concerning a device must the patient or subject accurately comprehend before his consent is genuinely informed? A quick glance at the literature of biomedical ethics will show that answers to these questions are still matters of much debate. Though progress has been made in understanding and settling upon the meaning of such concepts as informed consent, many ethically important concepts may continue to defy complete analysis. In any case, analyzing moral concepts as fully as possible and thus coming to understand as completely as possible the terminology of moral deliberation is crucial to the effort of deciding moral questions correctly.

Normative Ethics

Arriving at valid moral judgments requires knowledge of valid moral standards. How is such knowledge obtained? The efforts to answer this question comprise the second branch of ethical theory: normative ethics. Two competing and perhaps incompatible schools of thought currently dominate normative ethical theory: **utilitarianism,** a form of consequentialism, and **Kantianism,** a form of nonconsequentialism. Consequentialism holds that the morally right action is always the one among the available options that has the best consequences. An important implication of consequentialism is that no specific actions or courses of conduct are automatically ruled out as immoral or ruled in as morally obligatory. The rightness or wrongness of an action is wholly contingent upon its effects.

According to utilitarianism, the dominant form of consequentialism, there are two steps to determining what ought to be done in any situation. First, determine which courses of action are open. Second, determine the consequences of each alternative. When this has been accomplished, the morally right course of action is the one that maximizes pleasure, minimizes pain, or both; the one that does the "greatest good for the greatest number." Because the central motivation driving development and use of medical devices is improvement of medicine's capacity to protect and restore health, an obvious virtue of utilitarianism is that it assesses medical technology in terms of what many believe makes health valuable, the attainment of pleasure and the avoidance of pain.

Before discussing nonconsequentialist ethics, some of the considerations advanced against utilitarianism should be discussed. Jeffrie Murphy and Jules Coleman (1984) provide a compelling illustration of what many find unacceptable about utilitarianism:

> *Suppose that cancer and all other major diseases could be cured and the vast majority of human beings thus rendered much more happy and secure by rounding up a few persons against their will and subjecting them to painful and ultimately fatal medical experiments. (To avoid any complexities that might be raised by the suggestion that we search for volunteers, let us suppose that the experiments require a certain enzyme secreted by the brain only when persons are unaware that they are being coerced, hurt, and threatened with death.) Intuitively, most of us would be inclined to say that — even given the general good consequences that would flow from this experimental process — adopting the process would still be immoral. We might say that it is* ***unjust*** *to treat people in this way and say that they have a* ***right*** *not to be treated in this way and say that if utilitarianism cannot accommodate such rights (and thus agree with us in condemning the practice) then so much the worse for utilitarianism. But how can utilitarianism accommodate a respect for rights and justice and thus condemn the practice? Does not its commitment to "the greatest good for the greatest number" require that it approve of treating people in this awful way if the general welfare will be promoted, if happiness will be maximized? The moral is then clear: it* ***is*** *so much the worse for utilitarianism, and all morally sensitive people will thus reject it as an ethical theory.*

The point is that utilitarianism takes the end to justify the means and so allows, indeed requires, the use of any form of treatment that maximizes good consequences. To many people, though, it seems that the end does not always justify the means and that individuals have rights that are not to be violated no matter how good the consequences of violation might be. On this view, utilitarianism's downfall is its ability to justify injustice.

In opposition to utilitarianism stands the school of normative ethical thought known as **nonconsequentialism**. Proponents of this school deny that moral evaluation is simply and wholly a matter of determining the consequences of human conduct. They agree that other considerations are relevant to moral assessment and so reject the view that morally right conduct is whatever has the best consequences. Based largely on the views of the German philosopher Immanuel Kant (1724–1804), this ethical theory insists, as Murphy and Coleman (1984) note, that

> *there is something uniquely precious about human beings from the moral point of view. There are, for example, certain special moral requirements (rights) that attach to human beings that do not attach to any other animal, e.g., the requirement that we not kill and eat them for food, or hunt them for sport, or experiment on them for medical science. They are, in short, owed a special kind of respect simply because they are people.*

To understand the Kantian basis of this perspective, it is necessary to recognize that Kant's views are an attempt to capture in secular form a basic tenet of Christian morality. What makes human beings morally special entities deserving a unique type of respect? Christianity answers in terms of the doctrine of ensoulment. This doctrine holds that only human beings are divinely endowed with an eternal soul. According to Christian ethics, this unique human feature makes humans the only beings with intrinsic value and is the very reason they deserve rights that limit how they may be properly treated. Kant's secular version of the doctrine of ensoulment claims that human beings are made morally unique and deserving of special respect by their autonomy. Autonomy is taken by Kant to be the capacity to make choices on the basis of rational deliberation. The central task of ethics then is to specify what is required by respect for the unique dignity of human beings. For most Kantians, this means determining what limits human beings must observe in the way they treat each other and this, in turn, is taken to be a matter of specifying each individual's fundamental moral rights.

Beneficence, Nonmaleficence, and Technological Progress

Two moral norms have remained relatively constant across the various moral codes and oaths that have been formulated for health-care deliverers since the beginnings of Western medicine in classical Greek civilization, namely, **beneficence** — the provision of benefits — and **nonmaleficence** — the avoidance of doing harm. These norms are traced back to a body of writings from classical antiquity known as the *Hippocratic Corpus*. Although these writings are associated with the name of Hippocrates, the acknowledged founder of Western medicine, medical historians remain uncertain whether any, including the *Hippocratic oath*, were actually his work. Although portions of the *Corpus* are believed to have been authored during the sixth century B.C., other portions are believed to have been written as late as the beginning of the Christian era. Medical historians agree, though, that many of the specific moral directives of the *Corpus* represent neither the actual practices nor the moral ideals of the majority of physicians of ancient Greece and Rome.

Nonetheless, the general injunction, "*As to disease, make a habit of two things — to help or, at least, to do no harm,*" was accepted as a fundamental medical ethical norm by at least some ancient physicians. With the decline of Hellenistic civilization and the rise of

Christianity, beneficence and nonmaleficence became increasingly accepted as the fundamental principles of morally sound medical practice. Although beneficence and nonmaleficence were regarded merely as concomitant to the craft of medicine in classical Greece and Rome, the emphasis upon compassion and the brotherhood of humankind, central to Christianity, increasingly made these norms the only acceptable motives for medical practice. Even today the provision of benefits and the avoidance of doing harm are stressed just as much in virtually all contemporary Western codes of conduct for health professionals as they were in the oaths and codes that guided the health-care providers of past centuries.

Traditionally, the ethics of medical care has given greater prominence to nonmaleficence than to beneficence. This priority was grounded in the fact that, historically, medicine's capacity to do harm far exceeded its capacity to protect and restore health. Providers of health care possessed many treatments that posed clear and genuine risks to patients but that offered little prospect of benefit. Truly effective therapies were all too rare. In this context, it is surely rational to give substantially higher priority to avoiding harm than to providing benefits.

The advent of modern science changed matters dramatically. Knowledge acquired in laboratories, tested in clinics, and verified by statistical methods has increasingly dictated the practices of medicine. This ongoing alliance between medicine and science became a critical source of the plethora of technologies that now pervades medical care. The impressive increases in therapeutic, preventive, and rehabilitative capabilities that these technologies have provided have pushed beneficence to the forefront of medical morality. Some have even gone so far as to hold that the old medical ethic of *"Above all, do no harm"* should be superseded by the new ethic that *"The patient deserves the best."* However, the rapid advances in medical technology capabilities have also produced great uncertainty as to what is most beneficial or least harmful for the patient. In other words, along with increases in ability to be beneficent, medicine's technology has generated much debate about what actually counts as beneficent or nonmaleficent treatment. Having reviewed some of the fundamentals of ethics, let us turn to several specific moral issues posed by the use of medical technology.

DEFINING DEATH: A MORAL DILEMMA POSED BY MEDICAL TECHNOLOGY

Supportive and resuscitative devices, such as the respirator, found in the typical modern intensive care unit provide a useful starting point for illustrating how technology has rendered medical morality more complex and problematic. Devices of this kind allow clinicians to sustain respiration and circulation in patients who have suffered massive brain damage and total permanent loss of brain function. These technologies force us to ask precisely when a human life ends? When is a human being indeed dead? This is not the straightforward factual matter it may appear to be. All of the relevant facts may show that the patient's brain has suffered injury grave enough to destroy its functioning forever. The facts may show that such an individual's circulation and respiration would permanently cease without artificial support. Yet these facts do not determine whether treating such an individual as a corpse is morally appropriate. To know this, it is necessary to know or perhaps to decide on those features of living persons that are essential to their status as living persons. It is necessary to know or decide which human qualities, if irreparably lost, make an individual identical in all morally relevant respects to a corpse. Once those qualities have been specified, deciding whether total and irreparable loss of brain function constitutes death becomes a straightforward factual matter. For then one would simply have to determine if such loss itself deprives the individual of those qualities. If it does, the individual is morally identical to a corpse. If not, then the individual must be regarded and treated as a living person.

The traditional criterion of death has been irreparable cessation of heart beat, respiration, and blood pressure. This criterion would have been quickly met by anyone suffering massive trauma to the brain prior to the development of modern supportive technology. Such technology allows indefinite artificial maintenance of circulation and respiration and, thus, forestalls what once was an inevitable consequence of severe brain injury. The existence and use of such technology therefore challenges the traditional criterion of death and forces us to consider whether continued respiration and circulation are in themselves sufficient to distinguish a living individual from a corpse. Indeed, total and irreparable loss of brain function, referred to as "brainstem death," "whole brain death," and, simply, "brain death," has been widely accepted as the legal standard for death. By this standard, an individual in a state of brain death is legally indistinguishable from a corpse and may be legally treated as one even though respiratory and circulatory functions may be sustained through the intervention of technology. Many take this legal standard to be the morally appropriate one, noting that once destruction of the brain stem has occurred, the brain cannot function at all, and the body's regulatory mechanisms will fail unless artificially sustained. Thus mechanical sustenance of an individual in a state of brain death is merely postponement of the inevitable and sustains nothing of the personality, character, or consciousness of the individual. It is merely the mechanical intervention that differentiates such an individual from a corpse and a mechanically ventilated corpse is a corpse nonetheless.

Even with a consensus that brainstem death is death and thus that an individual in such a state is indeed a corpse, hard cases remain. Consider the case of an individual in a persistent vegetative state, the condition known as "neocortical death." Although severe brain injury has been suffered, enough brain function remains to make mechanical sustenance of respiration and circulation unnecessary. In a persistent vegetative state, an individual exhibits no purposeful response to external stimuli and no evidence of self-awareness. The eyes may open periodically and the individual may exhibit sleep–wake cycles. Some patients even yawn, make chewing motions, or swallow spontaneously. Unlike the complete unresponsiveness of individuals in a state of brainstem death, a variety of simple and complex responses can be elicited from an individual in a persistent vegetative state. Nonetheless, the chances that such an individual will regain consciousness are virtually nil. Artificial feeding, kidney dialysis, and the like make it possible to sustain an individual in a state of neocortical death for decades. This sort of condition and the issues it raises were exemplified by the famous case of Karen Ann Quinlan. James Rachels (1986) provided the following description of the situation created by Quinlan's condition:

> *In April 1975 this young woman ceased breathing for at least two fifteen minute periods, for reasons that were never made clear. As a result, she suffered severe brain damage, and, in the words of the attending physicians, was reduced to a "chronic vegetative state" in which she "no longer had any cognitive function." Accepting the doctors' judgment that there was no hope of recovery, her parents sought permission from the courts to disconnect the respirator that was keeping her alive in the intensive care unit of a New Jersey hospital.*
>
> *The trial court, and then the Supreme Court of New Jersey, agreed that Karen's respirator could be removed. So it was disconnected. However, the nurse in charge of her care in the Catholic hospital opposed this decision and, anticipating it, had begun to wean her from the respirator so that by the time it was disconnected she could remain alive without it. So Karen did not die. . . . Karen remained alive for ten additional years. In June 1985 she finally died of acute pneumonia. Antibiotics, which would have fought the pneumonia, were not given.*

If brainstem death is death, is neocortical death also death? Again the issue is not a straightforward factual matter. For, it too, is a matter of specifying which features of living individuals distinguish them from corpses and so make treatment of them as corpses morally impermissible. Irreparable cessation of respiration and circulation, the classical criterion for death, would entail that an individual in a persistent vegetative state is not a corpse and so, morally speaking, must not be treated as one. The brainstem death criterion for death would also entail that a person in a state of neocortical death is not yet a corpse. On this criterion, what is crucial is that brain damage be severe enough to cause failure of the body's regulatory mechanisms.

Is an individual in a state of neocortical death any less in possession of the characteristics that distinguish the living from cadavers than one whose respiration and circulation are mechanically maintained? Of course, it is a matter of what the relevant characteristics are, and it is a matter that society must decide. It is not one that can be settled by greater medical information or more powerful medical devices. Until society decides, it will not be clear what would count as beneficent or nonmaleficent treatment of an individual in a state of neocortical death.

EUTHANASIA

Whatever society's decision is as to what constitutes death, a long-standing issue in medical ethics, which has been made more pressing by medical technology, is euthanasia, the deliberate termination of an individual's life for the individual's own good. Is such an act ever a permissible use of medical resources? Consider an individual in a persistent vegetative state. On the assumption that such a state is not death, withdrawing life support would be a deliberate termination of a human life. Here a critical issue is whether the quality of a human life can be so low or so great a liability to the individual that deliberately taking action to hasten death or at least not to postpone death is morally defensible. Can the quality of a human life be so low that the value of extending its quantity is totally negated? If so, then Western medicine's traditional commitment to providing benefits and avoiding harm would seem to make cessation of life support a moral requirement in such a case.

Consider the following hypothetical version of the kind of case that actually confronts contemporary patients, their families, health-care workers, and society as a whole. Suppose a middle aged man suffers a brain hemorrhage and loses consciousness as a result of a ruptured aneurysm. Suppose that he never regains consciousness and is hospitalized in a state of neocortical death, a chronic vegetative state. He is maintained by a surgically implanted gastronomy tube that drips liquid nourishment from a plastic bag directly into his stomach. The care of this individual takes seven and one-half hours of nursing time daily and includes shaving, oral hygiene, grooming, attending to his bowels and bladder, and so forth.

Suppose further that his wife undertakes legal action to force his care givers to end all medical treatment, including nutrition and hydration, so that complete bodily death of her husband will occur. She presents a preponderance of evidence to the court to show that her husband would have wanted just this result in these circumstances.

The central moral issue raised by this sort of case is whether the quality of the individual's life is sufficiently compromised by neocortical death to make intentional termination of that life morally permissible. While alive, he made it clear to both family and friends that he would prefer to be allowed to die rather than be mechanically maintained in a condition of irretrievable loss of consciousness. Deciding whether his judgment in such a case should be allowed to carry the day requires deciding which capacities and qualities make life worth living, which qualities are sufficient to endow it with value worth sustaining, and whether their absence justifies deliberate termination of a life, at least when this would be the wish of the individual in question. Without this decision, the traditional norms of medical ethics, beneficence and nonmaleficence, provide no guidance. Without this decision, it cannot be determined whether termination of life support is a benefit or a harm to the patient.

An even more difficult type of case was provided by the case of Elizabeth Bouvia. Bouvia, who had been a lifelong quadriplegic sufferer of cerebral palsy, was often in pain, completely dependent upon others, and spent all of her time bedridden. Bouvia, after deciding that she did not wish to continue such a life, entered Riverside General Hospital in California. She desired to be kept comfortable while starving to death. Although she remained adamant during her hospitalization, Bouvia's requests were denied by hospital officials with the legal sanction of the courts.

Many who might believe that neocortical death renders the quality of life sufficiently low to justify termination of life support, especially when this agrees with the individual's desires, would not arrive at this conclusion in a case like Bouvia's. Whereas neocortical death completely destroys consciousness and makes purposive interaction with the individual's environment impossible, Bouvia was fully aware and mentally alert. She had previously been married and had even acquired a college education. Televised interviews with her portrayed a very intelligent person who had great skill in presenting persuasive arguments to support her wish not to have her life continued by artificial means of nutrition. Nonetheless, she judged her life to be of such low quality that she should be allowed to choose to starve to death deliberately. Before the existence of life support technology, maintenance of her life against her will might not have been possible at all and at least would have been far more difficult.

Should Elizabeth Bouvia's judgment have been accepted? Her case is more difficult than the care of a patient in a chronic vegetative state because, unlike such an individual, she was able to engage in meaningful interaction with her environment. Regarding an individual who cannot speak or otherwise meaningfully interact with others as nothing more than living matter, as a "human vegetable," is not especially difficult. Seeing Bouvia this way is not easy. Her awareness, intelligence, mental acuity, and ability to interact with others means that although her life is one of discomfort, indignity, and complete dependence, she is not a mere "human vegetable."

Despite the differences between Bouvia's situation and that of someone in a state of neocortical death, the same issue is posed. Can the quality of an individual's life be so low that deliberate termination is morally justifiable? How that question is answered is a matter of what level of quality of life, if any, is taken to be sufficiently low to justify deliberately acting to end it or deliberately failing to extend it. If there is such a level, the conclusion that it is not always beneficent or even nonmaleficent to use life-support technology must be accepted.

Another important issue here is respect for individual autonomy. For the cases of Bouvia and the hypothetical instance of neocortical death discussed above, both concern voluntary euthanasia, that is, euthanasia voluntarily requested by the patient. A long-standing commitment, vigorously defended by various schools of thought in Western moral philosophy, is the notion that competent adults should be free to conduct their lives as they please as long as they do not impose undeserved harm on others. Does this commitment entail a right to die? Some clearly believe that it does. If one owns anything at all, surely one owns one's life. In the two cases discussed above, neither individual sought to imposed undeserved harm on anyone else, nor would satisfaction of their wish to die do so. What justification can there be then for not allowing their desires to be fulfilled?

One plausible answer is based upon the very respect of individual autonomy at issue here. A necessary condition, in some views, of respect for autonomy is the willingness to take whatever measures are necessary to protect it, including measures that restrict autonomy. An autonomy-respecting reason offered against laws that prevent even competent adults from voluntarily entering lifelong slavery is that such an exercise of autonomy is self-defeating and has the consequence of undermining autonomy altogether. By the same token, an individual who acts to end his own life thereby exercises his autonomy in a manner that places it in jeopardy of permanent loss. Many would regard this as justification for using the coercive force of the law to prevent suicide, for instance. This line of thought does not fit the case of an individual in a persistent vegetative state because his autonomy has been destroyed by the circumstances that rendered him neocortically dead. It does fit Bouvia's case though. Her actions indicate that she is fully competent and her efforts to use medical care to prevent the otherwise inevitable pain of starvation is itself an exercise of her autonomy. Yet, if allowed to succeed, those very efforts would destroy her autonomy as they destroy her. On this reasoning, her case is a perfect instance of limitation of autonomy being justified by respect for autonomy and of one where, even against the wishes of a competent patient, the life-saving power of medical technology should be used.

Active versus Passive Euthanasia

Discussions of the morality of euthanasia often distinguish active from passive euthanasia in light of the distinction made between killing a person and letting a person die, a distinction that rests upon the difference between an act of commission and an act of omission. When failure to take steps that could effectively forestall death results in an individual's demise, the resultant death is an act of omission and a case of letting a person die. When a death is the result of doing something to hasten the end of a person's life (giving a lethal injection, for example), that death is caused by an act of commission and is a case of killing a person. When a person is allowed to die, death is a result of an act of omission, and the motive is the person's own good, the omission is an instance of passive euthanasia. When a person is killed, death is the result of an act of commission, and the motive is the person's own good, the commission is an instance of active euthanasia.

Does the difference between passive and active euthanasia, which reduces to a difference in how death comes about, make any moral difference? It does in the view of the **American Medical Association**. In a statement adopted on December 4, 1973, the **House of Delegates of the American Medical Association** asserted the following (Rachels, 1978):

> *The intentional termination of the life of one human being by another — mercy killing — is contrary to that for which the medical profession stands and is contrary to the policy of the American Medical Association.*
>
> *The cessation of extraordinary means to prolong the life of the body where there is irrefutable evidence that biological death is imminent is the decision of the patient and immediate family. The advice of the physician would be freely available to the patient and immediate family.*

In response to this position, Rachels (1978) answered with the following:

> *The AMA policy statement isolates the crucial issue very well, the crucial issue is "intentional termination of the life of one human being by another." But after identifying this issue and forbidding "mercy killing," the statement goes on to deny that the cessation of treatment is the intentional termination of a life. This is where the mistake comes in, for what is the cessation of treatment in those circumstances*

[where the intention is to release the patient from continued suffering], if it is not "the intentional termination of the life of one human being by another?"

As Rachels correctly argues, when steps that could keep an individual alive are omitted for the person's own good, this omission is as much the intentional termination of life as taking active measures to cause death would be. Not placing a patient on a respirator due to a desire not to prolong suffering is an act intended to end life as much as the administration of a lethal injection would be. In many instances, the main difference between the two cases is that the latter would release the individual from his pain and suffering more quickly than the former. Dying can take time and involve considerable pain even if nothing is done to prolong life. Active killing can be done in a manner that causes death painlessly and instantly. This difference certainly does not render killing, in this context, morally worse than letting a person die. Insofar as the motivation is merciful (as it must be if the case is to be a genuine instance of euthanasia) because the individual is released more quickly from a life that is disvalued than otherwise, the difference between killing and letting one die may provide support for active euthanasia. According to Rachels (1978), the common rejoinder to this argument is the following:

> *The important difference between active and passive euthanasia is that in passive euthanasia, the doctor does not do anything to bring about the patient's death. The doctor does nothing, and the patient dies of whatever ills already afflict him. In active euthanasia, however, the doctor does something to bring about the patient's death: he kills him. The doctor who gives the patient with cancer a lethal injection has himself caused his patient's death; whereas if he merely ceases treatment, the cancer is the cause of death.*

According to this rejoinder, in active euthanasia someone must do something to bring about the patient's death, and in passive euthanasia the patient's death is caused by illness rather than by anyone's conduct. Surely this is mistaken. Suppose a physician deliberately decides not to treat one a patient who has a routinely curable ailment, and the patient dies. Suppose further that the physician were to attempt to exonerate himself by saying, "I did nothing. The patient's death was the result of illness. I was not the cause of death." Under current legal and moral norms, such a response would have no credibility. As Rachels (1978) notes,*"it would be no defense at all for him to insist that he didn't 'do anything.' He would have done something very serious indeed, for he let his patient die."*

The physician would be blameworthy for the patient's death as surely as if he had actively killed him. If causing death is justifiable under a given set of circumstances, whether it is done by allowing death to occur or by actively causing death is morally irrelevant. If causing someone to die is not justifiable under a given set of circumstances, whether it is done by allowing death to occur or by actively causing death is also morally irrelevant. Accordingly, if voluntary passive euthanasia is morally justifiable in the light of the duty of beneficence, so is voluntary active euthanasia. Indeed, given that the benefit to be achieved is more quickly realized by means of active euthanasia, it may be preferable to passive euthanasia in some cases.

Involuntary and Nonvoluntary Euthanasia

An act of euthanasia is involuntary if it hastens the individual's death for his own good but against his wishes. To take such a course would be to destroy a life that is valued by its possessor. Therefore, it is no different in any morally relevant way from unjustifiable homicide. There are only two legitimate reasons for hastening an innocent person's life against his will: self-defense and saving the lives of a larger number of other innocent persons. Involuntary euthanasia does not fit either of these justifications. By definition, it is done for the good of the person who is euthanized and for self-defense or saving innocent others. No act that qualifies as involuntary euthanasia can be morally justifiable.

Hastening a person's death for his own good is an instance of nonvoluntary euthanasia when the individual is incapable of agreeing or disagreeing. Suppose it is clear that a particular person is sufficiently self-conscious to be regarded a person but cannot make his wishes known. Suppose also that he is suffering from the kind of ailment that, in the eyes of many persons, makes one's life itself unendurable. Would hastening his death be permissible? It would be if there were substantial evidence that he has given prior consent. He may have told friends and relatives that under certain circumstances efforts to prolong his life should not be undertaken or continued. He might have recorded his wishes in the form of a Living Will (below) or on audio- or videotape. Where this kind of substantial evidence of prior consent exists, the decision to hasten death would be morally justified. A case of this sort would be virtually a case of voluntary euthanasia.

But what about an instance in which such evidence is not available? Suppose the person at issue has never had the capacity for competent consent or dissent from decisions concerning his life. It simply cannot be known what value the individual would place on his life in his present condition of illness. What should be done is a matter of what is taken to be the greater evil — mistakenly ending the life of an innocent person for whom that life has value or mistakenly forcing him to endure a life that he radically disvalues.

TO MY FAMILY, MY PHYSICIAN, MY CLERGYMAN, MY LAWYER:

If the time comes when I can no longer take part in decisions about my own future, let this statement stand as testament of my wishes: If there is no reasonable expectation of my recovery from physical or mental disability, I, ________________________________, request that I be allowed to die and not be kept alive by artificial means or heroic measures. Death is as much a reality as birth, growth, maturity, and old age — it is the one certainty. I do not fear death as much as I fear the indignity of deterioration, dependence, and hopeless pain. I ask that drugs be mercifully administered to me for the terminal suffering even if they hasten the moment of death.

This request is made after careful consideration. Although this document is not legally binding, you who care for me will, I hope, feel morally bound to follow its mandate. I recognize that it places a heavy burden of responsibility upon you, and it is with the intention of sharing that responsibility and of mitigating any feelings of guilt that this statement is made.

Signed ________________________________

Date ________________________________

Witnessed by

____

____

Living Will statutes have been passed in at least 35 states and the District of Columbia. For a Living Will to be a legally binding document, the person signing it must be of sound mind at the time the will is made and shown not to have altered his opinion in the interim between the signing and his illness. The witnesses must not be able to benefit from the individual's death.

Should Voluntary Euthanasia Be Legalized?

Some argue that even if voluntary euthanasia is morally justifiable, it should be prohibited by social policy nonetheless. According to this position, the problem with voluntary euthanasia is its impact on society as a whole. In other words, the overall disutility of allowing voluntary euthanasia outweighs the good it could do for its beneficiaries. The central moral concern is that legalized euthanasia would eventually erode respect for human life and ultimately become a policy under which "socially undesirable" persons would have their deaths hastened (by omission or commission). The experience of Nazi Germany is often cited in support of this fear. What began there as a policy of euthanasia soon became one of eliminating individuals deemed racially inferior or otherwise undesirable. The worry, of course, is that what happened there can happen here as well. If social policy encompasses efforts to hasten the deaths of people, respect for human life in general is eroded and all sorts of abuses become socially acceptable, or so the argument goes.

No one can provide an absolute guarantee that the experience of Nazi Germany would not be repeated, but there is reason to believe that its likelihood is negligible. The medical moral duty of beneficence justifies only voluntary euthanasia. It justifies hastening an individual's death only for the individual's benefit and only with the individual's consent. To kill or refuse to save people judged socially undesirable is not to engage in euthanasia at all and violates the medical moral duty of nonmaleficence. As long as only voluntary euthanasia is legalized, and it is clear that involuntary euthanasia is not and should never be, no degeneration of the policy need occur. Furthermore, such degeneration is not likely to occur if the beneficent nature of voluntary euthanasia is clearly distinguished from the maleficent nature of involuntary euthanasia and any policy of exterminating the socially undesirable. Euthanasia decisions must be scrutinized carefully and regulated strictly to ensure that only voluntary cases occur, and severe penalties must be established to deter abuse.

HUMAN EXPERIMENTATION

Although the overriding aim of diagnosis and therapy is to provide benefits to individual patients, experimentation aims to expand the boundaries of scientific knowledge. As therapist, the clinician focuses upon the well-being of the patient, but as researcher, the immediate concern is to generate scientifically sound information. Accordingly, intention or aim rather than outcome differentiates therapy from experimentation. Even when a course of treatment fails to improve the patient's condition, it constitutes therapy if such improvement was the intent. This remains true even when the course of treatment yields exciting new medical knowledge as an unintended consequence. Similarly, even when a course of treatment does benefit a subject, it constitutes experimentation if its aim was primarily acquisition of new knowledge and it ranks as experimentation even when it fails to realize this aim.

At this point in discussions of the morality of human experimentation, the traditional move is to distinguish therapeutic from nontherapeutic experiments. As Fried (1978) wrote:

"In therapeutic experimentation a course of action (or studied inaction) is undertaken in respect to the subject for the purpose of determining how best to procure a medical benefit to the subject. In nontherapeutic experimentation, by contrast, the sole end in view is the acquisition of new information."

Again, the central difference is a matter of intention or aim rather than results. If the purpose of an experiment is to determine how best to benefit the patient, it is deemed therapeutic. If its purpose is to generate new knowledge, it is deemed nontherapeutic.

These distinctions between therapy and experimentation on the one hand and therapeutic and nontherapeutic experimentation on the other, however, can often be misleading. To define therapy in opposition to experimentation may lead to a failure to appreciate that therapy is only one kind of clinical practice aimed at generating patient benefits and so may lead to the mistaken conclusion that all nontherapeutic practices are experimental. Clearly, this is an error. In addition to attempting to heal patients and to mitigate the effects of illness, medical-care providers also seek, where possible, to prevent disease. In addition, therapy itself is generally preceded and to some extent dictated by diagnostic measures: efforts to discover the nature and source of the patient's ailment. Therapy, prevention, and diagnosis are all conducted with the aim of benefiting the patient. This applies to the distinction between therapeutic and nontherapeutic experimentation as well. Just as a course of action may be taken to determine what form of therapy will best benefit the patient, so can a course of action be taken to determine what will yield the best diagnosis or will best prevent illness in the first place. Although diagnostic and preventive measures are not themselves therapeutic, the primary motivation for using them is to benefit patients.

Practice and Research

Given these considerations, a distinction drawn in the mid-1970s by the **National Commission for the Protection of Human Subjects of Biomedical and Behavioral Research** is more appropriate for discussion of the morality of human experimentation. The commission offered a distinction between practice and research to replace the conventional distinction between therapy and experimentation. Quoting the commission, Alexander Capron (1986) writes:

"[T]he term 'practice' refers to interventions that are designed solely to enhance the well-being of an individual patient or client and that have a reasonable expectation of success." In the medical sphere, practices usually involve diagnosis, preventive treatment, or therapy; in the social sphere, practices include governmental programs such as transfer payments, education, and the like.

By contrast, the term 'research' designates an activity designed to test a hypothesis, to permit conclusions to be drawn, and thereby to develop or contribute to generalizable knowledge (expressed, for example, in theories, principles, statements of relationships). In the polar cases, then, practice uses a proven technique in an attempt to benefit one or more individuals, while research studies a technique in an attempt to increase knowledge."

Although the practice/research dichotomy has the advantage of not implying that therapeutic activities are the only clinical procedures intended to benefit patients, like the therapy/experiment distinction it is based on intention rather than outcome. Interventions constitute practices when they are proven techniques intended to benefit the patient. Likewise interventions aimed at increasing generalizable knowledge constitute research.

What about those interventions that do not happily fit into the dichotomy between research and practice? As Capron (1986) notes:

> *"[Not} every use of unproven techniques amounts to research; the way in which the technique is used must be designed as to permit generalizable knowledge to be gained — something more than just seeing what results from using the technique in one particular instance. Conversely, not every intervention carried out with the intent of benefiting the patient (or other subject of the intervention) thereby qualifies as an instance of practice; prior study of the technique must have provided adequate information about it, to give rise to a reasonable basis for believing that it will achieve the intended result.*

Nonvalidated Practice

To cover interventions that do not fit the research/practice distinction, practice must be further distinguished from nonvalidated practice. Like the term "therapeutic experiment," "nonvalidated practice" connotes that the selected course of action aims to benefit the patient. Unlike the term "therapeutic experiment," it explicitly encompasses prevention along with diagnosis and therapy. Additionally, the term "therapeutic experiment" seems to be at war with itself by implying that an intervention can be primarily intended to benefit the patient while also being primarily directed at generating sound scientific information. The term "nonvalidated practice" clearly connotes that the intervention's primary purpose is to benefit the patient while making clear that it has not been shown to be safe and efficacious.

An important difference between the therapeutic/nontherapeutic experimentation distinction and the concept of nonvalidated practice is that whereas the former limits attention to new and innovative interventions, the latter encompasses some interventions that are neither new nor innovative. Robert Levine, who coined the term "nonvalidated practice," writes (Capron, 1986):

> *"A practice might be nonvalidated because it is new; i.e., it has not been tested sufficiently often or sufficiently well to permit a satisfactory prediction of its safety or efficacy in a patient population. An equally common way for a practice to merit the designation "nonvalidated" is that in the course of its use in the practice of medicine there arises some legitimate cause to question previously held assumptions about its safety or efficacy."*

Whether an intervention's safety and efficacy are at issue because it is new or because clinical experience has posed questions about its value, the central moral issue is the same. Patients are subjected to a course of treatment for which there is no well-founded basis from which to assess its risks and benefits. Therefore, a well-founded basis upon which to determine whether the benefits sufficiently outweigh the risks is lacking.

The Ethics of Research on Humans

In order to appreciate the moral concerns raised by nonvalidated practice, it is first necessary to address the general topic of research on human beings.

> *"The basic ethical problem . . . is the use of one person by another to gather knowledge or other benefits that may be only partly good, if at all, for the first person; that is to say, the . . . subject is not simply a means but is in danger of being treated as a mere token to be manipulated for research purposes"* (Capron, 1978).

These remarks indicate that the major moral issue posed consists in the fact that research on humans is not intended to benefit the research subjects themselves directly. Instead, it is intended to provide knowledge that will be added to the stock of information possessed by medical science and in the long run will benefit humankind in general. Whether this is an important moral issue depends upon how the proper relationship between the well-being of distinct individuals and the social whole to which they belong is conceived.

> *"Those who regard individuals as parts of a collective whole which allocates rights and protects them, can justify a wide scope for experimentation that serves to advance the interests of the collectivity. Conversely, for those who emphasize the inviolability of human persons and the moral obligation not to treat them simply as parts related to a social whole, any human experimentation whose purpose is to benefit persons other than the subjects of the experimentation requires very strong justifying reasons"* (Capron 1978).

From an essentially utilitarian perspective in which the common good is conceived as greater than the good of particular individuals, the fact that a program of research sacrifices the interests of particular individuals for the greater good of society need not be problematic. According to this outlook, a program of research is justified solely to the degree that it poses a genuine prospect of general benefit and that the probability and level of benefit are sufficiently high to outweigh any losses to individual research subjects. The important consideration here is that research promises a net gain even if that gain does not accrue to its individual subjects. Accordingly, the worry that research always poses the danger of using individuals as mere resources for the good of others has little significance from this utilitarian viewpoint.

From a perspective that takes individual dignity to be paramount, an essentially Kantian perspective, what can be done to promote the general good is clearly limited. Although this perspective recognizes the importance of aiming to generate the greatest good for the greatest numbers, it insists that this goal must be sought only in ways that are not demeaning or dehumanizing. This means that pursuit of the common good must take place only in those ways that do not reduce individuals to mere resources for the good of others. Adhering to this moral imperative necessarily limits what can be done in the name of even clearly beneficial medical research.

The history of atrocities perpetrated against individuals in the name of research, especially those committed by the Nazis, is well known and need not be reiterated here. An important consequence of those atrocities, though, is that the Kantian perspective has become dominant in Western thinking about research on human subjects, and the protection of those who serve as research subjects has become a paramount priority. Numerous guidelines and codes of ethics for human experimentation have been formulated since World War II to promote limits on research that will maintain and respect the dignity of human subjects. (Perhaps the most famous is the Nuremberg Code, one of the first formal codes of ethics for research on humans. This code was deliberately developed in response to the horrors of Nazi research on human subjects.)

Although the differences between various codes are numerous, they generally converge on several requirements for ethically sound human experimentation (Capron, 1986). First, research on humans must be based upon prior laboratory research and research on animals as well as upon established scientific fact *"so that the point under inquiry is well focused and has been advanced as far as possible by nonhuman means"* (Capron, 1986). Second, research on humans should use tests and means of observation that are reasonably believed to be able to provide the information being sought by the research. Methods that are not suited for providing the knowledge sought are pointless and rob the research of its scientific value. Third, research should be conducted only by persons with the relevant scientific expertise. Fourth, *"all foreseeable risks and reasonably probable benefits, to the subject of the investigation and to science or more broadly to society, must be carefully assessed, and . . . the comparison of those projected risks and benefits must indicate that the latter clearly outweighs the former. Moreover, the probable benefits must not be obtainable through other less risky means"* (Capron, 1986). Fifth, participation in research should be based on informed and voluntary consent. Sixth, *"participation by a subject in an experiment should be halted immediately if the subject finds continued participation undesirable or a prudent investigator has cause to believe that the experiment is likely to result in injury, disability, or death to the subject"* (Capron, 1986). Conforming to conditions of this sort probably does limit the pace and extent of medical progress, but society's insistence on them is its way of saying that the only medical progress truly worth having must be consistent with a high level of respect for human dignity. Of these requirements, the requirement to obtain informed and voluntary consent from research subjects is widely regarded as one of the most important protections. Before discussing this requirement, however, a second important ethical issue regarding research on humans will be discussed.

This issue concerns the oldest norms of traditional medical morality: beneficence and nonmaleficence, the duty to benefit the patient and the duty to avoid harming the patient. The purpose of research is to provide new knowledge, and although research has benefits, these are not aimed primarily at the research subject. This means that any harm the subject suffers is justified, if at all, not by benefits to the subject but by benefits to others. So when the researcher is a physician and the subject is a patient, then the physician/researcher is not discharging his duty to concern himself primarily with the patient's well-being. If the patient benefits, these benefits are incidental to the aim of the research, and if the patient is harmed, that harm cannot be justified on the grounds that it was an unavoidable concomitant to benefiting the patient. Indeed, the intervention in question, if it is genuinely an instance of research, cannot be based upon well-founded beliefs about what harms or benefits it will pose for the patient. The testing needed to have such beliefs is itself the substance of the research. How then can physicians or researchers reasonably intend their actions to benefit or not harm their patients as research subjects? Clinicians may hope for this but cannot reasonably intend it. Can the aims of research be reconciled with the traditional moral obligations of physicians? Is the researcher/physician in an untenable position?

Answering these questions leads back to the requirement of informed and voluntary consent. The leading idea behind this requirement is that if the subject of an experiment agrees to participate in the research, then what happens to him during and because of the experiment is a product of his own decision. It is not something that is imposed on him, but rather, in a very real sense, something that he elects to have done to him. Because his autonomy is thus respected, he is not made a mere resource for the benefit of others. Although he may suffer harm for the benefit of others, he does so of his own volition, as a result of the exercise of his own autonomy, rather than as a result of having his autonomy limited or diminished. An extremely important difficulty here is knowing when consent is genuine, when it is truly voluntary and not the product of coercion. Not all sources of coercion are as obvious and easy to recognize as physical violence. A subject may be coerced by fear — by the fear that there is no other recourse for treatment of the ailment (even when it is known that any benefit the intervention will bring is incidental to its purpose), by the fear that nonconsent will alienate the physician on whom the subject depends for treatment, or even by the fear of disapproval of others. This sort of coercion, if it truly ranks a such, is often difficult to detect and remedy.

In any case, the mere absence of coercion is insufficient. Voluntariness can also be undermined by ignorance and misunderstanding. One's consent to something is not autonomous unless one understands to what he is consenting. A research subject must be given information sufficient to arrive at an intelligent opinion concerning whether to participate in the research or to continue to participate after research has commenced. In the absence of this information, the subject may agree to something that is not what one believes it to be, and here consent will not reflect one's own values and priorities.

Two difficulties arise here. The first and probably less worrisome is the issue of what constitutes sufficient relevant information for the subject to arrive at an intelligent opinion. Although a subject need not be given all the information a researcher has, how much should be provided, and what can be omitted without compromising the validity of the subject's consent? The second difficulty lies in knowing whether the subject is competent to understand the information given and to render an intelligent opinion based upon it. This renders research on children and the mentally handicapped especially suspect. It also makes research suspect when its subjects include patients whose ailments compromise their competence. In any case, efforts must be make to ensure that sufficient relevant information is given and that the subject is sufficiently competent to process it. These are matters of judgment that probably cannot be made with absolute precision and certainty, but rigorous efforts must be made in good faith to prevent research on humans from involving gross violations of human dignity.

How does the requirement of informed and voluntary consent speak to the tension between the goals of research and the traditional moral norms of medicine? Being concerned about the well-being of the patient is often crucial to prevent him from being dehumanized and treated as a mere resource. In recent years, Western societies have tended to regard respect for a person's autonomy as the most crucial aspect of respecting the individual's humanity. That is, the Kantian notion that what makes humans morally special is their capacity for autonomy has become widely accepted, as expressed in a strong and widespread rejection of paternalism. To treat a person paternalistically is to limit the person's liberty for his own good. Although many paternalistic measures would benefit those subjected to them, Western societies, especially the United States, have been exceedingly reluctant to take such measures. In medicine, this respect for individual autonomy has taken the form of limiting the traditional moral obligations of physicians. Increasingly, advocates of patients' rights have persuasively argued that there is no valid justification for not allowing patients to do as they please as long as they do not harm innocent others. Acceptance of this Kantian view has meant that physicians are expected to discharge their duties of beneficence and nonmaleficence within the limits set by the autonomy of the patient. Indeed, this is why it is widely accepted that before any intervention is undertaken, no matter how well validated, informed and voluntary consent must be secured. The patient who voluntarily and with adequate information chooses to become a research subject releases the physician from the responsibility of making the patient's well-being the paramount concern. The physician can then take on the role of researcher and attend to the goal that justifies research in the first place — benefit to humanity in general. Of course, this does not mean that anything goes. The physician is still obligated to pursue the ends of the research with as little risk to the subject as possible.

The Ethics of Nonvalidated Practices

> *"What should one's ethical response be to activities that fall within this region of nonvalidated practices? Since they are not carried out according to a research plan (or "protocol"), they cannot be justified by their benefit to science; since they lack*

a valid basis in science, they cannot be defended for the benefit they will provide to those with whom they are used. The solution, of course, is to employ the procedure in the context of an appropriate research plan or to substitute a proven treatment. Yet this will not always be possible, especially when attempting to cure problems (such as life-threatening conditions) for which no satisfactory therapy exists and when the need to intervene is too urgent to allow a formal research plan to be adopted" (Capron, 1986).

A nonvalidated practice thus lacks the justification available to ethically sound research, i.e., providing some benefit to science and thereby to society as a whole. It also lacks the justification available to practice, benefit to the patient, precisely because sufficient research to show that benefit can be reasonably expected has not occurred. Is nonvalidated practice therefore always unjustifiable? As the quotation from Capron above notes, this is not necessarily the case. In circumstances where life itself is at stake or where severe debilitation is highly probable and where validated practices have failed or cannot be deployed, nonvalidated practices may be morally acceptable. Of course, the requirement of informed consent must be met here as well. Indeed given the desperate nature of the circumstances, informed consent may well be more important here than in the circumstances of research or validated practice. The issue is why a patient who is in desperate circumstances, who is well apprised of the uncertainties of the proposed intervention, and who is competent to make his own choices should be deprived of the opportunity to have his life or health saved, however uncertain that opportunity might be. Of course, the great difficulty here is knowing whether the patient in desperate circumstances really is well apprised of the relevant information and is competent to process it.

Can an intervention be part of a research plan and be a nonvalidated practice at the same time? Clearly it can in certain circumstances. An intervention may be part of a research plan and thereby intended to provide generalizable knowledge and yet be used outside the plan on a patient who is not one of the research subjects if that patient is in a medical crisis where validated practices are not available or effective. It is important to note that this sort of use of an intervention as a nonvalidated practice occurs outside the research plan and on someone who is not a research subject. Therefore, it has a very different sort of purpose than use of the same intervention within a research plan. Whereas the latter aims at providing generalizable medical knowledge, with benefits accruing to research subjects being incidental to this purpose, the former use aims at providing a possibility of benefit to a patient for whom all other options are closed or have been exhausted, and any information thereby gained is incidental to this purpose. In this kind of circumstance, these different primary goals can be kept separate even when the physician conducting the research is also the physician conducting the nonvalidated practice because the intervention is applied to different persons — a research subject in the former case and a patient in the latter case.

Can an intervention be both a nonvalidated practice and part of a research plan in a meaningfully different situation? Can one and the same intervention when applied to one and the same person be both nonvalidated practice and research at one and the same time? This notion is highly problematic. The limits that research must observe to be scientifically sound might not be compatible with providing maximal benefit to the patient. When this is the case, if the physician observes the conditions required of legitimate research, he fails to do what is required of him as a physician. He does his duty as a researcher but not as physician. If he does his duty as a physician and violates the canons of legitimate research, he fails to do his duty as a researcher. His situation is thus ethically untenable. The ethical obligations of a physician with respect to nonvalidated practice are the same as those with respect to validated practice: to benefit and avoid harm to the patient. These are very different from and may be in irresolvable conflict with those of ethically sound research.

REGULATION OF MEDICAL DEVICE INNOVATION

Responsibility for regulating medical devices falls to the **Food and Drug Administration** under the **Medical Device Amendment** of 1976. This statute requires approval from the FDA before new devices are marketed and imposes requirements for the clinical investigation of new medical devices on human subjects. Although the statute makes interstate commerce of an unapproved new medical device generally unlawful, it provides an exception to allow interstate distribution of unapproved devices in order to conduct clinical research on human subjects. This investigational device exemption (IDE) can be obtained by submitting to the FDA "*a protocol for the proposed clinical testing of the device, reports of prior investigations of the device, certification that the study has been approved by a local institutional review board, and an assurance that informed consent will be obtained from each human subject*" (Bronzino et al., 1990a).

With respect to clinical research on humans, the FDA distinguishes devices into two categories: devices that pose significant risk and those that involve insignificant risk. Examples of the former included orthopedic implants, artificial hearts, and infusion pumps. Examples of the latter include various dental devices and daily-wear contact lenses. Clinical research involving a significant risk device can not begin until an institutional review board (IRB) has approved both the protocol and the informed consent form and the FDA itself has given permission. This requirement to submit an IDE application to the FDA is waived in the case of clinical research where the risk posed is insignificant. In this case, the FDA requires only that approval from an IRB be obtained certifying that the device in question poses only insignificant risk. In deciding whether to approve a proposed clinical investigation of a new device, the IRB and the FDA must determine the following (Bronzino et al., 1990a):

1. That risks to subjects are minimized.
2. That risks to subjects are reasonable in relation to anticipated benefit and knowledge to be gained.
3. That subject selection is equitable.
4. That informed consent materials and procedures are adequate.
5. That provisions for monitoring the study and protecting patient information are acceptable.

The FDA allows unapproved medical devices to be used without an IDE in three types of situations: emergency use, treatment use, and feasibility studies.

Ethical Issues in Feasibility Studies

> *Manufacturers seeking more flexibility in conducting investigations in the early developmental stages of a device have submitted a petition to the FDA, requesting that certain limited investigations of significant risk devices be subject to abbreviated IDE requirements* (Bronzino et al., 1990a).

In a feasibility study, or "limited investigation," human research on a new device would take place at a single institution and involve no more than ten human subjects.

> *The sponsor of a limited investigation would be required to submit to the FDA a "Notice of Limited Investigation," which would include a description of the device, a summary*

of the purpose of the investigation, the protocol, a sample of the informed consent form, and a certification of approval by the responsible IRB. In certain circumstances, the FDA could require additional information, or require the submission of a full IDE application, or suspend the investigation (Bronzino et al., 1990a).

Investigations of this kind would be limited to certain circumstances:

(1) investigations of new uses of existing devices, (2) investigations involving temporary or permanent implants during the early developmental stages, and (3) investigations involving modification of an existing device (Bronzino et al., 1990a).

To comprehend adequately the ethical issues posed by clinical use of unapproved medical devices outside the context of an IDE, it is necessary to utilize the distinctions between practice, nonvalidated practice, and research elaborated in the previous pages. How do those definitions apply to feasibility studies?

Clearly, the goal of this sort of study, i.e., generalizable knowledge, makes it an instance of research rather than practice. Manufacturers seek to determine the performance of a device with respect to a particular patient population in an effort to gain information about its efficacy and safety. Such information would be important in determining whether further studies (animal or human) need to be conducted, whether the device needs modification before further use, and the like. The main difference between use of an unapproved device in a feasibility study and use under the terms of an IDE is that the former would be subject to significantly less intensive FDA review than the latter. This, in turn, means that the responsibility for ensuring that use of the device is ethically sound would fall primarily to the IRB of the institution conducting the study.

The ethical concerns posed here can be best comprehended only with a clear understanding of what justifies research in the first place. Ultimately, no matter how much basic research and animal experimentation has been conducted on a given device, the risks and benefits it poses for humans cannot be adequately determined until it is actually used on humans.

The benefits of research on humans lie primarily in the knowledge that is yielded and the generalizable information that is provided. This information is crucial to medical science's ability to generate new modes and instrumentalities of medical treatment that are both efficacious and safe. Accordingly, a necessary but insufficient condition for experimentation to be ethically sound is that it be scientifically sound. (The three criteria of scientifically sound research are encompassed by the first three of the six requirements of ethically sound research enumerated by Alexander Capron above.)

Although scientific soundness is a necessary condition of ethically sound research on humans, it is not of and by itself sufficient. Indeed, it is widely recognized that the primary ethical concern posed by such investigation is the use of one person by another to gather knowledge or other benefits where these benefits may only partly or not at all accrue to the first person. In other words, the human subjects of such research are at risk of being mere research resources, as having value only for the ends of the research. Research upon human beings runs the risk of failing to respect them as people. The notion that human beings are not mere things but entities whose value is inherent rather than wholly instrumental is one of the most widely held norms of contemporary Western society. That is, human beings are not valuable wholly or solely for the uses to which they can be put. They are valuable simply by being the kinds of entities they are. To treat them as such is to respect them as people.

Respecting individuals as people is generally agreed to entail two requirements in the context of biomedical experimentation. First, since what is most generally taken to make human beings people is their autonomy — their ability to make rational choices for themselves — treating individuals as people means respecting that autonomy. This requirement is met by ensuring that no competent person is subjected to any clinical intervention without first giving voluntary and informed consent. Second, respect for people means that the physician will not subject a human to unnecessary risks and will minimize the risks to patients in required procedures. (These two requirements are derived from requirements 4, 5, and 6 of Capron's above account of the requirements for ethically sound human research.)

Much of the ethical importance of the scrutiny that the FDA imposes upon use of unapproved medical devices in the context of an IDE derives from these two conditions of ethically sound research. The central ethical concern posed by use of medical devices in a feasibility study is that the decreased degree of FDA scrutiny will increase the likelihood that either or both of these conditions will not be met. This possibility may be especially great because many manufacturers of medical devices are, after all, commercial enterprises, companies that are motivated to generate profit and thus to get their devices to market as soon as possible with as little delay and cost as possible. These self-interested motives are likely, at times, to conflict with the requirements of ethically sound research and thus to induce manufacturers to fail (often unwittingly) to meet these requirements. Note that profit is not the only motive that might induce manufacturers to contravene the requirements of ethically sound research on humans. A manufacturer may sincerely believe that its product offers great benefit to many people or to a population of especially needy people and so from this utterly altruistic motive may be prompted to take shortcuts that compromise the quality of the research. Whether the consequences being sought by the research are desired for reasons of self-interest, altruism, or both, the ethical issue is the same. Research subjects may be placed at risk of being treated as mere objects rather than as people.

What about the circumstances under which feasibility studies would take place? Are these not sufficiently different from the "normal" circumstances of research to warrant reduced FDA scrutiny? As noted above, manufacturers seek to be allowed to engage in feasibility studies in order to investigate new uses of existing devices, to investigate temporary or permanent implants during the early developmental stages, and to investigate modifications to an existing device. As also noted above, a feasibility study would take place at only one institution and would involve no more than ten human subjects. Given these circumstances, is the sort of research that is likely to occur in a feasibility study less likely to be scientifically unsound or to fail to respect people than normal research upon humans in "normal" circumstances?

Such research would be done on a very small subject pool, and the harm of any ethical lapses would likely affect fewer people than if such lapses occurred under more usual research circumstances. Yet even if the harm done is limited to a failure to respect as people the ten or fewer subjects in a single feasibility study, the harm would still be ethically wrong. To wrong ten or fewer people is not as bad as to wrong in the same way more than ten people but it is to engage in wrongdoing nonetheless. In either case, individuals are reduced to the status of mere research resources and their dignity as people is not properly respected.

Are ethical lapses more likely to occur in feasibility studies than in studies that take place within the requirements of an IDE? Although nothing in the preceding discussion provides a definitive answer to this question, it is a question to which the FDA should give high priority in deciding whether to allow this type of exception to IDE use of unapproved medical devices. The answer to this question might be quite different when the device at issue is a temporary or permanent implant than when it is an already approved device being put to new uses or modified in some way. Whatever the contemplated use under the feasibility studies mechanism, the FDA would be ethically advised not to allow this kind of exception to IDE use of an unapproved device without a reasonably high level of certainty that research subjects would not be placed in greater jeopardy than in "normal" research circumstances.

Ethical Issues in Emergency Use

What about the mechanism for avoiding the rigors of an IDE for emergency use?

> *"The FDA has authorized emergency use where an unapproved device offers the only alternative for saving the life of a dying patient, but an IDE has not yet been approved for the device or its use, or an IDE has been approved but the physician who wishes to use the device is not an investigator under the IDE* (Bronzino et al., 1990a).

Because the purpose of emergency use of an unapproved device is to attempt to save a dying patient's life under circumstances where no other alternative is at hand, this sort of use constitutes practice rather than research. Its aim is primarily benefit to the patient rather than provision of new and generalizable information. Because this sort of use occurs prior to the completion of clinical investigation of the device, it constitutes a nonvalidated practice. What does this mean?

First, it means that while the aim of the use is to save the life of the patient, the nature and likelihood of the potential benefits and risks engendered by use of the device are far more speculative than in the sort of clinical intervention that constitutes validated practice. In validated practice, thorough investigation, including preclinical studies, animals studies, and studies on human subjects, of a device has established its efficacy and safety. The clinician thus has a well-founded basis upon which to judge the benefits and risks such an intervention poses for his patients.

It is precisely this basis that is lacking in the case of a nonvalidated practice. Does this mean that emergency use of an unapproved device should be regarded as immoral? This conclusion would follow only if there were no basis upon which to make an assessment of the risks and benefits of the use of the device. The FDA requires that a physician who engages in emergency use of an unapproved device must *"'have substantial reason to believe that benefits will exist.' This means that there should be a body of preclinical and animal tests allowing a prediction of the benefit to a human patient"* (Bronzino et al., 1990a).

Thus, although the benefits and risks posed by use of the device are highly speculative, they are not entirely speculative. Although the only way to validate a new technology is to engage in research on humans at some point, not all nonvalidated technologies are equal. Some will be largely uninvestigated, and assessment of their risks and benefits will be wholly or almost wholly speculative. Others will at least have the support of preclinical and animal tests. Although this is not sufficient support for incorporating use of a device into regular clinical practice, it may however represent sufficient support to justify use in the desperate circumstances at issue in emergency situations. Desperate circumstances can justify desperate actions, but desperate actions are not the same as reckless actions, hence the ethical soundness of the FDA's requirement that emergency use be supported by solid results from preclinical and animal tests of the unapproved device.

A second requirement that the FDA imposes on emergency use of unapproved devices is the expectation that physicians *"'exercise reasonable foresight with respect to potential emergencies and . . . make appropriate arrangements under the IDE procedures.' Thus, a physician should not "create" an emergency in order to circumvent IRB review and avoid requesting the sponsor's authorization of the unapproved use of a device"* (Bronzino et al., 1990a).

From a Kantian point of view, which is concerned with protecting the dignity of people this is a particularly important requirement. To create an emergency in order to avoid FDA regulations is to treat the patient as a mere resource whose value is reducible to service to the clinician's goals. Hence, the FDA is quite correct to insist that emergencies are circumstances that reasonable foresight would not anticipate.

Also especially important here is the nature of the patient's consent. Individuals facing death are especially vulnerable to exploitation and deserve greater measures for their protection than might otherwise be necessary. One such measure would be to ensure that the patient, or his legitimate proxy, knows the highly speculative nature of the intervention being offered. That is, to ensure that it is clearly understood that the clinician's estimation of the intervention's risks and benefits is far less solidly grounded than in the case of validated practices. The patient's consent must be based upon an awareness that the device whose use is contemplated has not undergone complete and rigorous testing on humans and that estimations of its potential are based wholly upon preclinical and animal studies. Above all the patient must not be lead to believe that the risks and benefits of the intervention are not better understood than they in fact are. Another important point here is to ensure that the patient understands that the options he is facing are not simply life or death but may include life of a severely impaired quality, and therefore that even if his life is saved, it may be a life of significant impairment. Although desperate circumstance may legitimate desperate actions, the decision to take such actions must rest upon the informed and voluntary consent of the patient, especially when he is an especially vulnerable patient.

It is important here for a clinician involved in emergency use of an unapproved device to recognize that these activities constitute a form of practice, albeit nonvalidated, and not research. Hence the primary obligation is to the well-being of the patient. The patient enters into the relationship with the clinician with the same trust that accompanies any normal clinical situation. To treat this sort of intervention as if it were an instance of research and hence justified by its benefits to science and society would be to abuse this trust.

Ethical Issues in Treatment Use

> *The FDA has adopted regulations authorizing the use of investigational new drugs in certain circumstances where a patient has not responded to approved therapies. This "treatment use" of unapproved new drugs is not limited to life-threatening emergency situations, but rather is also available to treat "serious" diseases or conditions* (Bronzino et al., 1990a).

The FDA has not approved treatment use of unapproved medical devices, but it is possible that a manufacturer could obtain such approval by establishing a specific protocol for this kind of use within the context of an IDE.

> *The criteria for treatment use of unapproved medical devices would be similar to criteria for treatment use of investigational drugs: (1) the device is intended to treat serious or life-threatening disease or condition, (2) there is no comparable or satisfactory alternative product available to treat that condition, (3) the device is under an IDE, or has received an IDE exemption, or all clinical trials have been completed and the device is awaiting approval, and (4) the sponsor is actively pursuing marketing approval of the investigational device. The treatment use*

protocol would be submitted as part of the IDE, and would describe the intended use of the device, the rationale for use of the device, the available alternatives and why the investigational product is preferable, the criteria for patient selection, the measures to monitor the use of the device and to minimize risk, and technical information that is relevant to the safety and effectiveness of the device for the intended treatment purpose (Bronzino et al., 1990a).

Were the FDA to approve treatment use of unapproved medical devices, what ethical issues would be posed? First, because such use is premised on the failure of validated interventions to improve the patient's condition adequately, it is a form of practice rather than research. Second, since the device involved in an instance of treatment use is unapproved, such use would constitute nonvalidated practice. As such, like emergency use, it should be subject to the FDA's requirement that prior preclinical tests and animal studies have been conducted that provide substantial reason to believe that patient benefit will result. As with emergency use, although this does not prevent assessment of the intervention's benefits and risks from being highly speculative, it does prevent assessment from being totally speculative. Here, too, although desperate circumstances can justify desperate action, they do not justify reckless action. Unlike emergency use, the circumstances of treatment use involve serious impairment of health rather than the threat of premature death. Hence, an issue that must be considered is how serious such impairment must be to justify resorting to an intervention whose risks and benefits have not been solidly established.

In cases of emergency use, the FDA requires that physicians not use this exception to an IDE to avoid requirements that would otherwise be in place. This particular requirement would be obviated in instances of treatment use by the requirement that a protocol for such use be previously addressed within an IDE.

As with emergency use of unapproved devices, the patients involved in treatment uses would be particularly vulnerable patients. Although they are not dying, they are facing serious medical conditions and are thereby likely to be less able to avoid exploitation than patients under less desperate circumstances. Consequently, here too it is especially important that patients be informed of the speculative nature of the intervention and of the possibility that treatment may result in little to no benefit to them.

The Safe Medical Devices Act

On November 28, 1991, the *Safe Medical Devices Act of 1990* (Public Law 101-629) went into effect. This regulation requires a wide range of health-care institutions, including hospitals, ambulatory-surgical facilities, nursing homes, and outpatient treatment facilities, to report information that "reasonably suggests" the likelihood that the death, serious injury, or serious illness of a patient at that facility has been caused or contributed to by a medical device. When a death is device-related, a report must be made directly to the FDA and to the manufacturer of the device. When a serious illness or injury is device-related, a report must be made to the manufacturer or to the FDA in cases where the manufacturer is not known. In addition, summaries of previously submitted reports must be submitted to the FDA on a semiannual basis. Prior to this regulation, such reporting was wholly voluntary. This new regulation was designed to enhance the FDA's ability to learn quickly about problems related to medical devices and supplements the medical device reporting (MDR) regulations promulgated in 1984. MDR regulations require that reports of device-related deaths and serious injuries be submitted to the FDA by manufacturers and importers. The new law extends this requirement to users of medical devices along with manufacturers and importers. This act gives the FDA authority over device-user facilities.

The new regulation is ethically significant because by attempting to increase the FDA's awareness of medical device–related problems, it attempts to increase that agency's ability to protect the welfare of patients. The main controversy over this new regulation is essentially utilitarian in nature. Skeptics of the law are dubious about its ability to provide the FDA with much useful information. They worry that much of the information generated by the new law will simply duplicate information already provided under MDR regulations. If this is the case, little or no benefit to patients would accrue from compliance with the regulation. Furthermore, the new regulations, according to the skeptics, are likely to increase lawsuits filed against hospitals and manufacturers and will require device-user facilities to implement formal systems for reporting device-related problems and to provide personnel to operate those systems. This would, of course, add to the costs of health care and thereby exacerbate the problem of access to care, a situation that many believe to be of crisis proportions already. In short, the controversy over the new policy centers upon the worry that its benefits to patients will be marginal and significantly outweighed by its costs.

CONCLUSION: EQUITABLE ACCESS TO MEDICAL TECHNOLOGIES

Access to quality health care and thereby to validated medical technologies is often quite unequal. Currently, one's level of access is determined by a wide range of variables, e.g., personal wealth, employment benefits, eligibility for federal, state, or local welfare programs, geographic region, etc. Needy persons with low levels of access to validated medical technologies often have no recourse but to accept the charity of their fellow citizens. (Such appeals have often been made in recent years on behalf of individuals needing organ or tissue transplants.) Unfortunately, such charity is rarely sufficient. Is this sort of unequal access to medical technology and the other components of quality health care justifiable? Does society have an obligation to ensure some minimal level of access to everyone?

These questions challenge the widespread notion that medical technologies and health care are not different in morally significant ways from other kinds of goods and services. They challenge the notion that medical technologies are morally indistinguishable from automobiles, television sets, and compact disc players. Although these sorts of nonmedical technologies are highly valued by many people, the view that society has an obligation to ensure some level of access to them to all of its members has little support. The types of compact disc players, for example, that are produced, their distribution to the population, the means by which they are delivered, and the means by which they are financed are largely determined by the market, i.e., by the voluntary transactions of individuals using their own legitimately held resources. Although such exchanges occur within a framework of laws and regulations designed to protect the overall welfare of society, no one is guaranteed any level of access to the majority of nonmedical technologies thereby generated. What is produced, who gets it, and how it is paid for are left up to the decisions individuals make with their own resources. The result may be high levels of access to these technologies for all, low levels of access for all, or, more likely, varying degrees of unequal access. No particular pattern of access is ruled out as long as it is genuinely the outcome of voluntary exchanges between individuals using their own legitimately held resources in pursuit of their own aims and ends. Why shouldn't medical technology be treated the same way? Why shouldn't the types and quantities of medical technologies produced, their distribution, and the mode of financing them be determined by the market, that is, by the voluntary transactions of individuals pursuing satisfaction of their own preferences?

Commentators have noted several features of health care that give it special significance but perhaps none is more important in the context of a society like the United States than its effect on opportunity. This can be seen by focusing upon the nature and importance of health care needs. Of course, people do have needs for health care and thereby for medical technology but this alone does not indicate what is morally special about the practices and technologies of health care. Indeed, given one very common sense of "need," almost anything can legitimately count as a need. As ethicist Norman Daniels (1987) has noted, "*Without abuse of language, we refer to the means to reach any of our goals as needs. To reawaken memories of Miller's, the neighborhood delicatessen of my childhood, I need only the smell of pickles in a barrel. To stay at Cape Cod next weekend, I need a motel reservation.*"

In this sense, what an individual "needs" is a matter of one's wants and preferences, a matter of one's particular goals. On this understanding, needs are completely relative to the individual and the importance of a need is primarily, and perhaps wholly, a subjective matter, a matter of the intensity of the individual's wants and preferences. If X is wanted more intensely than Y, then those things that are required for the attainment of X are more important needs than those that are required for the attainment of Y. Thus, on this conception of need, whether needs for medical technology and health care in general are of special importance depends upon whether the wants that can be satisfied by medical technology and other instrumentalities of health care are more intense than wants satisfiable by other means. If this is the only acceptable sense of the term "need," then it is difficult to see how health care and its technologies can be regarded as importantly different from any of the other kinds of goods and services produced in a society. The wants that are satisfied by means of compact disc players, fur coats, and tennis rackets can be felt just as intensely and even more intensely than those that are satisfied by medical technology.

Although this sense of need is a legitimate one, it is not the only legitimate one, as illustrated by the fact that the notion of need does play a role in attempts to determine when individuals have some responsibility to provide others with the things they need. When we attempt to determine those needs of others that we, as individuals or as a society, have some responsibility to meet, we in fact do discriminate between kinds of needs on grounds other than the intensity of wants and preferences. Some needs are regarded as making valid claims on our resources. Others are not. As Daniels (1987) has argued,

> *not all the things we say we need are equally important. It is possible to pick out various things we say we need, including needs for health care, which play a special role and are given special weight in a variety of moral contexts. If I appeal to my friend's duty of beneficence in requesting $100, I most likely will get a different reaction if I tell him I need the money to get a root-canal than if I tell him I need the money to go to the Brooklyn neighborhood of my childhood to smell pickles in a barrel. Indeed, it is not likely to matter in his assessment of his obligation that I strongly prefer to go to Brooklyn. Nor is it likely to matter that I insist I feel a great need to reawaken memories of my childhood.*

In making this sort of distinction, according to Daniels, we are refusing to rely solely upon the individual's own assessment of his well-being as the basis for deciding which of his needs may obligate us to come to his aid. But what, other than the intensity of an individual's wants, could be the basis for regarding some of his needs as important enough to place responsibility upon others?

Daniels argues that the answer to this question depends upon an important distinction delineated by David Braybrooke. According to Braybrooke, all of the things an individual can need are either "course-of-life needs" or "adventitious needs" (Daniels, 1987):

> *Adventitious needs are the things we need because of the particular contingent projects (which may be long term ones) on which we embark. Their relative importance will reflect many idiosyncratic facts about our personal choice of a plan of life. Course-of-life needs are those needs people "have through all their lives or at certain stages of life through which all must pass." They include food, shelter, clothing, exercise, rest, companionship, a mate (in one's prime), and so on. Such needs are not themselves deficiencies, for example, when they are anticipated. But a deficiency with respect to them "endangers the normal functioning of the subject of need, considered as a member of a natural species." Thus course-of-life needs are important when we abstract from many particular choices and preferences individuals might make or have.*

Clearly, the notion of a course-of-life need is quite different from the notion of a need that is entirely related to an individual's wants and preferences, i.e., a notion of need that is captured by the concept of adventitious needs. A course-of-life need remains a need even when it cannot be connected to some particular aim or goal that an individual wishes to realize. Such a need is identified, not by looking to the individual's specific wants or particular goals, but rather by looking to a standard that Daniels has referred to as "species-typical normal functioning." This standard identifies needs that individuals will have all through their lives or in particular phases of life through which all individuals pass (if life is not prematurely ended), regardless of their particular aims and ends, wants or preferences.

What then is species-typical normal functioning? The basic idea is that for any given natural species, there are kinds and levels of functioning that are normal for a typical member of that species. What is normal for such an individual will be a matter of the species to which it belongs. Although an account of species-typical normal functioning can be given for an oak tree, a Dalmatian, or a Homo sapiens, clearly the account given will be different for each of these entities. The task of determining exactly what species-typical normal functioning is falls on the sciences that study natural species and thereby determine the defining properties. In the case of the human species, this includes the science of human biology and all of the biomedical sciences, and given that humans are intrinsically social and psychological creatures, at least some of the social sciences will also be relevant. As these sciences reveal more about human nature and thereby more about species-typical normal functioning for human beings, those things that are viewed as course-of-life needs will likely change. By whatever means the notion of species-typical normal functioning is specified, those things that are necessary to maintain and restore such functioning are course-of-life needs.

Species-typical normal functioning and the course-of-life needs that must be met to maintain or restore it constitute a dimension of individual well-being that is distinguishable from the intensity of the individual's wants and preferences, a dimension that is objectively specifiable. We intuitively recognize this objective dimension of well-being when we recognize that something a person is interested in, even very intensely, may not be in the individual's best interest. For instance, we recognize that while an individual might intensely prefer to consume large quantities of alcohol, satisfying this want would be to his detriment. Although he is truly interested in the pleasure such consumption would provide, it is not in his best interest to engage in such consumption because in so doing he would impair his ability to function in the ways and at the levels which are normal for human beings. Some such notion of well-being which can be identified apart from the individual's wants and preferences is presupposed when we judge a person's wants to be contrary to his interests.

Forms of health care and their technologies belong in the category of course-of-life needs. This follows from the very nature of health and disease. As Daniels (1985) has noted, *"The basic idea is that health is the absence of disease, and diseases (I include here deformities and disabilities that result from trauma) are deviations from the natural functional organization of a typical member of a species."*

Thus, health-care needs, by their very nature, are things we must have *"in order to maintain, restore, or provide functional equivalents (when possible) to normal species functioning"* (Daniels, 1987). Although this will include a diverse body of things, ranging from adequate nutrition to adequate rest to adequate sanitation, clearly it will include access to some level of validated medical technologies as well.

So far it has been argued that health-care needs are course-of-life needs, needs for things that are necessary for maintaining and restoring species-typical normal functioning and compensating for its loss. If this is correct, then medical technologies and health care in general are different from compact disc players, car alarm systems, and other similar nonmedical technologies. But how does this support the notion that medical technology and health care are special in some morally significant way? How is it relevant to the question of whether society has a duty to ensure some level of access to those goods and services to all of its members?

The relevance lies in the effect that disease has on opportunity. Consider Daniels' (1987) notion of a "normal opportunity range":

> *The normal opportunity range for a given society is the array of life plans reasonable persons in it are likely to construct for themselves. The range is thus relative to key features of the society — its stage of historical development, its level of material wealth and technological development, and even important cultural facts about it.*

Access to health care is surely one of the most important of the many factors that affect how the normal range of opportunity for a given society is actually distributed across its population. An individual who cannot function in the ways or at the levels that are normal for a typical human being will not have equal access to the range of opportunity available in the society to unimpaired fellow citizens. One of the most highly regarded norms of contemporary American society is equality of opportunity. According to this norm, any given individual's share of the society's normal opportunity range should be determined, as far as possible, by one's talents and skills. When determined by individual talents and skills, shares of that range of opportunities are not necessarily equal in the sense that every individual has exactly the same share as every other individual. Rather, they are equal in the sense that the share held by each person, no more or less than the share held by any other person, is determined only by the individual's skills and talents. Because individual skills and talents differ, the shares of the normal opportunity range held by different individuals will also differ even when those shares are fair. Some will have larger shares than others. Although opportunity will be unequal in this sense, it will be equal in the sense that everyone is constrained only by their own abilities.

Whereas disease is clearly one constraint that can cause an individual's share of the normal opportunity range to be less than the share his talents and skills would otherwise make available to him, it is not the only constraint (Daniels, 1987):

> *[S]kills and talents can be underdeveloped or misdeveloped because of social conditions, e.g. family background or racist educational practices. So, if we are interested in having*

> *individuals enjoy a fair share of the normal opportunity range, we will want to correct for special disadvantages here too, say, through compensatory educational or job-training programs. Still, restoring normal functioning through health care has a particular and limited effect on an individual share of the normal functioning range. It lets him enjoy that portion of the range to which his full array of skills and talents would give him access, assuming that these too are not impaired by special social disadvantages.*

In recent years, American society has gone to great lengths to identify and attempt to eliminate or mitigate social conditions that unfairly limit an individual's share of the normal opportunity range, and such efforts continue today. Although there has been and will continue to be much debate about which social conditions are relevant and which responses are appropriate to them, the commitment to ensuring that an individual's opportunities are, as far as possible, a function only of one's talents and skills is widespread and deeply held. The kind of commitment to equality of opportunity that underlies efforts to mitigate social barriers to such opportunity for all justifies similar efforts against those conditions that can be prevented, removed, or at least somewhat ameliorated by health-care and its technologies. This is ultimately the reason for regarding health care needs as special and for wanting to ensure some level of access to medical technology to all individuals, the reason for not wanting who gets what kinds and quantities of health care to be determined in the way these matters are determined for microwave ovens, for example.

Although the powers of modern health care and its machines far exceed those of the health care available only a few decades ago, even now there are diseases and impairments that cannot be prevented, cannot be cured, and whose effects can not be significantly ameliorated. No matter how great a society's commitment to equality of opportunity, it cannot be expected to do the impossible. The fact that some of its members do get ill, live impaired lives, or die prematurely does not show that society has failed to ensure that medicine is doing all that can be done to remove health as a barrier to equal opportunity. It may simply mean that what medicine can do is always limited. Whatever equitable access to medical technology may mean, it does not mean absolute protection against illness, impairment, and premature death.

But what does equitable access mean? What level of access to medical technologies and health care in general must society guarantee to all its members in order to provide equitable access? Insofar as the commitment to equality of opportunity is the basis for a social obligation to provide equitable access, society need not ensure access to all kinds of medical technology and care to all people. Not all kinds of medical technology and care function to maintain or restore species-typical normal functioning. An individual may desperately want a beautiful nose, and the technology to provide it exists. Yet providing such a nose does not necessarily maintain, restore, or compensate for loss of species-typical normal functioning. If it does not, then society has no obligation to provide access to this cosmetic surgery, no matter how intensely it may be desired. Only if some genuine course-of-life need is met by a form of technology can society have an obligation, given its commitment to equality of opportunity, to provide that form of technology or care. Only then does that form of technology have the kind of effect on species-typical normal functioning that is relevant to equality of opportunity.

Ideally, equitable access should mean equal access for all to any and all forms of medical technology that can prevent loss of species-typical normal functioning, restore such functioning, or compensate for impairments to it. But given that resources are finite and that society has other valued goals, access of this kind is probably impossible.

If the ideal in equitable access is not feasible, what would be a realistic sense of equitable access? In answer to this question, it should be noted that not all forms of medical technology or health care in general will have the same effects on species-typical normal functioning. Among preventive technologies, some will prevent more serious impairments than others. Among curative and rehabilitative technologies, some will restore more important kinds and levels of functioning than others. Among technologies that compensate for incurable impairment, some will compensate for more important losses than others. If society, given its resource constraints and other goals, cannot provide access for everyone to everything that can prevent, cure, or compensate for the effects of disease, then it ought to do as much as it can to ensure that everyone has a reasonable level of access to those technologies that have the greatest effects upon species-typical normal functioning, i.e., those technologies that meet the most important course-of-life needs. By definition these will be the technologies that do the most toward realizing equality of opportunity. These technologies will do the most to remove impairments that prevent an individual's share of the society's normal opportunity range from being as large as it would be if it were determined on the basis of skill and talent alone. Which technologies do in fact have the greatest positive effect on keeping individuals at the level of functioning normal for typical human beings is a matter to be determined by scientific judgment. What level of access to such technologies is reasonable and so the level that ought to be guaranteed is a matter for social decision in light of society's resource constraints. Although this question cannot be answered here, it is one that society is forced to face given its commitment to equality of opportunity.

What implications for efforts to contain the costs of medical care would follow from a commitment to provide all individuals with whatever level of access to validated medical technologies is mandated by fair equality of opportunity? First, it would mean that efforts to control the costs of care should initially be directed at those kinds of medical technology and care that do not meet course-of-life needs and that do not function to maintain, restore, or compensate for loss of species-typical normal functioning. Second, it would mean that if those efforts prove insufficient and if further savings are attainable only by utilizing cost-saving measures with respect to technologies that do affect species-typical normal functioning, before measures are taken that affect access, efforts should be made to eliminate all inefficient use of such technologies. Only then should access be restricted. Insofar as access is reduced, reductions should be aimed at those technologies that are least important for maintenance of species-typical normal functioning. Third, it would mean that society must ask whether, in order to contain the costs of health care, it is willing not to guarantee access for all to those medical technologies and forms of health care that are most important for keeping individuals functioning in the ways and at the levels that are typical of normal human beings. A decision of this nature would be a decision to be less committed to the equality of opportunity for some than for others. It would mean not ensuring that as much will be done to avert or neutralize the most severe limits on opportunity that disease and impairment can engender for some persons as would be done for others. Can society make that decision without thereby implying that it values some of its members more than others? If it cannot, one must wonder what reason such less-valued individuals could have for feeling allegiance to society. Is the moral cost of treating certain of its members as second-class citizens with respect to health care a moral cost that society can afford to bear? This question cannot be answered here, but it is unavoidable for a society that is committed to both the equality of opportunity for all and to containing the costs of health care.

Presently, although American society is committed to the equality of opportunity, it has failed to ask what this means in terms of access to medical technologies and other forms of health care. Failure to ask this question has left society unable to see that this commitment requires that a reasonable level of access to certain kinds of technology and care be provided to all or that it must face up to whether the financial costs of providing such access are preferable to the moral costs of not doing so.

EXERCISES

1. The branch of ethical theory concerned with the analysis of moral concepts is

   (a) normative ethics.
   (b) applied ethics.
   (c) metaethics.

2. The branch of ethical theory concerned with knowledge of valid moral standards is

   (a) normative ethics.
   (b) applied ethics.
   (c) mctacthics.

3. All moral judgments are

   (a) non-normative judgments.
   (b) aesthetic judgments.
   (c) normative judgments.

4. An act of euthanasia that hastens the individual's death for his own good but against his wishes is

   (a) active.
   (b) passive.
   (c) involuntary.
   (d) nonvoluntary.

5. Normative judgments can always be distinguished from non-normative ones simply by their characteristic terminology. True or False?

6. Ethics is itself a normative study of moral judgments. True or False?

7. A complete set of necessary and sufficient conditions probably cannot be provided for all moral concepts. True or False?

8. From a utilitarian perspective, human beings are morally unique and deserve special respect because of their autonomy. True or False?

9. Define the following terms:

(a)	Consequentialism	(b)	Utilitarianism
(c)	Nonconsequentialism	(d)	Beneficence
(e)	Nonmaleficence	(f)	Brain death (i.e., brainstem or whole brain death)
(g)	Chronic vegetative state	(h)	Euthanasia
(i)	Passive euthanasia	(j)	Active euthanasia
(k)	Species-typical normal functioning	(l)	Normal opportunity range
(m)	Adventitious need	(n)	Course-of-life need

10. State the defining characteristics of moral standards.

11. What are the fundamental differences between practice and research?

12. Discuss the importance and the limitations of a codes of ethics.

13. What are the fundamental differences between practice and nonvalidated practice?

14. Discuss the importance of informed and voluntary consent in ethical research on human subjects.

15. State the three types of situations in which the FDA allows unapproved medical devices to be used without an investigational device exemption (IDE).

16. State the requirements imposed upon health care institutions by the Safe Medical Devices Act of 1990.

17. Why are health-care needs different in a morally important sense from other kinds of needs?

REFERENCES

Bronzino, J., Flannery, E.J., and Wade, M.L. "Legal and Ethical Issues in the Regulation and Development of Engineering Achievements in Medical Technology," Part I *IEEE Engineering in Medicine and Biology*, 1990a.

Bronzino. J., Flannery, E.J., and Wade, M.L. "Legal and Ethical Issues in the Regulation and Dcvclopment of Engineering Achievements in Medical Technology," Part II *IEEE Engineering in Medicine and Biology*, 1990b.

Capron, A. "Human Experimentation: Basic Issues." in: *The Encyclopedia of Bioethics* vol. II. The Free Press, Glencoe, IL, 1978.

Capron, A. "Human Experimentation." in: (J.F. Childress, et al., eds.) University Publications of America, 1986.

Daniels, N. "Justice and Health Care" in: *Health Care Ethics: An Introduction*, (D. Vandeveer, and T.Regan, T., eds.), Temple University Press, Philadelphia, 1978.

Daniels, N. *Just Health Care* Cambridge University Press, Cambridge, 1987.

Fried, C. "Human Experimentation: Philosophical Issues," in: *The Encyclopedia of Bioethics*, vol. II. The Free Press, Glencoe, IL, 1978.

Murphy, J., and Coleman, J. *The Philosophy of Law*, Rowman and Allenheld, 1984.

Rachels, J. "Active and Passive Euthanasia," in: *Moral Problems*, 3rd ed., (Rachels, J. ed.), Harper and Row, New York, 1978.

Rachels, J. *Ethics at the End of Life: Euthanasia and Morality*, Oxford University Press, Oxford, 1986.

Valasquez, M. *Business Ethics* 2nd ed. Prentice-Hall, Englewood Cliffs, NJ, 1988.

Chapter 11

CLINICAL ENGINEERING: INTERNATIONAL COMPARISONS AND FUTURE DIRECTIONS

As the number of clinical engineers increased during the 1970s, professional groups began to form throughout the world. In Canada, for example, the first professional engineering group appeared in Montreal in 1974 with participating members coming from the provinces of Ontario and Quebec and even from the state of Vermont. In 1979, the **International Federation of Medical and Biological Engineering (IFMBE)**, a federation of biomedical societies from almost 30 countries, created a five-member Working Group on Clinical Engineering whose task was to foster the development of clinical engineering in various areas of the world. To accomplish this goal, the working group organized seminars and workshops in the United Kingdom, Greece, Germany, and Hungary and cooperated in local workshops organized in France, Finland, Sweden, and Italy. The discussions that ensued at these meetings permitted clinical engineers from all over the world to compare their activities and the organizational infrastructures in which they operated. In 1985, the IFMBE working group was dissolved, and the International Clinical Engineering Division of IFMBE was created in its place. This division initiated a newsletter entitled *Clinical Engineering Update* which is published two to three times a year to encourage the exchange of information and news among clinical engineers worldwide.

In France, a formal organization of clinical engineers, L'Association Française des Ingénieurs Biomédicaux (AFIB) was created in 1982. Since its creation, this association has organized annual workshops and also produces a regular newsletter, *Journées biomédicales* promoting the exchange of information between clinical engineers.

In the United States, the American College of Clinical Engineering (ACEE) was officially founded in 1990 (see Chapter 1) to do the following:

- Establish a standard of competence and promote excellence in clinical engineering practice.
- Promote safe and effective application of science and technology to patient care.
- Define the body of knowledge on which the profession is based.
- Represent the professional interests of clinical engineers.

The ACEE also publishes a newsletter, *ACEE News*, to facilitate communication among it's members.

Although the organizational structure and function of clinical engineering departments appeared very similar in the various industrialized countries in the mid- 1980s, there was little evidence to support this conclusion. A study by Pacela (1985) provided some quantitative information regarding the structure and function of clinical engineering in the United States; however, no hard data existed comparing the level of development of clinical engineering departments in other countries. In an effort to obtain such information, an international survey of clinical engineering departments was conducted to compare to the development of the field around the world (Frize, 1988, 1990a, b; Frize and Shaffer, 1991).

The first international survey, conducted in 1988, investigated the extent of functional involvement of clinical engineering departments in the equipment management process and compared results for teaching versus non-teaching hospitals, in four geographic locations: Canada, the U.S., three countries in the European Economic Community (France, the U.K., and the Netherlands) and two Nordic countries (Sweden and Finland). The questionnaire developed for this study also provided respondents the opportunity to express their degree of satisfaction with the reporting structure in their respective countries and their perceived level of recognition within their institution. This first survey was followed by a second one, three years later, to determine whether substantial changes had occurred in any of the factors affecting the development of the clinical engineering field. This chapter discusses the findings of both studies.

THE FIRST INTERNATIONAL SURVEY OF CLINICAL ENGINEERING DEPARTMENTS (1988)

Approximately five hundred questionnaires were mailed to clinical engineering departments in several countries; 122 replies (24 percent) were received as follows: Canada (41), the U.S. (37), the EEC (20), the Nordic countries (18). Results of this study were reviewed in the following categories: organizational setting; level of functional involvement for various clinical engineering tasks; resources provided to the department to sustain the level of activity; educational level and training of personnel; and perceived level of recognition achieved by the department within its institution.

Organizational Setting

The organizational setting included a number of factors, such as hospital type (teaching and non-teaching), hospital size, whether the clinical engineering department existed as a separate entity or not, the type of reporting authority, the education level of the staff, and the level of recognition achieved by the department.

Hospital Type. In the geographic areas surveyed, the proportion of respondents from teaching institutions was 65 percent in Canada, 47 percent in the U.S., 67 percent in the EEC, and 56 percent in the Nordic countries. Because it has been reported that teaching hospitals invest roughly six times as much annually as non-teaching hospitals and urban hospitals invest about four times as much as their rural counterparts (Cromwell et al., 1987), this factor appeared to affect significantly both the level of involvement of clinical engineering departments in the overall activity of the institution and the extent of the equipment base supported by these departments. Hospital equipment was divided into four types to quantify the extent of the technology base supported by clinical engineering departments. The equipment types considered included medical, radiological, clinical laboratory, and anesthesia. Comparisons were made using three main variables: (1) equipment replacement value, (2) the number of devices directly supported by the department, and (3) hospital size.

Figure 11.1a shows a geographic comparison of the value (in 1988 U.S. dollars) of the equipment base supported by clinical engineering departments in teaching hospitals in these four geographic areas. Figure 11.1b shows similar information for non-teaching hospitals. These results confirm that clinical engineering departments in teaching hospitals generally support a larger equipment inventory value than departments in non-teaching institutions. Because there is a higher proportion of beds for intensive care in teaching hospitals, there is a more technology-intensive environment in these teaching institutions in all four geographic areas. Geographically, the average value of equipment supported by departments in the EEC and the Nordic countries appears to be substantially higher than that supported by departments in the U.S. or Canada.

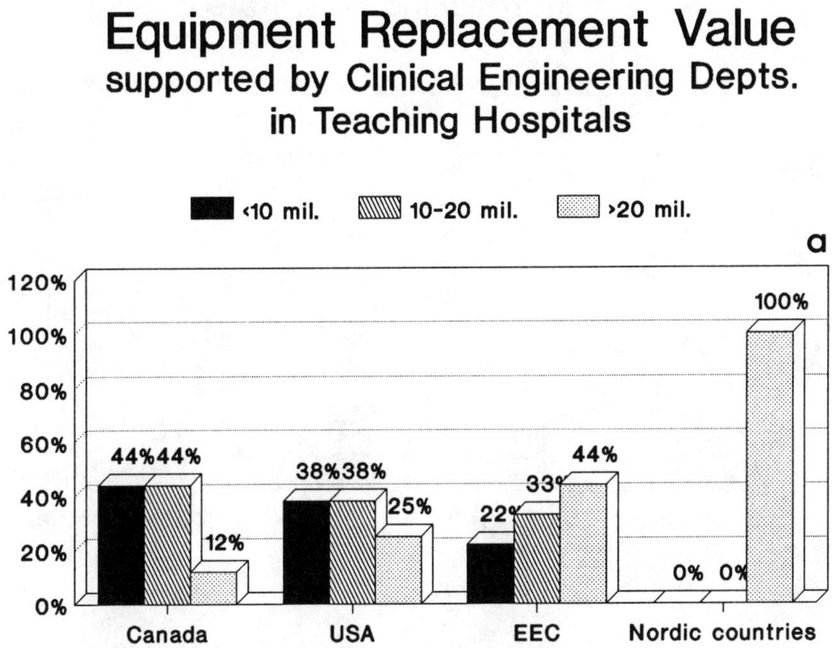

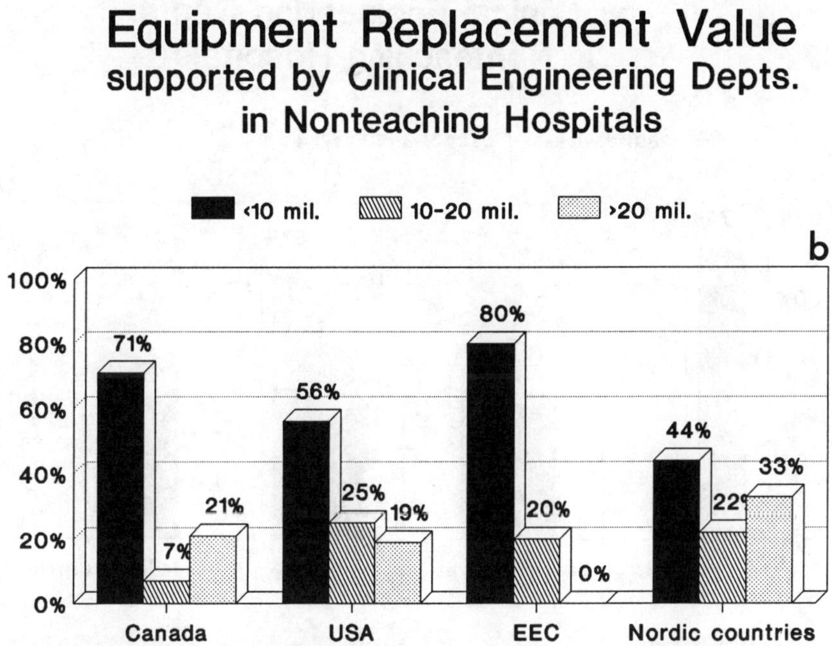

Figure 11.1: Equipment replacement value of devices supported by clinical engineering departments in teaching (a) and nonteaching hospitals (b).

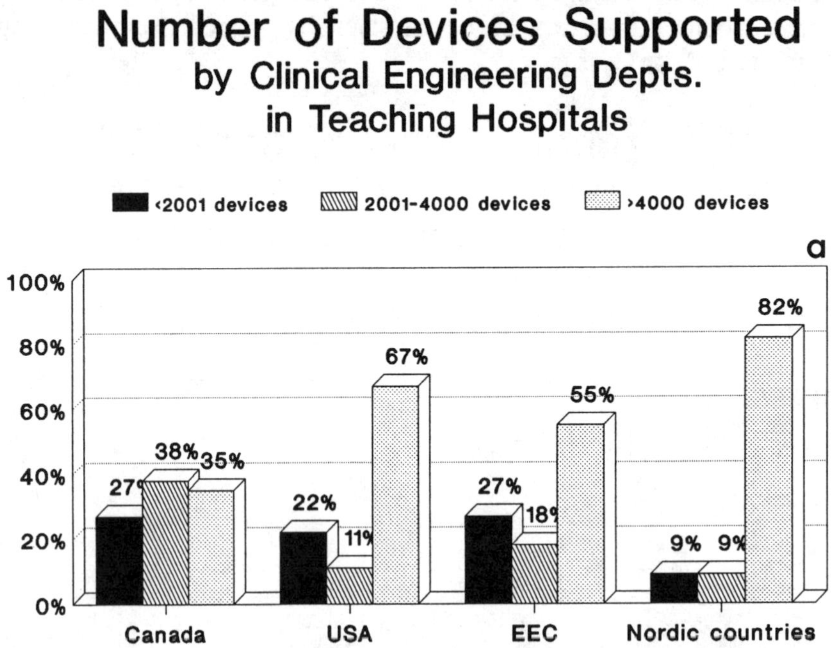

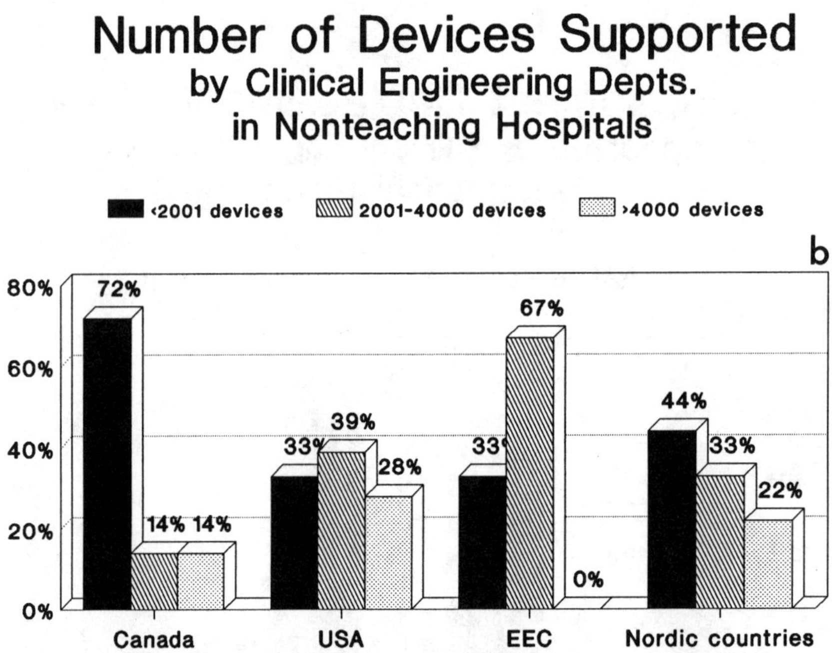

Figure 11.2: Number of devices supported by clinical engineering departments in teaching (a) and nonteaching hospitals (b).

In studying the number of devices supported by the clinical engineering departments (see Figure 11.2), teaching hospitals are significantly more equipment-intensive than non-teaching ones. Once again, departments in the EEC and Nordic countries generally support greater numbers of devices than their counterparts in North America. The geographic variations indicated by the survey can partly be explained by the size of hospitals found in each of the areas concerned. Figure 11.3 shows the distribution of hospital size in the various geographic areas. Hospitals in Europe and the Nordic countries tend to be large and equipped with vast numbers of devices with substantial replacement value that are supported by large clinical engineering departments. The opposite appears to be true in the U.S. and Canada.

The effect of hospital size on the value and number of devices supported by clinical engineering departments is further illustrated in Figures 11.4 and 11.5. By defining small hospitals as having less than 500 beds, medium-sized as 501 to 1,000 beds, and large as more than 1,000 beds, the relationship between hospital size and equipment replacement value was developed (see Figure 11.4) for three categories of value, i.e., capital investment in medical equipment: less than 10 million (U.S. dollars), 10 to 20 million, and more than 20 million. Figure 11.5, on the other hand, shows the relationship between hospital size and the number of devices supported by clinical engineering departments for three categories of numbers of devices: i.e., less than 2,000, 2,001 to 4,000, and more than 4,000.

After reviewing these figures, it is evident that clinical engineering departments in smaller hospitals generally support a smaller number of devices that have a lower replacement value than medium or large institutions. This correlation is fairly uniform across all regions, except that in the EEC where the equipment base in the small hospitals is large compared to the other geographic samples. Although there will always be exceptions in any sample (such as a 100-bed cardiac-care hospital, that is highly technology dependent), hospital size has a direct correlation with the number of devices and equipment value supported by clinical engineering departments. It is important to note that the technology base in the hospital may be much larger than the proportion supported by clinical engineers and thus, no conclusion is made in this study about the overall value and number of devices owned by the hospital.

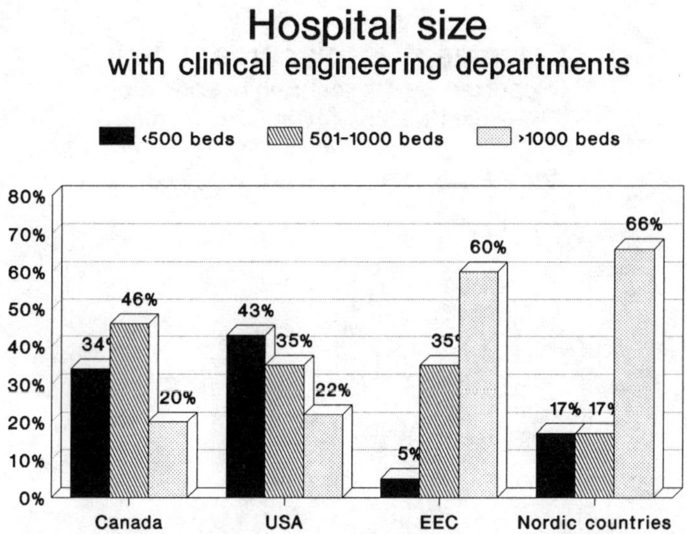

Figure 11.3: Percentage of hospitals having a clinical engineering department as a function of hospital size.

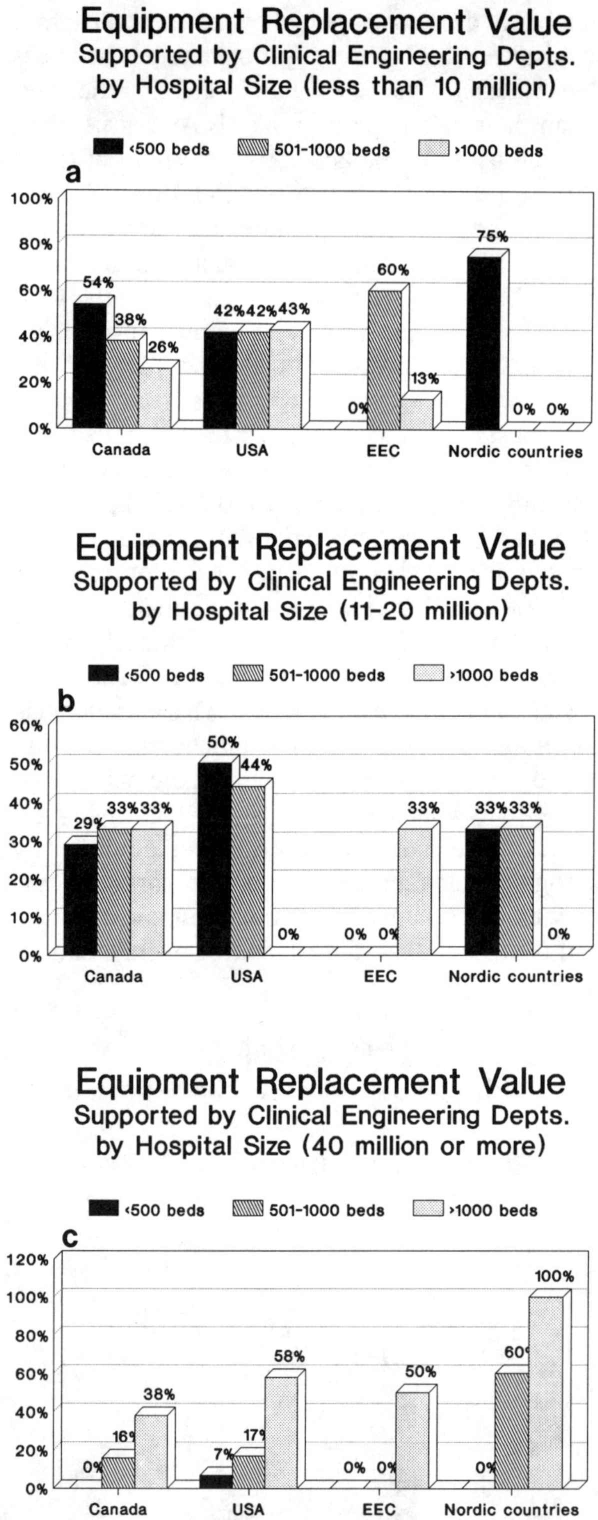

Figure 11.4: **Equipment replacement value of devices supported by clinical engineering departments as a function of hospital size, (a) less than \$10 million, (b) \$11 to 20 million, and (c) \$40 million and greater.**

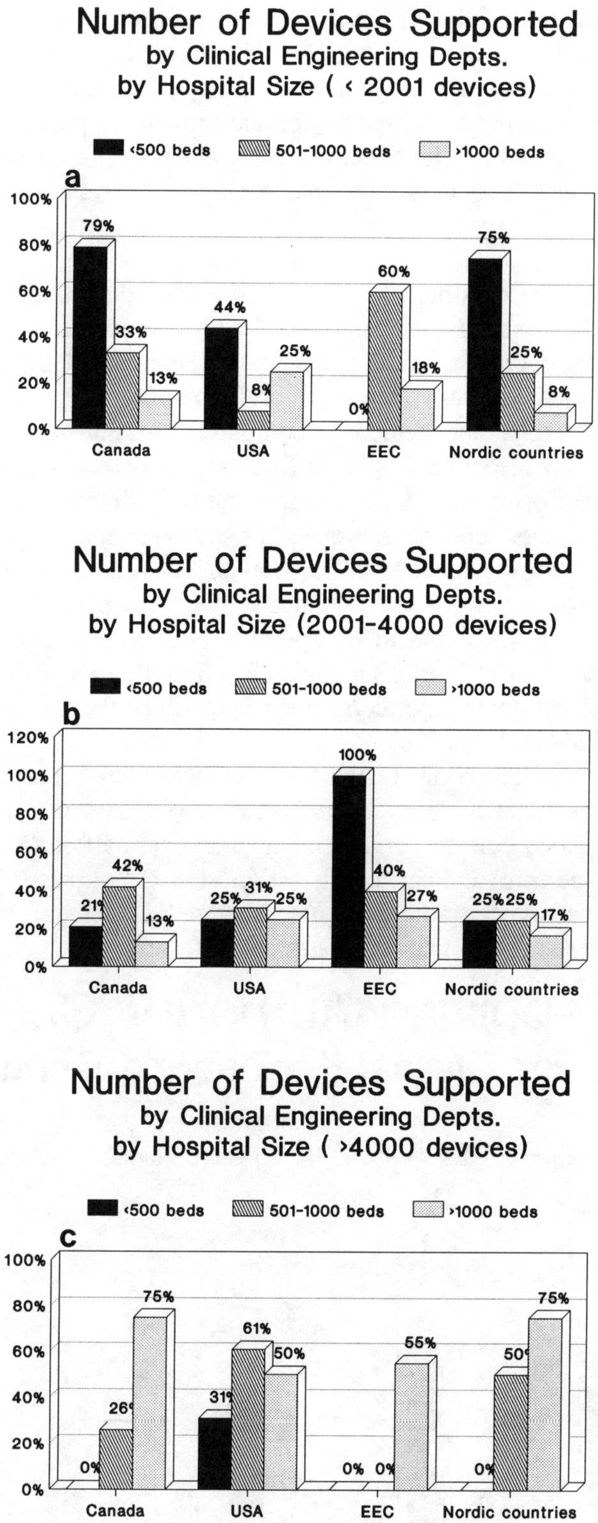

Figure 11.5: Number of devices supported by clinical engineering departments as a function of hospital size, (a) less than 2,000 devices, (b) 2,001 to 4,000 devices, (c) more than 4,000 devices.

If one assumes that staffing levels are matched to expected workloads based on service numbers of medical devices in the hospital, clinical engineering departments in Europe and the Nordic countries should be larger. It is not surprising that this is often the case. Large departments, in turn, create several subspecialties and provide support for equipment in other areas not traditionally tackled by clinical engineering departments, such as medical imaging (radiology) and the clinical laboratory. This has been found to be the case, especially in the Nordic countries.

Reporting Authority. The majority of clinical engineering departments responding in this survey reported that they existed as separate entities: 94 percent in the U.S., 83 percent in Canada and the Nordic countries, and 81 percent in the EEC. Others existed as part of another department, usually plant operations or a medical unit, and a few existed as subdivisions within materials management or computer operations departments.

Just over half of the respondents (54 percent) reported to a senior administrator; 29 percent reported to plant operations, 9 percent to a medical director and 8 percent to "other managers," mostly computer services and materials management. Figure 11.6 outlines the reporting authority choices as a function of geographic location. The predominant reporting authority in all geographic areas is a senior administrator. However, reporting directly to the medical director was more prevalent in Europe and the Nordic countries, and the "other" category was more common in North America. In all areas except the U.S., one-third of clinical engineering departments reported to plant operations; the proportion was lower (12 percent) in the U.S. sample.

In reviewing how satisfied clinical engineers were with their reporting authority choice, the results indicated that the majority of respondents (95 percent) reporting to a senior administrator were satisfied with this arrangement. Just over half of those individuals under plant operations, (58 percent) indicated satisfaction, and two-thirds (67 percent) of those reporting to other managers and more than three-quarters (82 percent) of those reporting to a medical director were satisfied with their arrangement.

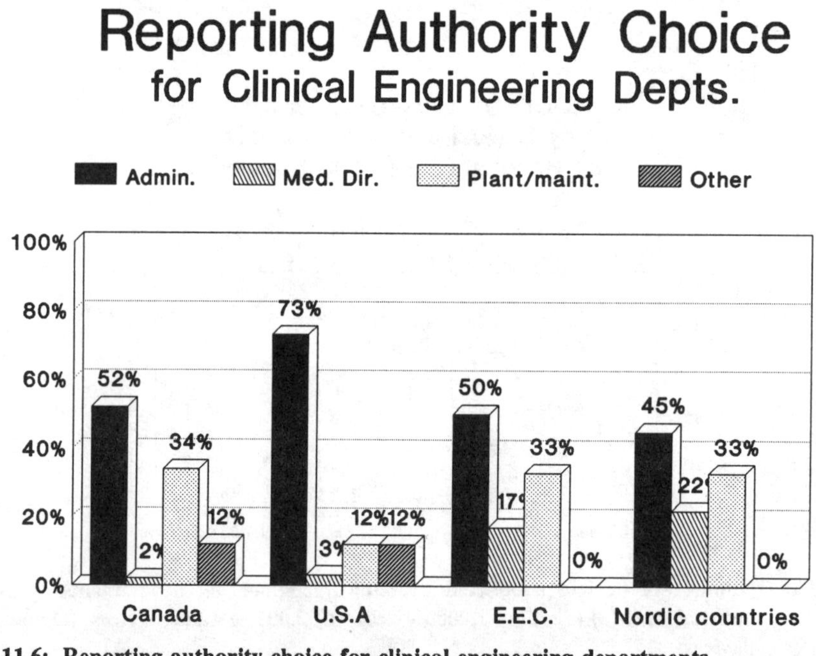

Figure 11.6: Reporting authority choice for clinical engineering departments.

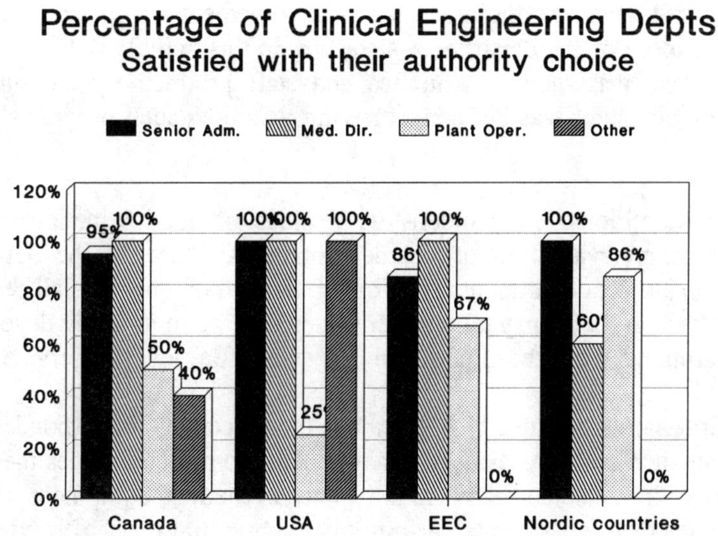

Figure 11.7: Percentage of clinical engineering departments satisfied with their reporting authority choice.

Figure 11.7 indicates the percentage of respondents satisfied with their reporting authority based on geographic location. It is evident from the data that the highest levels of satisfaction were obtained from those clinical engineers who reported to a senior administrator. However, the results varied widely by geographical location for the other authority choices. In Canada, the lowest satisfaction levels were obtained from departments reporting to "other" and plant operations categories, whereas in the U.S., only plant operations received a dissatisfactory rating. In Europe, plant operations also received a lower rating, and in the Nordic countries, the medical director choice was the least popular.

When the educational level of respondents was linked to reporting satisfaction, 67 percent of nonengineers were satisfied with their reporting authority choice, compared to 84 percent for engineers with a university degree. Thus, there appears to be a significant relationship between satisfaction with reporting authority and the education level of respondents.

Level of Functional Involvement

To study the level of functional involvement for each of the tasks normally performed by clinical engineering departments, respondents were asked what percentage of the equipment base in their institution was repaired and maintained by their department. A substantial in-house level of service was defined as departments performing corrective maintenance on 75 percent of this medical equipment inventory. Similar questions were asked about the level of corrective maintenance of anasthetic, radiological, and clinical laboratory equipment inventories.

For other types of tasks, a substantial level of service was defined as follows:

- For incoming inspections (acceptance testing), 75 percent or more of new equipment or equipment returning from an outside repair prior to its acceptance for patient use.

- For prepurchase consultation, being consulted for at least 75 percent of the equipment acquisitions of each of the four equipment types listed above.
- For research and development, a substantial involvement was defined as investing 10 percent or more of the department's staffing in this activity.
- For activities such as quality assurance and staff productivity measurements, a substantial involvement was defined as having instituted such programs within the last year.

Using these definitions, comparisons were made on an international scale. These comparisons permitted evaluation of the developmental stage of the department to be determined. For example, departments performing services on only a small percentage of the total equipment base in their hospital were considered to be in an early development stage, and mature departments were those performing a substantial level of service.

Corrective Maintenance. Figure 11.8 illustrates the percentage of respondents performing corrective maintenance on more than 75 percent of the four technologies mentioned above. The highest level of in-house corrective maintenance of medical equipment was found in the U.S., with 96 percent of departments performing a substantial level of service. In Canada, this number was 83 percent; it was 59 percent in the Nordic countries and 56 percent in EEC countries. Anesthetic equipment was the next most supported technology of clinical engineering departments, with 71 percent of respondents providing a substantial level of support in the Nordic countries, 56 percent in the EEC, 44 percent in the U.S. and 32 percent in Canada.

Incoming Inspections. As discussed in Chapter 3, new medical devices and those returning from either an outside or an in-house repair should be inspected for performance and safety. The survey indicated that the incoming inspection function has been well integrated into the activities and role of the North American clinical engineering departments; in the U.S., 100 percent of sampled respondents performed a substantial level of incoming inspection, in Canada, 91 percent, in the Nordic, 67 percent; and only 50 percent of departments in the EEC performed a substantial level of all incoming inspections (i.e., 75 percent or more of inspections to be done).

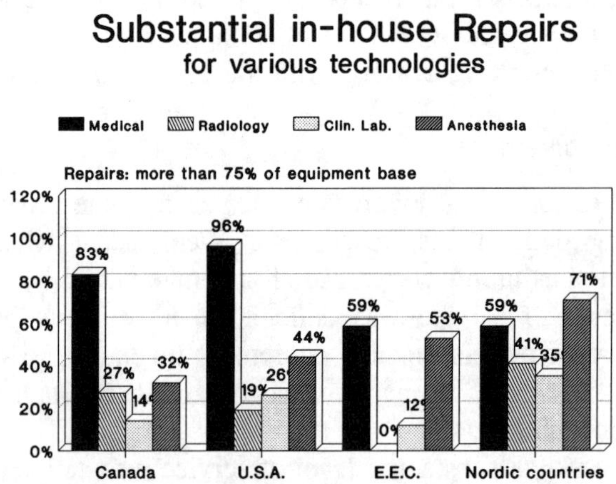

Figure 11.8: Percentage of hospitals performing in-house repairs on more than 75% of the equipment base.

User Training. As discussed in Chapter 1, one of the key functions of clinical engineering departments is to provide training to medical and nursing staff on the safe and effective use of medical equipment. Such training includes educating users about the equipment's limitations and hazards and how to avoid misuse or abuse of equipment. Because of the importance of this training function, the study assessed the percentage of respondents who were responsible for 75 percent or more of all equipment training needs within their institution. The results indicated that respondents from all geographic areas commit relatively little department time to this function. The largest commitment to this training activity was reported in the Nordic countries, where 44 percent of respondents stated that they provided at least 75 percent of all user training at their institutions, while 37 percent of respondents in the U.S., 12 percent in Canada, and only 6 percent in the EEC provided this level of training.

Prepurchase Consultation. Responses to the survey indicated that the number of prepurchase consultations involving the clinical engineering department varied with the type of technology and the geographic area. Figure 11.9 shows the percentage of respondents who were consulted for 75 percent or more of the equipment acquisitions in their hospitals. Clinical engineering departments in the EEC had the highest level of involvement in prepurchase consultations. This finding was surprisingly high, considering that these respondents reported relatively little involvement in the repair of this same equipment. This result indicates that these departments have established themselves in a consultative role rather than in a repair role. This factor is also a good indicator of the relative development of clinical engineering in the various countries surveyed. For example, in the U.S., more respondents were consulted at a high level for medical equipment than in any other geographic area tested (81 percent). In Canada, only 56 percent of respondents were consulted on medical equipment acquisitions at this high level, and in the Nordic countries, 65 to 69 percent of respondents reported being consulted at these levels.

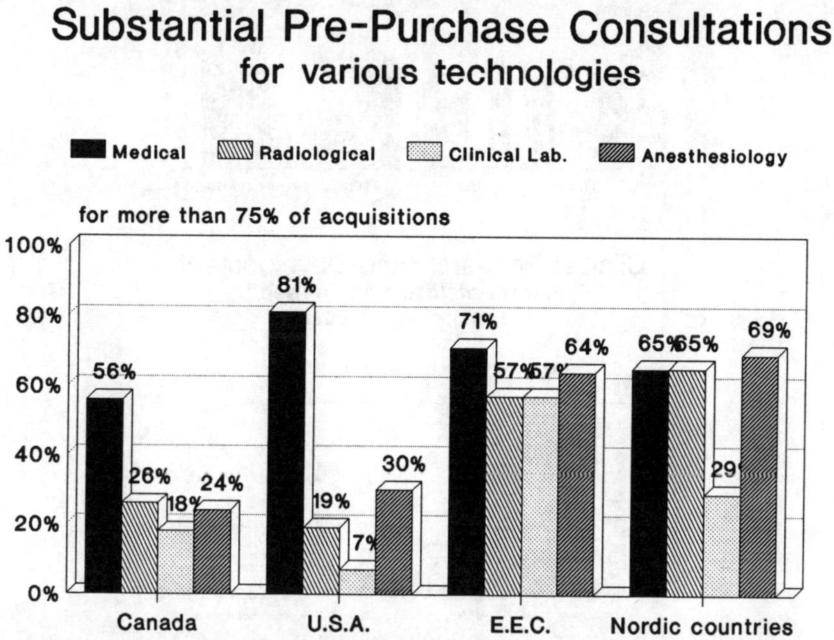

Figure 11.9: Percentage of clinical departments that participate in substantial (more than 75%) prepurchase equipment consultations.

The importance of prepurchase consultation cannot be overstated. The prepurchase period is the ideal time to negotiate manuals and service courses and to establish levels of standardization that facilitate future equipment support. Input from the clinical engineering staff is also helpful in ensuring that final choices are cost effective and that all operating and installation costs have been considered. Departments by-passed during this critical step of the equipment management process are often perceived as nothing more than "repair depots" that exist only to service the machinery.

Clinical Research and Development (R & D)

To assess clinical engineering department's role in research and development, activities related to signal acquisition and processing and equipment design and modification were considered. Figure 11.10 shows the percentage of clinical engineering departments involved in these research areas in teaching and non-teaching institutions. To ascertain the percentage of a department's commitment to this activity, departments were placed into one of four categories: (1) departments not involved in any research, (2) those assigning less than 5 percent of their staff to this activity, (3) those committing between 5 and 10 percent of staff to this activity, and (4) those assigning more than 10 percent of staff. A comparison of figures 11.10a and b indicates that departments in teaching institutions were more involved in research than those in non-teaching institutions for all regions except Europe, where more research was performed in non-teaching hospitals than in teaching ones.

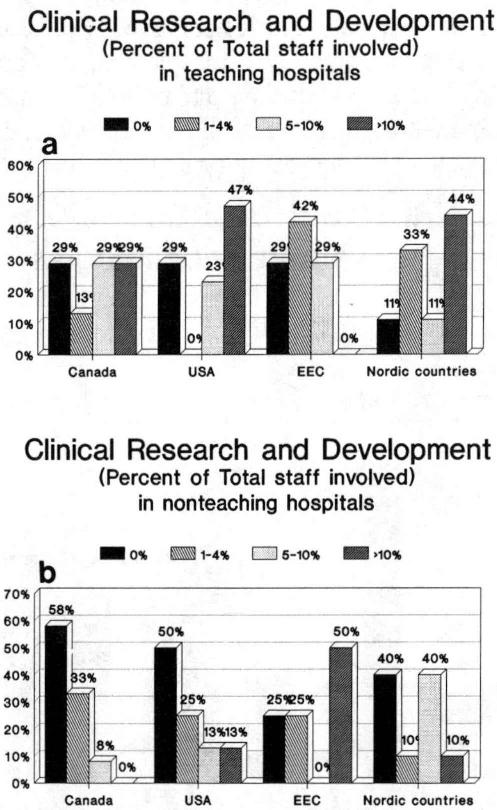

Figure 11.10: Percentage of total clinical engineering staff involved in clinical research and development in (a) teaching and (b) nonteaching institutions.

This result is not surprising (except in Europe) because teaching hospitals usually consider research as part of their mission. The surprising result in this study was that one-third of all surveyed departments in teaching institutions did no research at all. Geographic comparisons indicated that there was generally more involvement in R & D in the EEC and Nordic countries than in the U.S. or Canada. This fact confirms impressions gathered from international conferences that clinical engineering as practiced in the U.K. and Europe is primarily a service that is involved in direct patient care. Participation in clinical research is an excellent way to bring about this involvement.

Quality Assurance

Since the mid-1980s, hospital accreditation councils in the U.S. (**Joint Commission on Accreditation of Healthcare Organizations**) and Canada (**Canadian Council on Hospital Accreditation, CCHA**) have required that all departments in health-care institutions within these countries have a program to measure the quality of services provided. When the first international survey was compiled in 1988, several departments had not yet developed a quality assurance program. Of those departments with a QA program in existence for at least one year, the highest percentage was in the U.S. (53 percent), followed by 35 percent in Canada, 29 percent in the Nordic countries, and 15 percent in the EEC. Although hospital accreditation councils did not exist in Europe or the Nordic countries in 1988, the results indicated some involvement in this type of activity, suggesting that the QA trend was universal. The proportion of departments just starting a QA program in 1988 was 30 percent in the U.S., 37 percent in Canada, 25 percent in the EEC and none in the Nordic countries.

Although clinical engineering departments perform quality assurance to meet accreditation guidelines, the true objective of the JCAHO and CCHA requirement is to test the "quality" of services provided. These tests, therefore, should be designed in a manner to identify problems and weaknesses in the departments (Keil and Camplin, 1987). Of the departments that had QA programs, a number of them had not identified deficiencies through this process. In departments in North America with a quality assurance program, 74 percent had identified deficiencies through this process, while in the EEC and Nordic countries, all departments with a quality assurance program had been able to identify weaknesses or deficiencies.

Staff Productivity

Staff productivity can be defined as follows:

- By specifying the amount of time each technologist or engineer spends on each assigned task.
- By estimating the hours of work recorded and dividing this by the hours available for work (AHA, 1982).

Regardless of the method used to measure productivity, the intent of the 1988 study was to find out how (or if) various departments actually measured staff productivity. In the U.S. 56 percent of respondents indicated that they had been measuring productivity for at least one year, while in Canada this figure was 30 percent, 15 percent in the EEC, and 6 percent in the Nordic countries. The survey also indicated that computer accessibility was a significant factor in whether productivity assessment measures were made. Studying the relationship between productivity assessment and accessibility to a computer, it was noted that, of those departments with access to a computer, 73 percent in the U.S., 42 percent in Canada, and 31 percent in the EEC had begun to measure productivity. Only one of the Nordic departments was measuring this variable.

Budget, Staffing, and Other Resources

Budget. To assess the level of budget allocation, expressed as a percentage of the equipment replacement value supported by the department, budget allocation categories were defined as (1) less than 3 percent (2) 4 to 5 percent, and (3) more than 5 percent of the replacement value of equipment supported. Figure 11.11 illustrates the budget allocations for teaching and non-teaching hospitals. A comparison of these figures indicates that budget allocations for clinical engineering departments are generally higher in teaching than in non-teaching hospitals. This was true in most areas tested, the EEC being the only exception. As with the research activity level, the non-teaching departments in the EEC sample seem to have a high profile and be highly supported. They also show a substantial level of involvement in such "engineering" functions as prepurchase consultation and research and development. As for the remainder of the geographic locations, the majority of departments in non-teaching hospitals have a budget allocation of less than 3 percent of the equipment value they support.

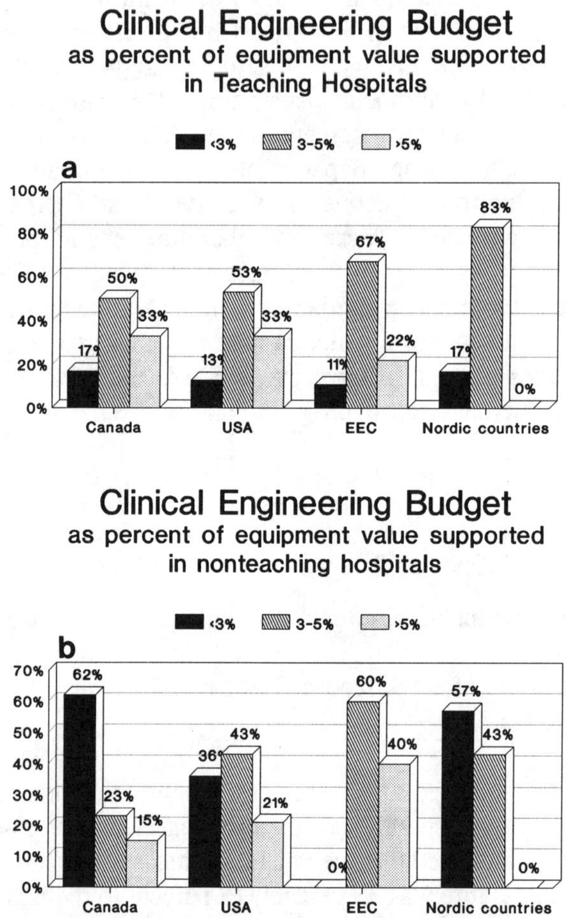

Figure 11.11: **Cinical engineering department budgets as a percentage of the value of supported equipment in (a) teaching and (b) nonteaching hospitals.**

Staffing

In the 1988 survey, the majority of departments reported being understaffed. To establish the adequacy of staffing levels, the following question was asked: Do you feel that your level of staffing is adequate to accomplish the role of your department? The next question asked how many additional engineers, technologists, or clerical personnel were needed. The percentage of departments responding that their staffing level was inadequate was 80 percent in the EEC, 72 percent in the Nordic countries, 63 percent in Canada, and 40 percent in the U.S.

Figure 11.12 shows the percentage of respondents indicating inadequate staffing levels and the percentage of additional engineers, technologists, and clerical personnel required. It can be seen from this figure that the highest proportion of additional staff needed was in the technologist category in all areas except the Nordic countries, where more engineers were needed. A substantial proportion of departments also needed clerical staff.

Other Resources. In assessing other resources available to clinical engineering departments, such as the availability of spare parts, test equipment, and physical space, comparisons were based on the level of spare parts and test equipment measured as a percentage of the replacement value of the equipment supported. Figure 11.13 shows the percentage of clinical engineering departments having a spare parts inventory value of (1) less than 0.5 percent (2) 0.5 to 1.5 percent, and (3) more than 1.5 percent of the equipment replacement value. Figure 11.14 shows similar information for test equipment. The majority of respondents from North America reported a spare parts inventory that was valued at more than 0.5 percent of the equipment base supported. The results are similar for their test equipment inventory. However, in the EEC and the Nordic countries, the majority of respondents reported less than 0.5 percent in spare parts, that may be explained by the lower level of corrective maintenance of medical equipment done by these departments. As for test equipment, the North American departments typically have more than departments in either the EEC or Nordic countries.

Space allocation, measured in square meters per person in the department, was also compared. Figure 11.15 illustrates the percentage of departments with (1) less than 15 square meters per person, (2) 15 to 20 square meters per person, and (3) more than 20 square meters per person. Space allocation appeared to be most generous in the Nordic countries, where 94 percent of departments reported having more than 15 square meters per person, while 71 percent of departments in the U.S., 63 percent in the EEC, and 55 percent in Canada reported having this same space allocation.

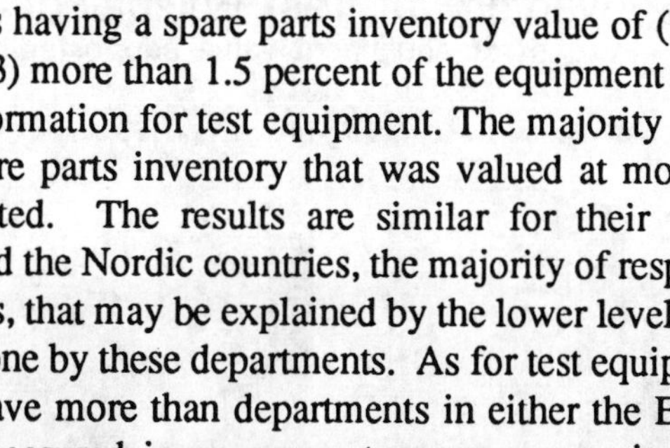

Figure 11.12: Adequacy of specific clinical engineering staff levels in the various sampled groups.

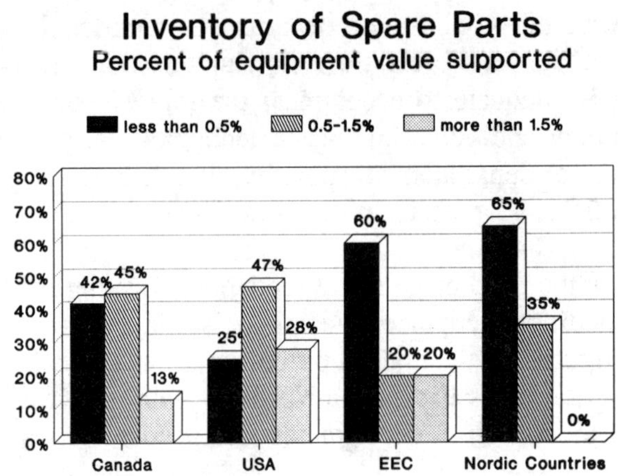

Figure 11.13: Spare parts inventory as a function of the value of supported equipment.

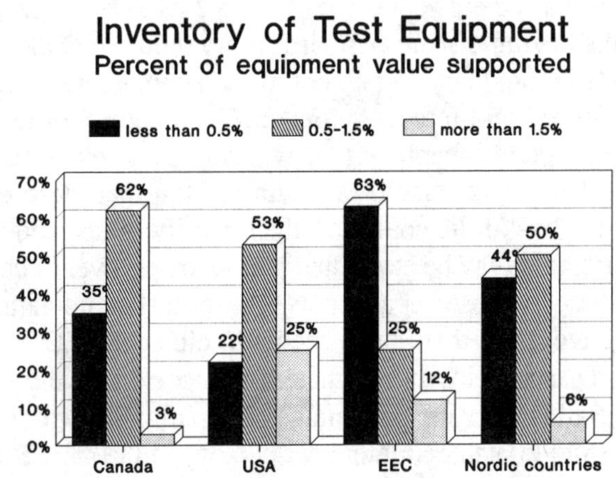

Figure 11.14: Test equipment inventory as a function of value of supported equipment.

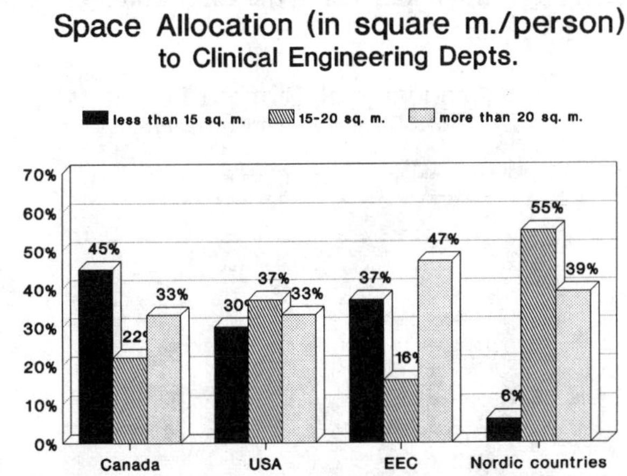

Figure 11.15: Space allocated to clinical engineering departments (in square meters/person).

Educational Level (Engineers and Technologists)

In assessing whether qualified clinical engineers and technologists had been hired or whether the clinical engineering departments were staffed only by technologists or technicians, comparisons of the highest educational level of departmental staff were also made. Figure 11.16 shows the percentage of respondents by highest educational level for each geographic area. The educational categories selected were (1) no engineers; (2) engineers with an undergraduate degree (B.Sc.); (3) engineers with a master's degree; and (4) engineers with a doctoral degree. In those departments with degreed engineers, the majority held a graduate degree (M.Sc. or Ph.D.). This represents a major change in hiring philosophy on the part of hospital administrators during the last decade. A 1977 study (Boxerman and Hooten) reported that 14.9 percent of administrators had been satisfied with technicians, 68.1 percent desired engineers with a bachelor's degree, 12.8 percent wanted engineers with a master's degree and none wanted engineers with a doctoral degree.

The education level of the technicians and technologists is depicted in Figure 11.17. The majority (65 percent) had completed a two-year study program at a technical college after earning a high school diploma. Almost a third (27 percent) had completed a three- or four-year program. Most of them had received their biomedical training on the job.

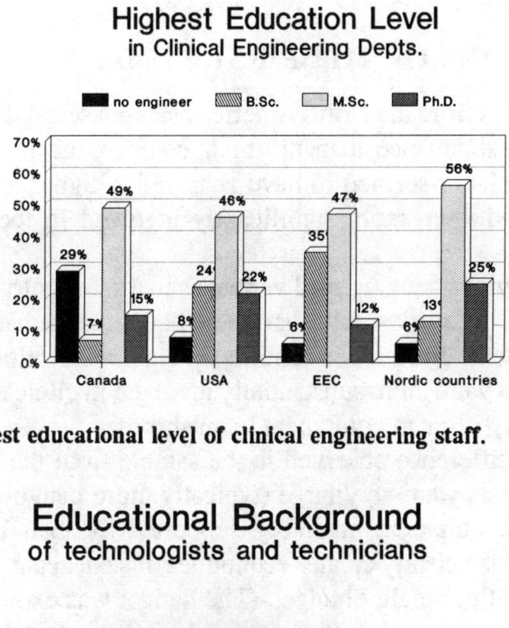

Figure 11.16: Highest educational level of clinical engineering staff.

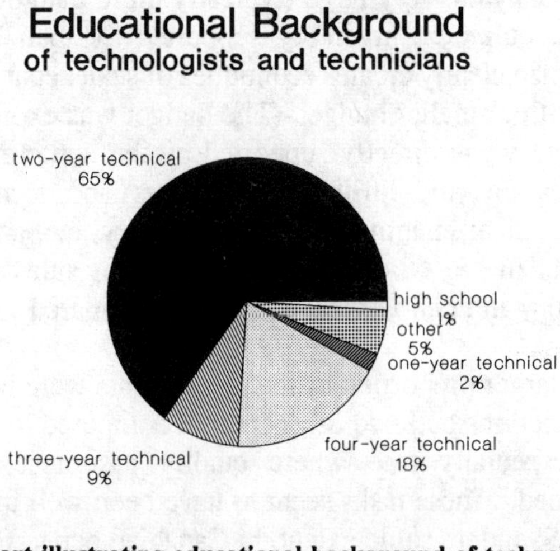

Figure 11.17: Pie chart illustrating educational background of technologists and tecnicians.

Recognition

Recognition was assessed by asking the question, Do you feel that clinical engineering in your hospital has reached its full recognition and status (*strongly agree, agree, disagree, strongly disagree*)? Replies were merged into two categories: agree or disagree. In Canada, only 38 percent of the respondents agreed with the statement, indicating that the majority did not think that their department was sufficiently recognized; 44 percent of respondents in the Nordic countries, 54 percent in the U.S. and 70 percent in the EEC perceived the level of recognition to be adequate. In linking this variable to reporting authority, the results showed that over half (52 percent) of respondents reporting to a senior administrator felt recognized, 55 percent reporting to a medical director or other manager also felt recognized, and just over a third reporting to Plant Operations felt recognized.

The high level of recognition perceived by respondents in the EEC sample may be linked to their involvement in the equipment purchasing process and in clinical research and development. Departments that are bypassed during the purchasing process but are expected to repair and maintain the devices once the warranty has expired are likely to feel that they have a "repair depot" image and that they are not recognized or supported. In fact, a correlation study between the variable "level of prepurchase consultation" and "recognition of the department" was highly significant.

MAJOR CONCLUSIONS OF THE FIRST STUDY

In general, respondents from the North American sample seemed to perform higher levels of in-house corrective maintenance than did their counterparts in Europe and the Nordic countries. However, the latter seemed to have achieved a higher level of support for other types of technologies and were more significantly involved in the equipment purchasing process.

Some of the most obvious geographical variances in the first survey included the fact that respondents in the EEC countries felt that they had have achieved a higher level of recognition than respondents from other countries. This observation may be linked to two factors: these departments were more substantially involved in clinical research and they were consulted more frequently prior to equipment acquisitions.

Another interesting difference observed in the sample from the Nordic countries is that the majority of the hospitals were very large (typically more than one thousand beds). This is reflected in the large equipment inventory supported by their biomedical departments (Oberg, 1990). Hospital size clearly creates economies of scale, enabling clinical engineering departments to operate with a smaller budget. (The budget was expressed as a percentage of the equipment replacement value directly supported by the department.) The large size of the department often justifies the hiring of engineers and technologists with various specializations, such as medical imaging, clinical laboratory, etc, and explains why a larger proportion of respondents in the Nordic countries perform substantially higher levels of repairs of clinical laboratory and radiological equipment compared to departments from other geographic areas.

In North America, a larger proportion of the respondents were involved in the full range of clinical engineering functions outlined in Chapter 1, compared to the EEC and the Nordic countries. This was especially true where quality assurance and staff productivity assessments were concerned. These tasks seem to have been well integrated into the role of the departments in the U.S. and, to some extent, in Canadian departments. This function was somewhat less developed outside of North America.

THE SECOND STUDY (1991)

In 1991, three years after the first study, a second questionnaire was sent to all 116 participants of the first survey; 59 replies were received, and these were matched with the same 59 respondents of the first survey. All of the variables were reanalyzed with the combined databases (1988 and 1991). The results provide a means of assessing changes in key variables that occurred during the three year-period between surveys. In view of the smaller number of respondents per geographic area in the second survey, however, no specific geographical comparisons were made. The resultant comparisons do serve to illustrate general global trends.

Organizational Setting

Hospital Type. The overall proportion of respondents from teaching hospitals was similar in both surveys. It is not surprising that the status of teaching hospitals does not appear to have changed during this three-year period. Similarly, the proportion of small, medium-sized, and large hospitals responding was one-third in each size category in both studies.

Table 11.1 Comparison of replacement value of supported equipment as a function of hospital type, 1989–1991.

TABLE 1

Replacement Value of Equipment Supported by CE Departments (US Dollars)	1988 Survey		1991 Survey	
	Teaching Hospitals	Nonteaching Hospitals	Teaching Hospitals	Nonteaching Hospitals
Less 10 million	9 (32%)	14 (52%)	7 (26%)	14 (44%)
10 - 20 million	9 (32%)	8 (30%)	4 (15%)	7 (12%)
more than 20 million	10 (36%)	5 (18%)	16 (59%)	11 (34%)

Table 11.2 Comparison of the number of supported devices as a function of hospital size.

TABLE 2

Number of Devices Supported by CE Departments (US Dollars)	1988 Survey		1991 Survey	
	Teaching Hospitals	Nonteaching Hospitals	Teaching Hospitals	Nonteaching Hospitals
Less 2000 devices	8 (27%)	12 (45%)	3 (11%)	10 (32%)
2001 - 4000	9 (30%)	9 (33%)	7 (26%)	10 (32%)
More than 4000	13 (43%)	6 (22%)	17 (63%)	11 (36%)

However, workload indicators, such as the number of devices and the equipment replacement value supported by the clinical engineering departments, showed a considerable increase between the first and second surveys. Table 11.1 shows the proportion of respondents supporting (1) less than 10 million (U.S. dollars) of equipment, (2) between 10 and 20 million, and (3) more than 20 million in teaching and non-teaching institutions in 1988 and 1991. A comparison between the two surveys shows that the proportion of departments supporting more than 20 million dollars of equipment value has increased significantly. This change is even more dramatic in the non-teaching hospitals where the percentage rose from 18 to 34 percent.

Table 11.2 shows the proportion of departments supporting less than 2,000, 2,001 to 4,000 and more than 4,000 devices in teaching and non-teaching hospitals in 1988 and 1991. Again, a dramatic increase has occurred in the proportion of respondents supporting more than 4,000 devices. The results illustrated in these two tables indicate a continuing upward trend in hospital equipment acquisitions.

Reporting Authority. The latest survey indicates that clinical engineering departments existing as separate entities are still the majority, with no change in status between the two studies (51 out of 59, or 86 percent). Table 11.3 compares the proportion of respondents reporting to the various authority choices for both hospital types and for both surveys. Although there was a small shift from reporting to plant operations or other managers to reporting to a medical director in teaching hospitals, the majority of respondents indicated no change in their reporting authority.

Level of Functional Involvement

Corrective Maintenance and Incoming Inspections. Table 11.4 shows a comparison of the corrective maintenance levels for each of the four types of equipment for both studies. The proportion of departments performing a substantial level of corrective maintenance of medical equipment is similar in both studies. The level of involvement in incoming inspections has also changed little from the previous study.

Table 11.3 Reporting authority as a proportion of respondents in teaching and nonteaching hospital.

TABLE 3				
Proportion of Respondents Reporting to:	1988 Survey		1991 Survey	
	Teaching Hospitals	Non-teaching Hospitals	Teaching Hospitals	Nonteaching Hospitals
Senior Administrator	21 (73%)	14 (50%)	21 (78%)	18 (58%)
Medical Director	1 (3%)	3 (10.5%)	2 (7%)	2 (6%)
Plant Operations	4 (14%)	8 (29%)	3 (11%)	8 (26%)
"Other" Managers	3 (10%)	3 (10.5%)	1 (4%)	3 (10%)

Table 11.4 Comparison of the proportion of equipment base repaired by in-house staff in (a) 1989 and (b) 1991.

TABLE 4 (a)

Proportion of equipment base Repaired by Respondents	1988 Survey Number (Percentage) of Respondents			
	Medical Equipment	Radiological Equipment	Laboratory Equipment	Anaesthetic Equipment
Less than 25%	1 (2%)	32 (60%)	26 (49%)	18 (34%)
26 - 74%	8 (15%)	10 (19%)	17 (32%)	10 (19%)
75% or more	43 (83%)	11 (21%)	10 (19%)	25 (47%)

TABLE 4 (b)

Proportion of equipment base Repaired by Respondents	1991 Survey Number (Percentage) of Respondents			
	Medical Equipment	Radiological Equipment	Laboratory Equipment	Anaesthetic Equipment
Less than 25%	2 (4%)	31 (62%)	30 (60%)	18 (36%)
26 - 74%	7 (14%)	7 (14%)	12 (24%)	7 (14%)
75% or more	41 (82%)	12 (24%)	8 (16%)	25 (50%)

User Training. Over the three-year period, a decrease in the level of involvement did occur in the already poorly supported user-training task. Table 11.5 shows a comparison of levels of involvement in user training for both studies. In the latest study (1991), only two departments indicated that they provide a substantial level of user training compared to ten in the earlier study.

Table 11.5 Comparison of the proportion of user training needs met by clinical engineering departments.

TABLE 5

Proporation of User-Training Needs Met by Respondents	1988 Survey	1991 Survey
Less than 25%	25 (49%)	31 (62%)
26 - 74%	16 (31%)	17 (34%)
75% or more	10 (20%)	2 (4%)

Prepurchase Consultation. There was a marked decrease in the proportion of respondents who were substantially consulted prior to equipment acquisitions. Table 11.6 shows the comparison of the level of prepurchase consultation for the various types of equipment for both studies. The decrease in the consultation level of the clinical engineering department may be interpreted as a loss of recognition of their role in their respective institutions.

Research and Development

Table 11.7 shows the proportion of departments (1) performing no research, and (2) assigning 1 to 4 percent, (3) 5 to 10 percent, and (4) more than 10 percent of their staffing to R & D activities, for teaching and non-teaching hospitals for both surveys. The latest survey (1991) shows a definite decrease in this activity for both hospital types, but the decrease is even more dramatic in the non-teaching hospitals. A decrease in the participation in clinical research indicates a decline in the "engineering" component of the clinical engineering role and probably less involvement in direct patient-care activities. Although this may not be a surprising result for non-teaching institutions, it is unfortunate to also observe a 15 percent decrease in the proportion of departments in teaching hospitals investing more than 10 percent of their staff to research in the three-year period between both surveys.

Quality Assurance

The overall proportion of respondents performing QA functions for at least one year increased significantly (up 14 percent), and the proportion of those respondents who had not yet started a program declined by 10 percent.

Staff Productivity

The proportion of respondents measuring staff productivity for at least one year increased significantly (up 12 percent) from 1988 to 1991, and the proportion of those who were not measuring this factor declined by 12 percent.

Table 11.6 Comparison of the proportion of equipment acquisitions that the clinical engineering department gave prepurchase consultation.

TABLE 6 (a)

Proportion of Equipment Acquisitions for which Respondents are Consulted	1988 Survey Percentage of Respondents			
	Medical Equipment	Radiological Equipment	Laboratory Equipment	Anaesthetic Equipment
Less than 25%	7 (14%)	30 (60%)	34 (68%)	24 (48%)
26 - 74%	9 (18%)	2 (4%)	4 (8%)	6 (12%)
75% or more	34 (68%)	18 (36%)	12 (24%)	20 (40%)

TABLE 6 (b)

Proportion of Equipment for which Respondents are Consulted	1991 Survey Percentage of Respondents			
	Medical Equipment	Radiological Equipment	Laboratory Equipment	Anaesthetic Equipment
Less than 25%	13 (26%)	31 (62%)	38 (76%)	24 (48%)
26 - 74%	8 (16%)	4 (8%)	2 (4%)	2 (4%)
75% or more	29 (58%)	15 (30%)	10 (20%)	24 (48%)

Table 11.7 Percentage of clinical engineering staff involved in research and development.

TABLE 7
Clinical Research & Development
Percentage of Total Staff Involved

Percentage of staff involved in research and development	1988 Survey		1991 Survey	
	Teaching Hospitals	Non-teaching Hospitals	Teaching Hospitals	Non-teaching Hospitals
none	6 (23%)	10 (44%)	6 (27%)	18 (62%)
1 - 4%	2 (8%)	7 (30%)	3 (14%)	3 (10%)
5 - 10%	7 (27%)	3 (13%)	7 (32%)	4 (14%)
more than 10%	11 (42%)	3 (13%)	6 (27%)	4 (14%)

Budget, Staffing, and Other Resources

Budget. Budget levels rose slightly over the three-year period. Table 11.8 compares budget allocations for respondents in teaching versus non-teaching hospitals, for both studies. Most respondents in the lowest budget category show similar results in the two surveys. However, there is a marked increase of departments in the budget category of 3 to 5 percent for non-teaching institutions.

Staffing. The reported staffing levels were similar for both surveys (Table 11.9). In the 1988 survey, 58 percent of departments stated that they did not need additional staff to accomplish their role; in 1991, this proportion was similar (57 percent).

Other Resources. The second survey indicated a slight rise in the number of respondents in the lower category of inventory value of spare parts compared to the previous study. However, there was also a slight increase in the number of respondents in the highest category of inventory value of test equipment. As for space, the same number of respondents have the smallest space allocation in both surveys (less than 15 square meters per person), but four additional departments are now in the largest space allocation category (more than 20 square meters per person).

Educational Level (Engineers and Technologists)

Table 11.10 shows the proportion of respondents for each education level for both surveys. The proportion of departments without engineers is similar (9 percent in 1988 and 10 percent in 1991), but the proportion of engineers with a B.Sc. went down by 8 percent, those with a M.Sc. went up by 2.5 percent, and respondents with doctoral degrees went up by 4 percent, indicating a slight increase in the education level of the clinical engineers. Regarding the technologists' education, most categories remained the same, but there was a 5 percent increase in the proportion of technologists completing a four-year program.

Table 11.8 Comparison of clinical engineering department budgets as a function of the value of supported equipment.

TABLE 8 Clinical Engineering Department Budget				
Budget level, as a percentage of equipment replacement value supported	1988 Survey		1991 Survey	
	Teaching Hospitals	Non-teaching Hospitals	Teaching Hospitals	Non-teaching Hospitals
Less than 3%	10 (36%)	13 (50%)	10 (37%)	11 (34%)
3 - 5%	11 (39%)	8 (31%)	7 (26%)	15 (47%)
more than 5%	7 (25%)	5 (19%)	10 (37%)	6 (19%)

Table 11.9 Comparison of perceived staffing needs in specific categories .

TABLE 9 Proportion of Respondents Needing Additional Engineers Technologists and Clerical Personnel						
	1988 Survey			1991 Survey		
	Eng.	Tech.	Clerical	Eng.	Tech.	Clerical
None needed	35 (61%)	29 (51%)	39 (68%)	42 (73%)	28 (48%)	44 (76%)
Need one	15 (26%)	10 (17.5%)	18 (32%)	13 (22%)	14 (24%)	14 (24%)
Need two	5 (9%)	8 (14%)		2 (3%)	10 (17%)	
Need more than two	2 (4%)	10 (17.5%)		1 (2%)	6 (11%)	

Table 11.10 Comparison of the education level of clinical engineering department staff.

TABLE 10		
Educational Level	Proportion of Respondents	
	1988	1991
No Engineers	5 (9%)	6 (10%)
BSc Engineers	12 (21%)	8 (13%)
MSc Engineers	28 (50%)	31 (53%)
PhD Engineers	11 (20%)	14 (24%)

Recognition

No change in the perceived level of recognition was found to have occurred over the three-year period. In 1991, just over half (54 percent) of the respondents perceived that their departments were recognized adequately.

MAIN CHANGES OCCURRING OVER THE THREE-YEAR PERIOD (1988–1991)

The comparison between the two studies points out that the majority of the parameters assessed changed very little. In a space of three years, minor variations have occurred except in the workload indicators, where a dramatic increase has been noted in the number of devices and equipment replacement value supported by clinical engineering departments was reported. Smaller changes (of the order of 6 percent) were noticed in the variables assessing resource allocations and level of functional involvement. Most of the parameters displayed variations of less than 5 percent. This indicates that clinical engineering departments have achieved a certain level of stability in developed countries around the world.

Such a study would be incomplete, however, without a discussion of the organizational climate in the hospitals surveyed and how this factor affects the level of functional involvement of clinical engineering departments. The organizational factors used to define the organizational climate were (1) choice of reporting authority; (2) hospital type (teaching and non-teaching); (3) whether the department was recognized; and (4) whether there were engineers with university degrees in the department. These factors were then correlated with the level of involvement of the department for each task previously described, and the results are presented in the form of tables described below (Frize, 1990b).

The Effect of Reporting Authority Choice

The degree of functional involvement of respondents placed under a senior administrator was compared to the degree of involvement of departments reporting to plant operations. Table 11.11 shows the proportion of departments substantially involved in each of the tasks and indicates the degree of significance of the correlation (p-value) for each variable. For example, 86 percent of respondents who report to a senior administrator and 60 percent of respondents reporting to plant operations perform in-house corrective maintenance on more than 75 percent of the hospital's medical equipment base.

A higher proportion of respondents reporting to a senior administrator also perform substantial levels of incoming inspections, user training, and clinical research and development functions than do those reporting to plant operations. In addition, far more of the former are involved in quality assurance and productivity assessment of their staff, that indicates their stronger commitment to quality and efficiency. The correlation study shows an especially high level of significance between the reporting authority factor and the following tasks: incoming inspections, quality assurance, and clinical research and development.

Table 11.11 Influence of reporting authority on the level of functional involvement of the clinical engineering department.

Clinical Engineering Function	Percentage of Departments Performing High Levels of Activity		Correlation Study	
	Reporting to			
Respondents Performing	Senior Administrator	Plant Operations	Correlation Coefficient	Significance Level (*p*-value)
More than 75 percent of medical equipment repairs	44/51 (86%)	15/25 (60%)	.13	.10
Incoming inspections on more than 75 percent of new equipment	45/51 (88%)	15/25 (60%)	.22*	.02
More than 75 percent of the user-training needs on the safe and effective use of equipment	13/49 (27%)	3/22 (14%)	.06	.29
Prepurchase consultation for more than 75 percent of acquisitions of medical equipment	34/49 (69%)	13/23 (57%)	.09	.20
Quality assurance programs since at least one year	27/58 (47%)	9/31 (29%)	.19*	.03
Staff productivity measurement since at least one year	23/57 (40%)	6/31 (19%)	.05	.30
Clinical resarch and development (10 percent or more of staffing assigned)	26/66 (39%)	24/33 (17%)	.15*	.09

* correlation highly significant

Table 11.12 Influence of hospital type on the level of functional involvement of clinical engineering departments.

Clinical Engineering Function	Percentage of Departments Performing High Levels of Activity Hospital Type		Correlation Study	
Respondents Performing	Teaching	Nonteaching	Correlation Coefficient	Significance Level (*p*-value)
More than 75 percent of medical equipment repairs	47/58 (81%)	27/38 (71%)	.11	.14
Incoming inspections on more than 75 percent of new equipment	46/56 (88%)	30/38 (79%)	.92*	.43
More than 75 percent of the user-training needs on the safe and effective use of equipment	14/53 (26%)	7/38 (18%)	.08	.22
Prepurchase consultation for more than 75 percent of acquisitions of medical equipment	40/54 (74%)	21/37 (57%)	.20*	.03
Quality assurance programs since at least one year	28/64 (44%)	14/45 (31%)	.18*	.03
Staff productivity measurement since at least one year	22/63 (35%)	14/45 (31%)	.10	.16
Clinical resarch and development (10 percent or more of staffing assigned)	16/53 (30%)	4/40 (10%)	.32*	.001

* correlation highly significant

Table 11.13 Influence of recognition on the level of functional involvement of the clinical engineering department.

Clinical Engineering Function	Percentage of Departments Performing High Levels of Activity		Correlation Study	
Respondents Performing	Departments Recognized	Departments Not Recognized	Correlation Coefficient	Significance Level (*p*-value)
More than 75 percent of medical equipment repairs	43/49 (88%)	32/48 (67%)	.24*	.009
Incoming inspections on more than 75 percent of new equipment	39/49 (80%)	38/46 (83%)	.002	.49
More than 75 percent of the user-training needs on the safe and effective use of equipment	15/49 (31%)	7/43 (16%)	.25*	.008
Prepurchase consultation for more than 75 percent of acquisitions of medical equipment	41/47 (87%)	21/45 (47%)	.40*	.000
Quality assurance programs since at least one year	23/56 (41%)	19/53 (36%)	.08	.21
Staff productivity measurement since at least one year	24/56 (43%)	12/52 (23%)	.24*	.006
Clinical resarch and development (10 percent or more of staffing assigned)	10/47 (21%)	10/47 (21%)	.14	.08

* correlation highly significant

Table 11.14 Influence of availability of an engineer on the level of functional involvement of the clinical engineering department.

Clinical Engineering Function	Percentage of Departments Performing High Levels of Activity		Correlation Study	
Respondents Performing	With Engineer	Without Engineer	Correlation Coefficient	Significance Level (*p*-value)
More than 75 percent of medical equipment repairs	66/92 (72%)	8/16 (50%)	.08	.22
Incoming inspections on more than 75 percent of new equipment	66/92 (72%)	10/16 (63%)	.10	.19
More than 75 percent of the user-training needs on the safe and effective use of equipment	19/92 (21%)	2/16 (13%)	.02	.43
Prepurchase consultation for more than 75 percent of acquisitions of medical equipment	57/92 (62%)	4/16 (25%)	.21*	.03
Quality assurance programs since at least one year	36/92 (39%)	4/16 (25%)	.14*	.08
Staff productivity measurement since at least one year	33/92 (36%)	3/16 (19%)	.17*	.05
Clinical resarch and development (10 percent or more of staffing assigned)	20/78 (26%)	none	.36*	.000

* correlation highly significant

Hospital Type

Table 11.12 shows a comparison of the level of functional involvement for teaching and non-teaching hospitals and the corresponding correlation coefficients and their significance level for the various activities. In teaching hospitals, more respondents perform substantial levels of service for each task described. The correlation was particularly significant for these tasks: pre-purchase consultation, quality assurance, and clinical R & D.

Recognition

The recognition variable was seen to have the most significant impact on the degree of functional involvement of clinical engineering departments. Table 11.13 shows a comparison in the level of functional involvement for respondents who felt recognized by their institution and for those who did not. The table also gives the correlation coefficients and corresponding significance level for each task type. Respondents who felt that their role was recognized showed a more substantial involvement in all of the tasks described except for incoming inspections and quality assurance, the results of which were similar for both groups. The correlation was significant for all other tasks and especially high in these engineering functions: consultation and user training.

Presence of University-Degree Engineers

Table 11.14 shows the level of functional involvement of departments with engineers and of those without engineers. Departments with qualified engineers are more involved in all aspects of clinical engineering functions. The correlation was especially significant for the tasks: prepurchase consultation, staff productivity measurement, and clinical R & D.

CONCLUSION

Based on the results of these surveys, it appears that the field of clinical engineering has reached a certain stability with regard to its organizational setting, role, and financial support. However, the profession of clinical engineering cannot be considered as mature until the value and importance of its role are recognized and supported by the majority of health-care institutions. The continued development of strong, committed clinical engineering associations or colleges can provide the framework to foster communication and cooperation between the various groups around the world. In this global economy, it is easy to imagine that three main international zones exist, with natural economic and geographic ties, where closer cooperation could be achieved:

- North, Central and South America.
- An extended Europe (East and West).
- Asia and the Pacific.

Clinical engineering associations and colleges would gain much by a unification process that, without being entirely global, would create closer links between groups of professionals with similar interests.

By clearly stating their mission, objectives, workloads, and resource requirements, clinical engineering departments can enhance their profile and raise the awareness of hospital administrators and other health-care professionals regarding their role and the benefits of supporting such services. As experience, skills, and resources are acquired, the basic role of the clinical engineering department can be expanded to support as much of the equipment as possible. In addition, well-designed quality assurance programs will be a key factor in the professional success of the department and, ultimately, in the financial success of the health-care institution.

In the 1990s, justification of the existence of clinical engineering departments is still a valid and necessary process, especially in this recessionary economy. Care must be taken not to focus entirely on the corrective maintenance role. The importance of in-house repairs is likely to decrease with the proliferation of the multilayered boards and VLSI circuits. User training and prepurchase consultation tasks should take on higher priority. Added to these two important tasks may be software customization for newly acquired equipment or for upgrading existing systems. Developing computer interfaces for patient data management will also become a major activity in the future.

Clinical engineering remains a fascinating profession with much room for both individual and departmental development. The degree of interest and motivation that will come to characterize its practitioners will depend directly on how clinical engineers and technologists define their roles and create and manage their activities within the health-care environment.

REFERENCES

A.H.A. "Medical Equipment Management in Hospitals." *American Society for Hospital Engineering* (of the American Hospital Association), Chicago, 60611, 1982.

Bauld III, T.J. "Productivity: Standard Terminology and Definitions." *J. Clin. Engin.*, 12(2):139–145, 1987.

Boxerman, S. B., and Hooten, C.J. "Clinical Engineering, the Administrator's Perspective." *IEEE Transactions BME*, 24:57–59, 1977.

Cromwell, J., Hewes, H.T., Kelly, N.L., and Franklin, S. "Comparative Trends in Hospital Expenses, Finances, Utilization, and Inputs, 1970–81," *Health Care Financing Review*, 9(1): 51–69, 1987.

Dalziel, C.R. "Electric Shock Hazard," *IEEE Spectrum* 9:41, 1972.

Fennigkoh, L. "The Clinical Engineering/Health Care Mismatch; It's Effect on Personnel Management," *Med. Biol. Comput.*, 22:113–114, 1984.

Frize, M. "The Clinical Engineer: A Full Member of the Health Care Team?" *Med. Biol. Engin. Comput.*, 26:461–465, 1988.

Frize, M. "Results of an International Survey of Clinical Engineering Departments. Part I: Role, Resources and Recognition," *Med. Biol. Engin. Comput.*, 28:153–159, 1990a.

Frize, M. "Results of an International Survey of Clinical Engineering Departments. Part II: Budgets, Staffing, Resources and Financial Strategies," *Med. Biol. Engin. Comput.*, 28:160–165, 1990b.

Frize, M., Shaffer, M. "Clinical Engineering in Today's Hospital: Perspectives of the Administrator and the Clinical Engineer," *Hospital & Health Services Administration*, 36(2):285–305, 1991.

Keil, O.R., Camplin, C.R. "Quality Assurance," *J. Clin. Eng.*, 12(2):153–158, 1987.

Neuhausel, D.J. "Productivity in Clinical Engineering," *J. Clin. Eng.*, 10(4):289–300, 1985.

Oberg, P.A. "Clinical Engineering in Sweden—Organization and Education," *Proceedings of the International Clinical Eng. Workshop*, Weimar, GDR, (Dept. of Biomedical Engineering, Linköping University, Linköping, Sweden), 1990.

Ouchi, W.G. "Theory Z. How American Business Can Meet the Japanese Challenge," *Avon Books*, New York, 1981.

Pacela, A. "Survey of Biomedical and Clinical Engineering Departments in the U.S. Hospitals," Quest Publishing Co., Brae, California, pp. 1–24.

INDEX

Design issues in medical facilities, 206–207
Device regulation, 118
Diagnostic and Therapeutic Technology Assessment (DATTA), 121
Diagnostic-related guidelines (DRGs), 120
Diagnostic support systems, 358–362; artificial intelligence (AI), 358
Diffusion, 113
Drug regulation, 117